sex: a lover's guide

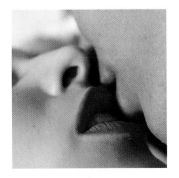

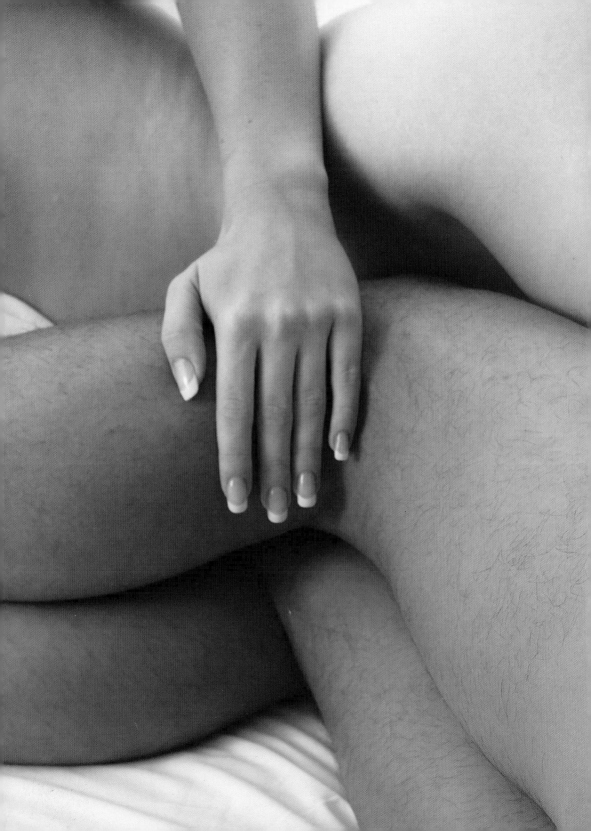

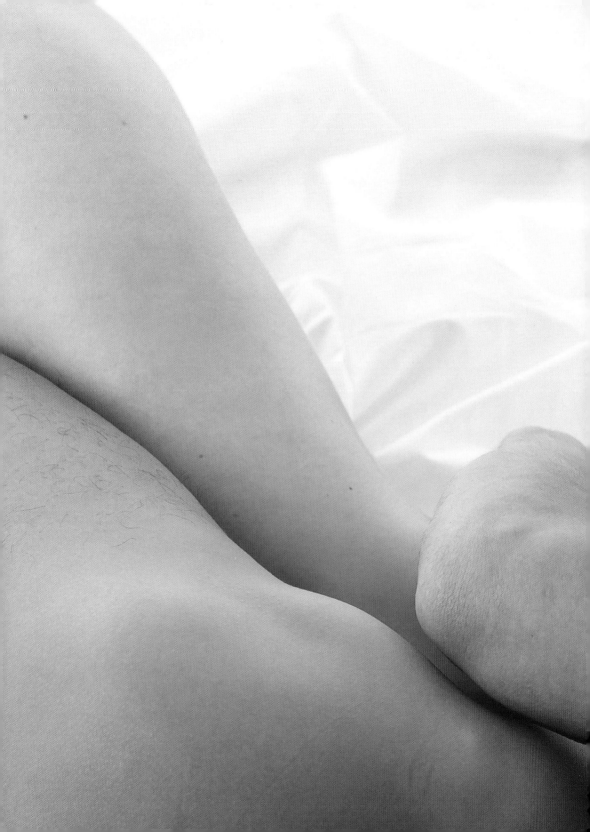

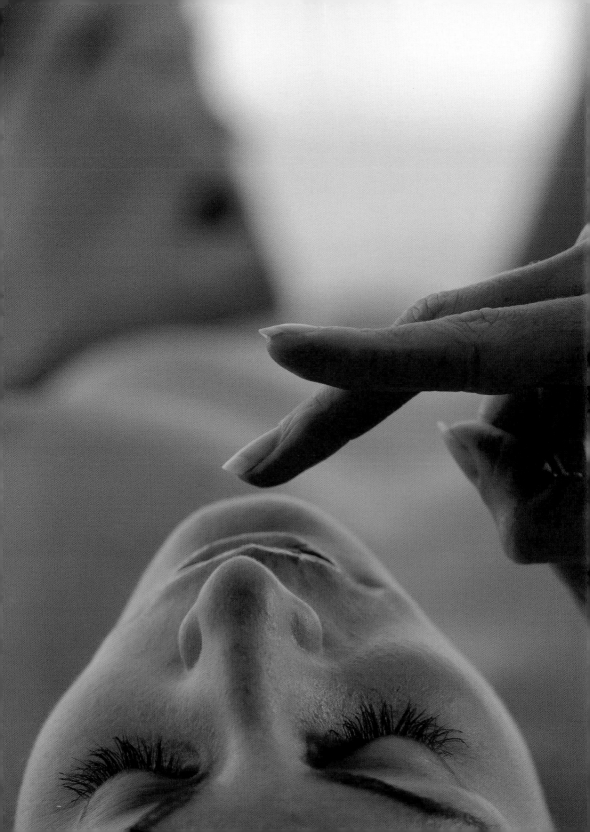

sex: a lover's guide

the ultimate guide to physical attraction,
lovemaking techniques and sexual relationships
with over 1000 photographs

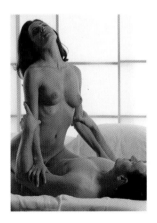

Judy Bastyra and Nitya Lacroix

Foreword by Ed Straw
Vice-President of Relate

southwater

This edition is published by Southwater, an imprint of Anness Publishing Ltd,
108 Great Russell Street, London WC1B 3NA; info@anness.com

www.southwaterbooks.com; www.annesspublishing.com; twitter: @Anness_Books

If you like the images in this book and would like to investigate using them for publishing, promotions or
advertising, please visit our website www.practicalpictures.com for more information.

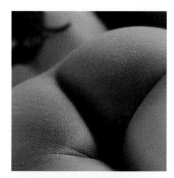

A CIP catalogue record for this book is available from the British Library.

Publisher: Joanna Lorenz
Senior Project Editors: Doreen Gillon and Katy Bevan
Copy Editors: Sarah Brown, Judy Cox and Linda Doeser
Designer: Whitelight and Bill Mason
Photography: John Freeman, assisted by Alex Dow; Alistair Hughes
Make-up Artist: Bettina Graham
Illustrations: Samantha Elmhurst
Production Controller: Ben Worley

Illustrations of the *Kama Sutra* by courtesy of The Art Archive/JFB
Extract from *The Butcher* by Alina Reyes used by permission of The Random House Group Limited.

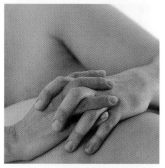

PUBLISHER'S NOTE
Although the advice and information in this book are believed to be accurate and true at the time of going
to press, neither the authors nor the publisher can accept any legal responsibility or liability for any errors
or omissions that may have been made nor for any inaccuracies nor for any loss, harm or injury that
comes about from following instructions or advice in this book.

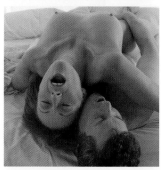

The authors and publisher have made every effort to ensure that all instructions contained within this
book are accurate and safe, and cannot accept liability for any resulting injury, damage or loss to persons
or property, however it may arise. Laws around the world are different and ever changing – it is the
reader's responsibility to ensure that what they do is within the law, and no responsibility can be taken
by the authors or publisher for any legal repercussions.

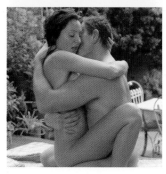

CONTENTS

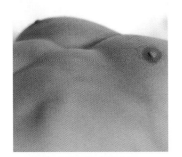
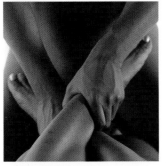
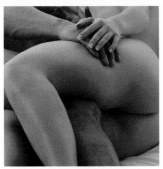
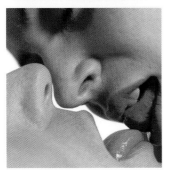

foreword

WHAT AN INTERESTING BOOK! We are all supposed to be experts, but I have certainly learnt a lot. This includes what coffee, Brussels sprouts and asparagus have in common, and a better understanding of anatomy. That the understanding of "why and where" improves skills and therefore motivation, and that sex is no different in this regard. Why smell matters; why post-coital is a part of seduction; and where the blissful sensation of orgasm comes from...

The advice starts at the beginning, with preening and cleaning, meeting places, chat-up lines that work (stick to the straightforward and avoid the search for the silver bullets: they are all dud), reading body language, and seduction. The book then gets down to the nitty-gritty of foreplay, finding the spot, coitus, oral and anal sex, and a splendid array of erotica. The difficult areas of dysfunction, health and safety are not ducked and the referral list is comprehensive.

The entire book is presented in a non-judgemental way, refreshing in a society smothered by rules. Choose from the banquet the dishes you feel like today: this is not about right and wrong, but the sexual menu that changes from day to day.

We are surrounded by images of sex in magazines, on film and in advertisements, but so much of it seems to miss the point. Sex is a set of sensations, and both an emotional trip and an exploration of self. This book can help you reach parts you did not even know you had. Dip in and dip out, read it from cover to cover, read it separately or together.

BELOW | There are a myriad of ways to be intimate with your lover, many of which you will discover in this book.

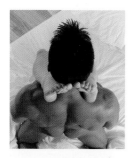

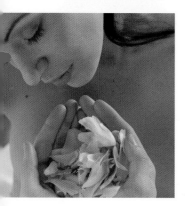

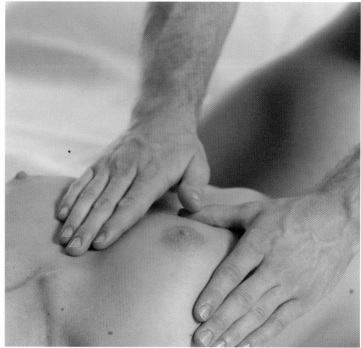

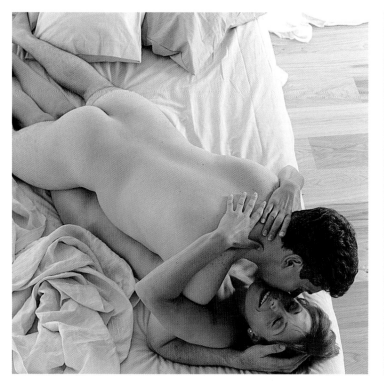

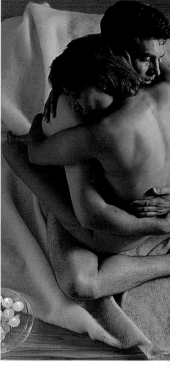

My experience is that people are becoming much more willing to discuss their sexual issues and are more likely to insist on a good sex life. Relate is perhaps best known for its relationship counselling. Less well known is that it has a long-standing sex therapy service as well. Sex therapy was developed in response to the realization that, in some cases, sexual problems were the source of the relationship difficulty. Of course, the reverse could be the case: poor emotional connections can cause poor sex. But in many cases, good sex can transform a relationship. And the beauty of it is that much of sex is behavioural: skills are needed and these can be taught and learnt.

This book presents and teaches the subject in an open, clear and affirming way, very much in keeping with a modern view, uncluttered by any inhibition or disapproval and sustained by the notion of sex as a gift that we can offer to each other.

For many, this will be a very personal read: curl up in your favourite place and enjoy a good cuddle before taking it further. A dose of sensuality can only be beneficial. Have a good time.

Ed Straw, Vice-President, Relate
(The UK's largest relationship support organization)

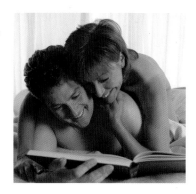

ABOVE LEFT AND RIGHT | Sex, at any age, can be intimate, fun and very sensual.

BELOW | Enjoy a good read with your partner – it may open the door for discussion and then action.

introduction

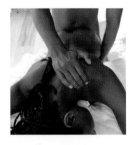

This inspirational reference book is indispensable for anyone intent on achieving a truly fulfilled and satisfied love life. It covers every aspect of a sexual relationship, from the heady days of courtship and romance through to expert advice on maintaining and rekindling the spark in a long-term relationship. We live in what is supposed to be a sexually liberated age, but we still often find it difficult to openly discuss sex and any questions or concerns we may have.

THIS PAGE | Experiment with the vast number of sexual positions to enhance your sex life and keep the spark in your relationship.

OPPOSITE | Discover each other's erogenous zones by using all your sensory organs, including taste, touch and smell.

The opening pages set the scene for the rest of the book, stressing the importance of a positive self-image and the need to love and care for yourself. This theme is taken up later with advice on physical fitness, diet and self-massage, making you feel confident in your own body and sexuality. Before embarking on a new relationship, you need to understand the subtleties of outward appearance and body language, so important in the early days when you meet and are attracted to someone. Again, confidence and a direct, friendly manner are the best approach to the art of

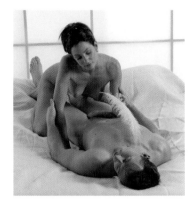

wooing. The first date and developing intimacy – holding hands, the first kiss – create valuable memories that you will look back on later.

The development of sexuality is traced from puberty to sexual peak, which is different in men and women. At this stage the male and female bodies are described and illustrated in detail, including the often mysterious internal sex organs. Armed with this knowledge, it is now time to explore your partner's body, discovering his or her erogenous and pleasure zones and delighting in sensual play, including the thrill of first undressing each other. Seduction is something to be lingered over in a new relationship, creating tantalizing discoveries and expectations. It is also valuable in a long-term relationship, whenever you have time to indulge in protracted kissing and foreplay, as if you were making love together for the first time.

The main body of the book details the full range of sexual positions to experiment with both in and out of the bedroom, enabling each couple to find the best recipes for orgasmic bliss and to add spice and variety so that sex never becomes routine. The explicit text deals in a frank and friendly way with all aspects of lovemaking, describing first the basic positions and illustrating their variations. A separate section is devoted to orgasm and to masturbation, both individually and

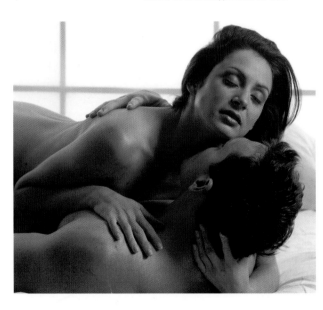

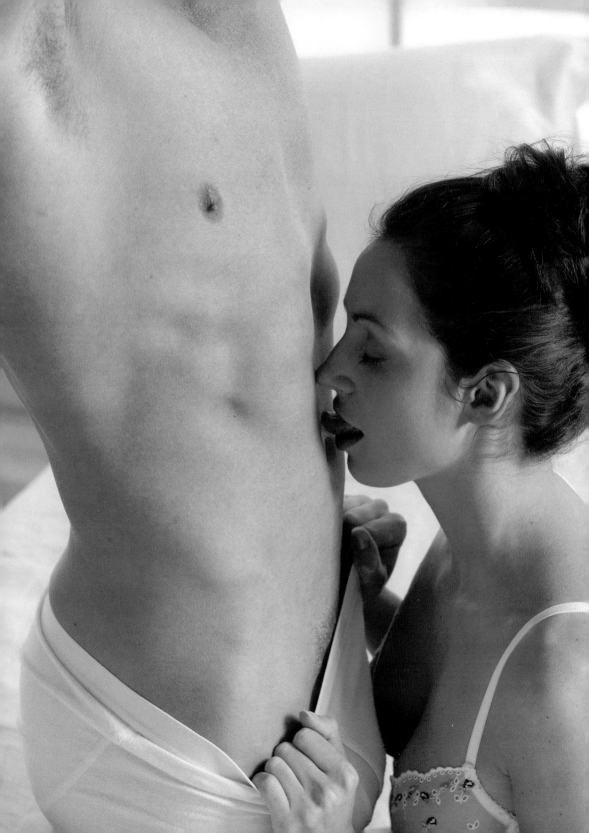

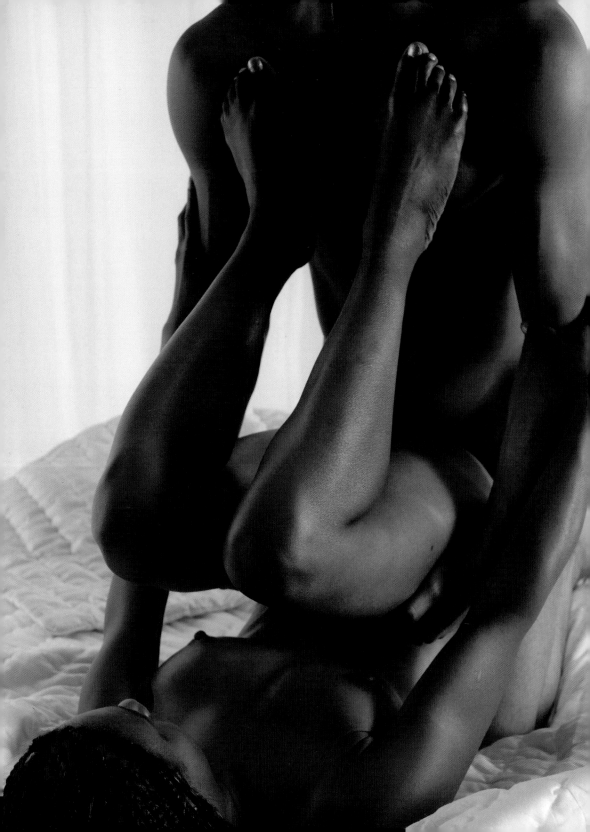

together, before returning to advanced sexual positions for the more adventurous. Tips are also given to help you become a better lover.

The next section describes erotica such as sharing sexual fantasies, dressing up, cross-dressing, dominance and bondage. A step-by-step sequence illustrates a long, slow strip-tease to make sure you get your partner's full attention. Subtle skin teasing aids such as feathers and silky fabrics will add an extra dimension to your love life, as may sex toys and reading pornography together.

Sensual massage can be a prelude to lovemaking and a detailed section gives full instruction on massage for various parts of the body. This loving way of expressing your feelings to your partner soothes away the stress of daily life as well acting as a form of foreplay. The chapter on divine sex reveals the art of tantric sex and the place of meditation in a relationship, opening the body's energy channels and honouring your partner's body as sacred; and Ananga ranga techniques are also explained. A short section on aphrodisiacs and the connection between food and sex follows.

A long-term relationship goes through different phases and you may need to adapt to changing needs and circumstances such as starting a family or growing older together. Special exercises will help strengthen the sexual parts of the body such as the pelvic floor. Due attention is paid to sexual health and hygiene, including safer sex and contraception.

The book closes with advice on any sexual problems you may experience. Experimenting with positions and techniques can revive a relationship but it is important to talk and listen to each other. Communication is key. In fact, the message of this whole book is that sex is something to be shared and enjoyed equally by both men and women. Different circumstances will call for different approaches but there is something here for every situation, to enhance your emotional and sexual relationships and your life.

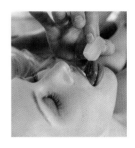

THIS PAGE AND OPPOSITE |
Touching doesn't just have to be with hands – use your feet, legs, lips and even the heat of your breath to touch and feel.

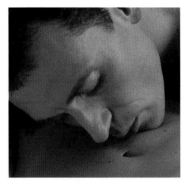

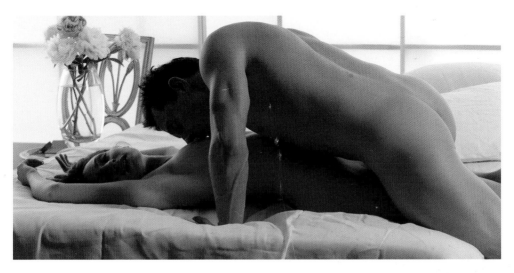

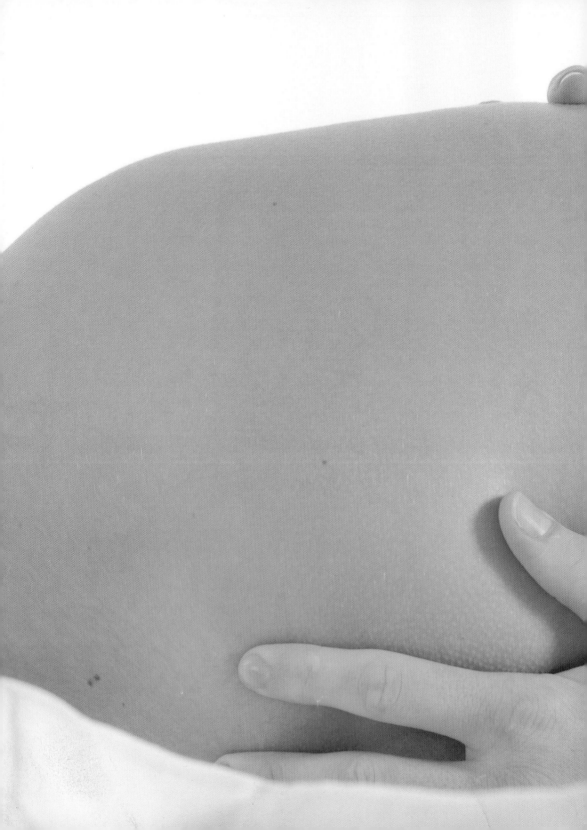

attraction

There is no accounting for the way individuals are attracted to each other.
Although there are many theories, no one has managed to write a
successful formula. Meanwhile, we are all susceptible to that certain
indefinable special something, that *je ne sais quoi*, that creates a tingle
when the right person comes along. When that happens, there are a few
practical things you can do to give nature a helping hand.

first impressions

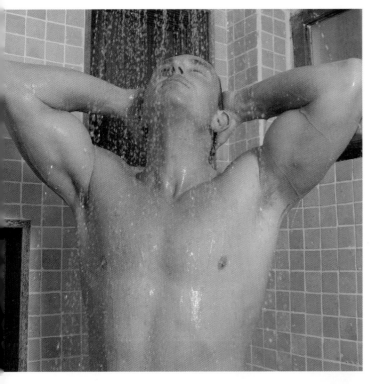

THE SOCIAL SCENE IN MANY WAYS matches the competitive environment in the workplace – too many people applying for the same job. So it's only common sense that the same amount of effort should be put into seeking your perfect partner as you put into finding your perfect job. For this you need preparation and a game plan.

First impressions are crucial, as you rarely get a second chance. People form their first impressions within four seconds of meeting, so appearances do count: hair, nails, teeth, smell, clothes, all the usual things. Women are usually better organized about this than men but it works both ways.

Nails, for example. It's not necessary to have weekly manicure sessions, but at least make sure that you give the undersides of your nails a really thorough scrub. There are few things more off-putting than unclipped and dirty-looking fingernails. Never mind where your hands have been: concentrate on where they are about to go.

Men, check that your beard, moustache or goatee is trimmed and tamed. Remember that women have sensitive skin. Scratchy facial hair not only gives them stubble-rash, but is also quite a turn-off. A recent survey has shown that 90 per

ABOVE | One of the main ingredients in a man's armpit sweat is androsterone, which helps to create that musty all-male smell – the same substance in truffles that makes pigs go crazy. However, it is best to continue washing until you find someone who loves you just the way you are.

RIGHT | Grooming is all-important for men and women alike, although the latter tend to be more naturally conscientious.

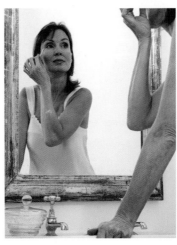

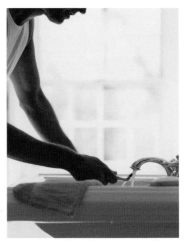

cent of women prefer clean-shaven men of any age. At the same time, take note of those unwanted hairs in the nose and ears. Check other areas such as your eyebrows. Hairs between the eyebrows can make a face appear severe, unapproachable, so undateable. A robust set of tweezers can solve this, and put you back in the running. Women, too, need the occasional battle with tweezers and the odd rogue hair.

Your teeth are important, as they will be checked out by anyone thinking of kissing you. If your teeth are stained from smoking or drinking coffee, then invest in some tooth whitener. Make sure your breath is inviting – carry mints with you. Bad breath is the *ultimate* turn-off.

the sweet smell of attraction

Make sure you have a shower before you go out, especially if it has been a hot day. There is nothing more attractive than meeting a man or woman who smells fresh and clean.

However, natural body scents have proved to be a big turn-on as relationships progress. Biologist Claus Wedekind of the University of Bern, Switzerland, published some interesting findings linking attraction with body odour and the immune system. In his study, a group of men were given plain T-shirts and instructed to wear them for two nights running without using artificial fragrance or cologne. The sweat-soaked articles were then given to a group of women for a sniffing session to rate the scents in levels of attractiveness. Both the men and the women were blood tested to discover the make-up of their major histocompatability complex (MHC). MHC is a brand of molecule, unique to each individual, which is involved in the immune system. Procreating with an individual with a different MHC results in offspring that inherit both parents' immune systems, and thus stronger immunity.

Wedekind's results showed that the women found the men's smell to be pleasant if the men had a different MHC from their own. This means that they were attracted to men who would produce stronger, more viable offspring with them.

No one can be certain whether people genuinely do fall for a particular individual purely because of their subtle scents, but have you ever said of someone, "It's not that they're particularly attractive, but there's just something about them…"?

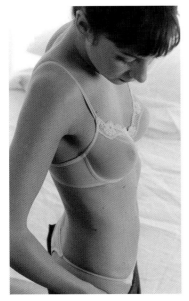

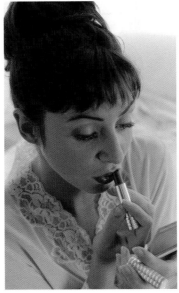

LEFT | Dressing and applying make-up for a date is an age-old ritual for women, but grooming shouldn't be ignored by men.

the language of clothes

THE CLOTHES YOU WEAR CAN SAY MUCH about your emotional state and feelings of confidence. Both men and women use clothes to broadcast aspects of their personalities, or to create a certain persona with which to impress other people. That slinky "little black number" can bring out many aspects of a woman's character that might otherwise have remained dormant. "Power dressing" inspires respect in others and so gives the individual's own confidence a major boost. In comfortable trousers, or jeans and a sweatshirt, on the other hand, a person presents a much more relaxed and easy-going image.

BELOW | The couple below are dressed to go on a romantic date but they are comfortable with their clothes and each other.

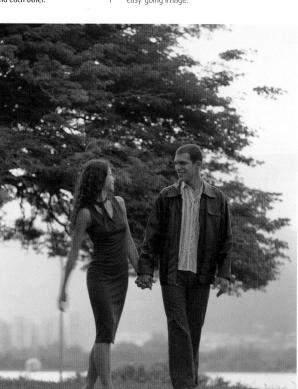

dress to express

Women often wear more revealing clothes when they are feeling confident about their sexuality. Some researchers claim this is most likely to be around the time of ovulation, when a woman is at her most fertile. However a woman can feel sexy at any time, and the clothes she wears will often reflect this mood, accentuating her most attractive characteristics.

It is a common misunderstanding, though, for a man to assume that a woman dresses purely for the effect her clothes will have on the opposite sex. Very often a woman chooses a certain style, even one that is overtly appealing, because she enjoys feeling attractive in her own right and expects to have the freedom to express it. A woman who chooses to wear a figure-hugging dress or even a revealing mini-skirt may be doing so because she favours the style and wants to feel good about the way she looks, and may be just as concerned about making an impression on her female friends as on men. In other words, if a woman is wearing clothes that reveal her body, it does not necessarily signal that she is wanting or expecting to receive uninvited male attention.

Nowadays, a women has a greater sense of her personal freedom, and her wish to express her sexuality without being perceived as a sex object means that men must decode her availability signals without simply basing them on the way she is dressed. This can be difficult to grasp for a man who is conditioned to believe that a woman's desire to look attractive is only designed for a male response. These days, if a woman wishes to attract the attention of a man, she is likely to give more direct signals to him. Men, then, can no longer afford to make automatic assumptions on a woman's intentions simply because she is attractively dressed to kill.

The ability to be able to change the style of the clothes to match the mood is a positive one, and gives a woman a greater flexibility in being

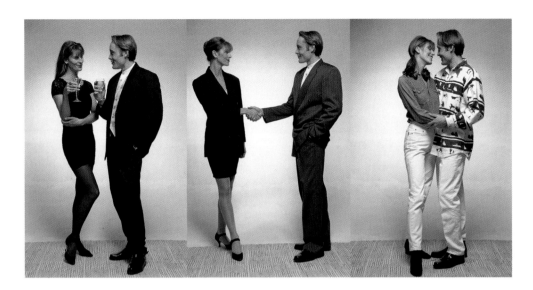

able to express herself as a more all-rounded person rather than being fixed into a specific image. On the whole, a woman will probably be more clothes-conscious than her men friends, or her partner, but it is important for her to select her clothes to suit her colouring, height and size rather than to try to emulate a particular style simply because it is fashionable.

When going out, a short, figure-hugging dress says a woman is in the mood for some fun and is not ashamed to broadcast the message. The dress is often shaped to reveal the sensual curves of her body, while the high heels accentuate the length of her legs. If she chooses black she is also showing she feels confident and in control. While revealing clothes can be fun to wear, and can certainly make a woman turn heads, sometimes the look can have a reverse effect on a man and actually scare him off. He might perceive the woman as a predatory man-hunter, and if he is not confident in his own sexuality, he may feel unable to cope with what he imagines will be her demands, and will miss an opportunity to meet a future partner.

A woman's size is not a barrier to her looking good if she takes the time to pick the clothes that flatter her particular body shape. She should forget about trying to copy any look that happens to be in vogue. Feeling comfortable in what she wears is the most powerful way for a woman to be attractive, and most men respond to a woman who is relaxed and confident in herself, rather than only to the clothes that she happens to be wearing.

a casual approach

A woman may prefer to dress in such a way that she camouflages her more obvious sexual attributes, because she prefers men to be drawn to her because of her personality rather than her obvious feminine assets.

She may prefer to wear comfortable clothes, such as a shirt and jeans, that do not reveal too much of the shape of her body. In doing so, she may feel that she is more able to relate to men on an easy, equal and friendly basis rather than an immediately sexual one. This does not necessarily mean that she has switched off her sexual signals, but she is drawing attention to herself as a complete person with a mind and personality, as well as a feminine body. She is sending out the message that any relationship must be serious and must include an appreciation of her as a person, not just as a sex object.

ABOVE LEFT | This short dress says the woman is in the mood for some fun.

ABOVE CENTRE | This is a style of suit that means business. Sex is definitely secondary to ambition. However, there are enough feminine touches – the open neck and length of skirt – to show that the wearer has not sublimated her sexuality. She is saying, "I have got where I am because I am a woman – not in spite of my sex."

ABOVE RIGHT | In tight white jeans and denim top, open at the neck, this woman can present herself as feminine but is making it clear she is meeting the man on equal terms.

dressed to impress

A man's clothes are likely to reflect his financial status and the power he commands as much as his sexual availability. A business suit, like a uniform, can indicate dominance and assertiveness and so conveys an air of confidence and achievement. For some women, this aura of power is very sexually attractive, particularly if they seek a partner with whom they will feel secure and who is a successful and reliable provider. So a well-cut suit from a famed fashion designer, suggesting financial security and career success, could have definite appeal to these women. Even a man's casual clothes will often have an expensive branded trademark if he likes to dress to impress.

When a man is feeling sexually confident his clothes are likely to reflect the fact. Most men who keep themselves fit look good in jeans and T-shirts and although this is a common masculine attire, it is usually very attractive to women. Many find that the sight of well-shaped buttocks, accentuated by the cut of a tight pair of jeans, is an extremely powerful turn-on. Men, like women, have increasingly broken the gender mould when it has come to dress, and a lot of men like to experiment with softer textures such as silk shirts and brighter colours, moving away from the more traditional choice of dull grey and blue. This gives them the opportunity to express the more flamboyant, artistic or sensitive sides of their nature.

Both men and women dress to please and attract the opposite sex, but there is far greater freedom of expression nowadays for them to explore and project their own personality through what they wear without being inhibited by the constraints of gender conditioning.

BELOW | If you are single, a party or social gathering is a great opportunity for both sexes to get together, dress up and try to attract new friends or a partner.

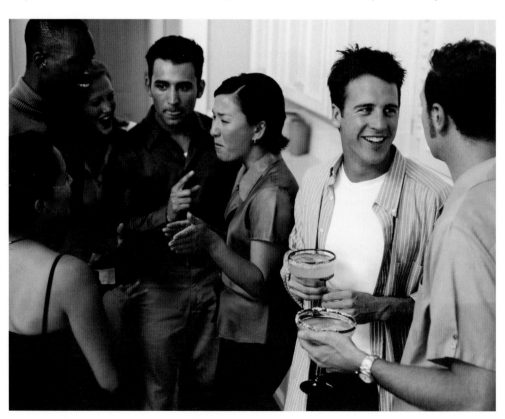

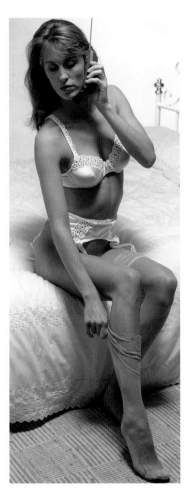

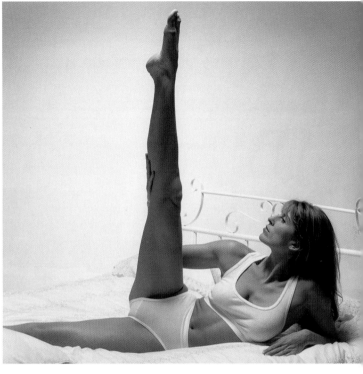

under your clothes

The choice of underwear or lingerie a woman picks to put on before going out on a social or business engagement can make a major difference to the way she feels about herself. What items of clothing she has next to her skin, and that only she knows she is wearing, can do much to enhance her confidence and sense of attractiveness.

The colours can also affect her own mood, and definitely those of a lover if he sees her when she gets undressed. For instance, a red bra-and-panty combination can send a passionate message. In

fact, for an overtly sexual statement you can't beat scarlet. It states that the woman is sexually confident and that she knows what she wants and plans to get it.

Black lacy underwear makes a sophisticated but feminine statement, and is flattering to any body shape. It is sultry and sexy while being practical, and shows the woman feels confident and in control. Sexy silk underwear in virginal white creates a wonderful contrast when worn under a smart but severe business suit. The soft material on the skin will feel very sensual and feminine. Silk underwear, in particular, is so smooth and teasingly flimsy that it gives a woman the daring impression that she is wearing nothing at all.

In contrast, sporty underwear that is comfortable and supportive helps a woman feel relaxed, knowing she can move easily and that her body looks and feels firm and secure.

LEFT | Silky virginal white underwear will make you feel sexy and special – no matter what the day holds in store.

ABOVE | Comfortable and sporty, this combination is not designed just for exercising to keep trim: it can make you feel relaxed and well-supported under leisure clothes.

psychological exercise

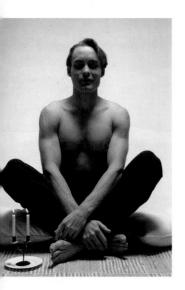

ABOVE | Take time to meditate each day to help you unravel the tensions caused by the daily stresses and strains and to restore your spirit to a state of equilibrium. Find a quiet place where you will not be disturbed, and light candles to enhance the meditative atmosphere. Then sit with your back straight and breathe naturally, focusing your awareness on your breathing as you inhale and exhale.

RIGHT | The first step towards finding a loving and fulfilling relationship is to have a positive attitude towards yourself. How can you expect someone else to love you if you don't love yourself?

A MAJOR STEP TOWARDS FINDING a partner with whom you can truly relate as an intellectual, sexual and emotional being is to have confidence in your own mental outlook, physical attractiveness and emotional status. Before you can develop your self-esteem you must first identify and eliminate the negative patterns of behaviour formed by past experiences and replace them with positive and self-enhancing thoughts and attitudes.

Negative patterns of thought and behaviour can often become etched into the unconscious mind as a result of unhappy childhood experiences, broken relationships and unfulfilled hopes and desires. These harmful facets of the human psyche represent a heavy burden, holding us back in our attempts to form loving liaisons based on mutual respect and esteem. Yet we are often totally unaware of the unwelcome mental baggage we are carrying around with us.

The effect that the mind has on our psychological make-up can be likened to an iceberg. It is only our conscious mental processes that we are fully aware of yet these actually play a small part in the development of our psychological profile. It is the unconscious, an unseen force lurking below the waterline of our awareness, that has the most profound influence on our behaviour patterns, our self-image and our ability to form lasting and meaningful relationships. Negative patterns of thought that have formed in the unconscious can damage our self-esteem and hinder our attempts to form lasting relationships. By following a daily pattern of psychological exercises we can get in touch with our unconscious selves and repair the damage caused to our sense of self-worth.

breathing and meditation

To form a loving and giving relationship with another person you must first learn to be at peace with yourself. Pressures at work, the demands of friends and relatives, as well as the constant reminders of international tensions, make this increasingly difficult. However, it is vital for your mental equilibrium that you try to set aside some time each day for quiet contemplation in order to relax your mind and body completely.

You have to cut yourself off totally from the turmoil of the outside world until you are able to restore your physical and emotional nature to a state of peace and harmony. You will then be able to return to the pressures of the daily routine feeling revitalized and replenished in body, mind and spirit.

The first step on this road is to learn the correct breathing techniques. Breathing powers the brain cells so that you become more open and alert, it provides the vital nutrients required by the tissues, and it removes harmful wastes. Correct breathing will recharge your batteries when you are feeling tired and will soothe you when you are feeling anxious or under stress. Don't force your breathing. Inhale and exhale through your nose, letting the air flow smoothly down into your lungs and

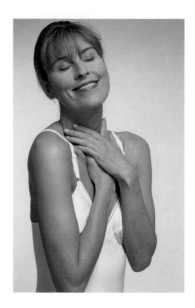

feeling it spread throughout your body, replenishing its cells. Close your eyes and focus on your breathing, feeling the rise and fall of your abdomen as you breathe.

Breathing can then combine with meditation to help you relax totally and get in touch with your inner being. Seek out a quiet place to sit and meditate for 20 minutes and make it a daily routine of relaxation. To enhance the atmosphere of contemplation, close the curtains, turn down the lights and let candlelight cast a gentle glow.

Make sure you have a comfortable, straight-backed chair to sit on so you can maintain a good upright posture, or sit cross-legged on a cushion on the floor, keeping your back straight. Take a few minutes to relax and then start to breathe regularly, as above. Clear your mind of all thoughts and just concentrate on your breathing, focusing on the slow and regular movements of your abdomen. Now direct your breathing to all areas of the body, relaxing each part in turn with every exhalation. Work slowly from your toes to the top of your head, paying special attention to the legs, pelvis, back, shoulders, arms, neck and head.

By developing these meditation skills you will find a way to get in contact with the innermost

reaches of your mental processes and help your psyche to be more receptive in preparation for the next stage of your programme of mental self-improvement – to develop a loving attitude towards yourself.

positive thinking

Negative feelings about your physical or psychological self, and indeed whether you are even worthy of forming a good relationship, can act as a self-fulfilling prophecy, either blocking attempts to enter into new liaisons, or ensuring that any relationship that develops is full of disharmony and discord and so bound to fail. By following a psychological exercise programme each day you can eliminate negative thoughts and accentuate positive ones. You will not only feel good about yourself but also encourage others to feel the same way about you too, fostering a sense of love and equilibrium in any partnership that develops.

A low self-image can often become deeply ingrained as a result of the negative messages we have received from friends, relatives and loved ones, particularly in our early formative years when we were at our most vulnerable and impressionable. Therefore, if you are to develop a positive image of yourself you must first find a way to counteract these negative feelings. The first step is to try to identify those aspects of your thoughts and feelings about yourself that embody your negative mental patterns and to write them down as a list on one side of a piece of paper.

These may be, for example: "I am not attractive", "I am not sexually desirable", "I am not worthy of a relationship", "Nobody could love me", "My relationships don't last". Next, on the opposite side of the paper, write down the positive affirmations that counteract these negative images. Write "I AM attractive", "I AM sexually desirable", "I AM worthy of a relationship", "I CAN be loved", "My relationships WILL last". Say these things to yourself every day and this continual reinforcement of your positive nature will change the negative patterning of your subconscious mind, creating a direct effect on your conscious actions, and your attitudes to others.

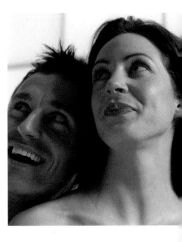

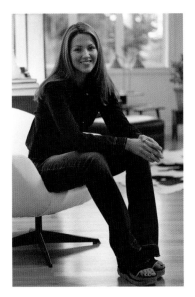

ABOVE | Never under-estimate the importance of smiling and laughter to lighten up your life. If you make the effort always to look for the joyful aspects of every situation, rather than being suspicious of happy feelings, you will encourage others to share your sparkling mood.

LEFT | Feeling comfortable and happy within yourself is vital if you want to portray a positive image to others.

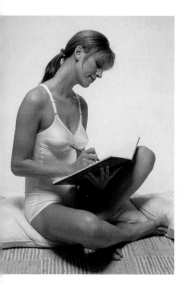

ABOVE | You can turn negative thoughts into positive ones by following a programme of exercises for making positive affirmations. Write down those thoughts and judgements you have on yourself, and then counteract them with positive affirmations. Repeat this regularly to yourself to counteract the negative patterning of your thoughts.

RIGHT | Self-discovery is an ongoing process. Take time to study self-improvement books and learn to expand your consciousness so that you can release all the potential that is lying dormant deep inside your psyche.

visualization techniques

When individuals have endured a very painful experience in a relationship, or have been left deeply scarred as a result of psychological trauma or a broken family background, it can leave them feeling disillusioned with themselves and lacking confidence in their ability to form loving relationships. In such cases they will often have to reach deep down inside their subconscious to undo the damage that has been caused.

One way to achieve this is to use the technique of positive visualization. Sit in front of a large mirror, and make yourself comfortable. You need to be very relaxed and at ease, so use the deep-breathing and meditation techniques you have already learnt to get into a relaxed and receptive frame of mind, ensuring that you keep your eyes closed.

Once you feel physically and mentally at peace, cast your mind back to a time when you felt truly loving towards another person, recalling the situation in minute detail. Try to remember where you were, who you were with, and what had happened to make you feel this way. Recapture the feelings of love that you experienced at the time and fill your mind and body with them.

Now, open your eyes and look at the image of yourself with the feelings of love, tenderness, warmth and joy you have just re-evoked. Think about the various aspects of yourself that you most admire; not just the physical characteristics that you are happiest with – your attractive eyes, perhaps, your shapely legs, or your long hair – but also the personality traits that you think are most worthy of appreciation – maybe your intelligence, loyalty, perseverance, or affectionate nature.

Once you have begun to see yourself in this new and affirming light, concentrate on those aspects of your character that you would like to improve. Perhaps you would like to be more relaxed, or more energetic, more forgiving, or more loving. Repeat this exercise every day. You may not get spectacular results immediately, but slowly these positive affirmations will print themselves over the negative patterning that

existed before. By enhancing this positive self-image, you give out a confident, contented aura that encourages others to think highly of you as well, and so increases your chances of forming a successful and fulfilling relationship.

Once you are in a relationship, it is important to continue with these exercises to reinforce your positive thinking patterns and to counteract any discordant feelings that might arise. You can use these techniques with your partner to reinforce each other's self-image and your loving feelings towards one another.

Take it in turns to make positive loving statements about each other while gazing deeply into your partner's eyes. Combine this with mutual breathing and meditation sessions to help bring you closer on an emotional and spiritual level.

seeking friendship

To achieve true contentment, it is important to feel fulfilled on all levels. If you are in a committed relationship it is all too easy to look to your partner to satisfy all your emotional and psychological needs. In fact, though, it is rarely possible for one person to gratify another's wants and desires in this way. For example, it might be a very loving and contented partnership on a domestic level, but there may also be major intellectual differences. Perhaps one of you is interested in

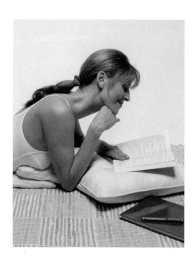

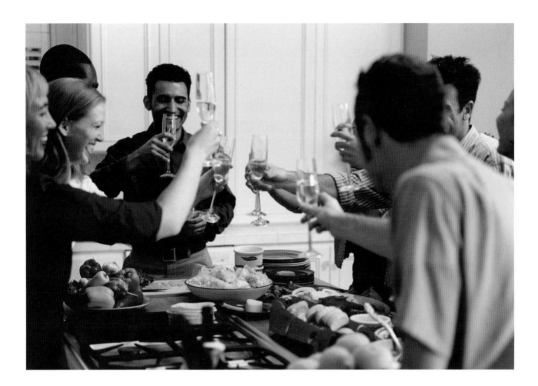

opera or philosophy and the other prefers to talk about sport and listen to pop music.

If you keep looking to each other to fulfil your needs on every strata it can quickly drain the relationship, leading to disharmony and conflict. For this reason it is vitally important to have a wide circle of friends to act as a natural resource from which you can gather all the mental and spiritual stimulation you need and also to share parts of yourself that perhaps do not flourish within the partnership.

These friends should include members of the same sex to satisfy other aspects of the relationship that your partner cannot give you. The nourishment that comes with this form of close bonding can be very important. In any relationship, certain issues crop up, whether of a sexual or emotional nature, that you cannot talk over with your partner, or indeed any member of the opposite sex. In these situations you can benefit from talking to someone of the same sex

who will have a natural empathy to your situation. Men and women can more easily relate to their own sex and have a common outlook, and a meeting of minds, that can rarely be achieved with a partner, no matter how close. Women are usually much better at forming these sympathetic same-sex relationships, but men, too, can benefit from having friends who will provide insights and experiences from which they can learn.

Discovering yourself is an ongoing process and one that could never be fully achieved even if you devoted your entire lifetime to the task. But there are a wide range of self-improvement books that help you achieve greater insights into your mental and emotional condition and enable you to fulfil more of your potential. Books on relaxation, visualization, meditation and positive thinking, for example, can help to reveal dormant abilities and find new ways to accentuate your latent active and creative sides, while at the same time eliminating the negative aspects of your nature.

ABOVE | It is important to have a wide circle of friends outside a sexual relationship. Friends can provide communication, empathy, and support that comes from shared interests and a similar outlook, and can often satisfy needs that cannot be fulfilled within the sexual relationship itself.

flirting

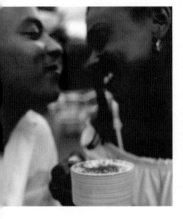

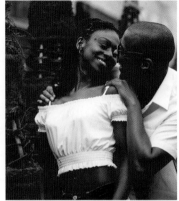

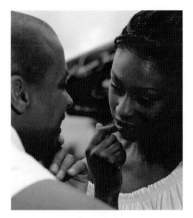

ABOVE | Flirting is a natural skill everyone can learn. Making body contact, and touching the face while maintaining eye contact, are classic ways of displaying interest in someone.

BELOW | Keeping eye contact while smiling is a great way to get someone's attention.

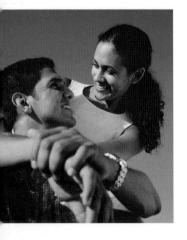

MANY THINGS ARE CHANGING in our society, but there are certain things that remain constant. One of those, fortunately, is flirting. Flirting is a fun and exciting game that comes naturally, but like any game it takes practice, skill and determination.

the game begins

A lot of people find it difficult to attract members of the opposite sex. You may feel that you are too shy for flirting, or not confident enough to approach anyone who may interest you. It should be a comfort, therefore, to know that it doesn't matter how confident or outgoing the individual – everyone finds this tricky and there are some simple things you can do to improve your prospects. The best advice is to remember to be yourself.

Flirting begins once you've established eye contact. This is how the game begins. The eyes are said to be the windows of the soul and are the most powerful weapon in your arsenal.

Once you have noticed a person you think looks promising, try to catch his or her eye as he or she walks past. If your gaze is returned, try to hold on to the contact for a couple of seconds. For the more adventurous, this is a good time to use that charming smile (but please check that you don't have spinach between your teeth beforehand).

It is easy to affect someone's first impressions of you. It is important to smile, as it says that you are friendly and approachable. Your smile can completely alter your face. When you think of someone you love, you often imagine them smiling. Backing up a smile by saying hello is one step further. A wink is a really cheeky opener, if you are brave enough.

When you are in a large crowd, surrounded by friends or colleagues, you can seem quite unapproachable, especially to anyone who is not confident enough to penetrate your group and talk to you. If you have seen someone that you like the look of, then try to make it easy for him or her to approach you. Offer to go to the bar to get the next round of drinks, or go around topping up people's glasses at a party – anything that takes you away from the crowd and gives you an opportunity to sidle past him or her.

Sometimes, you might really like the look of someone you may be standing next to while waiting in line for the cinema or some other form of entertainment. Lines and queues are perfect opportunities for flirting, as you can easily strike up a conversation about the poor service, what film you are waiting to see or what time it is due to start.

women are natural flirts

Most women, for one reason or another, are more natural about flirting than men. Women tend to have a more flirtatious manner and will often flirt with both men and women. To add to the confusion, women who flirt are not necessarily doing it because they are attracted to whoever they are talking to, but more as a means of assessing how a person responds to them.

Austrian anthropologist Karl Grammer, the Director of the Ludwig Boltzmann Institute of Ethology in Vienna, conducted a study on 45 pairs of male and female strangers. They were secretly monitored through a two-way mirror to analyse how they interacted with one another. The majority of the women attracted male attention using flirtatious gestures and chatting easily, regardless of whether they later admitted to finding the men attractive. The subconscious flirting methods they used, such as nodding with encouragement, were merely a means of assessing the men's suitability. Grammer concluded, "You can predict male behaviour from female behaviour, but not the other way round."

Although this is an interesting insight into female behaviour, it is important to remember that this was a study of group interaction and not one-to-one. If, as a man, you are not sure whether a woman is interested in you when you are in a group environment, try to get to talk to her on her own. If she continues to flirt more directly at you alone, you could be in with a chance.

first moves

Once you have made eye contact and smiled, the next step is to take a deep breath and go over for round one – the chat. Remember, this is the 21st century and it's no use sitting idly twisting the straw in your drink and waiting for him (or her) to make the first move. It's up to you to get off your chair and introduce yourself. If you don't, someone else will beat you to it.

Your opening line is paramount. This will decide whether you end up pulling up a chair or doing the walk of shame. A study involving 1,000 women, conducted by leading psychologist

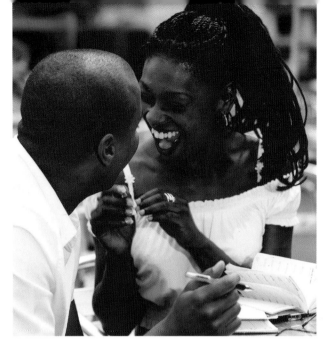

Chris Kleinke, showed that the straightforward approach is best. Charlene Muehlenhard of Texas University did a similar study on men with the same result, so keep it simple.

Kleinke's women's study showed that some of the most successful lines were simple and inoffensive openers, such as, "Do you want to dance?" or "Can I buy you lunch?" The least successful lines were those that were either smug or flippant, such as, "You remind me of a woman I used to date", or "Bet I can out-drink you!"

It's important to remember to give the object of your desire your undivided attention. This person is now *the* most fascinating you have ever met and they need to feel like it. Psychiatrist Danilo Ponce advises people to concentrate on personal attributes rather than material ones. He warns, "Don't compliment a woman's earrings – compliment her beautiful smile."

The most important thing to remember is that flirting is usually innocent and light-hearted. Try to avoid going into any situation with the thought that "this could be the one" at the back of your mind. Keep relaxed about it; at the end of the day, he or she is usually just another person looking for love. Enjoy the excitement of meeting a totally new person, keep an open mind and have fun.

ABOVE | Once you get to this stage, make sure you take the time to write future assignations in your diaries so neither of you forgets.

dating

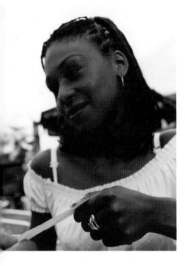

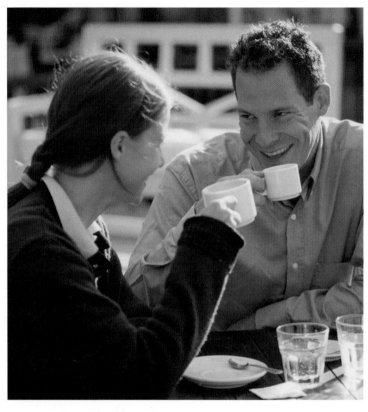

ABOVE | Don't fight over who pays – better to give in gracefully and then you can pay the next time.

RIGHT | Keep the conversation light until you know each other better, steering away from politics or subjects that you feel strongly about.

A DATE IS AN OPPORTUNITY for you and your new acquaintance to get to know each other more fully, work out if you seem to be compatible and, perhaps more importantly, if you would like to see each other again.

Going on a date with a new person can be nerve-racking; it is exciting, but ultimately you each want to come across in your best light. Choosing where to go on a date relies a lot on the circumstances. If the decision has been left to you, try to find a place that is neutral and keep it relatively simple. You should aim to be in an environment where you can talk easily and that makes you both feel at ease. The cinema is not ideal as a first date, as you can't really talk to each other. However, it is a good option for a second date, especially if you have dinner afterwards as the film provides an ideal subject for discussion, helping you determine the depth of someone's character. It also provides insight into whether you have the same opinions about things, or if you can respect each other's differences.

meeting places

A daytime coffee or a drink after work is a good option for starters, as you can make it as short or long as you like. When going to a bar, remember to drink in moderation, as it's always a bonus if you can remember whether you would or wouldn't like to see him or her again the next day. It can also prevent you from making the mistake of sleeping with them on the first date, when you might not necessarily have done so had you been sober. (If you do choose to sleep with someone after the first date, then make sure that you are equipped to protect yourself using condoms.)

A walk in the local park is pretty romantic. The fresh air and natural surroundings can help you both feel comfortable and makes conversation flow more easily. Obviously you need fair weather, as shouting over gale-force winds with your freshly blow-dried hair flying around your head can really put a damper on proceedings, although it could provide comic entertainment if nothing else.

Alternatively, you could do something a little different, such as ice skating or bowling. Having an actual activity to do together is a fantastic option. While it provides a topic of conversation instantly, it also reduces the pressure to talk constantly, and can be hilarious fun if a sense of humour in a partner is important to you.

The crucial thing to remember is to do something that you will both be comfortable doing. Imagine a really good evening or day out with your best friend, and mimic that. Where you both go should be a mutual decision so if, for example, you are a Formula One racing driver, a

blind date

Many single people have to go through a relentless trawl in search of their perfect mate. You don't have to go on television to get a blind date; these days there are a multitude of ways to meet people.

There are online dating agencies, holiday clubs and singles columns in newspapers and magazines. Why not choose a specialist publication you are interested in? You may find someone with like interests.

Speed dating is a refreshing addition to the singles scene, available at some special singles functions. Participants have the opportunity to date up to ten people in one evening. Each person is given a name badge and a score card before being paired up. After seven minutes, a bell is rung and the men move on to the next date. If there is a mutual interest, then the speed-dating organizers will give them each other's phone numbers.

Seven minutes may not be enough time to get to know someone, but they do say that most people gain an impression of a stranger within the first few minutes of meeting them.

day at the race track may make you look great, but could be a dull, or at worst uncomfortable, experience for them.

dating etiquette

There are certain things to consider before a date, such as who pays. The best option is to assume that you are going to pay half-and-half. If you are a woman, your date may be particularly chivalrous and insist on paying. You may be fine with this or it may make you feel uncomfortable, so the best way of dealing with it is to accept his generosity graciously and then suggest that next time you will pay – you shouldn't be made to feel that you owe him anything in return.

Keep the conversation light. There are some obvious no-go areas, such as discussing your ex-partners too much, or other potentially touchy subjects. Ideally, you want to give your date an idea of what makes you tick. The time to discuss more volatile subjects is when you get to know each other better, but for now, just keep it simple. It's always an idea to maintain an air of mystery; you want them to leave feeling like they have just touched the surface of you and would like to delve deeper. Don't be frosty – just don't give them too much personal information too soon. There will be plenty of time for that later.

BELOW LEFT | Some people are lucky enough to meet potential lovers at dinner parties hosted by friends.

BELOW RIGHT | Many people spend most of their days at work, so this also may be a meeting place for like minds.

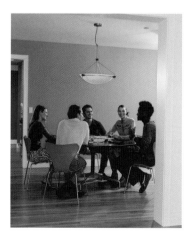

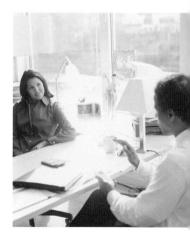

body language

ACCORDING TO PSYCHOLOGISTS, up to two-thirds of communication between humans is non-verbal. The way you sit or stand and the gestures you make broadcast a powerful message to the people you meet.

While some of these signals may be given consciously, most body language is involuntary, either instinctive behaviour or unconsciously learned through watching others. Even if you try to hide it, this secret code can reveal the way you truly feel. Understanding these subtle signs can

indicate whether the person you feel drawn to is going to reject your overtures – or already feels the same way about you.

Our innermost thoughts trigger chemical and emotional changes in the body and we respond on a physical level by unconsciously altering our posture, expression and mannerisms. These responses may be subtle movements of the eyes and mouth, or more obvious statements, such as the way we fold our arms. Individually the signals may not amount to very much, but they all

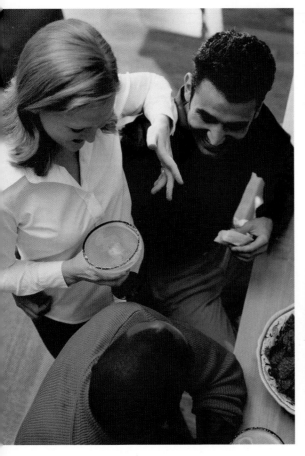
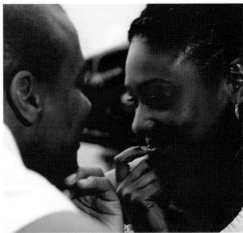
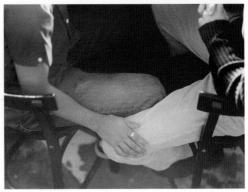

represent little clues, like pieces in a jigsaw, that can fit together to reveal a picture of our true feelings. Most people have a radar or sixth sense that tells them when another person is interested, but some people give away little and can be very hard to read. This is when an understanding of body language is invaluable.

sexual signals

Women tend to use body language more than men, but many signs are used by both sexes.

Charles Darwin said, "In the most distinct classes of the animal kingdom, with mammals, birds, reptiles, fish, insects, and even crustaceans, the difference between the sexes follows almost

BELOW | Feet directly pointed at you show positive interest.

BOTTOM | People-watching. Use the signals in the box opposite and see how many signs you can recognize.

people-watching

If the man or woman you are interested in displays some of these signals, you may be in luck. It is not a form of consent, but means you might stand a chance.

males and females – biting of lips, wetting of lips and showing the tongue, touching the front teeth.

males and females – gazing into the eyes with interest and dilating pupils.

females only – blinking more than usual, fluttering eyelashes and then looking up through them.

usually females only – twirling long hair around fingers.

males and females – he or she touches an arm, thigh or hand while talking.

males and females – matching your voice, speeding up and slowing down speech patterns in imitation.

males only – standing with legs apart, and often with hands on hips, he puffs out his chest like a cockerel.

males and females – pointing feet directly. This is a classic indication of interest.

males and females – mirroring movements; as one person leans back to sip on a drink, the other does the same.

males and females – leaning forwards and decreasing personal space.

males and females – skin tones reddening slightly, particularly on the face.

males and females – exposing the palm of the hand while facing you, or cupping an elbow in one hand and holding the other hand out, palm up.

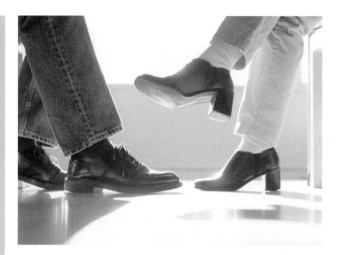

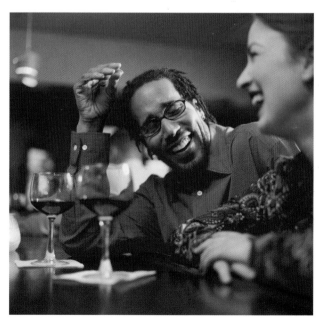

exactly the same rules; the males are always the wooers." Roughly translated, this means that the male will use all his sexual prowess in order to copulate, whether it's the peacock raising his elaborate fan and wafting it in the direction of the peahen, or a man dancing suggestively in the female's line of sight.

The females of the animal kingdom will, in turn, emit scents and signals to show either interest or lack of it. The peahen, for example, may coyly turn her back, and in some cases, so may a woman.

You should start reading body language even before the first approach. When talking to someone, watch how he or she sits, how he or she looks at you, and be aware of even the smallest gestures, because they all mean something. If you notice that you are, in fact, getting the opposite of these signs, it's time to stop talking and start walking so as not to waste your valuable time on a lost cause. You don't care; they weren't your type anyway, right?

Our body language is most expressive when we are with a member of the opposite sex. Men and women may not always be conscious of their feelings, but if they are genuinely attracted to another person, their bodies will broadcast the message loud and clear. Some responses are due to the fact that sexual attraction causes the body

to release chemicals such as adrenaline, the "fight or flight" hormone, which causes the heart and breathing rate to quicken and so prepares a person for sudden hectic physical activity.

This leads to feelings of tension and restlessness, makes the mouth go dry and produces other signs associated with nervousness and embarrassment, such as a flushed face and sweating, reactions impossible to suppress.

As society becomes more complex, so does non-verbal communication. Body language now must cope with the subtle interplay of relationships between busy working men and women, both in their social lives and while pursuing demanding careers.

confused signals

Women complain that men often misread their signs. One reason for this may be that much of a woman's body language is concerned with creating a good impression generally, perhaps to a colleague, or to acquaintances. In crowded work or social situations it may not even be clear who, if anyone, has caught the woman's interest, or she may give conflicting signals because she is unsure of herself or has other things on her mind. Her signals may not even be aimed at a single individual.

A woman who is unsure about the response she will get from a man may at first look at everyone else in the room rather than the man

BELOW | The body language of this couple shows a relaxed, trusting intimacy, with her head resting on his shoulder.

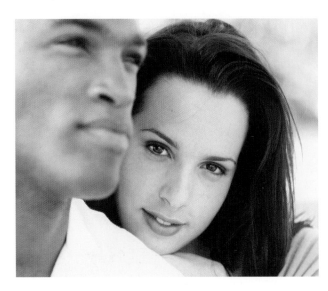

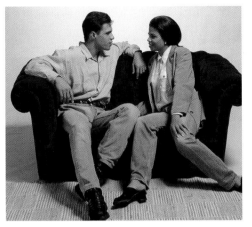 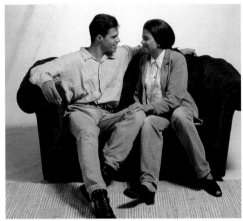

she is attracted to, apart from an occasional glance. This is a signal that men frequently misread as indicating a lack of interest.

Differences in background can also lead to confusion. For example, a woman raised in an overly protective environment, or one where contact with males has been limited, may give out seemingly provocative signals when talking to men. She might be shocked to discover her behaviour was seen as a sexual invitation. On the other hand, the signals given out by a woman who is well used to male attention may be too discreet. Careful to avoid giving a false impression, her subtle signals might appear remote or even unfriendly.

A woman's natural fluency in body language means she can often spot when another female is attracted to a man before he can. He may even be unaware of being the focus of a female's attention, in the office or at a party, for example, until his partner points it out to him.

Men, too, must be careful about the signals they broadcast. As women tend to use delicate non-verbal cues with members of their sex, they can mistakenly believe that men are equally subtle and so get a false impression. What seems to be a brush-off may simply be a sign that a man is preoccupied with his thoughts.

Alternatively, a man may be thought to be showing genuine interest in a woman when, in fact, he is just being friendly, or going through the motions of flirting without any real intention of taking it further.

Complete rejection is usually easy to comprehend, but there are other more subtle signals which may suggest doubt or shyness. So never try to read body language in isolation or be too quick to jump to conclusions. It is important to weigh up all the signals before making a judgement. A man might be indicating a lack of interest if he evades your eye or he may just be shy. A slumped posture could be a sign of rejection or that a man is feeling depressed.

At times, what seems like rejection might actually indicate confusion. If a woman sends out conflicting signals, seemingly interested but also defensive, it might be because her body is saying one thing but her mind is over-riding it. Such a situation may arise when a woman is in a long-term relationship with one man but is strongly attracted to another, and may be playing for time.

If your instinct tells you that a man is attracted to you, but he is not responding, there may be reasons for his negative body language. He may be recovering from a relationship in which he was hurt and so is wary of getting involved again. He may already be in a relationship and so unable to show his feelings openly, or he may be incapable of making a commitment. Or perhaps he considers you to be unattainable, even though he desires you.

OPPOSITE TOP | Negative signals: These body postures signal protection and defence. The arms are folded, closing off the emotional centres – the heart and belly – there is a distance between the couple, their eyes are averted and they are wearing bored expressions. There is no interest, and no chemistry.

ABOVE CENTRE | Opening up: The body language here is starting to convey availability. Their bodies are leaning towards one another, and their arms and legs are in a more open posture, showing they are beginning to feel sexually at ease. A knee is extended to make that initial, exploratory touch.

ABOVE RIGHT | Making contact: They feel safe enough in each other's company to really open up. They are smiling and making eye contact.

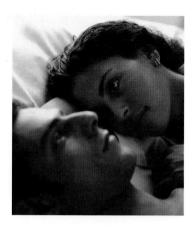

RIGHT | Learning to read
negative body signals
will help you understand
each other and begin
a relationship.

RIGHT | Learning to read
negative body signals
will help you understand
each other and begin
a relationship.

BELOW | Both people are
uncomfortable in this situation.
The woman has her legs
tightly crossed and her arms
protectively cover her lap and
genital area – an indication
that this is off limits.

A round-shouldered stance, whether seated or
standing, indicates that a man or woman is not
feeling at ease. This message is often reinforced
by a typical protective posture – arms folded
defensively, knees held tightly together and legs
or ankles crossed – in a subconscious desire to
guard vulnerable parts of the body.

Sometimes a woman will sit or stand with her
legs tightly entwined, with one foot locked behind
the calf of the other leg, and she may place her
hands protectively in her lap, unconsciously
indicating that her genital area is off limits. A man
may signal rejection by turning right away from

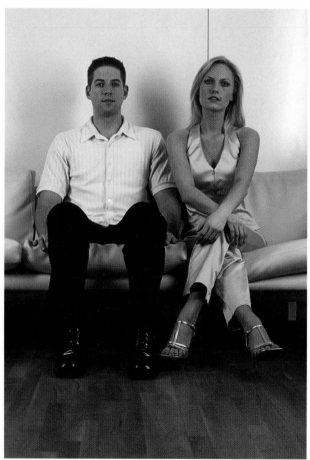

the other person, but in social situations it is
usually only the lower half of the body that
indicates the true state of affairs. For example,
a man's head and torso are turned towards the
woman and he appears to be concentrating on
what she says, but his legs and feet point towards
the exit door, indicating where his thoughts are
leading him.

Men and women also use eye language to
indicate rejection. These messages, known as "cut-
off signals", indicate the desire to withdraw from
a situation through lack of interest, or shyness. A
woman will often glance round the room, as
if calling out for someone to rescue her. It is an
unspoken plea to be taken away from her
companion, or for others to join the group, and
so diffuse the situation.

Men and women may indicate stress through
rapid blinking, or a blink that lasts longer than
normal. They may also signal their unease by
glancing rapidly to and fro, as if looking for
someone, unable to settle their gaze on you.

Our social conditioning makes it difficult to be
deliberately rude to people we meet, no matter
how much we may dislike them. To avoid causing
insult we are sometimes forced into telling "white
lies". This can cause a conflict between what we
say and how we feel, which is reflected in our
body language. Small children automatically put a
hand to their mouths when they tell a lie. In adults
the gesture is much more subtle. A person who is

being evasive will often rub his nose, or hold a hand up to his cheek in an unconscious attempt to hide the falsehood.

If a man stands with his arms crossed and his thumbs pointing upwards he is communicating that someone is getting too close for comfort and is invading his body space. A similar defensive gesture is to sit with one arm placed across the body at waist level.

accentuate the positive

While body language is mostly involuntary, simple changes may improve the way you appear to others. If you are nervous or insecure you may give out negative signals, such as folding your arms, even when you want to be friendly. There are positive steps you can take to make yourself more inviting to other people, particularly members of the opposite sex.

It is vital to relax, particularly when meeting a man or woman for the first time. When you are tense your muscles tend to stiffen and this limits your repertoire of facial expressions and makes your movements seem jerky, awkward and ungraceful. It also makes you seem much older. You can reduce the tension in work or social situations, for example, by learning a relaxation technique such as deep, regular breathing whenever you feel nervous. A natural smile, on the other hand, relaxes the facial muscles and has

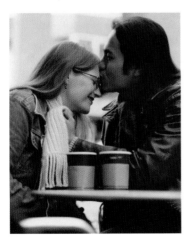

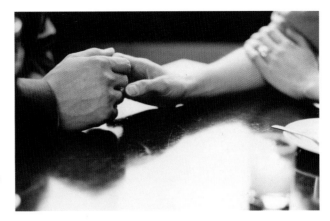

an instant effect on those around you, immediately putting them at their ease. If the smile is genuine, a small group of facial muscles will make the skin form characteristic little crinkles around the eyes. These muscles are impossible to control consciously. In contrast, a false smile looks stiff and lasts longer than is natural.

It is also important to adopt an erect posture. Sitting or standing in a slumped, round-shouldered way creates a negative impression. For women in particular, it tends to be seen as a defensive posture that suggests you have put up barriers and are not inviting anyone to take the trouble to get to know you. Try to adopt a more open posture and you will seem more approachable.

A man should aim to hold the woman's gaze directly, without furtively glancing away, even if he is feeling nervous. Otherwise he can appear rather shifty. His gaze should be friendly, rather than deeply penetrating, which can appear fierce. An open, steady look that is softened with a smile can work wonders.

A major turn-off is a look that seems to linger over a woman's body, studying every curve. A man's urge to look at a woman's body is natural, but he should do it in a respectful way otherwise she will feel as if she is under a microscope. The man who is most popular with the opposite sex is the one who makes each woman he talks to seem special by concentrating his gaze exclusively on her, without glancing at other females.

ABOVE | Holding hands is the beginning of establishing trust, confidence and openness in your relationship.

BELOW LEFT | The intimacy and trust is clear as they lean in towards each other.

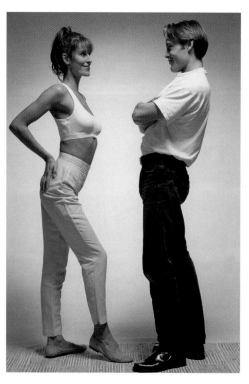

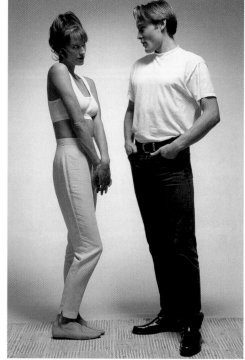

BELOW LEFT | This couple may look as if they are getting on well, but the pose is quite defensive. The woman's pulled-back pelvis indicates a withholding of her sexual energy. He is the opposite. His pelvis is forward, indicating sexual willingness, but his chest is pulled back and his arms are folded, suggesting emotional withholding.

BELOW RIGHT | Here, the woman plays helpless and vulnerable, her defenceless posture signalling "I need to be rescued". He plays the macho super-hero always in control, coming to her rescue.

relaying availability

Men have a more limited non-verbal vocabulary than women when it comes to signalling interest in the opposite sex. Men often think they are making the opening moves in the mating game and so have less need of subtlety. In fact, it is a woman's more expressive body language that encourages the man she has chosen to make that first approach. Females have such a wide range of body postures, movements and actions in their sexual armoury that males are often powerless to resist.

The way that males and females signal their availability is – initially – very similar in both sexes. When men and woman feel strongly attracted to someone they have seen for the first time, in the office or at a party, for example, the first sign is usually a change of posture. They will immediately sit or stand much straighter, which has the effect of making their tummy and neck muscles tighter

and flatter, thereby giving a taller, leaner and more youthful outline.

A woman may arch her back so that her breasts are pushed out. She will often tilt her head back or to the side, exposing her sexually sensitive neck and making it seem longer and more elegant – a universal symbol of beauty. Preening actions, such as smoothing the dress down and patting the hair, are typical gestures and, if walking, the sway of the hips may become more exaggerated. If a woman is holding an object such as a wine glass she may begin to stroke it rather suggestively.

A man may push his shoulders back and thrust his chest out, too, making his shoulders seem much broader, and his torso more muscular. Some sexually aggressive males may stand with both hands arrogantly placed on the hips and the chin jutting forward. If they are fairly assured of success they may lounge back in the chair with their hands behind their head. These gestures are designed to

mirror images

Psychologists say that an important sign of whether a couple are forming a rapport is a type of behaviour called "mirroring". Here the man and woman unconsciously copy each other's actions or posture. For example, at a party if two people are sitting on a sofa deeply engrossed in conversation, the man may turn sideways and lean towards the woman, perhaps resting an arm on the sofa back. Almost immediately, this action is likely to be copied by the woman. If the woman crosses her legs the man will cross his too, or they will both raise their wine glasses and take a sip of their drinks at the same time. To observers these copy-cat actions will seem like mirror images.

emphasis. This pose is particularly common among adolescent males who have not learned a more subtle approach. A less blatant way of indicating the genital area is to stand with one hand inside a trouser or jacket pocket.

A woman's eyes will open much wider, giving her a welcoming yet rather vulnerable appearance. She will look for an opportunity to move closer to the man, even if she is currently engaged in talking to a friend or client. If this is not immediately possible she will often turn towards him slightly to reduce the distance between them. If he is close by, this may draw him into the group, so providing an opportunity to initiate a conversation. She may glance over her shoulder, or lower her eyelids and glance sideways until the man notices, and then look away. If a woman lacks self-confidence she may only give sidelong glances. A more overtly sexual gesture is to toss her head, flicking the hair out of her face, or run her hands through her hair.

enlarge the man's outline, so making him look bigger and more powerful, and to create an air of confidence.

If a man and a woman are strongly attracted to each other they may stand with their legs wider apart than normal. In women this stance makes such a powerful sexual statement that it is regularly used by fashion models to make clothes look sexier. A relaxed, open stance also makes a woman seem friendlier and more approachable, so inviting the man to make contact.

At a party, a woman may sway in time to the music and glance at the male of her choice, inviting him to suggest that they dance together. This can be such a subtle gesture that men often feel that they instigated the approach without any prompting from the woman.

Male body language tends to draw attention to the genital region as the most overtly sexual signal. For example, a man will often sit with his legs spread apart to display his crotch, or he will stand with his pelvis thrust forward. One or both thumbs may be hooked into his belt or the waistband of his trousers, with the fingers pointing downwards towards the genitals to give extra

BELOW | Sitting close to each other allows for foot signals and touching each other's feet and legs.

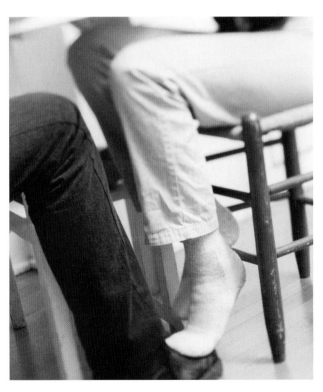

first encounters

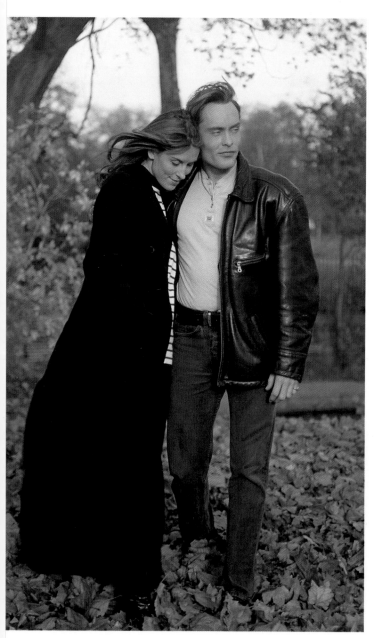

THE FIRST MOMENTS IN A RELATIONSHIP are very important. You are both nervous, unsure of yourselves and of how the other will react, yet desperately eager to create the right impression. You are aware that there is something special between you – the butterflies in the pit of your stomach and the light-headed feeling confirm that. But you are also worried that a careless move or a thoughtless word can spoil the mood and cause irrevocable harm to this budding relationship. Fear not, you must seize the moment. Remember, "Faint heart never won fair lady" – or man.

How a man and woman interact when they meet for the first time can set the seal on a relationship, or may crush a fledgling romance before it can take flight. A certain gaucheness now is understandable and acceptable. A slip of the tongue, a clumsy action – like knocking over a wine glass, or tripping over your feet – is to be expected when you are nervous about the way you will appear.

You are both eager to seem attractive, informed, interesting and sexy, but try to keep control of yourself – and the situation – and not let your tongue run away with you. You are keen to create a good impression, but don't start babbling on about yourself and stop the other person from getting a word in. At best, this can make you seem rather self-obsessed and conceited, and it may even appear that you have no interest in him or her but are simply looking for an available audience.

To avoid creating this impression, you should take every opportunity to draw the other person into the conversation. If you have been talking about a movie you saw recently, ask your companion what he or she likes to see. If you have a favourite sport or pastime, try to find out about the other person's interests.

This approach is particularly important if your companion seems tongue-tied, perhaps through shyness or because he or she is unsure of the situation and anxious not to make a wrong move.

Try to find areas of shared interest and keep to those, avoiding controversial topics, or subjects that seem to bore or irritate the other person. This will help you to discover whether you are compatible and may build a springboard from which you can launch the next stage of the relationship.

the first date

No matter how well this first interaction with your new companion has gone, the relationship can still be nipped in the bud unless one of you plucks up the courage to ask the other for a date. Traditionally the man has been expected to make this first move. But now that women want to become more assertive in a relationship, this rule need no longer apply. Indeed, many men would be extremely flattered to be asked out by a woman.

However, no matter how confident some women are about other aspects of their lives, they may be reluctant to initiate the first approach. In that case they should steer the conversation in such a way that the man is encouraged to suggest a date. For example, a woman might mention in passing that there is a movie she has been keen to see, or she could ask if he knows anything about a rather cute little restaurant that has just opened. Whoever makes the suggestion, the venue should be chosen with care on this all-important first date. You are still in the process of finding out about each other and need to select somewhere that will let you relate in an intimate atmosphere that is free from distractions.

the first touch

Now that you are sure there is a developing bond between you, try to open up and reveal something about yourself, your hopes and aspirations, as well as your likes and dislikes. But don't just communicate your feelings verbally. Body language continues to play an important part in the way a couple interact, even after the initial meeting. On this first date, try to avoid creating barriers, such as placing a handbag or umbrella

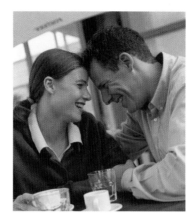

between you, or folding your arms across your chest. Walking with your hands behind your back can also be taken as a defensive posture – that you are withdrawing into yourself.

People react differently when courting, according to their personality type, perhaps appearing very restless or withdrawn. Watch out for signs of tension or anxiety in your companion, such as tightly crossed ankles, or fidgeting with jewellery or cutlery, and look for ways to put her or him at ease.

OPPOSITE | The meeting place for that special first date will be special wherever you choose. But make sure it is somewhere you can talk and really get to know each other. A simple walk in the park will give you the time and space you crave, without the fear of irritating interruptions.

LEFT | Meeting in a restaurant gives you plenty of time to get to know each other.

give the first date a chance

Avoid choosing a nightclub or pop concert for the first occasion. The noise and the crowd will make it difficult for you to hear each other, let alone talk, and you will probably have learnt little more about each other by the end of the evening than you knew at the beginning.

If you choose a movie, allow plenty of time to chat beforehand and conclude the evening with a visit to a bar or a restaurant so you have another opportunity to get to know each other.

Remember, though, the most idyllic settings are usually the simplest. If you are in reach of the coast, there is nothing like walking along a sandy seashore, as the setting sun casts golden reflections in the sea, to create an atmosphere of enchantment in which a relationship can flourish.

You could take a stroll in the park together – when there is an autumnal carpet of russet leaves covering the ground, or as the first buds of spring are peeping into view. Whatever the season, it is up to you to create the magic mood to match the moment. If the love affair develops these early trysts will always have an important place in your memories.

public gestures

A simple touch of the hand can be very comforting, if it is done lightly, in a non-threatening way. Allow your fingers to brush against his, or take her hand in yours and give it a little squeeze. But don't make a sudden grab for the other person's hand before they are ready or it can be viewed as a show of power rather than a sign of affection.

By holding hands as you walk along you are providing a clear sign of your feelings. Many men are reluctant to display such a simple show of affection in public, yet to women it can mean a great deal. Women have often said that it was when their partner first held their hand in public that they realized the depth of their love.

If, perhaps out of shyness, the man does not make this move, it gives the woman an opportunity to take the initiative. This touching gesture from her reveals her feelings for him and can give his confidence a tremendous boost.

A comforting, protective arm round her shoulder is a simple enough gesture, too, but says far more than words can ever do. But the timing has to be right – watch for an instinctive flinching or tensing up on her part to indicate you have moved too soon. If you sense this, don't remove your arm too quickly as this will show you have noticed her reaction and may embarrass her. Instead, wait a few minutes to take your arm away and then try again when your instincts tell you the gesture will be appreciated. If the relationship develops as you hope, you will soon be moving on to one of the most significant aspects of a new romance – the first kiss.

sealed with a kiss

It is natural to be over-anxious about the first kiss. Advertisements on television and in the glossy magazines are designed to make us feel insecure about the way we smell and taste to others. Provided you have followed the basic rules of oral hygiene you can rest assured that your companion will be feeling just as nervous and insecure, and with as little reason.

However, if you are going to have a meal it is a good idea to avoid foods with really pungent aromas, such as curry, garlic or onions, unless you know your companion is going to be eating the same thing.

A really confident, extrovert male may throw his arm round a woman and kiss her passionately on their first date. But with most women this rather proprietorial gesture is likely to lead to embarrassment and even hostility. Her body language will indicate this. She will tense up and look away, while her hands remain at her side showing no sign of returning the gesture. A better

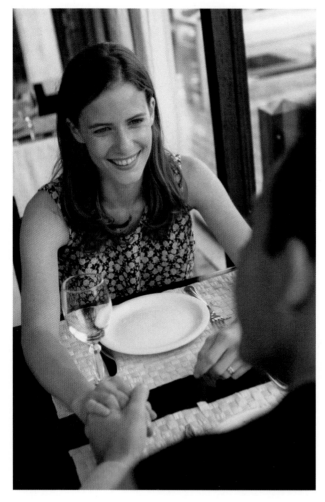

BELOW | Holding hands is an important first step in showing your feelings.

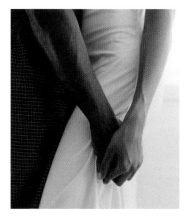

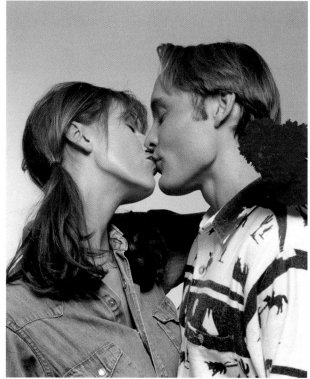

approach is to kiss her gently on the cheek, perhaps accompanied by the lightest of touches on the arm or shoulder.

Once you detect that a rapport has developed between you, the time will come to show your affection with a kiss. Unless you are sure that your partner is in the grip of an all-conquering passion – and that you feel the same way – it is best to keep this first mouth-to-mouth kiss as light and affectionate as possible. Again, the man is usually expected to make the first move – although there is no law that says this has to be the case.

A man will be looking for a sign from his companion that his advances will not be rejected. As he slowly edges forward he will notice whether she stays in the same place, or edges back defensively, or whether she mirrors his movements and leans forward too. She may lift her face to meet his and purse her lips slightly. If a woman closes her eyes as she kisses a man she is showing a clear sign of trust and affection, but this may not come until much later in the relationship. At this early stage, he should be guided by her reaction.

Kissing can remain friendly and affectionate like this, or it can build up to become passionate and arousing. It takes sensitivity to know when the change is appropriate. It is not a good idea to plant a wet slobbering kiss on the lips, or to put your tongue in someone's mouth before you receive a tacit invitation to do so.

At the same time, too much hesitation and uncertainty can be equally off-putting. If you are beginning to explore a sexual relationship with a new friend, let the kissing experience build up its own momentum.

Try to stay relaxed and calm so that your mouth and lips remain soft and yielding. That will help you to avoid the embarrassment of clashing teeth that so frequently occurs during the teenage days of early sexual exploration.

In many ways, the sexual kiss reflects the sexual act itself, because it involves a close and intimate exchange of physical contact, and in the case of deep kissing, a mixing of body fluids as the tongue enters the warm, moist mouth. The contact of mouth, lips and tongue, all highly sensitive and erogenous areas, can be an initial and safe way to discover whether there is a sexual chemistry and compatibility between you.

ABOVE LEFT | Don't just hold hands palm to palm in the conventional way – intertwine your fingers, or give the hand a little squeeze, and gently stroke the highly sensitive skin on the inside of the wrist. These actions carry powerfully charged messages that can increase the electricity of the moment.

ABOVE RIGHT | When two people become sexually attracted to each other, the first mouth-to-mouth kiss usually signifies the change in the relationship from friends to potential lovers.

the next step

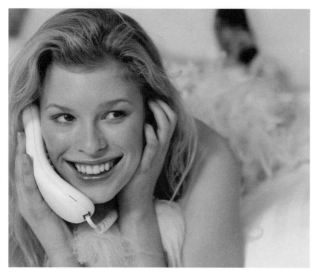

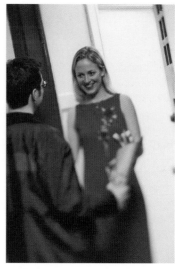

ABOVE | Making the next date. It can be difficult to get the correct balance between looking too keen and playing it too cool.

ABOVE RIGHT | Being given flowers – or even a single, perfect bloom – melts the heart of most people. A good tip, however, is not to buy them at the filling station.

SO YOU'VE MET SOMEONE you like, been out together and would love to see them again. But who should make the next move? If you are a phone person, a call the next day is always good, either to say thank you or to make sure they got home safely – both reasons are fairly innocuous and won't compromise you. If you want to play it cool, leave it for a couple of days before you pick up the phone, but not too long, as you may well freeze yourself right out of the picture.

If you are unsure of your reception and would prefer to protect yourself, a card or letter is always a good bet. With technology forging ahead, letters are fast becoming obsolete; a huge amount of correspondence is now sent through the computer and so for many people the only mail they receive is brown envelopes demanding payment. It is so exciting, therefore, to receive a crisp, hand-written envelope through the post. It's much more personal than a text message and you have the added advantage of the sensuousness of the whole experience, opening the envelope, feeling the paper, analysing the handwriting. Plus you can re-read it

as many times as you like. If you don't want to be too serious, a postcard is always good – a "thank you" card or "thinking of you" card or even a silly card about something you have in common.

You could send a bunch of flowers. Flowers are one of the traditional symbols of romance. But how often are men given flowers by women? It would certainly make a change. However, a red rose sent to his office could produce a few unwanted blushes and comments from his not-so-fortunate colleagues.

hi-tech approaches

If you are firmly fixed in the 21st century and prefer to use modern technology, you can always use your mobile phone (cellphone) or email to send a message. Mobile phones are all fitted with the text message service, which provides a great alternative for passing on short messages and greetings. Text messages have become common currency among the younger generation and can be less potentially embarrassing than a phone call. Sending a text does alleviate the heart-thumping sessions next to the phone, dialling the number, while at the same time praying the line will be busy. Simply write a few words, swallow and send. If you get a response, you can even propose another date to see each other again.

Some people think that sending an email or text message is a little cowardly and that the phone is always better, but it does let you think about what you want to say and you won't be flustered by his or her questions. Plus you can think of amusing one-liners, thus emphasizing what a fantastically interesting and witty person you are. It's certainly more casual than a phone call, definitely less embarrassing and can be flirtatious and playful. Statistics show that 42 per cent of people aged between 18 and 24 use text messages to flirt, 20 per cent of them have used a text message to ask someone out on a date and, horrendously, an unbelievable 13 per cent have ended a relationship by text message. Message received, over and out.

continuing courtship

Gifts such as chocolates or a topical book won't cost too much, and it's wonderful when you receive a gift to know that your date has been thinking about you and has taken the time and trouble to find something that they think you will like. Sometimes an inexpensive gift is more thoughtful than one that costs loads of money, but timing is everything. A naughty or suggestive present in the early stages of a relationship may not have the desired effect – so save it until later.

cyber sex

In a sense, technology has replaced and reinvented the love letter and other more creative forms of romantic communication. People today are so much busier with their careers that finding the time to get to know new people is often difficult.

Many potential couples begin (and end) their courtship by emailing each other. Some never actually come face-to-face in the real world. Dating chat rooms have been set up specifically for people to meet other like-minded individuals.

tantalizing text

Shall I compare U 2 a ~0~'s day? U R mo luvlE & mo temperate.

Confused? This is the new language of love used by romantic text messagers. Some people use texting as a form of foreplay, making provocative suggestions, to keep their partners "simmering" before they meet. It's even possible to get texting dictionaries (dxnres) and Internet web sites provide translators so that you can type in what you want to say and you will receive an abbreviated version for your message. Here are some examples to get you started.

Hot4U – Hot for you
RUF2T – Are you free to talk?
PCM – Please call me
Un4gtebL – Unforgettable
IluvU (2) – I love you (too)
Sxy – Sexy
CU l8er – See you later
26E4U – Too sexy for you
ATB – All the best
LOL – Laugh out loud
MbRsd – Embarrassed
CU@ – See you around
F2F – Face to face
ILYQ – I Like you
URA*- You are a star
URAQT – You are a cutie

However, it is important to remember that people are rarely who they say they are: the beauty of the Internet is that it lets people reinvent themselves into an idealistic version of who they really want to be. Some people are also opting for the Internet for sexual gratification, a process known as "outercourse". These chat rooms are for people who have the same erotic fantasies in common. Cyber sex can be relatively harmless, recreational fun if kept in context but there are a few pointers to remember to keep it that way. You should never give out your identity or address, and just keep the experience firmly where it should be... on the net.

BELOW | Some people like to send text messages to their date. They are quick and simple, and don't come across as being too heavy or serious.

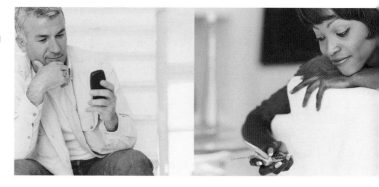

the art of wooing

BELOW | Find an interest that you have in common, such as jogging, and make it a regular part of your weekly schedule. Finding a sport or pastime you can share is the quickest way to cement a friendship.

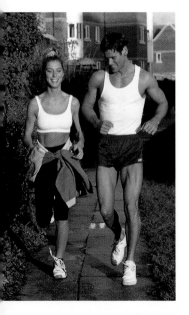

BUOYED UP BY THE SUCCESS of that first romantic meeting, you feel as though you are floating on air, and the signs are that your new friend feels the same. No matter how well that first date seemed to go, the start of a new relationship is a nerve-racking period filled with opportunities for misunderstandings. At this critical juncture, your next steps may decide whether you will part merely as friends or whether the relationship will develop into a lasting love affair. If both sides are honest and say how they feel, there is more chance that the relationship will be successful.

This is an anxious time as you wonder whether the person you have fallen for also feels the same way about you and would welcome another meeting. Waiting for someone to telephone to arrange another date can be agonizing, so, if you have had a good time, pick up the telephone and tell him or her how much you enjoyed the evening.

Suggest a second date within the next few days to judge whether your feelings are reciprocated. If you get the brush-off you must be philosophical; there is no easy way to deal with disappointment other than to hope to meet someone else soon. But if your companion is keen to see you again give plenty of encouragement.

It is important to nurture the friendship by keeping in contact and setting regular dates to meet. Try to vary the venues and activities to keep the relationship fresh and alive. Look for shared interests and try to capitalize on them by arranging activities you can take part in together. For example, if you both enjoy jogging, or have just talked about starting an exercise programme, arrange regular running sessions together. If you both enjoy the movies, set aside one night a week to see the latest releases.

Even if your pastimes are different, try to take an interest in the other person's pursuits. It won't hurt you to attend a classical music concert or a football game occasionally, and you may even enjoy it.

At the same time, try not to be over-enthusiastic. Give your new friend the space to continue with his or her own life and to maintain other friendships. This will avoid giving the impression that you are trying to push the relationship on too quickly. If you spend time away from each other, it will ensure your days together are even more vibrant.

keeping romance alive

Just because you are getting to know one another, don't take the relationship for granted and let the romance of those heady early days begin to slide. Look for ways to show your feelings, for example by giving a present when you next meet. This should be a simple token of affection and not an expensive gift loaded with expectation, as though you expect something in return.

Flowers such as roses, especially red ones, the colour that more than any other signifies love, still represent one of the most romantic statements a man can make. A woman, too, should play her part in the art of wooing by presenting the man with little gifts, such as a bottle of his favourite wine. As well as being a touching gesture in itself, this shows she has taken the trouble to discover his tastes.

Showing consideration and an awareness of the other person's moods and feelings can also enhance the loving feelings between two people. For example, a simple gesture such as helping a woman on with her coat, or complimenting her on her hair or dress, shows you really care.

Notice that your friend is tired after a busy day at the office and suggest that you cancel or postpone the date you had planned that evening, or leave early, even though you may have been looking forward to it. Your companion will really appreciate the fact that you are so finely attuned to his or her emotional wavelength and are willing to put another's best interests and needs before your own.

food of love

Once the relationship is at a stage where you feel confident enough to do so, it is natural to want to invite your new friend to your home for a meal. A sultry candlelit dinner is still one of the most romantic settings for a couple during the early stages of a relationship. It provides just the right ambience to open up to your new friend.

This does not have to be an exclusively female gesture. Males are just as capable of preparing a meal and a woman will be enchanted by this sign of a man's thoughtfulness. Cook only what you can comfortably handle. If the menu is too elaborate you will be tired before the meal starts and are likely to be spending all your time fretting about the next course, rather than enjoying your friend's company. You may also feel resentful if he or she shows less appreciation for your efforts than you think you deserve.

The atmosphere, rather than the food, is the most alluring aspect of the dinner, so aim to set the right mood. Low lighting is important to create the feeling of closeness, so you can relax and reveal your innermost thoughts. But don't rely on candles alone for the lighting.

If the room is too dark it can seem forbidding rather than comforting. The room should be pleasantly warm but not stifling, or you will both feel sleepy rather than romantic, so leave a window ajar to ensure there is adequate ventilation.

A vase of fragrant flowers adds a spring-like touch, and romantic music playing softly in the background will help enhance the mood, but make sure it is quiet enough for you to hear each other without raising your voices. Your aim is to create an island of intimacy, cut off from the cares of the outside world.

BELOW | A romantic meal can set the seal on a developing love affair. Bathed in the warm glow of candlelight you can lose yourselves in the magic of the moment and enjoy just being with your companion.

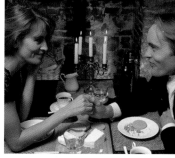

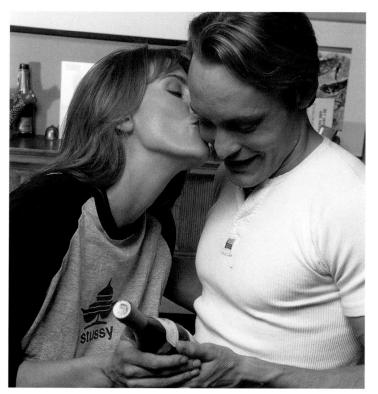

LEFT | A romantic gift should show some thought and consideration for the other person. A bottle of his favourite wine suggests that you have taken the trouble to discover his preferences.

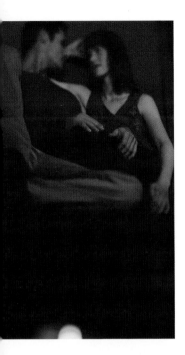

expectations

This can be a crucial time in a relationship. The romantic atmosphere can make your dinner date seem the sexiest companion in the world. Once you have opened up on an emotional level you will be better able to judge whether you want to take the relationship on to a more physical stage. Whether that means passionate kissing and heavy petting, penetrative sex, or any of the sexual possibilities in between, this is a very personal decision that individuals must make between themselves according to their own moral codes and social mores.

The question of when to sleep together for the first time has always been fraught with ethical and practical worries. In the past, the main concern has been the fear of pregnancy. The greater availability of effective contraception has largely removed that fear for many couples (although, on religious grounds, it may still not be an option for other people) but this concern has been replaced by the risk of HIV infection.

It is not unusual for some couples to have sex on the first date, while others prefer to reserve it for after marriage, or ensure that it is part of a clearly committed long-term relationship. For most modern couples, however, the change of pace from simple friendship to sexual intimacy is likely to occur at some point between these two extremes. However you feel about the issue, it is your decision and you should not feel pressurized into having sex before you are ready, nor should you coerce others to do so.

No matter how aroused you become, you will need to remain attuned to your partner's signals, ready to slow the tempo, or stop altogether, if there are any signs of nerves or hesitation. A man, in particular, is making a grave error if he assumes that his sexual technique is so irresistible he will be able to get a woman into a state of sexual arousal in the face of her signs of reluctance.

A woman's right to say "no" to sexual intercourse must always be respected, regardless of whether a couple have had sex on previous

ABOVE AND RIGHT |
A romantic night in is a very good time to talk and share and be as one with each other. How much of yourself you reveal in these intimate encounters is entirely up to you, but it is better to be as open as possible, rather than holding back and risking creating an emotional distance between you.

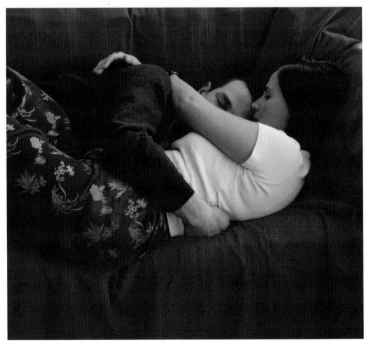

occasions, or have been enjoying a highly arousing session of kissing and petting. Her cooling off need not imply that the woman is a "tease" or that she has lost interest in the man, merely that she is not ready to let the relationship develop to that stage.

Just as men have always been expected to make the opening moves in a sexual encounter, a woman should also be free to take the initiative and invite the man to stay overnight if she chooses. And if the man declines, for whatever reason, or no reason at all, this should not be taken as a rejection or a lack of sexual interest. It may simply be that he is not ready to make that commitment, or is tired or has drunk a little too much alcohol, and is worried that his sexual performance will prove to be a disappointment to her. A sensitive lover is one who can read his companion's mood and knows how far to go. When two people are attuned to each other's needs and desires, eager to give pleasure as well as receive, and ready to consummate the relationship with a physical display of their love – the sky's the limit.

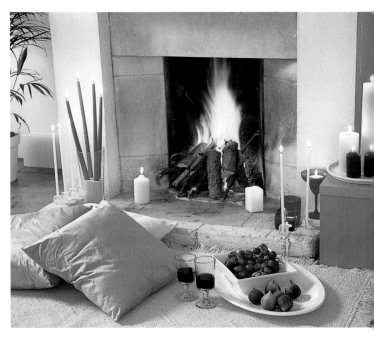

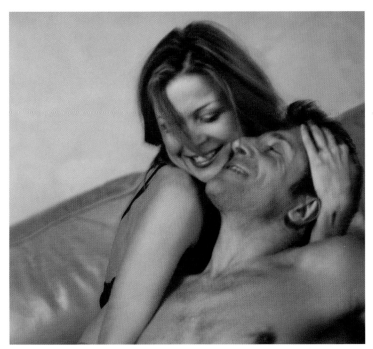

ABOVE AND LEFT | To set the scene for a romantic and intimate night in, think soft and warm. Candles, cushions and an open fire are traditional favourites for creating the right atmosphere; if you don't have an open fire, turn up the heating.

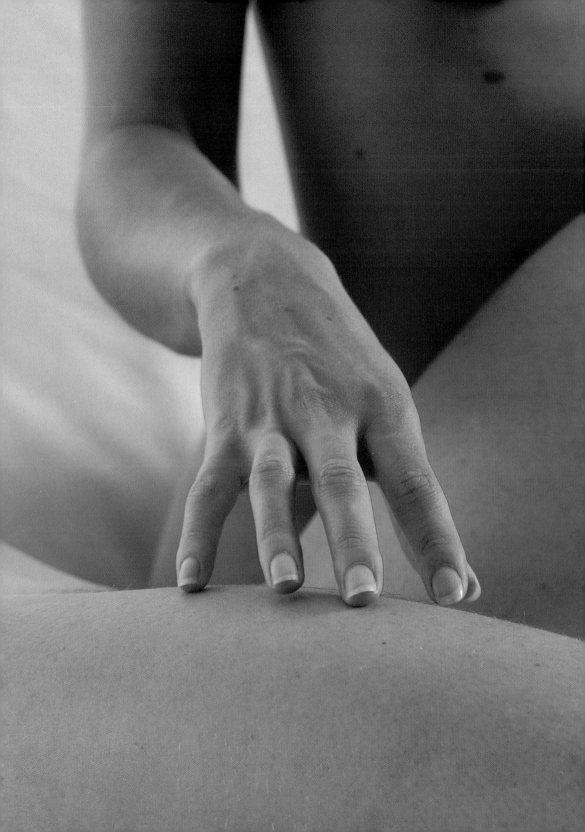

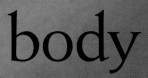

body

In order to achieve sexual harmony with your partner, you must have an understanding of both your lover's body and your own. Explore each other by touching and tasting different areas. After all, doing your sexual homework together is never going to be a chore.

caring for yourself

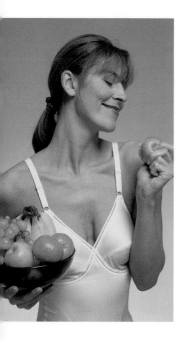

THE GIFT OF ANOTHER PERSON'S LOVE is a satisfying, fulfilling and nurturing force, but it is also important to gain that degree of caring and respect for yourself. We are not conditioned to love ourselves, but are encouraged to put our own well-being in second place in order to consider others. To create a secure sense of self-esteem involves a conscious drive towards self-awareness, and that is an ongoing process throughout our whole lives.

nurturing yourself

Building up your sense of self-worth will empower your life, and enable you to become less dependent on another person for your own feelings of personal value. This will sustain you in the times when you are on your own, and will also enrich any relationship you are involved in because you will have sufficient emotional resources to share.

You can start by planning a lifestyle that shows a real concern for the basics – a good diet, healthy exercise, and plenty of rest and relaxation. As well as enhancing your health and well-being, this will help you manage the tensions in your daily life so that stress becomes a power for good, for positive action and achievement, rather than a negative force that blocks and withholds your vital energy.

To have the confidence and enthusiasm you need to embark on a new relationship you have to feel good about yourself, and this means nurturing the essential you. This process of self-appreciation starts by ensuring you feel good internally and externally, so that your body is relaxed and full of energy and vitality, and your complexion is clear and glowing with life. Self-appreciation involves feeling good about your body so that you are content about yourself and life in general, as well as being very alive and spontaneous. It is also about preparing your physical self so that you are better able to fight disease and stay healthy, because ill health is a state of mind as well as

body, and will dampen the enthusiasm and self-confidence you need to seek and sustain a loving relationship.

Ensuring you have adequate rest is an important part of this process. Never neglect your sleep routine because without sufficient rest and relaxation, your body is unable to replenish its resources, and you are unlikely to achieve the mental harmony you need to fulfil your potential.

diet and nutrition

Diet can often have the most direct and immediate effect on your well-being, and yet it is the one aspect of the average person's lifestyle that is most likely to be neglected. A healthy body must start with a healthy diet. That "you are what you eat" is an old adage – yet it is literally true, because the cells in your body are constantly being replaced by the molecules in your food. Food supplies the building blocks, in the form of amino acids and essential fatty acids, which repair and replenish your tissues, and ensure the normal functioning of the basic bodily processes. It also provides the vital energy you need to power you through the day and it will certainly add zest to your sexuality.

Mealtimes should be an important part of your daily activity. Instead of rushing your food, take time to sit down and relax as you eat. Turn your mealtimes into an occasion for mental relaxation as well as physical renewal. In this high-speed, high-pressure world it is tempting to forsake a good diet in favour of high-fat fast foods and sugar-rich snacks. This can only be a short-term solution and can have disastrous long-term consequences.

Eating too much of the wrong kinds of foods leads to a much higher risk of digestive disorders, heart disease, and certain types of cancer, as well as risking obesity and tooth decay. The body also needs adequate levels of essential nutrients, including vitamins and minerals, to stay healthy.

ABOVE | Eat plenty of fresh fruit, at least five pieces a day, as part of a healthy diet.

Only by eating a balanced diet with a wide range of foods can you ensure that you are getting all the major nutritional components you need.

Highly processed foods invariably contain an excess of animal fats and refined sugars, while much of the goodness, in the form of fibre and vitamins, is removed. These foods represent empty calories that add to your waistline but provide little else of benefit.

Physical well-being starts with a well-balanced diet. Normally, a person should aim to increase the percentage of complex carbohydrates, such as bread and potatoes, in the diet, and reduce the amount of refined sugars, such as cane sugar. Complex carbohydrates provide energy at a steady, sustainable rate, while simple sugars give a quick-acting energy surge that can make you edgy, hyperactive and irritable, and then leave you feeling drained and lethargic.

You should also try to cut down on saturated fat, obtained from meat and full-fat dairy products such as butter and cream, which clogs up the arteries and increases blood pressure levels.

ideal daily diet

The daily diet for a healthy adult should include:
- Up to eight glasses of pure water a day. This helps keep the kidneys functioning properly and flushes out the toxins and waste products that can build up in the body. You should also reduce your intake of stimulant drinks, such as tea and coffee. These drinks can disrupt the body's fluid balance and over-stimulate the central nervous system, leading to insomnia, high blood pressure and raised heart rates, and aggravating stress disorders.
- Eat plenty of fresh fruit and vegetables, to provide the vitamins, minerals, and soluble and insoluble fibre you need.
- Have at least four servings a day of complex carbohydrates, such as bread (especially whole-wheat), pasta, rice, breakfast cereals, and potatoes.
- Include in your diet low-fat dairy foods, such as skimmed or semi-skimmed milk, yogurt or fromage frais. These provide the calcium and vitamins you need without significantly increasing your intake of saturated fats.

- Your daily intake of food should include two servings of protein foods such as lean meat, chicken, fish, eggs, nuts, seeds, beans, peas and lentils. This gives the vital proteins needed to replace worn-out and damaged tissues. By including oily fish, such as salmon, herrings and mackerel, in your diet you will also be getting the essential fatty acids your body needs. A vegetarian diet can also be healthy and sustaining, but take care to ensure it contains the right balance of amino-acids. A balanced diet will ensure you get all the vitamins and minerals you need for health and well-being.

BELOW | Sleep relaxes the mind as well as the body by helping to uncoil the cares and tensions that have been building up throughout the day. It also refreshes and revitalizes you for the day ahead.

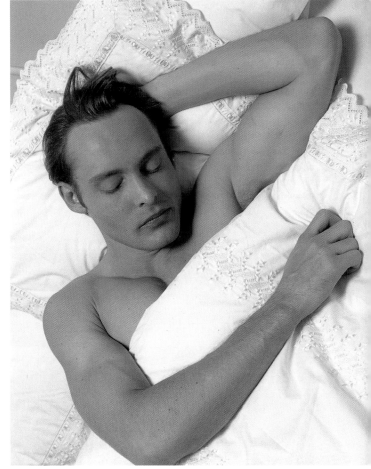

skincare

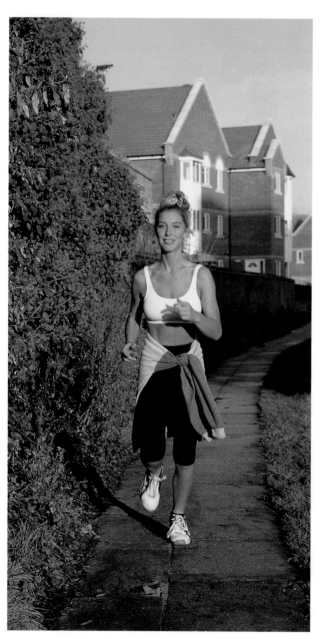

AS WELL AS BRINGING ABOUT internal physical changes to enhance your self-esteem, a health and self-awareness routine can also take into account your outward appearance. Good grooming and a concern for your appearance are just as important for men as for women.

Helping to keep your skin clean and youthful-looking does not need to involve expensive bills at a beauty parlour, or costly cosmetic preparations, as a simple daily regime is usually sufficient. A nutritious and balanced diet, of course, is the best way to have a healthy skin. Skincare is mainly aimed at counteracting the harmful effects of the sun and wind, and preventing the pores becoming blocked by removing dirt and excess grease along with the outer layer of dead skin cells. You should avoid wearing heavy make-up and use a cleanser to remove all cosmetics before you go to bed.

moisturizing your skin

Using creams and lotions to moisturize and revitalize your skin can make you feel sensual and help you to get in touch with your body. The insidious effect of advertising and its constant encouragement to achieve unrealistic perfection can often lead people, particularly women, to develop a negative body image. By massaging your own body with a good-quality moisturizing cream or lotion to help nourish your skin, you can take the opportunity to explore your body so you learn to appreciate yourself, lose your negative feelings, and feel more positive, as well as caring for your skin at the same time.

Starting with your face, spread upwards and outwards from your nose, working the cream into your forehead and then sweeping out to the temples. Slide your fingers along the sides of the nose and out over your cheekbones, then use your fingertips to stroke upwards and outwards from your chin over the jaw and up to the ears. Finish this area by rubbing the cream into your neck, using an upward motion to tone the muscles.

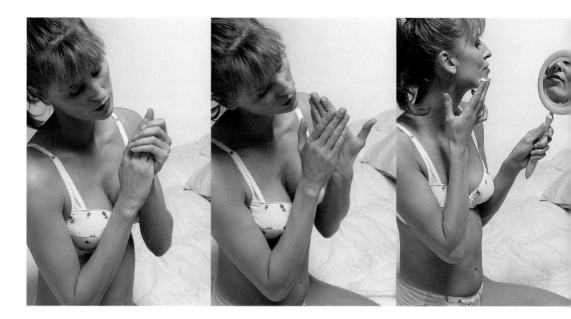

Now use light sensuous touches of your fingers and palms to spread the cream over your body. Working outwards from your heart, spread the cream across your chest, using an upward motion on your breasts, and then rub it over your shoulders and down your arms. Work from your lower breastbone over your belly and down your legs to your feet. Take time to rub the cream in well, particularly into the top and undersides of the feet, to squeeze out the muscular knots and tensions that can accumulate here.

Alternatively, spread a rich massage oil over your body. A man should pay attention to the muscles around the shoulders and arms and in the legs, kneading the flesh with the fingertips to loosen and invigorate the muscle fibres.

To enhance the feeling of relaxation, blend one or more aromatherapy oils into your massage lotion. Lavender is a safe and attractive oil for relaxation and harmony, which can also ease tired, stiff or aching muscles, but there are many more you can choose. By using these soothing caresses on your skin, you will begin to know and love your body, as well as nurturing your skin with the lotion to leave it soft and glowing.

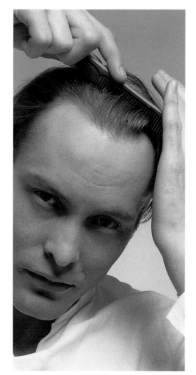

ABOVE | Apply a good-quality moisturizing cream to nourish your skin, and explore your face and body at the same time, so you can learn to appreciate yourself as you care for your complexion.

LEFT | Good grooming is just as important for men as it is for women. By taking some care over your appearance you encourage others to take an interest in you.

OPPOSITE | Aerobic exercise, such as jogging, will boost the heart and lungs and draw oxygen into the tissues to improve your health, well-being and mental alertness.

BELOW LEFT | Spread a
massage oil over your body,
working it into the muscles of
the shoulders, arms and legs.
Knead the flesh with the
fingertips to loosen and relax
the muscle fibres.

BELOW CENTRE | By making
your hands into a loose fist
you can gently pummel the
body to release tension in the
tissues and boost the blood
circulation, leaving you
feeling restored and
invigorated.

BELOW RIGHT | Use a skin
brush to remove the dead
outer layer of skin cells. It will
revitalize and refresh the skin
and also leave your body
tingling and glowing with
health and vitality.

self-massage

A regular self-massage programme makes you
look and feel more relaxed, as well as stimulating
the circulation and enlivening your skin so that you
can become more sensually responsive. It can
help you develop an awareness of your outer
self, as well as dispelling negative thoughts and
improving your body image.

Start off by massaging the head, using tiny
circular movements as if shampooing your hair,
and feel the scalp move under your fingers. Now
massage the temples, using two fingers of each
hand in a circular motion to relieve mental
tension, and then work on the fleshy areas of your
cheeks, using the flats of your fingers in large
circular movements.

The next stage is to follow an invigorating
sequence of massage strokes to refresh and
revitalize your skin and muscles. Start with the
face, and use the tips of your fingers to tap all
over the facial muscles, jaw-line, forehead,
temples and cheeks. Next, work on the shoulders
and neck. Make a loose fist and use the flat
surface of your fingers to pummel the muscles

gently. Use the same technique to pummel the
arms and down to the backs of the hands. Now
do the same thing on the inside of the hands and
arms, before using alternate strokes to pound the
ribcage vigorously. Finally, use a hacking motion
with the side of the hands on the legs and feet to
tone up the muscles and boost the circulation.

A very invigorating massage can be obtained
by using a skin brush. Available from health stores
and chemists (drugstores), this is used dry and
stroked over the skin. It removes the outer layer
of cells and allows the underlying cells to
regenerate themselves. It revitalizes and tones
the skin and enhances the body's ability to
eliminate toxins, as well as leaving the skin soft
and smooth to the touch.

Starting at your feet, work up your legs and
then your arms, and then over your body towards
your heart, following the direction of your
circulation. Follow it up with a shower to wash
off any remaining dead skin cells. If you do this
several times a week you will leave your skin
glowing with health and vigour, and silky soft
to the touch.

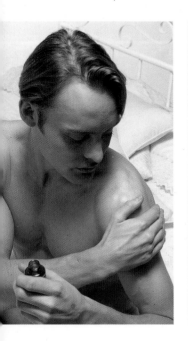 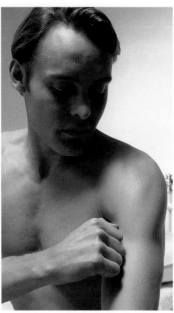 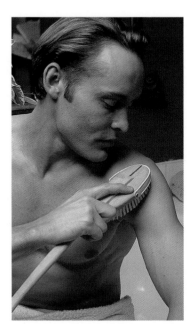

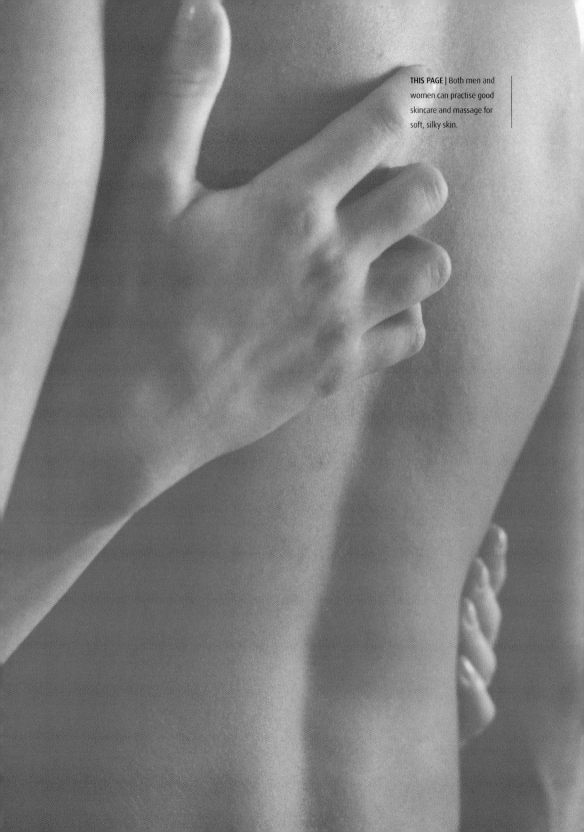

THIS PAGE | Both men and women can practise good skincare and massage for soft, silky skin.

the male body

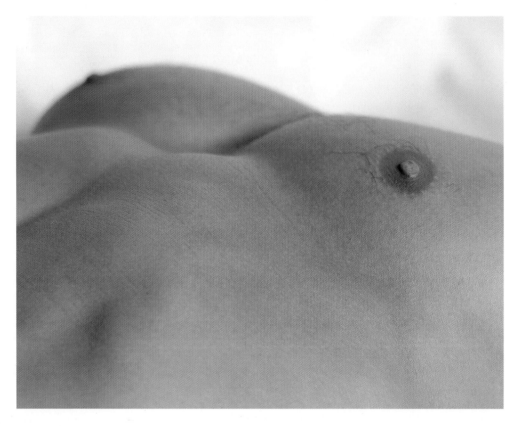

ABOVE | Many men love having their nipples played with. If they have been working out in the gym and have good pectoral muscles, lavish some time on that area to show your appreciation.

THE MALE BODY is a landscape that is well worth taking the time to explore. A body that is better known and understood will give improved and increased pleasure to its owner.

the penis

Forget dogs – the penis is man's best friend. Most men stroke and pet their penises at varying degrees of regularity. Some talk to their penises and even see it as a separate individual with its own identity and brain. So what is so special about it? Well, in some senses it does seem to have a mind of its own, especially during puberty, when it is liable to give a standing ovation at any given

opportunity. The subtle whiff of perfume from the new teacher, a hint of thigh from the woman on the bus, a pile of succulent melons in the supermarket – for young men these are trying times, a constant battle of mind over matter.

In spite of the apparent complexity and perplexity of its character, the penis is a remarkably simple organ in both structure and function. Biologically it only has two roles, those being the safe passage of urine and of sperm.

The penis has a variety of different components, all of which are made from erectile tissue, similar to that of the clitoris. In basic terms, there are four main parts making up the penis. The head, or glans, is the bulbous mushroom-shaped part at the end of the penis. The second is the shaft which makes up the length of the penis from the glans to the pubis (pelvic bones). The third is the urethra, which is the tube that runs through the shaft, and facilitates the passage of sperm and urine. Finally, the frenulum is the small piece of hypersensitive skin connecting the head to the shaft.

the glans or head

In the centre of the glans is the meatus, or urethral opening, which looks like a little slit. Sperm is ejaculated and urine expelled through this opening. The glans is the end point for a lot of nerves, making it one of the most sensitive areas on the penis.

In the uncircumcised man, the flaccid penis is covered with a thin membranous layer of skin called the prepuce or foreskin. When an uncircumcised man gets hard, this layer of skin slips back to display the glans and, during sex, it retracts further so that the glans is fully exposed. This dispels the myth that uncircumcised men have less sensitivity in that area compared with their circumcised counterparts. Circumcised or not, all the relevant areas are stimulated in exactly the same way. The only difference is that uncircumcised penises have to come outside to play first.

the shaft

The spongy erectile tissue that aids the stiffness of an erection is composed of three cylinders. The corpus spongiosum surrounds the urethra on the underside of the penis and expands at one end to form the glans. During erection and for a short time afterwards, the urethra is compressed so that it is not possible to pass urine, only semen. The other two vessels are called the corpora cavernosa, and lie at the top length of the penis.

When a man is sexually aroused, it is these three vessels which become engorged with blood, resulting in erection. Both the corpus spongiosum and the corpora cavernosa extend back inside the body towards the anus, underneath the prostate gland, to form the root of the penis, and are kept in place by ligaments.

the urethra

This is the tube that carries both urine and sperm down through the penis. The urethral sphincter muscles contract to allow either urine or semen to travel down the urethra, but not both at the same time.

the frenulum

This is located on the underside of the penis where the head meets the shaft in a puckering and folding of skin which tethers the foreskin to the head. It is an area of particular sensitivity, so it should never be ignored during lovemaking.

the corona

This is the ridge around the base of the glans where it meets the shaft. It is so sensitive that some say that light pressure around it can suppress orgasm and lengthen lovemaking. This is the area where smegma may collect, so wash regularly.

the testicles

Also called the testes (among many other less clinical names) the testicles are the most delicate and vulnerable part of the male body. Although they appear to be a pair, the testicles live in one sac which is called the scrotum. Externally, there is a very fine ridge around the centre of the scrotum called the median raphe. Inside, the septum divides the scrotum in two, so that the testicles each have their own compartment.

The job of the scrotum is to keep the testicles at the correct temperature for the production of sperm. This is a lower temperature than that of the rest of the body. You will probably have noticed that when they're warm, they hang lower and looser than when they're cold.

Each testicle is about the same size as an ovary, about 4cm/1½in long by 3cm/1¼in deep and 2.5cm/1in thick. Their main job is to produce and nourish sperm, but they are also responsible for producing the male sex hormones that control hairiness, muscularity and aggression. Each testicle produces nearly 150 million sperm every 24 hours, but after ejaculating several times it can take up to seven days to replace the sperm.

BELOW | The testes hang away from the body in one sac called the scrotum. Here the median raphe can be clearly seen.

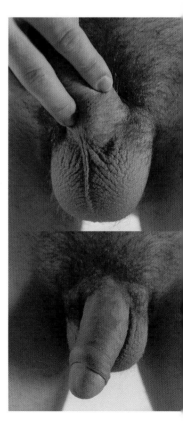

the anus

The anus is the tight, puckered hole located between the buttocks which, apart from its obvious function, can be seen as the gateway to the male G spot, the prostate. It is a tight muscle that many feel is impenetrable, but with the correct stimulation and enough lubrication, you can find it to be far more accommodating than you initially thought.

the perineum

This is the area of sensitive skin that covers the stretch between the anus and the testicles. It is often considered a flat, barren area with little purpose but to act as the frontier between the penis and anus. However, when you realize that it is located in an area of heightened sensitivity, it makes sense that here, too, is a miniature playground of pleasure, complete with its own delicious mixture of nerve endings, hot spots and endless possibilities.

sperm

The term sperm is often used to describe the milky substance produced when a man ejaculates. In truth, spermatozoa comprise only 10 per cent of this fluid, which is more correctly termed semen. In that 10 per cent, there are, on average, 200–500 million sperm, although the young adolescent male tends to produce more. This is owing to the production of androgen hormones, such as progesterone, during puberty. These hormones are also involved in the production of body and facial hair and the breaking of the voice.

BELOW | A man's body has many sensitive areas, both inside and out. All men should take time to explore their own bodies.

BELOW RIGHT | Male bodies come in all shapes and sizes.

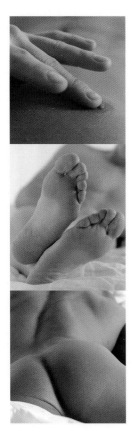

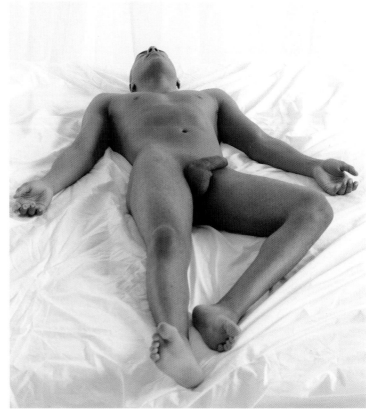

The remaining 90 per cent of the semen is composed of some 30 different substances and is referred to as seminal plasma. (Plasma is a fluid that carries solids suspended in it – in this case, semen carrying sperm.) These substances include calcium, cholesterol, fructose (a sugar that provides energy for the sperm) and lactic acid (a by-product of muscular activity). The amount of each substance varies in each ejaculate, depending on a number of different factors. For example, levels of lactic acid will increase after any form of muscular exercise. What has been eaten in the previous few hours also affects the chemical composition of the sperm and will have an effect on the taste too.

The production of semen marks the beginning of puberty and usually occurs around the ages of 12 and 13, when young males experience the emission of sperm during sleep – what is known as a "wet dream". This disposes of old sperm to allow for the production of new sperm. The emissions become less frequent as the boy starts to indulge in sexual activity.

semen – did you know?

- Semen is an eye irritant, so manual stimulation and oral sex need accuracy.
- Good for the skin, semen contains a lot of vitamins and minerals. Forget expensive creams and get your own private dispenser!
- Semen has a faintly metallic taste as it contains zinc.
- Per teaspoonful, semen contains around seven calories. For women watching their weight, there is no conflict between those love juices and that extra slice of pecan pie.
- Asparagus, Brussels sprouts and coffee all make semen taste unpleasant, while fresh mint, mangoes, green tea and confectionery all make for good-tasting sperm.
- Diabetics have sweet-tasting sperm owing to the excess amount of sugar in their bodies.

The quantity of semen produced varies from person to person. Most men ejaculate about one teaspoon of semen, although this amount can increase if a long period of time has passed since the last ejaculation. Extended foreplay and prolonged arousal time also increase the amount of semen produced, as reproductive glands, such as the prostate, are working harder.

The consistency and colour of semen is also variable. It is usually milky or pearly in colour but if it has been a while since the last ejaculation, then it may take on a slight yellowish tinge.

the big debate

For some reason men have it in their heads that women love huge penises. The reality is that a large penis can be difficult and even painful to accommodate. Remember, the average vagina is only around 10cm/4in in length. Although it is true that a small penis has its downside too, it is easier to accommodate by using different positions, fingers and sex aids, than a penis that is just too big. No matter how small or large, there's a solution for all eventualities. Anyone in a relationship having to deal with one or the other of these problems will know that half the fun is getting under the sheets and working out what to do about it.

erectile dysfunction

A quarter of all penises have a slight bend, either downwards or to the side, even when hard. Unless this causes pain or discomfort, it is completely normal. Some women report that a curved penis can heighten their experience and is easier to fellate.

Many men suffer other forms of erectile dysfunction, that is they are unable to keep an erection long enough to satisfy themselves or their partner. As many as 10 per cent of the male population have erectile problems, many suffering in silence as only 5 per cent tend to seek professional help. If you think you may have an erectile problem, try not to keep it to yourself – consult your regular doctor, a urologist or a psychosexual counsellor who can help.

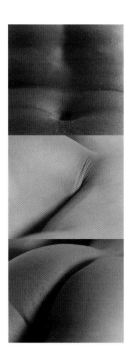

ABOVE | The landscape of the male body is often derided as holding fewer charms than the female physique – but beauty is very much in the eye of the beholder.

the internal male sex organs

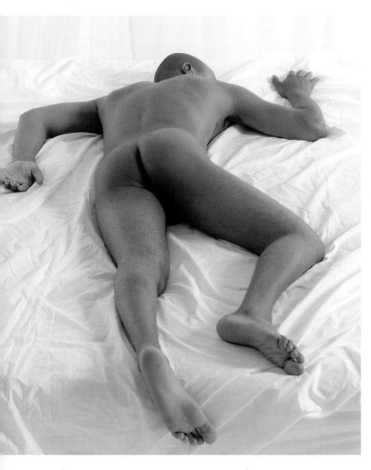

ABOVE | What's inside is just as important as the stuff you can see.

THESE ARE THE PARTS that you can't see from the outside, but understanding them is crucial to getting to know your own body.

the epididymis

This is a canal that leads from each testicle to the vas deferens. It is in the epididymis that sperm learn to swim before they make their long and perilous journey along the vas deferens and past three different glands on their way to the urethra before being ejaculated.

the vas deferens

"Vas" is Latin for vessel and "deferens" means bringing. The vas deferens are the ducts that transport the sperm up from each testicle to the penis through the epididymis. Sperm then travels through the vas deferens, which can be felt under the skin of the scrotum running up towards the groin. Most men have two, and some have three. The vas deferens is the part that is cut when a man has a vasectomy. Sometimes when a vasectomy doesn't work, it's because a man has three vas deferens and the surgeon has missed the third one.

As the vas deferens don't have any hormonal function, having a vasectomy does not affect a man's virility or the production of sex hormones and is often a good solution to the matter of long-term contraception.

the seminal vesicles

These glands are responsible for secreting seminal fluid that makes up the majority – about two thirds – of the semen. The fluid contains fructose, which provides the sperm with loads of energy for their arduous journey, and prostaglandins, which help break down the mucous lining of the woman's cervix to ease the way for them.

the bulbourethral glands

Also known as Cowper's glands, these pea-sized glands secrete most of the pre-seminal fluid that escapes from the penis before orgasm. The clear fluid protects the sperm from the acidic environment of the urethra.

the prostate gland

This little gland is about the size of a walnut. It is responsible for about a quarter of the fluid that makes up the ejaculate. It is located about 5cm/ 2in inside the anus on the front wall of the rectum, just below the bladder. The prostate gland is also known as the male G spot as, if it is stimulated, it

the male sex organs

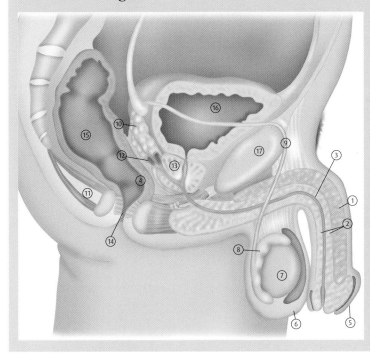

1 Corpora cavernosa
2 Corpus spongiosum
3 Urethra
4 G spot
5 Foreskin
6 Scrotum
7 Testicle (testis)
8 Epididymis
9 Vas deferens
10 Seminal vesicles
11 Puboccygeus muscle
12 Bulbourethral glands
13 Prostate gland
14 Anus
15 Rectum
16 Bladder
17 Pubis

produces a much more intense orgasm for the man. At the beginning of the 20th century, quite a few women used a steel device that was sold at the time to massage their husband's prostate during intercourse. During World War II, military medics gave prostate manipulation to soldiers who hadn't been with a woman for months to relieve them of pelvic congestion. This is called milking the prostate. Many men still feel shy about having their prostate touched, as the only route to it is via the anus. However, once they've overcome this hurdle, they will wonder how they could have missed it.

the puboccygeus muscle

Known as the PC muscle, this helps support the pelvic floor and is responsible for the fierce contractions that are felt during orgasm. It is well worthwhile keeping it in trim by flexing regularly.

the rectum

The anal sphincters are the two powerful muscles that control the entrance to the anus. The rectum is the passage through which the faeces are expelled, although, in fact, they just spend a very short time there, as they are stored further up inside the colon.

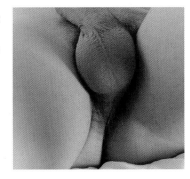

LEFT | The Leydig cells in the testes secrete testosterone and androsterone, male hormones which regulate hirsuteness and aggression, among other things.

sexploration and health

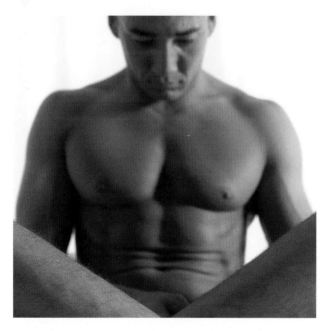

ABOVE | Take some time, in private, to become familiar with your own body.

COMPARED TO WOMEN, very few men tend to have hang-ups about their bodies. Having said that, there is one part of the male body that often causes concern – the penis. Very many men are obsessed with their penis and there are very few who haven't, at one time or other in their lives, worried about whether it is long enough, thick enough or hard enough.

The penis can be a tremendous source of anxiety to men. If it doesn't shape up in the sack, they can feel very embarrassed. Women, on the other hand, don't have to worry about things like that. They can always have sex as long as they are well lubricated.

It is more than likely that most men have examined their penises extremely thoroughly. Certainly, they know how they work and which part is the most sensitive as they often touch themselves. The first thing a male infant discovers on his body is his penis and from then on they

could be described as inseparable. However, men may not have examined themselves properly from different angles using a mirror, so why not try it? There are quite a few parts you might have overlooked and you may discover areas of sensitivity that you have previously ignored.

Lie on your back, bend your legs and put your feet flat on the bed. Separate your knees, so you can get a good view of your sex organs. Using a hand-held shaving mirror with a magnifying side and a regular side, look at all the different parts. As well as being informative, this procedure is also something that you should get into the habit of doing to check that everything is in good health.

cleanliness and health

Keeping your foreskin clean and smegma-free is essential to a successful sex life. If you wouldn't want it in your own mouth, then you can't expect anyone else to put it in theirs – or anywhere else. While washing, cradle your testicles in your hand and massage them to check for bumps and abnormalities. Explore your sensitive areas, such as the perineum and anus.

Prostate cancer is the most common form of cancer in males between the ages of 15 and 34 and, for unknown reasons, is four times as likely to occur in white males than it is in black males. The good news is that it is very easy to identify through self-checks and, over the last couple of decades, advances in therapeutic drugs and improved diagnostics have boosted the survival rate, making prostate cancer often completely curable if caught and treated early enough. Most tumours are discovered through self-examination. They usually present as an enlarged painless lump that can vary from the size of a pea to that of an egg. Other abnormalities may include an enlarged testicle, feelings of heaviness or sudden collections of fluid in the scrotum. Aches in the lower abdomen or groin, or enlarged or tender breasts can also indicate a problem.

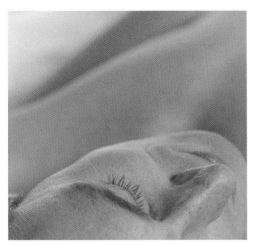
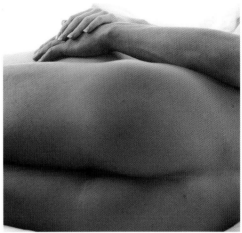

measuring up

The average erect penis is about 15cm/6in long. Ninety per cent of penises are between 13cm/5in and 18cm/7in. The smallest functioning penis stood tall at a proud 1.5cm/⅝in, and the largest soared at 30cm/12in.

When measuring your penis, always make sure that it is, first and foremost, erect. Then gently angle it down, so that it is perpendicular to your body. Use a regular ruler (metre rules are not usually necessary) to measure from the pubic bone at the base of your penis to the tip. Measuring the underside of the penis will give you a better result than measuring the top side.

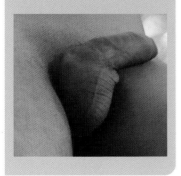

self-examination

It is best to try testicular self-examination (TSE) after a warm bath or shower, as the heat will relax the scrotum, making it easier to feel the full area. The National Cancer Institute recommends that all men, not just those in "at risk" groups, do the following at least once a month:

• Standing in front of a mirror, use both hands to check for swellings or abnormalities on the skin of the scrotum. Placing your index and middle finger under your testicle and your thumb on top, roll the testicles between your thumbs and fingers. If one seems bigger than the other, this is perfectly normal – don't panic.

• The soft, tube-like structure behind the testicle is the epididymis, which carries and collects sperm. Find this and become familiar with how it feels so that you don't mistake it for an abnormal lump. Cancerous lumps are most commonly located at the sides of the testicle although they sometimes appear at the front.

It is imperative that you contact your doctor should you find any lumps or bumps that you are concerned about. Many men feel embarrassed about a stranger handling their genitals but testicular cancer is a harsh reality. A lump does not automatically mean cancer, but it is better to be safe and most doctors will congratulate you for your preventative actions.

ABOVE LEFT AND RIGHT | The more familiar and comfortable you are with yourself, the more at ease you will be with others. Self-examination should not be considered as vanity, but as a necessary precaution against illness.

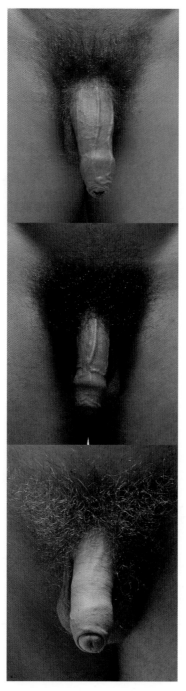

penis sizes

Most men have worried about the size, shape and performance of their penis, at one time or another. This is hardly surprising since men are constantly being subjected to the concept of the mythical penis – rock hard, huge and with immense staying power. This, of course, has very little to do with the performance of a real penis, which – like the person to whom it belongs – has its good days and mediocre days.

Quite often, though, men develop a distorted idea of their penis size. Comparisons with other men are inevitable but not always reliable. When men see each others' bodies, in communal showers or changing rooms, they see the full dimensions of the penises on display in a flaccid state. However, when a man looks down at his own penis, he is going to see it from a different and rather foreshortened angle. The best way to gauge your true penis size is to look at it sideways in the mirror.

Another anxiety for a man is whether a small penis will make a difference to the pleasure he can give a woman, although some men who are very well endowed can also be embarrassed about the size of their penis. It should be remembered that width or girth is more important than length in stimulating the lining of the vagina, and thereby giving sexual satisfaction to a woman. The vagina is around 10cm/4in in length, so it is the right size for most penises.

In exceptional cases, where an erect penis is very small, it may produce less stimulation. The woman, however, can still be stimulated orally, manually, and in lots of other exciting ways. The vast majority of women would say they fall in love with the man and not his penis. The skill with which a man uses his penis in lovemaking, his degree of sensuality and his sensitivity to her body's responses is what matters the most. The better a couple know each other and like each other initially will help overcome any difficulties.

penile erection

A full penile erection, commonly known as a "hard-on", is due to blood being pumped into the erectile tissues at a much faster rate than it can

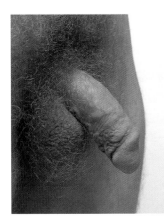
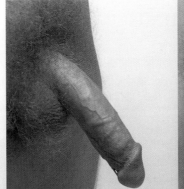
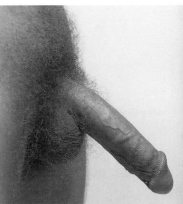

escape. This causes the tissues to swell and the penis to enlarge. Also, there are hundreds of nerves in the perineum – the triangle of flesh between the base of the penis and the anus, which when pressed, can send a many into orgasm.

circumcision

A circumcised penis is one in which the foreskin has been surgically removed. This is usually performed for religious reasons, particularly within the Jewish and Muslim communities, or for medical or health reasons. In the case of Jewish children, circumcision is usually carried out when a boy is eight days old. It is usually performed later with Muslim children, between the ages of three and 15 years. In western countries, circumcision is more likely to be performed for its perceived health benefits – some people believe the removal of the foreskin reduces the risk of infection as the penis can be more easily kept clean.

Circumcision is sometimes carried out for medical disorders such as phimosis, a condition in which the foreskin is too tight to retract properly, or balanitis, in which the tip of the penis becomes inflamed as a result of a build-up of secretions under the foreskin.

ABOVE | The size of the penis does not affect the pleasure a man can give to a woman.

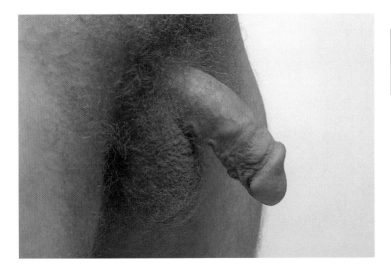

LEFT | Circumcision may be carried out on medical grounds, but more often it is for reasons of hygiene or religion.

the development of male sexuality

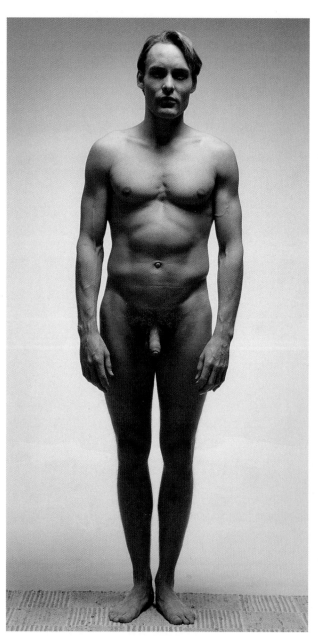

PUBERTY IS THE TIME when the male sexual characteristics become fully developed, leading to many changes in a young man's body. The first signs of puberty usually appear later in males than in females, between the ages of 12 and 14 years, although in some individuals it may be slightly earlier or later than this.

As with girls, the initial changes are triggered by chemical and nerve signals in the hypothalamus, a region of the brain. These signals trigger the release of gonadotrophins, which, in turn, instruct the testicles to start releasing increasing levels of male hormones, or androgens, such as testosterone, into the blood stream. These hormonal changes bring about a sudden spurt in bone and muscle development.

The initial signs of puberty in a boy are an increase in the size of the scrotum and testes, followed by the growth of pubic and facial hair. Sperm begins to develop within the testes, and other structures, such as the seminal vesicles and the prostate gland, begin to mature. Around the age of 13 years the penis begins to enlarge, taking around two years to reach its full adult size. The voice also begins to "break" as the larynx enlarges and the vocal cords thicken and lengthen, causing the voice to drop in pitch.

Body hair appears under the arms and on the chest, and the skin becomes coarser and may darken a little. The increased levels of testosterone tend to overstimulate the oil-producing glands in the skin, leading to acne. This can usually be treated medically and will improve with age. It is not uncommon for an adolescent male to experience temporary breast enlargement. This normally subsides within a few months, though the episode may embarrass him.

LEFT | The masculine form traditionally symbolizes strength, and this depiction of the athletic manly physique has been a popular theme in classic sculpture and art.

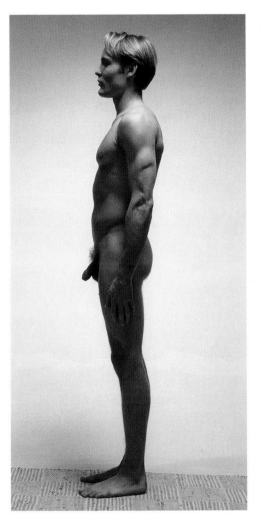

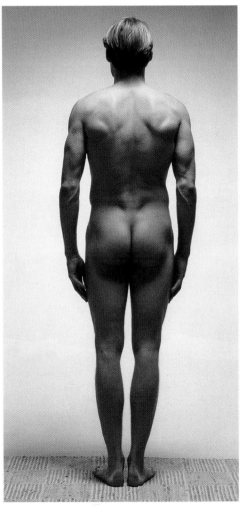

ABOVE | The development of the man's secondary sexual characteristics is triggered by signals from the hypothalamus, inside the brain, and by hormones from the pituitary gland, just underneath. These stimulate the production of the male sex hormones, such as testosterone. The physical changes are slight at first, but they speed up during the adolescent years, before stabilizing by the time the male has reached his early twenties.

ABOVE | During the adolescent years the male body develops its characteristic shape. Bones lengthen and strengthen, muscles enlarge, and the shoulders broaden as the youth begins to exhibit the physical strength of the adult male. There is usually a dramatic growth spurt between the ages of ten and 16 years, sometimes as much as 17cm/7in in a single year.

becoming a man

Puberty can be a difficult time for a young man: he has to come to terms with physical changes in his body, in addition to defining his role as a male in society. He experiences peer group pressure, while trying to live up to the expectations of parents and teachers, yet at the same time he is trying to determine his own beliefs and goals. During this period he may start testing or challenging authority figures as he struggles to assert his own identity. At this stage of a young adolescent's development he will greatly benefit from the friendship and guidance of older men who can act as role models and be prepared to advise him through this difficult, demanding and changing period of life.

male sexual experience

In addition to physical changes, a young male will probably start to experience exciting but somewhat frightening new sexual feelings. Erections occur frequently, and often at the most inopportune times. In his early teenage years, the adolescent may start to ejaculate during his sleep. These nocturnal emissions are commonly known as "wet dreams".

He will probably also engage in frequent masturbation, fuelled by his awakening desires and his growing fantasies about sex. It is not uncommon for adolescents to engage in sexual play with other boys of the same age. They may compare penises and frequency of ejaculations, and even masturbate together. For most boys this is only a passing phase, and can provide an

BELOW LEFT AND RIGHT | It is likely that after some sexual experimentation, a young man will want to form a more permanent and emotionally bonding sexual partnership. However, like women, men are now more likely to want to live with their partners for a time before making a commitment to marriage.

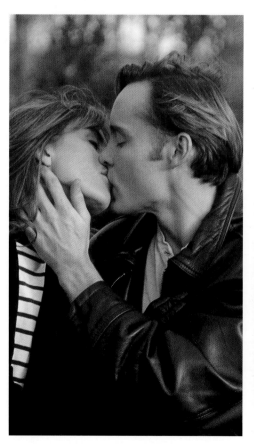
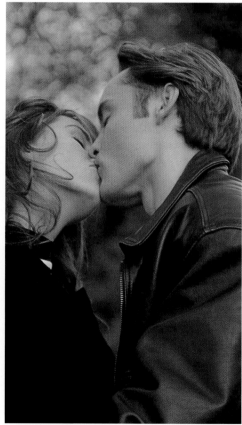

important means of gaining knowledge about their own bodies and of comparing their development with others. For some boys it can lead to an interest in same-sex relationships.

As a young man gains confidence in himself, he will start to develop an interest in the opposite sex and begin to form relationships. It is just as important for young men to be well informed on subjects such as contraception, safer sex, sexually transmitted diseases, and the relationship between sexuality and emotional happiness as it is for their female counterparts.

Adolescence is usually a time of sexual experimentation and normally, while the emotions involved may be intense, these relationships do not always last long. In western cultures particularly, young men often feel under peer-group pressure to lose their virginity as soon as possible. According to recent studies of sexual behaviour in Britain, the majority of men claim to have lost their virginity at around the ages of 16 or 17 years. This, of course, is not true for all men, and many males remain virgins until they are much older.

As a boy becomes a man he has to cope with demands made upon him from many different directions. During early adulthood his prime concerns will centre around his studies or career, and establishing himself in his chosen lifestyle, but his relationships with women or men will also be of great importance.

man's sexual peak

If a man's sexual peak is measured in terms of frequency of orgasm (either through masturbation or lovemaking) and the amount of resting time he needs between each ejaculation, he is at his most sexually potent in the years of late adolescence and early twenties. Generally, after that age his virility stabilizes, and then declines slightly in later years as he requires longer periods of recovery between each ejaculation. However, most men improve their lovemaking skills as they get older and become more sensitive to their partner's sexual needs. So, in fact, age can make a man a better lover, with more staying power during coitus. This undoubtedly enhances his sexual satisfaction, both physically and emotionally.

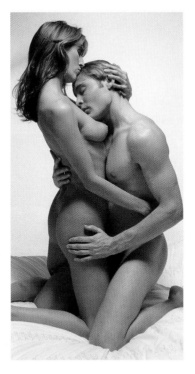

LEFT | During adolescence, a young man may want to experiment with a number of relationships, and this can help him to build up a broad range of sexual and emotional experiences. As he grows older, however, he will be more inclined to seek his true mate.

BELOW | As a young man gains confidence in himself, he will start to develop an interest in the opposite sex and begin to form relationships.

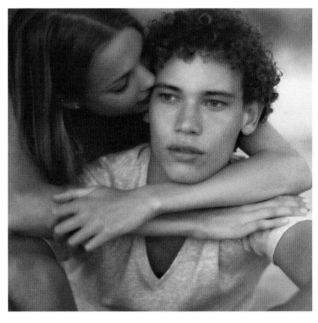

the female body

THE GEOGRAPHY of the female genitalia can be a source of much confusion and frustration to both men and women. Compared to the male genitalia, where what you see is pretty much what you get, it takes a greater basic understanding of the structure to find your way around the female body. An improved understanding of how everything works and where it is located greatly improves the love life of most couples.

minora, are a lot thinner, less fleshy and much more sensitive, as they are rich in nerve endings. They contain numerous oils and sweat glands, which help to keep the vulva hygienic and healthy. Inner labia vary in shape and size. In some women, they are small and hidden from view. In others, there is more skin and sometimes the folds of skin protrude beyond the outer labia, which is perfectly normal.

the labia

The vulva is the outside part of the female genitalia that the eye can see. The protective folds, or lips, that make up the vulva are called the labia. The outer labia, or labia majora, are usually covered in pubic hair. The inner labia, or labia

the mons pubis

The pubic mound, or mons pubis, is the mound of fatty tissue that protects the pubic bone during sex. Also known as the Mount of Venus, this area has many nerve endings, and at puberty, becomes covered in pubic hair.

BELOW | There is much more to the female body than meets the naked eye.

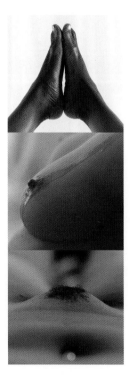

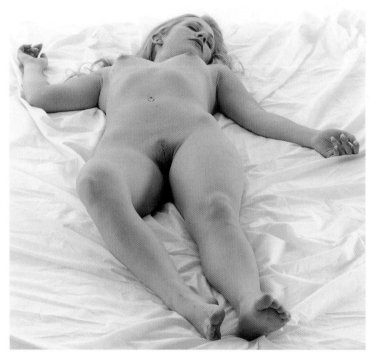

the clitoris

The magic button, die Kitzler, le cli cli or the clitoris – all women have one. On close inspection, the head, or glans, of the clitoris can be seen underneath the clitoral hood. Recent research has shown the clitoris to be a much larger organ than the part that can be seen externally.

Clitorises vary in shape and size from woman to woman, but in all women they are the only organ in the body whose sole purpose is to provide sexual pleasure. The clitoris is located just below the pubic bone so it can be gently manipulated and stimulated through intercourse, although this is often dependent on the sexual position. The head is only about the size of a pea but has between 6,000 and 8,000 nerve endings, which is why some women find direct stimulation too intense. Under the hood, the erectile tissue that makes up the rest of the clitoris forks off towards the back of the pelvis. The surrounding protective clitoral muscles are also extremely sensitive and their contraction aids a woman's sexual response.

On 1 August, 1998 Helen O'Connell, a urology surgeon at the Royal Melbourne Hospital, noted that the clitoral nerve system extended further than the visible tip of the clitoris, causing a media frenzy of speculation about the mystery of the giant female sex organs, some subsequent reports claiming that the clitoris was over 5m/15ft long.

The reportage of Ms O'Connell's article, in spite of its inaccuracies, was the first time it was acknowledged that there was more to the clitoris than meets the eye. Anatomists now state that the clitoris is made up of three parts: the glans, the shaft and the crura.

By pulling back the clitoral hood, you can clearly see the glans, which is comprised of erectile tissue that enlarges during arousal. Under the hood is a flexible cord known as the shaft, which feels rubbery to the touch. The majority of the clitoral structure is inside the body but the head, or glans, is clearly visible from the outside too. The third part of the clitoris is a wishbone-shaped structure comprising two crus, or crura, located where the shaft of the clitoris divides.

It is made of two extending wings of erectile tissue, the crura. You cannot see them, as they are internal structures, but they also contribute to sexual arousal and orgasm. In total the clitoris is about 9cm/3½in long. The two crus are covered by the inner labia but stretch back through to the muscles of the perineum between the vagina and anus.

The clitoris and the penis are one and the same structure in the first eight weeks of foetal development. However, although the clitoris is made up of erectile tissues, it does not form an erection but it does swell and engorge with blood.

the bulbs of vestibule

These bulbs lie on either side of the vaginal opening within the labia minora, are surrounded by muscle tissue, and fill with blood during arousal and contract during orgasm. It is thought that these bulbs facilitate intercourse by stiffening the walls of the vaginal opening, thus making entry of the penis easier.

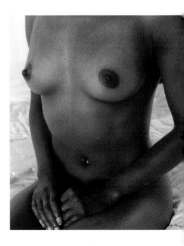

ABOVE | Sometimes inhibition can be a hindrance to learning about your own body.

the female sex organs

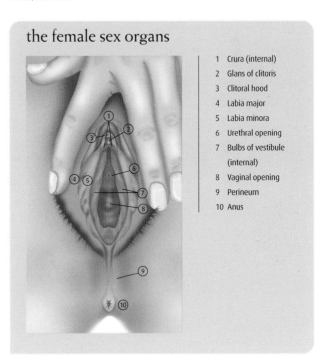

1   Crura (internal)
2   Glans of clitoris
3   Clitoral hood
4   Labia major
5   Labia minora
6   Urethral opening
7   Bulbs of vestibule
    (internal)
8   Vaginal opening
9   Perineum
10 Anus

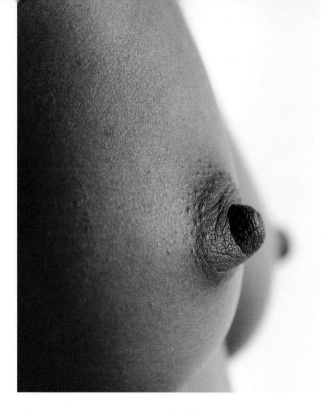

ABOVE | It is very common to have one breast larger than the other. Around 40 per cent of women have breasts of different sizes, but variations are generally minor. One breast tends to grow faster than the other and by the age of 20 they are usually fully formed.

urethral opening

For a long time people thought that women's urine came out of the vagina but in fact it comes out of a tiny hole just below the clitoris, called the urethral opening. The vaginal opening is found further below this, and is covered by a thin membranous layer called the hymen. This only partially covers the vaginal opening to allow for the flow of menstrual blood. The hymen is usually broken, either through exercise or using tampons, long before a girl loses her virginity.

the perineum

The flat area between the bottom of the vulva and the anus, the perineum, has a multitude of nerve endings that are very sensitive to touch. Some women like this area to be gently massaged during sexual arousal. The perineum is quite supple, making it possible for a woman to feel her partner's penis if she presses this area gently during penetration. Midwives recommend massaging the perineum with a mild oil, such as almond oil, to improve elasticity before childbirth.

the anus

The tight muscular opening to the rectum, the anus, is a very sensitive area that some people like to incorporate into their lovemaking. But beware, permission should always be asked first, and hands, fingers, dildos and anything else should be thoroughly cleaned before they are put back into the vagina after being in the anus.

breasts

Whether you own big, voluptuous bosoms or a smaller more compact pair, you will know that breasts are the ultimate toys for most men, regardless of shape and size. Playstations, football and Formula One all take a back seat in male priorities when set against a pair of breasts.

The breasts are composed of a mass of milk gland tissues that lie in a bed of fat and are attached to the muscular wall at the front of the chest. The milk ducts from the glands lead to milk sinuses, which are collecting areas, found just behind the nipple. Fibrous tissue runs between the ducts, providing the breasts with their firmness and structure. Breast size is wholly dependent on the amount of fat and glandular tissue, which is to some extent hormone-controlled and may vary throughout a woman's life.

A lot of people assume that larger breasts are better than smaller ones. Breast size and shape is inherited from both your parents. Women with large breasts often complain that people stare at their chests and feel that they are judged initially solely on their breast size, rather than their personality and intelligence, while other women have based their careers on the size of their chest. Either way, women must resist the pressure to look like everybody else – learn to love your assets, whatever their size.

Breasts are important to women psychologically, as they are a symbol of fertility and ability to feed offspring. Women can suffer huge grief if they must have a breast removed or if they reach adulthood without developing breasts. Plastic surgery is now available, with some degree of success, although it is important to weigh up the problem against your quality of life before taking any radical steps.

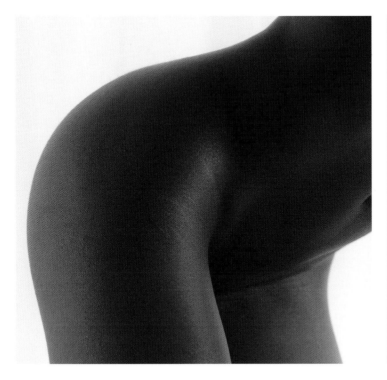

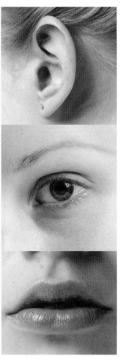

It is important to be measured for the correct size bra at a reputable store, especially if you are on the large side, to gain good support. Too many women wear the wrong size foundation garments. Take some time to become familiar with your breasts and learn to love them, using moisturizing cream to care for the thin skin that covers them.

The odd hair on the nipple is completely normal. If it is a real problem, your doctor can advise you on electrolysis or other hair-removal techniques, but the odd one here or there just needs plucking with your tweezers.

Inverted nipples, those that turn inwards instead of outwards, can be a cause for concern as they look different from those of other women. This condition affects about 10 per cent of women and is, in most cases, not a problem. During arousal or breast-feeding, the inverted nipple usually pops out. If breast-feeding is a problem, consult a doctor or midwife who will be able to advise you on how to rectify the situation.

the nipples

The term nipple only actually describes one part of the pigmented area of the breast. The protruding bud in the centre is the nipple. The surrounding circular area is the areola, the colour of which depends on the woman's skin colour, but in most cases it is pink, brown or black. Again, the size varies from woman to woman, but some are as large as 12.5cm/5in in diameter. The small nodes scattered on the surface of the areola are called the tubercles of Montgomery and are perfectly normal. The nipple has up to 20 milk duct openings which are active during the later stages of pregnancy and throughout the breast-feeding period. These ducts are directly linked to the brain and so the suckling of a baby or the attentions of a partner can have a very profound emotional effect on a lactating woman. The nipple is one of the most sensually sensitive areas on both men and women, and some women claim to be able to reach orgasm from nipple stimulation alone.

ABOVE | Total arousal starts with the senses: the taste of skin mingled with good wine, the sound of breathing against soft music, the sight of face and body in a candlelit room. Satisfaction involves sight, hearing, taste and smell as well as touch sensations.

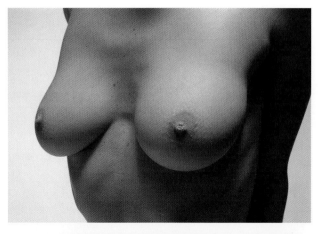

breast size and shape

Breast shape and size varies greatly between women. The way a woman with a 34 inch bust (the average breast size) feels about her breasts may partly depend on the era and culture she is born in. Fashions in what is considered an attractive breast size change constantly, from the buxom and curvaceous style favoured by Hollywood in the 1950s to the boyish, almost androgynous shape of many of today's top models.

It is important for a woman to love and accept her body – particularly the shape of her breasts – the way it is, for it is an expression of her own unique femininity. If the breasts are large and causing discomfort it will help to wear a good support bra. Small breasts cannot be enlarged directly by exercise as they do not contain muscle, but good posture (a lengthened spine, and straightened shoulders) can lift the ribcage to give the breasts a more pronounced shape. Likewise, you can develop the underlying pectoral muscles, which may help increase the lift and support the weight. A difference in size between the left and right breast is very common.

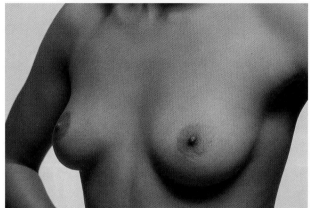

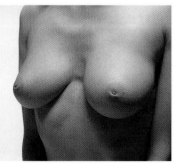

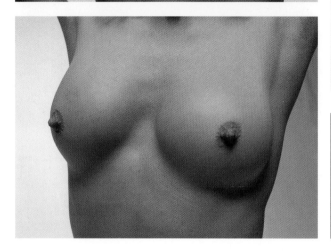

LEFT AND ABOVE | Nipple shapes and sizes are also very varied. Some nipples are naturally inverted – the nipple is pulled inwards and hidden behind a fold in the skin. In most cases, inverted nipples should not prevent successful breastfeeding. If, however, a nipple suddenly becomes inverted during adulthood, it is important to consult a doctor immediately, as this may indicate breast cancer.

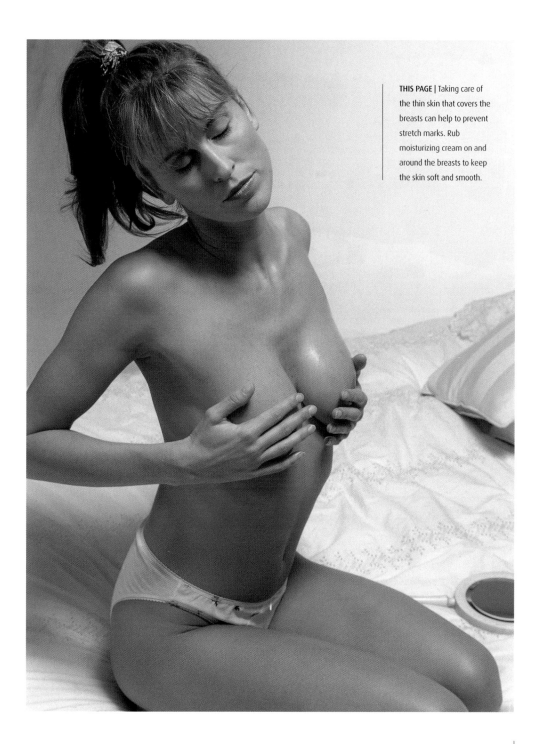

THIS PAGE | Taking care of the thin skin that covers the breasts can help to prevent stretch marks. Rub moisturizing cream on and around the breasts to keep the skin soft and smooth.

the internal female sex organs

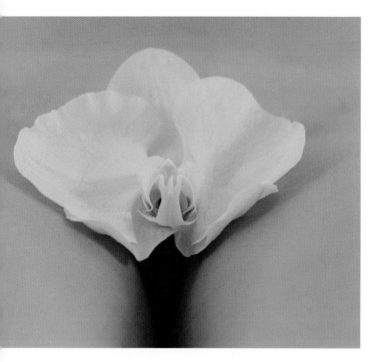

American sex researchers found that the vaginal walls are also responsible for the secretion of the love juices that are released during arousal. These juices lubricate the movements of sex, minimizing friction, which might be painful. Some women secrete more juice than others, and some even climax with the same liquid ferocity as men.

the cervix

Commonly known as the neck of the womb, the cervix connects the vagina and the uterus via a narrow tunnel that runs through the cervix and into the opening of the uterus. During intercourse the cervix drops down to help the sperm travel up the canal, into the uterus, on its way to the egg. The cervix is sometimes blocked with a mucous plug to protect the uterus from infection. This mucus thins during ovulation to allow sperm to enter the uterus. In the last stages of labour, the cervix has the ability to open wide enough to allow the passage of the baby.

It is important that women are aware of their cervixes and problems that may occur. Regular Pap or smear tests are vital in sexually active women.

the uterus

Also called the womb, the uterus is about the same size as a woman's clenched fist. It is composed of several layers of tissue and muscle. The inner lining, or endometrium, builds up over a month and then sheds during menstruation, keeping the environment clean and regenerated. The myometrium lies next to the endometrium and comprises powerful muscular tissue that contracts during both labour and orgasm. As oestrogen levels dwindle away during the menopause, the uterus decreases in size.

the fallopian tubes

The fallopian tubes link the ovaries to the uterus, branching out to lie symmetrically next to the outer wall of the uterus. They are about 10cm/4in

ABOVE | The female sexual organs, especially the vulva, have often been described as a flower. Women artists such as Georgia O'Keeffe and Judy Chicago have used the flower as a metaphor for the female pudenda in their work.

THESE ARE THE PARTS of a woman's body that are not immediately visible, but understanding them is crucial for health and sexual satisfaction.

the vagina

"Vagina" in Latin translates to mean sheath. True to its name, the main purpose of the vagina is to fit snugly around the penis, encouraging the safe passage of sperm to their final destination. The average vaginal canal is between 7.5cm/3in and 10cm/4in in length, although it is sometimes slightly longer in women who have had children. The muscular tissue inside the vagina allows for expansion and contraction, as it has to be able to open wide enough for a baby's head to pass through. During sexual excitement, the walls of the vagina balloon and extend, as well as contracting around the penis during orgasm.

in length and, at one end, they have finger-like projections which stroke the surface of the ovaries in order to pick up an egg before drawing it down the tube. If fertilization occurs, the first stage usually develops in the fallopian tube.

Until fairly recently, women needed at least one healthy tube to have a baby, although now microsurgery to unblock the tubes and IVF have helped to overcome these problems.

the ovaries

The ovaries are small, pinkish-white organs that lie in the pelvic area. They are about 3cm/1¼in long and 2cm/¾in wide and contain around 100,000 eggs each (formed before birth), but release only one a month, during ovulation. The ovaries are also responsible for the release of oestrogen and progesterone, hormones that play a vital role in the menstrual cycle.

the pelvic floor muscle

This is the powerful pubococcygeus muscle that supports the pelvic floor and the reproductive organs. During orgasm it contracts. By keeping your pelvic floor muscles well exercised you will reap the benefits in the bedroom, as deliberately contracting them during sex induces a pleasant "milking" sensation around your partner's penis.

Maintaining strong pelvic floor muscles also helps with childbirth and a speedy recovery. Pilates classes teach women to exercise their pelvic floor muscles, although there are numerous exercises that can be done independently. The beauty is that you can do them any time, anywhere and no one can tell what you're up to. To test your pelvic floor muscles try to stop your flow of urine for ten seconds and then continue. If you can achieve this, your pelvic muscles are quite strong; if not, a few minutes' exercising a day may save problems later.

BELOW | Regular exercise of the pelvic floor muscles will be a benefit now, as well as in later life.

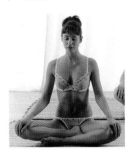

the internal female sex organs

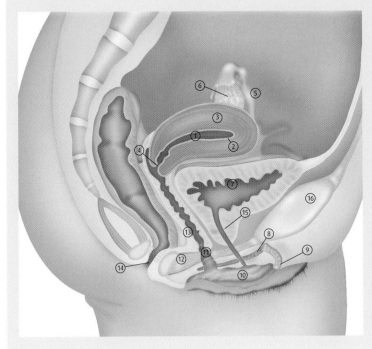

1 Uterus
2 Endometrium
3 Myometrium
4 Cervix
5 Fallopian tubes
6 Ovaries
7 Bladder
8 Crus
9 Clitoral shaft and glans
10 Labia majora and minora
11 Vagina
12 Pubococcygeus muscle
13 G spot
14 Anus
15 Urethra
16 Pubic bone

sexploration and health

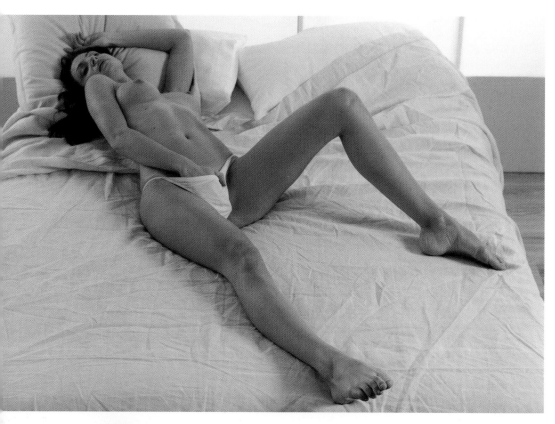

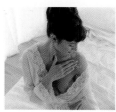

TOP | It is a natural progression to explore and take things further.

ABOVE | Look after your skin by using body moisturizers.

IT IS AMAZING how many women are unaware of where their organs are and how they work. This is where some intimate personal inspection with a small hand-held mirror in a quiet, undisturbed room becomes invaluable.

By asking your partner to join you, you can also introduce him to your personal playground, not only educating you both, but setting the perfect scene for some fun. Not only will this benefit you in understanding more about yourself as a sexual person, but it is also an excellent exercise that can help you to recognize the signs and symptoms that may indicate health problems in the future.

mirror image

An empty house and some free time provide the perfect opportunity to introduce yourself to yourself. Stand in front of a full-length mirror for a long time and look at your naked body. Acknowledge your unique sexiness. Notice the creases, the lines, the roundness and touch of your skin.

Compliment yourself on your attributes and concentrate on what looks good. Instead of grimacing at the parts you are not so keen on, try to view them in a positive light. A round protruding belly, for example, can either be seen as fat and unattractive, or a sign of femininity and fertility. Move your body around, sitting, kneeling and standing. Watch how your body moves and how your muscles and tendons work together. Gently touch your nipples, run your forefingers around them, pinch them gently between your forefinger and thumb, gradually increasing the pressure to see if you enjoy the sensation.

Grab the trusty hand-held mirror and find a comfortable position to sit. Spread your legs, with the mirror angled so that you can clearly see and examine yourself. You will need to separate your labia in order to access your clitoris. To see your

clitoris more clearly you may also need to pull back the clitoral hood, but remember this is a sensitive area, so handle with care.

Move your hands and fingers around your vaginal area, working out which areas are more sensitive than others. Don't ignore your anus and perineum, as for some women these are really exciting hot spots. Soon you and your delicate sexual organs should be thoroughly acquainted and you may then feel that you want to take the relationship a step further.

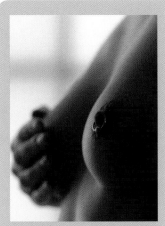

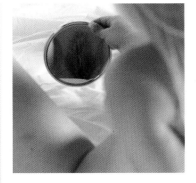

LEFT | Get that mirror out and have a look.

BELOW | Get to know how you like to be stimulated by trying it out for yourself.

breast checking

Lie flat or stand with one arm raised above your head. With your opposite hand, use the pads of your fingertips to massage the breast area, using small circular movements to check for any bumps or other abnormalities.

Put your raised arm back by your side and, using the opposite hand again, check the armpit area for lumps or swellings. Then repeat the whole process on the opposite side.

If you do find something *don't panic*. Visit your doctor for advice and remember that not all lumps are a sign of something sinister: often they are just fatty tissue deposits, but it's better to be safe than sorry.

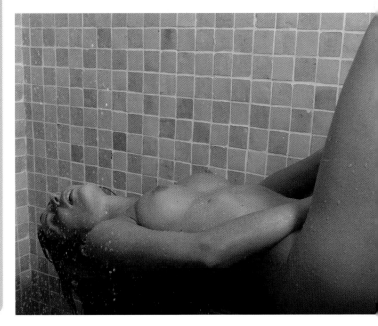

the development of female sexuality

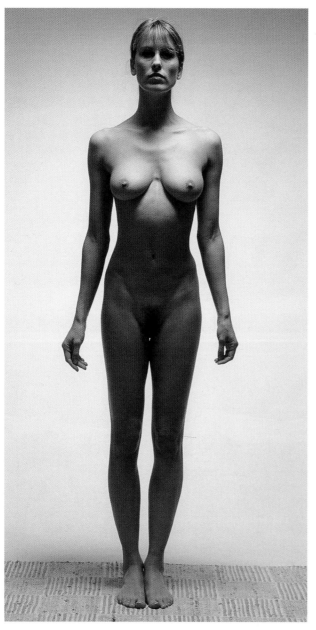

PUBERTY IN FEMALES STARTS at around the age of ten, triggered by an upsurge in the level of sex hormones secreted into the bloodstream, and can take up to five years to complete. The start and rate of development of a girl's sexual maturity differs from one individual to another, but may be influenced by hereditary factors, nutrition and health. The improvement in diet and living standards in industrialized nations is thought to be mainly responsible for the earlier onset of the first menstrual cycle in girls today.

The initial changes in puberty, between the ages of ten and 12, are triggered by chemical and nerve signals from a region in the brain called the hypothalamus. These signals cause the pituitary gland, just below the brain, to release hormones called gonadotrophins. These, in turn, instruct the ovaries to start releasing the hormones oestrogen and progesterone. The various hormonal changes at this time bring about a sudden spurt in growth, including increased height and muscle weight, changes in the distribution of fat around the body, and the development of the reproductive organs.

The first changes may be the budding of the breasts, one often earlier than the other, and the darkening of the pigment of the areolae. This is usually followed by the appearance of pubic hair, and then underarm hair. The uterus, Fallopian tubes and ovaries start to mature, the vagina enlarges, and the labia begin to swell. There may also be an increase in vaginal secretions, and the oil and sweat glands become highly active, often leading to acne and pimples.

The characteristic female shape now begins to develop, as the pelvis widens and fat deposits are

LEFT | The beautiful symmetry of a woman's body, its rounded contours and sensual shape, has inspired thousands of great sculptures, paintings, songs, poetry, and many works of literature.

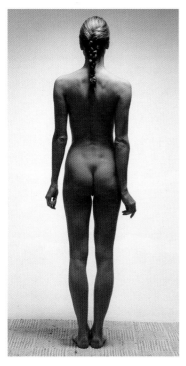

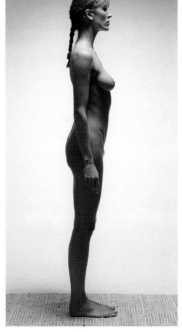

FAR LEFT | During the second decade of a female's life, her body undergoes a transformation, both internally and externally, as it begins to take on the full, rounded contours of the adult womanly shape. The pelvis widens, and fat distribution increases throughout the body, especially on the breasts, abdomen, pubic area, buttocks and hips.

LEFT | In the later stages of puberty, a female's menstrual cycle usually becomes more regular, on average settling at between 26 and 32 days' duration. Her breasts develop to their adult size, her pubic hair becomes thicker, and underarm hair appears. By now, her voice may have become slightly deeper. A woman's growth in height slows down soon after puberty.

laid down under the skin of the breasts, buttocks, hips and thighs. The first menstrual period, the menarche, occurs on average between the ages of 12 and 13 years, but usually not until at least a year after the secondary sexual characteristics have begun to develop. The start of regular periods marks the completion of puberty.

from girl to woman

An adolescent girl may welcome the dramatic changes in her body as evidence that she is entering womanhood. Equally, she may be distressed or alarmed by them, feeling that her body is out of control, or being reluctant to relinquish her childhood so soon. She is likely to go through intense mood swings, partly due to hormonal fluctuations, but also because she must

adapt psychologically as well as physically to her new identity.

She is no longer a little girl and, in various ways, she may demand that her changing identity is recognized by her family. A young teenage girl may need to assert her developing womanhood, separating herself temporarily from the close bond she had previously shared with her mother. Her relationship with her father may alter as they both try to find a new way of acknowledging and adjusting to her developing sexuality. At this point, a father may stop showing his normal displays of physical affection, unsure of exactly how to relate to his daughter. In spite of these difficulties, the adolescent girl will need a great deal of emotional support from her parents, even though she appears to challenge them on every issue.

sex education

It is important that a girl is fully informed about the physical changes her body will undergo during puberty, and has adequate knowledge about menstruation, and related hygiene matters, before her periods begin.

It is not always easy for parents to discuss sexual issues with their children although, nowadays, families do tend to be more open about such topics. If the mother, or guiding parent, feels unable to discuss these subjects with the daughter (girls may also find it embarrassing to discuss sexual matters with their parents), it is important to find someone the girl can trust and who will answer her questions, or provide her with suitable books from which she can gather accurate information. Informed sex education is not a green light for promiscuity.

A teenage girl will benefit from knowing that during adolescence she is likely to feel attracted to boys, and even experiment in sexual play with them, and that sometimes her emotions and sexual feelings will be overwhelming. She needs to understand the importance of defining the boundaries of her sexual behaviour so that she is able to resist male or peer group pressure to engage in any sexual activity for which she does not feel ready. By discussing these issues with an understanding adult, she will be better equipped to take control of her body and emotions.

Studies show that adequate sex education for young people (males and females) about contraception, sexually transmitted diseases, and the complexities of emotional and sexual feelings in relationships, can help reduce cases of premature sexual intercourse and teenage pregnancies.

BELOW LEFT AND RIGHT | On the whole, women of all ages consider intimacy, love and emotional bonding to be an important part of forming a sexual relationship.

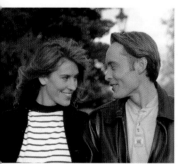

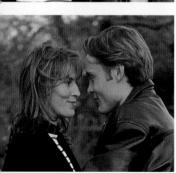

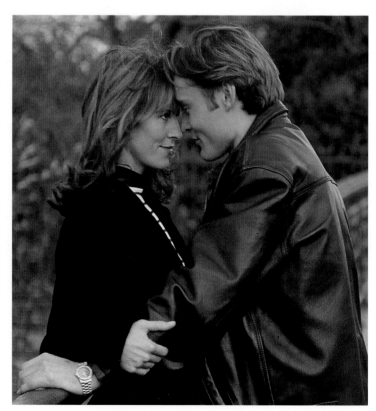

sexual experience

Young women masturbate, for sexual release and to explore their bodily responses, although slightly less often than males of the same age. According to research, the average age for the loss of virginity in young women in the United States and Great Britain is between 16 and 18. There are still many young women who, for religious, romantic or moral reasons, or through fear of pregnancy or sexually transmitted disease, prefer to remain virgins until they meet a man with whom they can develop a committed relationship.

However, in most western cultures there is no longer the same pressure on females to remain virgins until their wedding night, and many young women will have had several sexual partners by the time they reach their twenties.

These days, women expect to compete equally with their male colleagues in the academic and work environment, and for most women marriage and children are no longer seen as their only goals. The wider availability of contraception has given women greater freedom in all areas of their lives.

Increasingly, women are choosing to live with a partner before marriage, and to delay starting a family until established in a career or they have paid off student loans and have a settled home. It is not unusual for women to wait until their thirties before having their first baby – and some are now leaving it until their forties to start a family – and most expect to return to work within a few months or years after giving birth.

women's sexual peak

A woman's capacity to achieve an orgasm appears to increase with age and sexual experience. Women tend to reach their sexual peak during their thirties and can continue at this level for many years.

In part, this may be because as a woman gets older and becomes more confident and relaxed in her sexuality, she is better attuned to what will bring her sexual satisfaction during lovemaking and is more inclined to tell her partner what stimulates her.

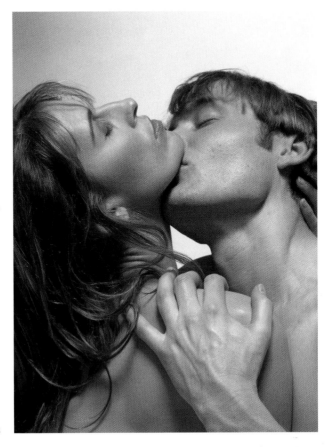

Younger women may be more preoccupied with trying to please their partners during intercourse, while, in general, women are more sexually responsive and confident when they are involved in a secure, intimate and loving relationship.

Although women are becoming more sexually assertive, active and better able to initiate relationships with the opposite sex, often they still suffer from western society's double standards over the morality of multiple sexual experience. Whereas it is acceptable for a man, and often expected, to "sow his wild oats" as evidence of his virility, a woman can still be regarded in many circles as promiscuous if she has had several sexual partners.

ABOVE | As a woman's sexual experience increases, so does her orgasmic capacity. When she is fully relaxed in her body, and is aroused lovingly by a sensitive and knowledgeable partner, her sexual pleasure is almost boundless.

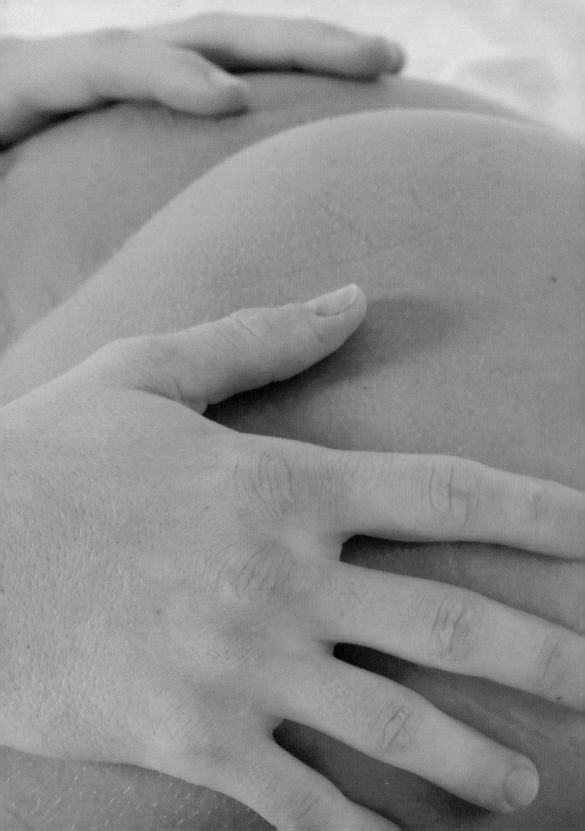

seduction

Seduction is the subtle art of exploring the chemistry that exists between you and then using it to the best possible advantage. It includes romance, persuasion and temptation, and doesn't stop after the first thrills of a relationship. The art of seduction also includes the post-coital afterglow – the comfort of lying together after sex – as well as recognizing that you may want to seduce a member of the same, rather than the opposite, sex.

the importance of seduction

A BOOK ON SEXUAL TECHNIQUES focuses a great deal on the physical aspects of sexual relationship, making it easy to ignore other essential elements such as romance and seduction. But sex is not just about the physical. Unlike most animals, humans have sex not just for procreation, but for relaxation, comfort, recreation and love.

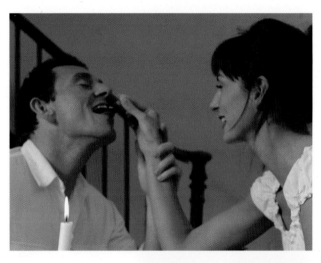

ABOVE AND RIGHT | In the first stages of a relationship you think of little else but each other. Senses are alive with anticipation and you lavish each other with romantic and thoughtful gestures.

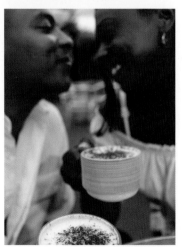

As the most complex organisms in the animal kingdom, humans need to have the erotic epicentre of the body – the brain – stimulated when preparing themselves for sex. Forget the clitoris, the G-spot, the penis and the prostate; if you're not in the mood, you're not in the mood, and this is controlled by the brain.

The true foundations of sensuality, sexual enjoyment and fulfilment are laid in the brain; the attic of your body rather than the basement. Preparation, anticipation and relaxation all start in the head, making mental stimulation an essential component of foreplay.

irresistible temptation

Dating, romancing, courting and flirting may seem a bit old-fashioned to some people, but even the most hardened cynic melts when a certain tune is played on the radio, igniting an old memory of a past relationship or a particularly memorable episode of a present one.

It is at the start of the relationship, when you are in love, that the senses are at their most heightened; the sky seems bluer, flowers seem to smell sweeter, everything tastes better and even jokes are funnier. Great memories are made during this period of getting to know one another. Smells are particularly evocative: the scent someone uses, the aroma of freshly baked bread when you first went shopping together, even the smell of a certain brand of coffee can all have an effect. Let's face it, the thrills and delights of sex are about much more than physical pleasure alone, however wonderful that may be.

Romance doesn't have to be all flowers, teddy bears and soppy letters, but at the beginning of a relationship, it is the grounding from which all your other memories with that person will blossom. It is a sad fact that the better you get to know someone, the more complacent you are likely to become about romantic gestures, so the scope for these gestures is quite limited.

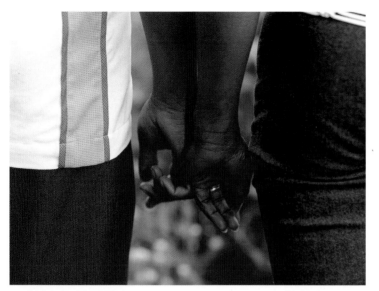

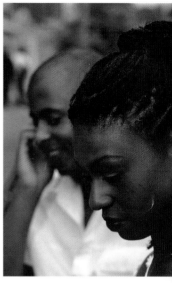

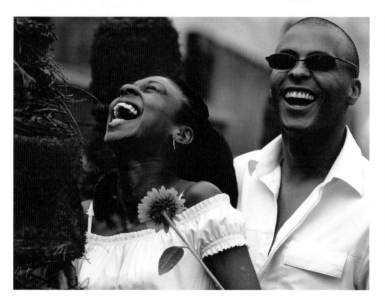

ABOVE LEFT | In the first flush of mutual attraction, simply touching hands or intertwining your fingers can send shivers of delight through you.

ABOVE RIGHT | Don't make the mistake of ignoring your date – they deserve your full attention.

LEFT | Giving a small token such as a flower may seem old-fashioned, but shows that you care.

Romancing can start before you have even become established partners, let alone had sex, with phone calls, text messages, notes, letters and emails. Small, thoughtful gestures often have a far greater impact than large, lavish ones. Show that you are getting to understand your new partner and potential lover, that you listen to what they say and that you care about what they want and like by buying the CD that you heard them mention, or an interesting book, her favourite flowers, his favourite beer, or some other small token just "because it reminded me of you".

kissing

rubbing noses

Although Europeans have been kissing for a couple of thousand years, it's believed that the practice may well have originated in India. Vedic Sanskrit texts from about 1500BC describe the custom of rubbing and pressing noses together. This type of greeting, often called "Eskimo" kissing, is also associated with the Inuit and with Pacific islanders. The lips don't actually touch; what is really happening is that each person literally inhales the odour of the scent glands on the cheeks of the other person. Animals do it all the time. Have you ever noticed that cats often rub their faces against their human pals as well as their feline friends?

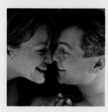

YOU CAN USUALLY TELL what sort of lover someone will be by the way they kiss. After all, kissing is usually your first moment of real sexual contact. While kissing, you literally get to taste and smell what is on offer. Kissing is not a universal custom; many remote cultures hadn't a clue about it until Europeans arrived and showed them what to do.

The tongue and lips are two of the most sensitive erogenous areas of the body, packed with nerve endings. When you kiss with passion, it releases a chemical in the brain similar to those engendered by extreme sports, such as skydiving or parachuting. Called neurotransmitters, these chemicals attach to pleasure receptors in the brain, resulting in euphoria, fluttering in your belly and a feeling of elation. Even if there isn't a grand passion when you kiss, it may still create an enjoyable physical sensation.

There's a whole repertoire of kissing you can try out while you explore your lover's erogenous zones. Not all passionate kisses have to involve tickling each other's tonsils. An almost imperceptible brush of the lips can be just as exciting.

lip sync

Most people like the idea of kissing someone with smooth and shapely lips, a generous smile and good teeth. Bad teeth are one of the ultimate turn-offs. Lip size doesn't indicate whether someone is a good kisser or not, but some mouths are just so kissable. It could be the shape, the smile or the fullness of the lips or even the way the person wets their lips with their tongue.

A survey carried out on kissing showed that women like kissing better than men and enjoy the whole long, lingering embrace, without it

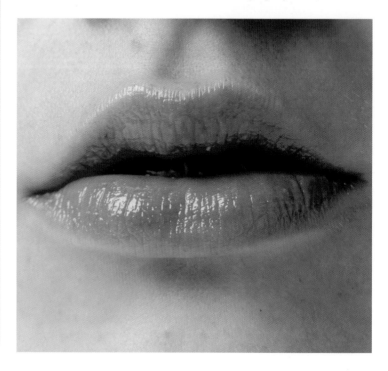

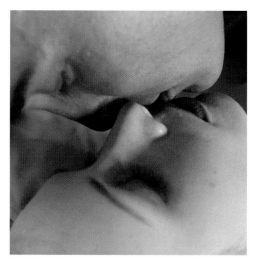
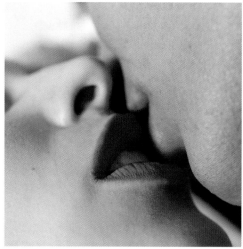

necessarily leading to anything else. In fact, some women have said that they find kissing the most erotic part of sex and have often had an orgasm just from a passionate session of kissing.

Men, on the other hand, do enjoy kissing but seem to see it as a necessary part of the ritual required to get to intercourse. Of course, lots of men, especially British and American men, hate public displays of affection. Mediterranean men seem to love kissing in public, though. They kiss their wives, mothers, girlfriends, kids, fathers and male pals with equal fervour. They even kiss three times on the cheek in greeting, instead of two.

Apart from the mouth and cheeks, there are loads of other places on the body that are just begging to be kissed – eyelids, nose, ears, neck (delicious), armpit (yes really), insides of wrists, fingertips, backs of knees, ankles, soles and toes, and lots more places in between. The best way to find out is to go on a kissing tour of your lover, working your way around the whole body.

kissing asides

What differentiates an average kisser from an exemplary kisser? That's the million dollar question. A relaxed mouth and an open mind are good places to begin. As to where to go from there, here are a few suggestions:

French kissing Gently caress the inside of your partner's mouth with your tongue. As he or she responds, you can quicken the pace and intensity, going for a fuller thrust.

chicken kisses Great for relaxation and moments of tenderness. Purse your lips and then plant a light kiss, a little like a peck, but at the rate of about three a second. It's between a kiss and a tickle really, but feels good. A good nose wrinkler.

silent but deadly Some of the sexiest kisses are the silent ones, lips and eyes closed, caressing each other's hair, face and neck with your hands.

stereophonic kiss Moan or slurp while you're kissing. Some people adore the sound and sensation of the inside of their ears being kissed – the sloshing sound really turns them on.

talking kiss Hold your partner's face between your hands and kiss different parts of their face, first each eyebrow, then eyelids, nose and so on, and between each kiss say something erotic. Describe what you are going to do to them, how you want them to kiss or lick you, where, and what position you want to try.

nibbling Don't bite, it hurts. Nuzzling, on the other hand, is delightful.

callcards Don't. Love bites are not exciting.

butterfly kiss Tried and tested. Use your eyelashes to brush against your partner's face or body.

ABOVE | A kiss has so many facets: security, love and comfort, as well as passion.

BELOW | Exploring the many different ways to kiss your new partner, from deeply passionate to lightly teasing or blowing, is a totally thrilling experience.

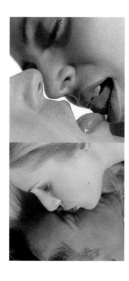

undressing each other

WHETHER YOUR RELATIONSHIP is new or well established, there is always a delicate moment of transition when it moves into a more intimate and sexual dimension and you both know that you want to make love. Men and women have developed all sorts of signals, both subtle and overt, to convey to their partners that they are ready for sex. So now is the moment to get undressed, to expose and reveal your bodies to each other, to explore one another and to become naked in body and desire.

Getting undressed with your lover is an important part of foreplay, an art in itself, and a vital scenario in the theatre of love. Of course, you can tear off your clothes, or each other's, throw them into a heap and leap into bed. Sometimes, when passions are running high, that uninhibited approach is all part of the fun. Or you may be shy about your body, have judgements about it, and end up trying to get undressed surreptitiously in the bathroom or under the bed clothes. Getting

undressed and being naked in front of a lover can be very traumatic for some people.

You may prefer to take off your own clothes and present yourself naked in front of your partner. But if you are shy, and your relationship is new, then you could choose to get undressed alone, and slip on an attractive dressing gown before returning to the bedroom.

dressing for undressing

For the bold and uninhibited and for couples who like to bring a little fantasy into their love lives, why not try a tantalizing strip-tease for your partner? However, undressing each other, slowly and lovingly, letting each part of the body reveal itself when the moment feels right, is a romantic way to become unclothed in your prelude to making love.

If the love scenes in movies are anything to go by, undressing your partner is guaranteed to be a smooth and graceful operation. Clothes slip like silk

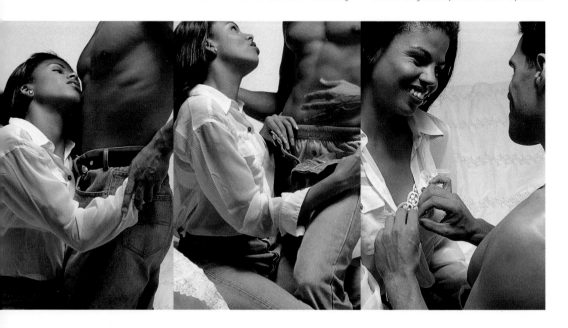

off the skin, buttons undo themselves and, most certainly, the bra fastener pops open with the greatest of ease.

It is rarely like that in real life, and most people have had embarrassing moments of fumbling and fiddling with fasteners, zips that stuck, or jeans and skirts which simply refused to budge past the thighs. If any of these situations happen then you may need to give your lover a hand or take off the awkward item of clothing yourself.

You do not always know when you are going to make love but if you have a suspicion that sex is on the agenda, dress with undressing in mind. Simplify your clothing so it can be removed easily, and avoid wearing items that leave marks on your skin. Don't be caught out wearing your oldest and most ragged piece of unattractive underwear, your woollen thermals, baggy Y-fronts, string vests, socks with holes, or immovable bra. What you have on next to your skin should add to your allure, and that applies both to men and women.

If you have time to prepare, put on soft lighting. Low-light lamps or candlelight will spread a more flattering and romantic glow in the room, softening your skin tones and body shape.

Background music at a reasonable volume can help you and your partner to relax, so have your favourite CDs close at hand.

slowly does it

Try to make the act of undressing part of your love play. Slowly undressing each other and allowing your mutual nakedness to reveal itself, stage by stage, will intensify your desire for one another. As each item of clothing slips from the body, pay your partner a compliment, mentioning not just the obvious sexual areas, but also the eyes, hair, mouth, skin, hands, feet and so on. If you have been hugging and kissing each other, you may need to signal that you are ready for more. It is sometimes a relief for the man when the woman decides to take the initiative, giving him signs that she wants to go further. Slowly undoing his belt buckle and trouser zip should really do the trick!

Then it is his turn to make a move. Take things slowly and let your mutual anticipation of pleasure build up gradually. Open the buttons carefully one by one, and joke about it if one gets stuck. Telling her just how much you have been looking forward to this moment of love will help to put her at ease.

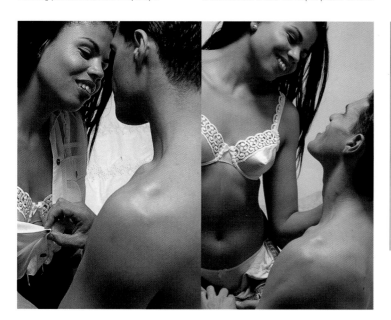

FROM LEFT TO RIGHT |
Undressing should be part of the whole lovemaking experience rather than a means to an end. As the clothes begin to slip from her body, continue to touch and kiss her. Part of the fun of undressing each other is to constantly exchange the active and passive roles. As her body becomes more exposed, stay sensitive to her signals so that she feels happy and relaxed about what is happening.

baring it all

Removing the top layer of clothing is an art to master, but even more sensual skill is needed when you start to take off each other's underwear. You are going to be naked and vulnerable and also, very turned on.

There is something very erotic about starting your foreplay with your underwear still on. At this point, you know you want to make love, but the presence of this scant clothing against your skin makes the whole situation more tantalizing. It creates an exciting sense of seduction as if you are saying to each other: "I want you and I know you want me but let's not take anything for granted."

Some couples like to make love while still wearing an item of clothing because a half-exposed body is more exciting to them, or they find certain types of underwear or lingerie inspire their sexual fantasies and hot up their sex lives.

The Esquire Report, Men on Sex reveals that many men find it more arousing to see their partners partially clothed rather than seeing them totally naked. The reason given was that it added to the air of expectation and anticipation even in a long-term relationship.

Also, keeping some clothes on encourages you to extend your time of foreplay, allowing you to embrace, kiss and caress longer before intercourse which gives your bodies more time to warm up and tune in to each other's mounting sexual feelings. If either one of you is shy or nervous about being seen naked or of making love, the lingering presence of these clothes will give you the extra time you need to relax.

fun of unfastening

Wearing a front-fastening bra will make the undressing manoeuvres easier for him. If it closes at the back, lean into his body and snuggle up to him, whispering some sexy words while he focuses on the job in hand. As you stroke and touch one another, the brush of the cloth against your breasts and genitals can be very arousing. Only you will know the point when you are ready to remove all your clothes.

voyage of discovery

As her bra falls from her body, and her breasts are exposed, cradle them in your hands to acknowledge their soft, sensual beauty. Touch

BELOW FROM LEFT TO RIGHT | Make the most of undressing by slowly removing each piece of underwear, taking it in turns to finally peel off his briefs and her panties. Standing behind her makes it easier to undo a back-fastening bra.

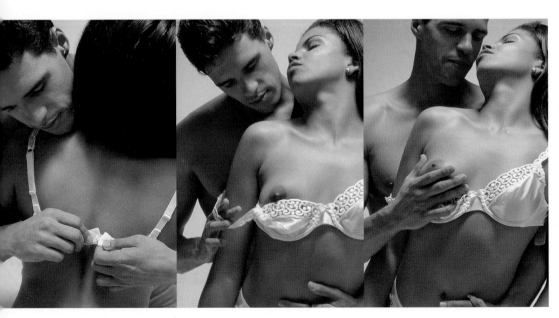

and stroke and caress her naked belly, letting your fingers slip slowly under the panty line with just a hint of exploration.

unpeeling her panties

When you remove her panties, try not to do so with indecent haste! She'll enjoy the feeling of having them peeled away from her like the skin of a forbidden fruit. Edge them down little by little, stroking and squeezing her buttocks gently. In certain positions, you can pull her close to your body to kiss and caress her at the same time.

Once the clothes are removed and there's nothing more to hide, your foreplay enters into a new and exciting stage. The whole body is available for all the touches of love that you can lavish on each other. Take some moments just to be there with each other, savouring and enjoying your own and your lover's nakedness.

brief encounter

Your man will be thrilled if you show your desire for him by removing his underpants. Roll them down slowly over his buttocks, allowing him to touch you while you do so.

getting undressed

Jane, aged 42, a nurse: "I've always been a little shy about undressing in front of a man, and I prefer to make my appearance in the bedroom already undressed but covered with a slinky, silk kimono. I feel most relaxed about it when I'm involved in a deeply trusting relationship, then somehow, if I feel relaxed, sensual and sexy enough, my skin just seems to have a special glow and I lose my inhibitions."

Lucy, aged 26, a production assistant: "I'm all for the bodice-ripping stuff and getting on with it the first time around. If I undress too slowly, then I'm afraid the man is going to be checking out my body too much. My fantasy, though, is to find a relationship with a man I trust enough, and who knows my body well enough, that I can undress for him by doing a slow strip-tease."

Ernie, 32, a photographer: "I prefer mutual undressing because it is less threatening. It's more playful and the power is shared. I find it very sexy."

Don, aged 28, a courier: "When I am going to have sex with my girlfriend, I like it best if we undress slowly and start doing it with some of our clothing on. I think it adds something 'naughty but nice' to the whole thing. It adds a bit of extra excitement as if we shouldn't really be going the whole way – though we both really know that we are."

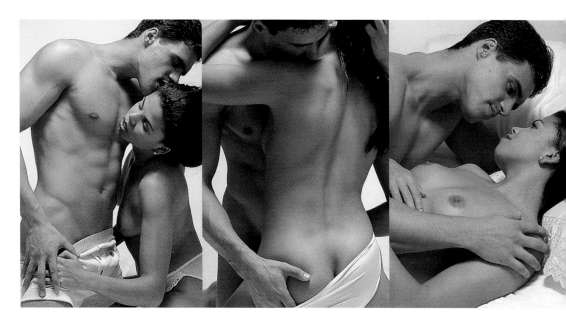

erogenous zones

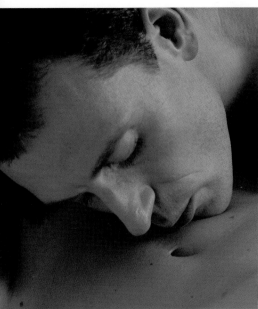
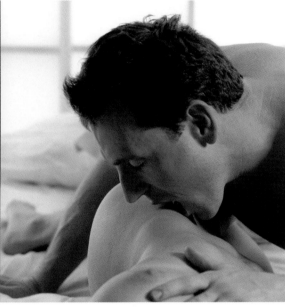

ABOVE | Together, map all your erogenous zones.

BELOW | Foot fetishists, also known as "shrimpers", have always known that toes are among the most erogenous zones on the human body.

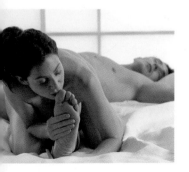

HOW OFTEN HAS YOUR partner absently stroked the back of your neck while watching television, sending electrifying spasms through your body? For a truly sensual experience, take yourself on a body voyage, concentrating more on the journey than the destination. Consider your partner's body as a luscious and varied landscape with an array of areas yet to be explored.

With sex it's all too easy to concentrate on the obvious: the testicles, clitoris, penis and breasts, but these make up a relatively small proportion of the bigger picture. It's often the less obvious areas that yield the most heated results. Touching and caressing all of each other's bodies can produce feelings that are not just sexual. The right touch can make you feel warm all over and reaffirm the deep-rooted feelings of love and care that you have for one another. Focusing on other parts of the body during foreplay shows that you find your partner sexy all over and not just at the hotspots.

the navel

The skin around the navel is a lot thinner, making it an extremely sensitive area. Belly buttons have taken on a new lease of life since they have begun to be decorated with tattoos and navel rings or studs. Some people are a bit squeamish about their belly buttons, but others enjoy having their navels caressed by a soft tongue. It may make them giggle a bit, but after all, this is meant to be fun.

the toe job

This is one of those things you either love or hate. Some people find the idea of placing a set of toes anywhere near their lips revolting, whereas others find it a real turn-on. If cleanliness is an issue for you, then why not treat your partner to a pre-toe-job pedicure? Providing he or she is not too ticklish, the pedicure process can be very relaxing. Alternatively, encourage your partner to have a bath and a good scrub beforehand and then

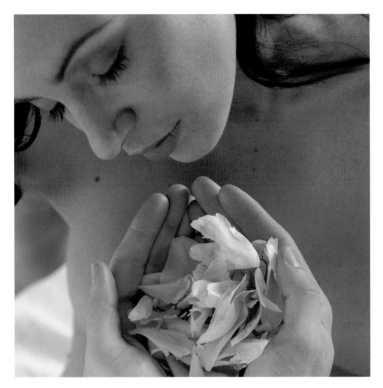

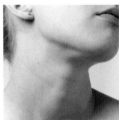

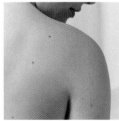

ABOVE | Stroking your partner's neck creates a tingling feeling of warmth along the spine.

ABOVE LEFT | Smell is one of the most powerful senses. Use the beautiful fragrance of flower petals or scented candles to create the mood.

BELOW | The male nipple is a sensitive erogenous zone that responds to a delicate touch.

moisturize their feet. It's surprising how you can begin to see feet as a seriously sexy zone, once you start to take care of them. It will start to look as if all those foot fetishists can't be wrong.

instep

For those who can bear to have their feet touched without collapsing in hysterics, the instep of the foot is a sensitive, nerve-rich area that can be licked and stroked. Many people love to have their feet massaged and pampered and the feet can also be used as an interesting and different way to stimulate other areas, but make sure they're warmed up first.

back of neck

There is something strangely comforting and at the same time sensually delightful about having the back of your neck stroked. It sends a mixture of warm and thrilling shock waves along the entire

length of your spine, leaving you feeling energized and loved. This is a very relaxing and loving place to caress your partner, as it has a mysterious link to his or her sensual centres.

armpit

No one is suggesting that you bury your face in your partner's armpits just as he or she leaves the gym, but think just how sensitive your armpits are. They are a veritable minefield of nerve endings and after a bath or shower they respond well to some gentle caressing and tingling licks.

fingers

The fingers are an understandably popular focus of attention, not least because the tips are so sensitive. During a romantic meal you may feed each other, licking and sucking the juices from fingers and wrists. The act of sucking fingers is so erotic because it is loaded with innuendo.

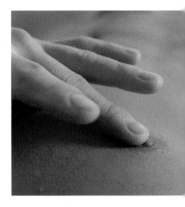

finding the pleasure zones

THERE ARE MANY PLEASURE ZONES in the sexual geography of the human body. When directly stimulated by touching, kissing, nuzzling, nibbling, sucking and licking they can awaken and heighten sexual response. Most sexually experienced adults know about the principle erogenous areas, such as a woman's lips, neck, breasts and clitoris, and a man's lips, penis and scrotum. But a considerate and caring lover also takes time to discover the more secret and mysterious pleasure sites on a partner's body.

It is important to think of your lover's body as a complete and integrated organism, of which every inch is worthy of loving attention and caresses, rather than as a map where specific areas are singled out for erotic arousal. Nothing is more of a turn-off than a text-book lover who has read all the information, and then proceeds to focus on a few selected parts of the body, to twiddle and fiddle with the expectation of scoring a sexy result.

Knowing the erotic physiology of the body is just one aspect in understanding and satisfying your lover's sexual needs. Whatever part of the anatomy you stimulate with your fingers, tongue, lips, breasts or penis, you simultaneously touch and arouse the emotional psyche of your partner.

The body's pleasure areas differ from one person to another, so the best way to discover the most erotically susceptible places on your partner's body is with foreplay and gentle exploration, when you can lovingly, teasingly and sensitively explore each other from top to toe.

Do not be afraid to ask how and where your lover most likes to be touched, and what kind of stimulation brings the greatest sexual thrill. You should also try to learn more about your own body's erotic responses, for this can be a changing and ongoing process of discovery. Tell your lover which parts of your body are most sensitive, to lips or fingers.

Touch games and sensual massage techniques are also excellent ways to become familiar with one another's physical needs and responses, while regular tactile stimulation of the skin's sensory system will heighten its erogenous reactions. The entire body is a potential pleasure zone for you to have fun exploring.

the miracle of the skin

The skin is our largest sensory and erotogenic organ. It houses our sense of touch, and its sensitivity and importance to our survival is second only to the brain and the central nervous system.

BELOW LEFT | Nibbling and nuzzling the soft sensual areas of the face is very sexy. Include the ears, nose and lips.

BELOW RIGHT | Trace the fullness of the lips with your tongue, and kiss the mouth gently, allowing the passion to increase before penetrating with your tongue.

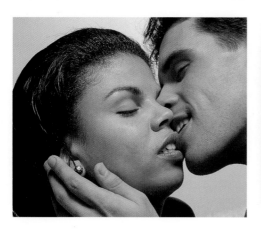

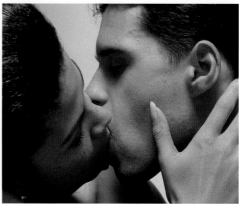

In fact, during our initial development in the womb, the skin, the sense organs and the central nervous system are produced from the same ectoderm tissue, the outermost of the three layers that make up the early embryo form. In this way the skin can be seen as the external, feeling surface of the internal mental processes of the brain. It has a vast network of nerve endings that responds to all manner of stimuli, from pain to pleasure. These impulses are transmitted through the nervous system to the brain.

Some areas of the skin, such as the breasts, nipples, lips, and genitals, as well as other more surprising parts of the body, are richly supplied with a high density of exquisitely sensitive and erotogenic nerve endings, sending signals of

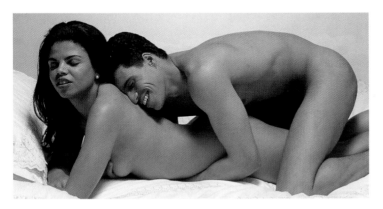

LEFT | Tuning in to your partner's body is like learning to play a fine musical instrument. You need to become sensitive to all its subtle nuances.

BELOW | Words of love, praise and affirmation, the look of appreciation in your eyes, your patience and understanding of your lover's unique sexuality, are as important to the art of lovemaking as your knowledge of a partner's erogenous zones.

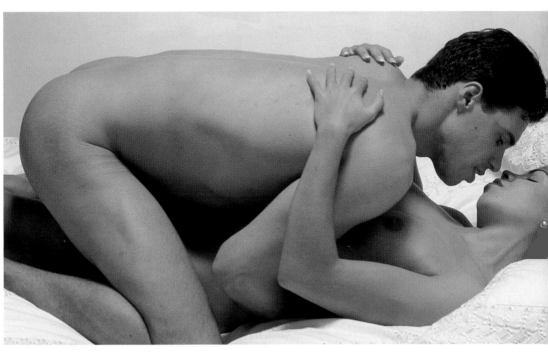

BELOW | Toe nibbling is a
playful pursuit and, especially
when concentrated on the big
toe, can be a major turn-on.

BOTTOM | Stroke the belly
gently as you cover it with
slow and teasing kisses,
then run your tongue around
his nipple.

sexual pleasure to the brain and back to the entire body. Women, in particular, respond to their partner touching and caressing their bodies.

As sexual arousal grows during foreplay and intercourse, the breathing becomes deeper and the tissues get infused with oxygen. This increases the excitability of the nerves at the surface of the skin, especially around the genitalia, so that the body becomes even more sensitive to touch. It is through this process of tactile stimulation, particularly to the most erogenous areas of the body, that men and women are brought to the very peak of sexual pleasure and so reach orgasm.

common erogenous zones in both sexes

Men and women differ in the way they respond to erotic tactile stimulation. Women tend to need more whole body touch to reach the height of sexual arousal, and they are generally more sensitive to skin sensations than are their male partners.

It is highly possible for a woman to reach orgasm purely through the oral or tactile stimulation of her breasts, nipples or mons pubis (Mount of Venus). Men, on the other hand, are greatly aroused by visual stimulation, and are much less likely to reach orgasm without direct physical contact with the penis, their most erogenous zone.

Some of these differences are the result of Western cultural conditioning; often women are much more encouraged to enjoy their total sensuality, while men are taught to focus purely on their genital sexuality.

Most men who allow themselves to experience and enjoy a much softer and more sensual approach to lovemaking will also discover the sheer joy and eroticism that exists in whole body touch.

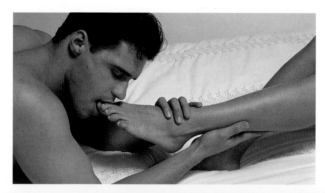

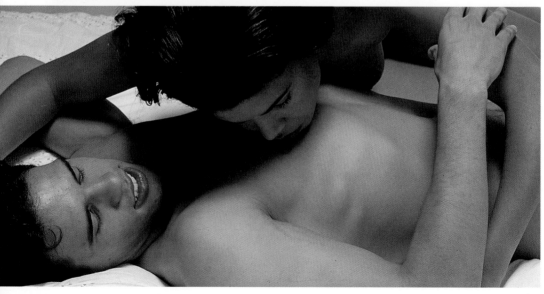

a woman's erogenous zones

The arms and hands: Kiss her hands and wrists tenderly and then suck gently on the fingertips. Pay attention to the soft skin on the underside of the arm, letting your mouth slowly move up towards the armpit.

Breasts and nipples: Treat them gently and with great respect. The breasts are glands, not muscles. This intimate area is packed with highly erotogenic nerve endings, which are directly connected to the emotional centres of her brain. Slowly and deliciously stimulate them with your fingers and tongue.

Thighs: Lick, kiss or stroke the thighs, especially along the soft skin of the inner thigh muscles and around the groin.

Mons pubis: The pubic area is a highly erotogenic area on a woman's body, with a rich supply of nerve endings at the base of the hair follicles. Gently rub or tug on the pubic hairs.

Clitoris: Every man should know more about a woman's clitoris as it is undoubtedly the most sexually important organ in her body, packed with highly erotogenic and sensitive nerve endings to the same extent as a man's penis. Focus on the clitoris only when her whole body has become sexually alive and receptive, and then caress it with your tongue and fingers to bring her to the peak of sexual arousal. Watch out for her signals indicating whether she wants you to change from gentle caresses to more vigorous stimulation.

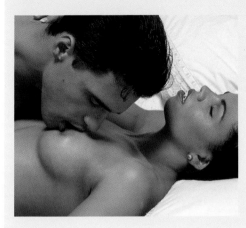

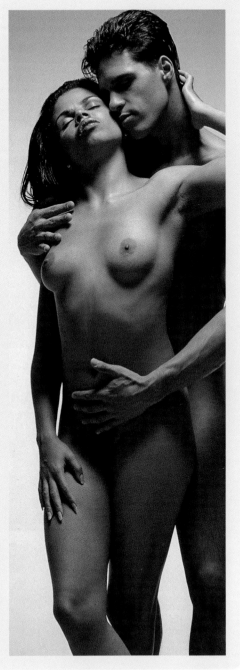

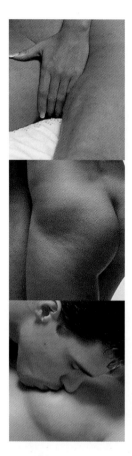

sensitive areas

Both sexes will respond well to loving attention on the following parts of the body:

Head and face: Tenderly caress and kiss the forehead, brows, eyelids, tip of the nose and the chin. Comb your fingers through the hair and plant tiny kisses along your partner's hair-line.

Neck and shoulders: Nibble and kiss along the sides and down the back of the neck and shoulders to send electric shivers through the whole body.

Belly and navel: The belly is a vulnerable but sexually exciting area because of its close proximity to the genitals. Rub your face softly against the belly and then blow gently over it. Cover it slowly and teasingly with kisses, and slide your tongue around the navel, before travelling slowly down to the pubic area.

Perineum: This area extends from the external genitalia towards and including the anus. It is richly served with highly erotic nerve endings and sensitive hair follicles. Stroking over the perineal skin and around the anal rim can greatly enhance sexual excitement.

Legs and thighs: Stroke the legs to awaken the sensuality of the lower half of the body. Focus on the thighs, particularly the inner leg, trailing your fingertips towards the groin. The back of the knees are surprisingly sensitive to erotic touch. Brush your lips against the skin, and let your tongue travel over it in circular movements.

Feet and toes: Squeeze and knead the feet to activate their many nerve endings and so bring them alive. Toe sucking, and rolling your tongue over the webs of soft skin between the toes can be a powerful sexual turn-on. (Always make sure that the feet are clean and the skin is healthy first.)

ABOVE | Explore your partner's body by touch.

RIGHT | Do not stop kissing and caressing the face and neck.

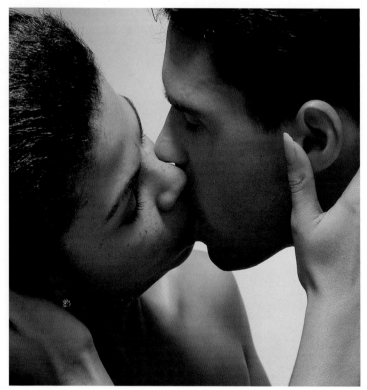

a man's erogenous zones

Chest and nipples: Stroke his chest and pectorals with your hands, and run your tongue around his nipples before sucking them gently. As with a woman, this area is sensitive to erotic arousal.

Penis and scrotum: Too much premature attention here could bring him to ejaculation too soon, as this is the most sexually charged area of a man's body. Run your hands and tongue playfully over his penis and scrotum, and cover them with tender and tantalizing kisses, before moving further down his body.

Buttocks: Focus attention on his buttocks, a very sexually charged zone for men, packed with erogenous nerve endings. Knead and squeeze the fleshy area firmly with your hands.

Back of the body: Men are aroused by sensual touches on the back of the body. Stroke his shoulders and run your fingers down his spine, and then caress his calves and the back of his thighs.

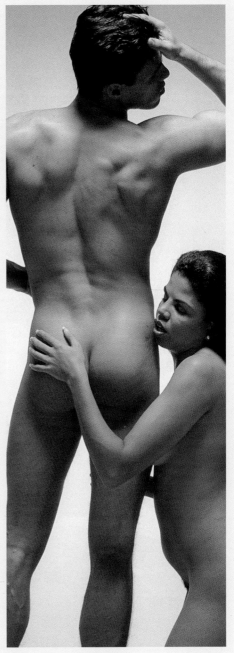

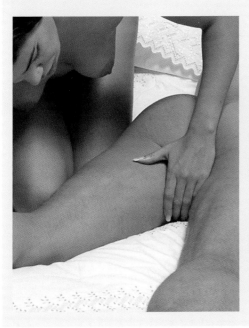

foreplay

REMEMBER THOSE TIMES growing up, before penetrative sex was *de rigeur*? Those steamy sessions in the car or cinema, the way you stroked each other's hands, walking along totally absorbed and wrapped up in each other? Those emotions and sensations were very exciting, in some ways better than sex itself. Foreplay is like looking through a keyhole and seeing how you will both fit together as lovers. It's a means of exploring each other physically and sensually, setting guidelines and maybe even boundaries, likes and dislikes, wants and needs. You are learning and working out ways to relax and please one another.

Asking what feels good and what your partner wants is the only way to fulfil both yourself and your partner sexually. When you indulge in foreplay, imagine you are a tourist on a body tour, asking directions to various destinations. Many people begin by caressing in a way that they would like to be caressed themselves, which is a good starting point as long as you are flexible enough to adapt to the preferences of your partner.

RIGHT | Take the time to undress each other slowly if you can bear the anticipation.

BELOW | Stroke and kiss using bold and confident movements and you will arouse your partner to fever pitch.

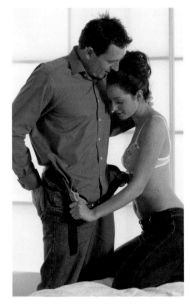

talking dirty

The idea of talking dirty fills some people with disgust. Others love it and actively incorporate it into their sexual repertoire. Still more people think that they might quite like it but would feel rather silly doing it.

Talking dirty doesn't necessarily mean putting your mouth up against your partner's ear and shrieking a string of four letter expletives. You can start with some encouraging oohs and ahhs when he or she is doing something particularly pleasurable to you. When you feel comfortable with this, progress to whispering things like, "You make me feel so sexy when you do that," or, "You taste so good." Fundamentally, talking dirty is an excellent form of sexual communication, in which you actively praise your partner for what he or she is doing.

If you feel stupid saying that this or that feels great, remember how you feel when he or she says it to you. The likelihood is that you don't cringe, but feel good that you are the source of so much pleasure. If you speak a foreign language, you might lose your inhibitions talking dirty in French or Spanish.

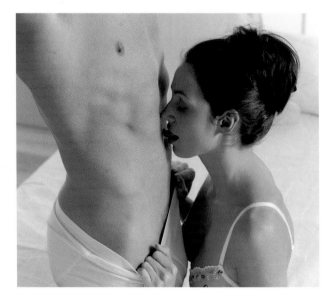

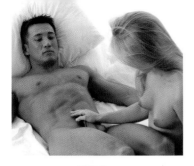

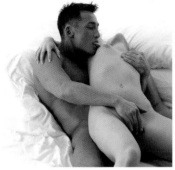

tried and tested

Foreplay doesn't have to start in the bedroom but can begin hours before. It could be a knowing look at a party, a naughty text message while you are at work or even an unexpected note in your pocket saying, "You're going to get some tonight."

As foreplay is in many ways the most exciting part of sex, it's fun to prolong it for as long as possible. Your partner and you should take time over this opportunity to indulge each other, caressing each other's bodies and enjoying the time you have together. You and your partner will enjoy sex so much more if the body is fully aroused, and moist, before coitus.

Start with the undressing. All too often, couples see clothes as an awkward barrier that must be removed quickly. However, it's very sexy to watch your loved one remove his or her own clothes. If you're feeling cheeky, put some music on and treat your partner to a long, slow, sexy striptease. He is guaranteed to adore it and she is bound to find it highly amusing, especially if he uses a hat at the end. It's also erotic to remove each other's clothes, taking it in turns to remove an item.

Kissing can set the pace for the type of lovemaking you both want to indulge in. Try a slow, loving kiss, caressing each other's mouths

with your tongues, or a more passionate, frenzied kiss where you are slightly rougher and more urgent with each other. Small kisses all over your lover's body will make him or her go wild with desire.

Try not to go straight for each other's genitals, but explore other parts of each other's bodies – fingers, toes, armpits and belly buttons – first. Really tantalize each other with massaging hand strokes and tender licks and kisses. Eventually you may end up stimulating each other almost to orgasm, until you cannot stand it any more, and then one thing can lead to another, if and when you are ready.

Foreplay should not just be a means to an end, but enjoyed for the pleasure it gives in its own right. This includes emotional foreplay as well as sexual. Touching, undressing and small kindnesses throughout the day are just as important as your wrist action.

The strokes and techniques you and your partner prefer are as individual as you are and will vary, depending on your mood, what sort of day you have had, and even the weather. The secret to good foreplay is simple. Take your time, and don't rush yourself or your partner. If you take half an hour to massage your partner's inner thigh, don't expect reciprocation. You should enjoy doing it as much as he or she enjoys receiving it. It will be your turn to be pleasured the next time.

tantric sex

These ancient teachings appreciate the differences in arousal times between men and women and aim to harmonize these differences by focusing on the female right to reach sexual arousal and teaching men to curb their passion.

One of the main teachings is the retention of the male orgasm, which according to Tantra weakens the life energy with each ejaculate. Men are taught to moderate their breathing and draw orgasmic energy towards the brain, thus allowing for a greater sense of spiritual realization. Extended foreplay is at the forefront of tantric loving, encouraging strengthened emotional connection through holding, caressing and eye contact.

a private conversation

Talking dirty is fun beyond the bedroom too. There's something really sexy about being in a crowded room, when your partner whispers something so incredibly naughty that you can't help but blush. The excitement lies in the knowledge that all the other people think you are just engrossed in a conversation, when really you are mentally ripping each other's clothes off.

ABOVE LEFT | Of course, touching each other's genitals is not off-limits, but bring your other senses, such as sight and taste, into play as well.

BELOW | Who could possibly have guessed that the film *The Full Monty* would have got quite so many hats off the hatstand?

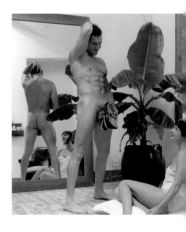

sensual play

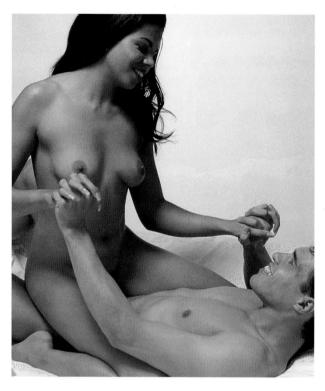

attracted to each other. It manifests in body language signalling a desire to become more intimate with each other. It includes holding hands, cuddling, hugging, kissing and the exchange of sweet words.

It plays a part in the way partners choose to spend time together – listening or dancing to music, going to the theatre or cinema, playing sport, walking in the woods, arranging candlelit dinners, and the exchange of small but meaningful gifts. Sensual play acknowledges the special relationship, both sexually and emotionally, that you have developed with your chosen partner, whether that person is a new or long-term lover.

It is not a set programme of techniques but more a response to, and an acknowledgement of, the whole person – body, mind and spirit – which makes you and your partner unique and special to each other.

It is important to give sensual play the time and space it needs, both outside and inside the bedroom, for it will benefit, nurture and enhance your emotional and sexual relationships, so that they remain caring and sensual, warm and erotically alive.

ABOVE | Sensual contact may be as simple as a cuddle for comfort and closeness, a massage for relaxation, kisses to show affection, caresses to soothe or pamper, or moments spent looking tenderly into each other's eyes. All of these can be the start of a sexual journey, but they can also be relished purely for their own sake.

THE TERM "SENSUAL PLAY" is probably more apt than "foreplay" to describe all the many wonderful, caring, romantic, sensual and sexual activities that a man and woman can engage in to express their attraction to and love for each other. "Foreplay" usually refers to those sexual techniques that lovers can use to arouse each other to ensure satisfactory intercourse and orgasm. As such, it implies an activity with a goal in mind, something that comes before the real thing, a little like the hor-d'oeuvres before the main meal – a nice taster but not quite substantial enough in itself.

While this section mostly focuses on sensual play in the context of lovemaking, it can actually start from the moment two people become

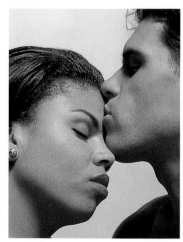

kissing

This is one of the most intimate aspects of sensual foreplay and lovemaking because, in addition to being sexually arousing, it reveals the degree of affection and tenderness which exists between you and your lover. Attitudes towards kissing change from culture to culture, and in some parts of the world it plays a very small role, if any, in the sexual relationship. Most of us, though, regard it as a highly personal part of our lovemaking which reflects emotional closeness. From our earliest memories, kissing is associated with warm and caring contact, and some people find it easier to have full penetrative sex for purely physical sensation and release than to kiss mouth to mouth without a certain depth of loving feeling.

Kissing usually plays a big part in the early stages of romance as a way of exploring sexual compatibility and expressing attraction. However, it can become a sadly neglected activity once the relationship has become established and is taken for granted. One of the most common complaints made by women in long-term relationships is that their men do not kiss them often enough, either as a purely affectionate gesture, or as part of their sexual lives. Too often, a sexual relationship can settle down to the basics, where arousal techniques are focused purely on intercourse and orgasm, while the subtler expressions of love and tenderness, such as kissing, are overlooked. Let kissing remain a part of your physical interaction outside the bedroom, as well as an integral part of your foreplay and lovemaking.

kiss and tell

Jacqueline, aged 28, a secretary, has been married for four years: "To be honest, kissing is the best part for me. If my husband doesn't kiss me enough, I just don't get that turned on. When he takes the time to kiss me properly, I feel he is appreciating me rather than just my body."

Roger, aged 27, unemployed, has a long-term girlfriend: "I used to be an action man, you know, straight to the point. When I met Louise, she was keen on lots of kissing and foreplay. I started to really enjoy it too, and sometimes now we just kiss and cuddle for ages before going on to anything else. It's great."

Avril, 31, a model, is currently single: "I love kissing, but I hate it when I've just met someone and he tries to stick his tongue in my mouth straight away. I prefer to be seduced into a full French kiss, and even then, only after the first few dates. How a man kisses me tells me a lot about how he is going to make love to me."

Fred, 62, a taxi driver, has been married for 32 years: "We are from the old school, and we didn't have a full sexual relationship until we were married. We were courting for several years and it was very romantic, but all we did was pet and kiss. Those kisses were lovely and so full of promise. Even now, we make sure we kiss each other every day."

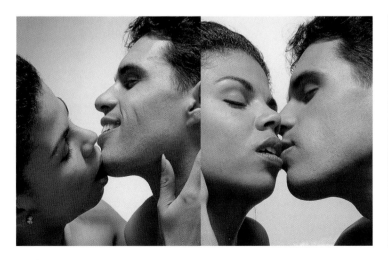

LEFT | Kissing during a sexual episode can change from being tender and sweet to deep and passionate. It can start with the gentle brushing of the lips over the face. Kissing the forehead is an affectionate gesture. So is planting kisses on the nose and cheeks. Playful kisses are also exciting. You can lift his face towards yours and teasingly kiss him on his chin and jaw, moving down to the erotically sensitive areas of the neck and throat.

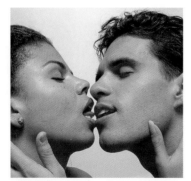

gentle kisses

When you first begin to kiss, let your mouths and lips relax together so that they become soft and yielding to one another. Don't rush into a deep, passionate kiss too soon. The longer you can delay before inserting your tongue into your partner's mouth, the more sensual and stimulating the kissing will be as it slowly begins to build up into an erotically charged embrace. Try kissing all around the edges of the lips, then run the tip of your tongue over them, as this can also be very sexy.

RIGHT | Tease your partner with your tongue on his or her lips.

BELOW | Continue to kiss when you finally embrace.

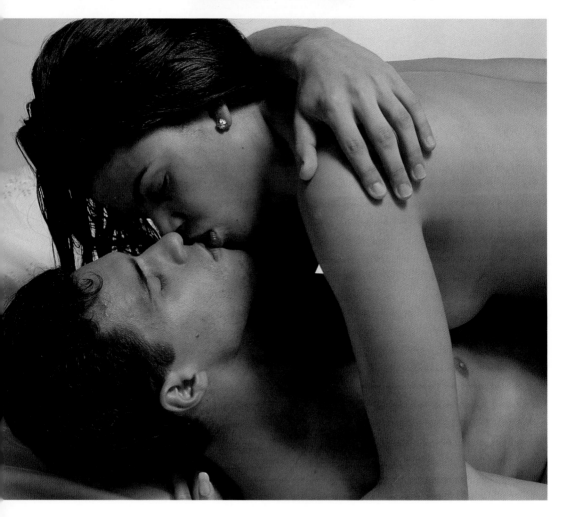

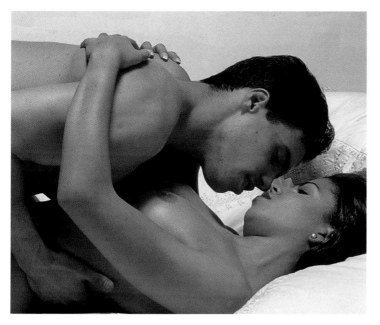
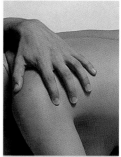
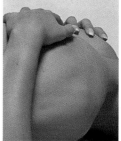

passionate embrace

The chemistry between you and your partner will heat up once the tongue enters the mouth – but don't thrust it immediately towards the throat. Instead, roll it languidly over the teeth and trace the moist contours of the mouth's interior. Then, let your tongues move and dart together to initiate a sexual rhythm, starting to setting the pace for what is to follow.

The act of kissing each other, gently and slowly, or passionately and urgently, can involve you both so deeply that you can begin to feel as if you are dissolving together and you can lose track of time. It can keep you attuned and responsive in both body and mind, while increasing your sexual arousal.

thrusting tongues

During intercourse, kissing can become very exciting if it imitates the movements of lovemaking. As you hold each other tight, your lips may meet with a new sense of urgency and your tongues will seek each other to dance together to the tempo of the pelvic thrusts.

be spontaneous

Sensual play is tremendously important to your emotional happiness and your sexual life. Forget the pre-conditioned programmes and learn to pleasure each other's bodies in ways that acknowledge the needs of the heart, mind and emotions of your partner at any particular moment. Also, become more aware of your own physical and emotional needs which will require different degrees of tactile stimulus depending on your own shifts in mood.

Acknowledge that there are times when either of you may want to be hugged and held, kissed and stroked, but may not necessarily be ready for full sexual intercourse. Couples often hold back from comforting physical contact because they are afraid it will lead to sexual intercourse for which they are not ready. If either you or your partner are under stress and simply not in the mood for sex, or if you have an infection or disability that would make intercourse unwise or undesirable, there is no need to abstain from loving physical contact. In its broadest sense physical contact answers a huge spectrum of human needs, sexual and non-sexual.

ABOVE | Sensual celebration: Sensual play can achieve something greater and more holistic than foreplay. It can be a wholly satisfying experience in itself, an expression of love, and a celebration of the playful, sensual and erotic capacity of the human body.

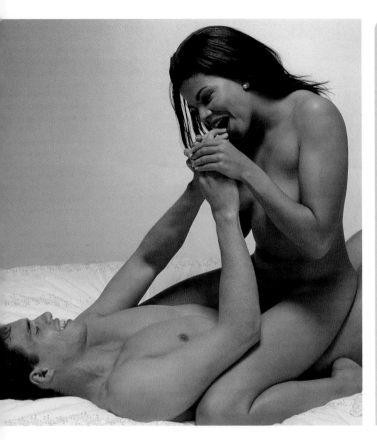

hygiene matters

Sensual foreplay means close physical contact with every part of your body, so take special care of your hygiene so that your body is fresh, clean and smelling good. Nothing is quite such a turn-off as unpleasant body odours, bad breath, smelly feet or dirty nails. Bathe or shower beforehand, alone or – even better – together, and try adding a few drops of luxuriant aphrodisiac essential oils, such as jasmine, ylang-ylang, patchouli or sandalwood, to the bath water. If you have eaten a spicy meal, garlic or onions beforehand, smoked a cigarette, or drunk alcohol, make sure that you clean your teeth and rinse out your mouth.

Some people enjoy "rimming" in foreplay, the term used for anal stimulation. If you do practise this, make sure you wash your fingers before inserting them into the vagina as you risk spreading bacterial infection to its delicate tissues. Taking special care about your hygiene is a statement of your self-esteem and also shows you care about your partner's well-being.

ABOVE | Sucking a man's fingertips will playfully arouse him.

becoming sexually alive

Play with each other's bodies in such a way that you enjoy each touch for its own sake, and try not to worry about achieving an orgasm, because that will create a subtle tension. Every person has different sexual responses, so explore with each other what turns you both on.

There is no specific programme of foreplay techniques that will be able to guarantee sexual success. What pleased and thrilled a previous partner may not be as exciting or acceptable to a new one. Also, sexual responses vary, not just from person to person, but at different psychological and biological stages of life and even day to day.

Learn to recognize your own sexual needs and those of your partner, and enjoy experimenting so you do not fall into boring patterns. It is not always easy to guess what a partner wants at any particular time, so be prepared to talk to each other about your likes and dislikes.

When something feels good, say so or make appreciative sounds. If it does not feel good, there is no need to criticize. Just say to your partner something like: "I would really like you to do this to me," and then be prepared to explain or demonstrate exactly how you want to be touched. Rather than focusing your whole attention on the most obvious sexual areas, such as the genitals or breasts, read the section on erogenous zones to appreciate how the whole body can be responsive to erotic touch. Enjoy the exploration so that you can turn your foreplay into a delightful variety of sensual play.

making it last

Take time to include sensual play as foreplay so that your lovemaking lasts longer and is more luxurious, making every cell of your body come alive and more responsive while letting yourselves become emotionally open and relaxed with each other. In this way your sexuality can envelop your whole being.

stoking the fires

Sensual play includes all forms of touch, such as stroking, caressing and holding, or oral contact, such as kissing, nibbling, sucking and licking. It can involve every part of the body. Sucking on his fingertips or rolling your tongue around them will certainly fire up his imagination.

fun and foreplay

Humour is an important part of foreplay and sensual play. It takes away the seriousness and tension of performance-related sex and helps you both to unwind and relax so your bodies feel completely at ease with each other. Play fighting, gentle bites, giggling, making sounds and rolling on the bed together can all be part of the fun.

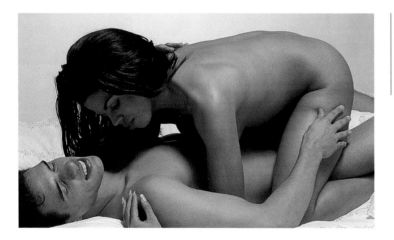

LEFT | Make foreplay and your sensual play last as long as possible, enjoying each new sensation and becoming really relaxed with your partner.

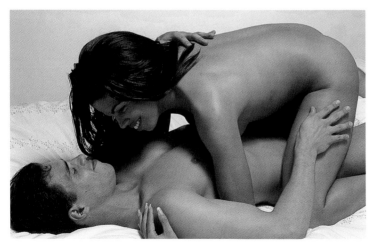

LEFT | Maintain eye contact and talk to your partner while enjoying your sensual foreplay, letting them know how you feel and what you want.

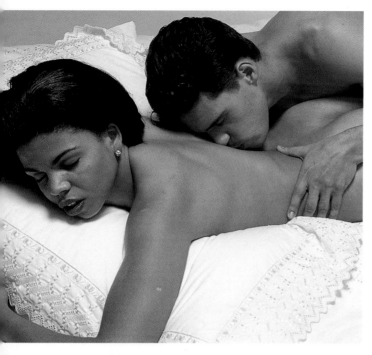

It would be a great mistake, though, to believe that foreplay is primarily a "woman's thing", and that it is something a man should learn to do just to satisfy his partner and be deemed a good lover. Men are sensual beings too, and like women can enjoy body stimulation, loving and playful strokes, kissing, licking and all kinds of erotic tactile contact.

A man who is relaxed in his sexuality will enjoy extended foreplay for its own sake, for his pleasure as well as his partner's. It will help him to be less genitally orientated so that he can feel all kinds of sensations throughout his body. Another important effect is that he will then be more emotionally in tune with his partner.

If he relaxes into full-body sensuality, a man can be more spontaneous and less programmed to performance. He will be less anxious about all the sexual pressures to which men are invariably subjected. Many men worry about performing well, maintaining an erection, fear of a premature ejaculation, fear of emotional vulnerability, concern about whether their woman will have an orgasm before they ejaculate, and so on. Sensual play will be an emotionally nourishing experience for them as well.

Text-book lovers, male or female, may achieve the sexual responses they seek from their lover, but their partner will know that the touches and techniques are more mechanical than loving, and geared to an ulterior motive. He or she may feel personally abandoned or used, even while being turned on. Most women dislike the experience of having a man immediately zone in on their breasts or clitoris, and having them rubbed or stimulated purely to achieve sexual stimulation.

Similarly, a sensual man may not be keen on having a woman grab for his crotch as a way of achieving an instant turn-on. Bodies are not separate from the feelings of the person within them and they cannot be turned on like light switches. They are not machines to be geared to results, regardless of their intrinsic emotional and subtle responses. Sensual play gives time for both men and women to warm up and tune in to each other, on all levels, physical and mental.

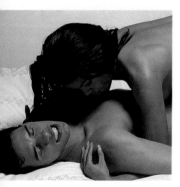

touching the whole person

There are no rules to sexuality except what feels good or right to the people involved. There are times when the passion is high or you haven't much time, and the "quickie" way of having sex is exciting and welcome to both parties. More often, though, extended loving foreplay is important to a sexual relationship, because it enhances the emotional bond, and helps the man and woman become sufficiently aroused so that the ensuing lovemaking is compatible and deeply satisfying to both people.

This is particularly important for a woman, who needs more time than a man to become sexually aroused, and whose sexual responses are heightened when she feels emotionally and physically cherished. Also a woman's whole body is erotically sensitive to loving touches, not just the most obvious erogenous zones, such as her genitals and breasts. The entire surface of a woman's skin, as it is smooth and delicate, is highly sensitive and responsive

TOP | The spine is especially sensitive to caresses.

ABOVE | Men as well as women enjoy being touched all over.

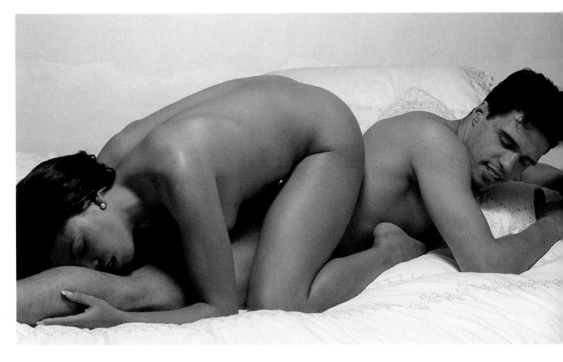

tools of arousal

Any part of the body can become a sensual tool in foreplay. The sweep of your hair, the soft brush of your nipples and breasts against his body, or the warmth of your breath on his skin will be extremely arousing to him. Trailing your fingertips or nails lightly over his skin will heighten its sensitivity. Try to involve your whole body in sensual play, so that even while kissing one part of his body, you are aware of the impact of your thighs, belly and pubic area as they press gently against him.

body worship

A woman's whole body, not just her most obvious sexual areas, is an erogenous zone. Take time to let your kisses and touches worship her total sensuality. Focus your attention not just on the front of her body, but on her arms, legs and back. Cover her back with a carpet of delicate kisses, following its sensuous curves and lines. Then stroke and gently squeeze the muscles in her buttocks and thighs.

loving touches

Your man will also enjoy having your touches and kisses on the back of his body. This can include massaging the legs, kissing and licking the highly sensitive soft skin at the back of the knees, stroking, pummelling and squeezing the buttocks, and lightly scratching your fingernails over his skin to excite sensory nerve endings. In this way, the whole body will be suffused with delicious sensual feelings.

tongue and toe

The feet and toes are remarkably sensitive to tactile stimulation if your partner is not too ticklish. Rubbing and massaging the feet can be followed by deliciously erotic toe sucking. Run your tongue around her toes, sucking on them playfully one by one. Special attention can be given to the big toe which, according to zone therapy, has a special connection with the pituitary gland, which regulates the sex hormones.

ABOVE | The skin at the back of the knees is one of the less obvious sensual areas.

sexual arousal

Extended foreplay allows the whole body to become flooded with sex hormones so that the correct physiological changes can occur to ensure harmonious lovemaking. For a woman, sufficient arousal will allow her vagina to undergo changes which enable successful and comfortable penetration during intercourse. The outer and inner lips of her vagina will swell and secrete lubricants, to give off her own special sexual scent. The shape of her vagina will change, so that the outer third becomes narrower and better able to grip the penis to ensure adequate friction, while the inner two-thirds of the vagina expands. It, too, will secrete a sexual lubricant as she becomes excited. Her clitoris also enlarges, as it becomes engorged with blood, and its nerve network becomes erotically sensitized.

As a woman's arousal increases, her breasts may increase slightly in size, and her nipples become erect. If the sensual play which has preceded intercourse has acknowledged her whole person, then physically and emotionally she should feel vibrant and receptive and ready to receive her man.

Loving and sensuous foreplay benefits the man because it can take the sexual charge away from his genital area so that it streams through his whole body, enabling him to become more relaxed and better able to enjoy full body pleasure without the fear of ejaculating too soon. If intercourse is to be the result of the foreplay, when the excitement grows the right tactile stimulation will enable him to achieve a full erection. As his arousal increases, the scrotum skin thickens, and the testes draw up closer to his body. In some men, nipple erection during arousal is also common.

wave of passion

Your extended foreplay should give you time to relax together emotionally, as well as becoming sexually aroused. If you enjoy it for its own sake, rather than proceeding headlong towards a goal, you can savour moments of tenderness purely to enhance your intimate connection. Do not be afraid to let your states of arousal rise and fall like waves in the ocean. Once you are in harmony, both physically and emotionally, you can ride those waves together, letting one peak of excitement ebb to give way to another. Touching, stroking, caressing and eye-contact will keep you closely attuned to each other.

secret zones

A woman's body has many surprising and hidden areas of sexual sensitivity. Sensual play allows you to unravel its mysteries, so that you both can discover new and exciting pleasure places. The underarm and armpit can be very responsive to your loving attention. Try rolling your tongue over its soft skin while gently stroking her breast.

breast care

A woman's breasts are one of her most erogenous areas, but their responsiveness to tactile stimulation may vary, depending on her mood or the phase of her menstrual cycle. Always be sensitive to them and to her responses, and do not zone in on them before she is ready for such intimate contact. Gentle palpation of the breasts can feel great, but remember her breasts are glands and not muscles, so handle them with care.

When your woman is sexually aroused, you will notice changes to the shape of her breasts as they begin to swell; the areola darkens and the nipples become erect. Licking and trailing your tongue around the areola at this point will be highly exciting to her, increasing her eager anticipation as your lips move closer to her nipple.

When sexually excited, the nipples seem magically connected to her whole nervous system, sending waves of pleasure down through her body to her genitals. Kissing, licking, sucking and flicking your tongue over the nipple will bring her to a peak of arousal. Pay loving attention to both breasts, moving from one to the other, and tell her how beautiful and special they are to you.

Many men love to have their nipples kissed, licked and stroked during foreplay. In some men, just as in women, the nipples will also become erect when they are sexually aroused.

BELOW | Men also enjoy having their nipples kissed and licked.

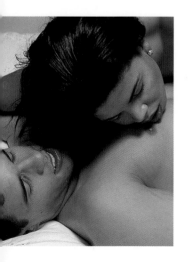

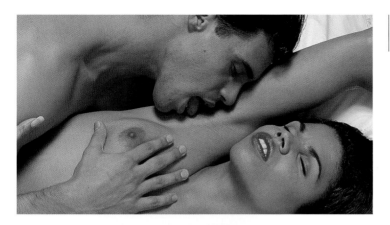

LEFT | Begin by licking the sensitive armpit, at the same time stroking her breast.

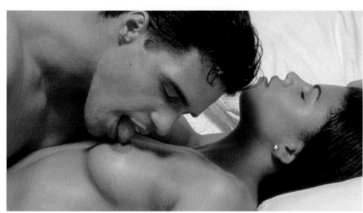

LEFT | Then lick her nipples and trail your tongue around the areola.

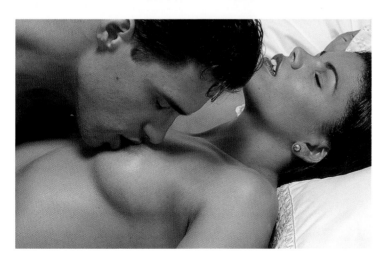

LEFT | Sucking and gently biting the nipples will bring her to full arousal.

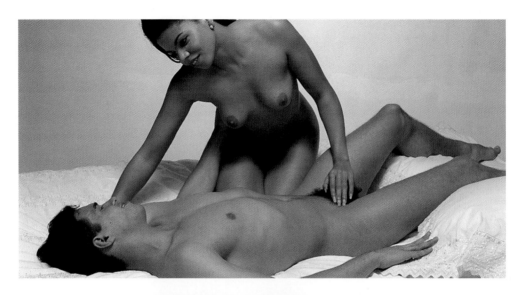

ABOVE AND RIGHT | Tell your lover how and where you like to be touched and kissed.

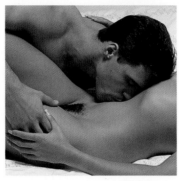

understanding each other

Even in close relationships, both men and women can be remarkably shy about discussing their sexual needs with each other, including what turns them on and what turns them off. This is partly because the sexual ego is very fragile and it is easy to feel rejected or to take any comments, other than highly positive ones, as criticism.

Talking about sexual issues requires delicate negotiation, being able to choose the right moment, a willingness on both sides to experiment and explore new methods, and a readiness to change old patterns. The latter can be particularly difficult if your methods have worked

perfectly well on previous occasions or with another partner.

However, by not disclosing your sexual needs and preferences, there is a danger that you may become resentful and gradually withhold your sexuality altogether from your partner, or deaden your sensory responses so that your sexual life becomes more of a functional duty rather than a joyful celebration of your relationship.

Sexuality should not be imposed on the other person regardless of how he or she may feel. Much of the pleasure can be in the mutual exploration of each other's bodily responses. It is a two-way interaction, involving many subtle nuances and variations. You can jangle along together, or you can compose a symphony of love, touch, sensuality and eroticism which will always hit the right note, depending on your changing needs and moods.

How most men and women touch and want to be touched in their most erotically charged areas – the penis and clitoris – reveals quite opposite male and female needs. A man will often long to receive firmer touches to his penis during manual stimulation, while a woman generally prefers a more subtle approach to the stimulation of her clitoris, usually after she has become aroused. You can help each other by showing exactly how you like to be touched. Many men and women experiment with genital touching during masturbation and usually perfect their technique in doing so. Watch each other masturbate, or guide your partner's hand or fingers with your own, showing the different pressures and strokes that you most enjoy and that are most likely to help you reach your peak of arousal.

warm and welcoming

The soft roundness of her belly will welcome your loving kisses as your lips slowly move down her body. This vulnerable area needs your attention so it can become charged with sexual energy. Kiss it tenderly all over, run your tongue teasingly around the navel, and warm the skin with your breath. Work slowly down to her pubic area. Stroking and

rubbing her mons pubis with your fingers and tugging gently on the pubic hair will enhance clitoral stimulation. Kissing along her groin and the tops of her thighs can also produce wonderful sensations.

guiding hand

Ask your man to show you exactly how he likes his penis to be touched. Stroking, rubbing and kissing his penis is all part of your sensual play. Being comfortable about touching this part of his body enhances your mutual satisfaction in lovemaking.

thighs and sighs

Don't focus your attention solely on her clitoris, but regularly return your sensual touches to other parts of her body, especially the areas close by, so that the erotic sensations can stream through her body.

BELOW | The inside of her thighs and belly are a very erogenous area. Cover the soft skin with kisses, bringing your lips a little closer each time to these most intimate parts of her body.

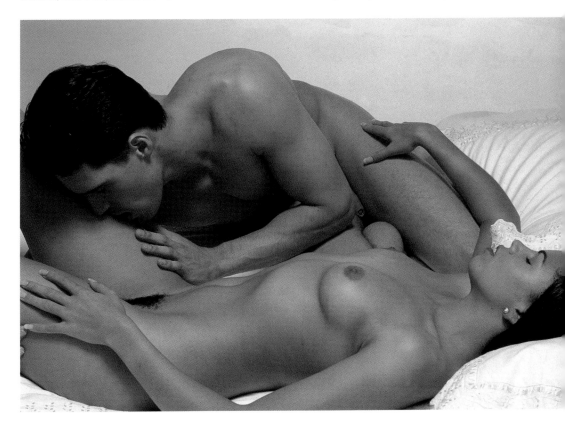

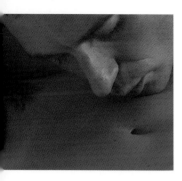

clitoral stimulation

Most women dislike having their clitoris roughly handled; it is an exquisitely sensitive part of their sexual anatomy. Correct stimulation of the clitoris is very important to a woman's sexual satisfaction and to her achieving an orgasm. Too much, too soon can be irritating and even painful.

Once your woman is aroused by more loving and sensual foreplay, and she is naturally producing her vaginal secretions, stroking and rubbing with a finger or fingers, licking, flicking the tongue back and forth and gentle sucking on the clitoris can create euphoric sensations throughout her whole body.

However, she may not want you to focus stimulation directly on to her clitoris for a prolonged period of time, but would prefer it if you also touched and palpated the surrounding areas, such as the vaginal lips and mons. Also, from time to time, return your attention to other sensual parts of her body which will be pulsating with pleasure and demanding your caresses.

ABOVE, LEFT AND BELOW | Gently stimulating each other together is a good way to find out your lover's desires.

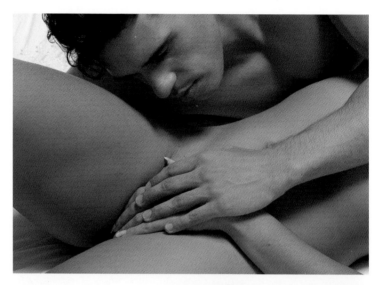

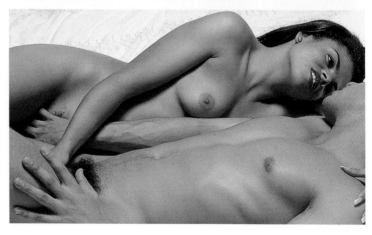

If you are using your fingers to stimulate the clitoris, then lubrication is important. It is best to spread some of the sexual juices from her vagina on to her clitoris. Otherwise, use your own saliva, or if necessary, an appropriate cream, gel or oil (make sure it is hypo-allergenic as the tissues here are very sensitive and delicate – scented creams should never be used).

Vary your rhythm, vibrations and movements, but remain alert to her responses, which she will indicate by the movements of her pelvis, and her sighs, moans and words of encouragement. Do not be afraid to ask her what, exactly, she likes best.

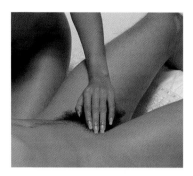

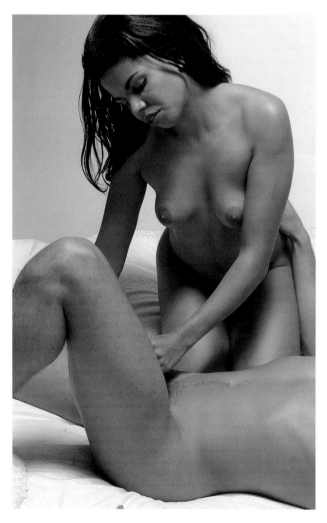

LEFT AND BELOW | Ask your lover to tell you how he likes his penis to be stimulated.

penile stimulation

A man most definitely wants his penis to be handled with care, but he may well prefer firmer pressure and strokes than he is actually getting from you. Many women err on the side of being too timid in the way they handle their lover's penis. Ask your man to show you exactly what he likes. Watch him stimulate himself, and then let him put his hand over yours to move it up and down the glans and shaft. This way you can learn whether he likes short or long strokes, rapid or more sensual ones.

Remember, though, that if you want to extend your foreplay, do not overstimulate his penis at this point, or you can bring your man to orgasm too soon. During sensual play, kissing and licking the penis and testicles tenderly, flicking your tongue over them, and saying appreciative things about this treasured part of his body, will make him feel especially good.

just connect

Foreplay can bring you both to a state of arousal, where intercourse is the desired conclusion. As sensual play, it can also be complete in itself without penetrative sex. Just pleasuring each other, exploring every part of the body with loving oral and tactile stimulation can create a deep and mutual sexual and emotional connection, whether or not it eventually leads to orgasm or sexual intercourse.

sensual massage

RESEARCH HAS SHOWN that the art of massage and touch has therapeutic effects on people, both physically and emotionally. The skin is the largest organ in the body, feeding the brain with information on our external environment, and if it is caressed gently and lovingly, then the brain will also relax and unwind. After a stressful day, massaging your partner allows you some time to wind down and enjoy each other's company.

Being massaged in a brightly lit room with blaring rock music may appeal to some, but for true sensuality it is better to dim the lights or even use candles, prepare some aromatic oils and put on some relaxing background music.

Have a warm, not hot, shower beforehand and make sure the room is warm enough. Both you and your partner must be comfortable, so the bed or the floor are usually the best places for a massage. Massaging in front of – but not too close to – an open fire is also extremely sensual, as the warmth and flickering light from the flames, combined with the soft crackle of burning wood, ignite the earthy and primal instincts in you.

basic technique

The secret to a good massage is to maintain a constant confident touch, using flowing unbroken strokes. Experiment with different pressures and

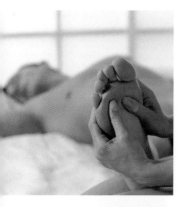

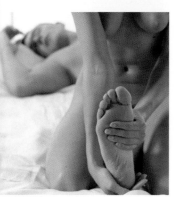

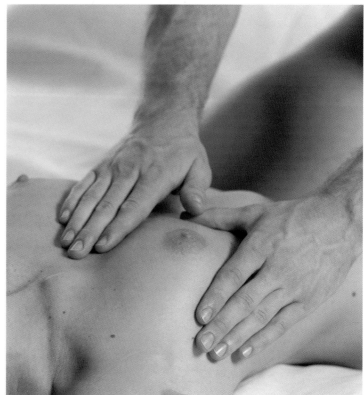

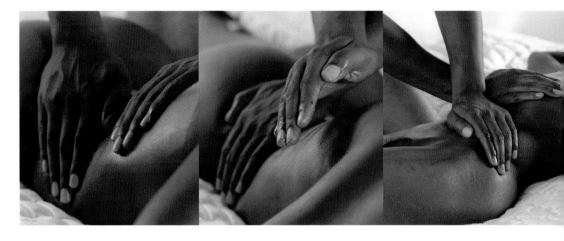

speeds, exploring a range of different techniques and communicating with each other as to what feels most delightful.

To lubricate the areas that you intend to massage, pour some blended oil in your hands, rubbing them together to warm them up. Apply enough oil so that your hands glide smoothly over the surface of your partner's body, but remember that a little goes a long way.

circle strokes

These stretch out the muscles, releasing tension from the soft tissues. They are best applied to broad surfaces, such as the back, thighs, chest and belly. Place both hands on the body, flat and side

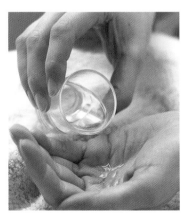

by side. Lead with your right hand and move them in a clockwise direction, using a constant, fairly gentle pressure.

fanning strokes

These strokes also release tension from the soft tissue and are ideal on the back, as it is a large broad surface. To fan upwards, place both hands flat at the base of the spine on each side of the spine. Glide them both up, concentrating pressure in your palm before fanning out to the sides of the body. From here, mould your hands around the sides of your partner's body and drag them down to the base again.

kneading strokes

These are ideal for fleshy areas, such as the buttocks and thighs, releasing tension from the larger muscles. Imagine that you are kneading dough by squeezing a portion of flesh in your fingers and then rolling it from one hand to the other and back again.

percussion strokes

Rapid strokes that create a vibrating sensation help to improve skin tone and circulation to nerve endings. Hacking involves a series of chopping movements, with alternate hands concentrating on the same area. The wrists must remain relaxed, so the action is bouncy rather than stiff.

ABOVE | With circle strokes, keep both hands next to each other, so your right hand will have to pass over the left.

BELOW LEFT | Warm some oil in your hands to avoid the shock of a cold touch.

BELOW | Percussion strokes can be fun, but be gentle.

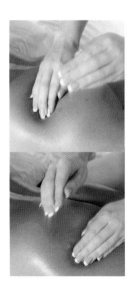

post-coital

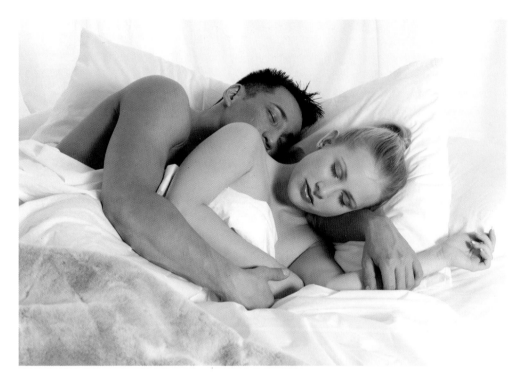

ABOVE | That glorious post-coital nap when you are both totally satisfied and spent is just another way to prolong the delights of lovemaking.

SEDUCTION DOESN'T STOP when the sex does. After sex is a time for cuddling, snuggling up and also sleeping – a time of lying together, perhaps talking, and certainly still enjoying each other's bodies. You continue to make love by caressing each other. The orgasm isn't the end of the process: touching is the ultimate way to complete the act of making love.

On the other hand, there is the thorny question of men who fall asleep immediately after sex. Most women find it exasperating if their partners roll over with their backs towards them and start snoring because, for them, the moments after sex are particularly precious and loving, when, lying in their partner's arms, they feel most relaxed and contented. It seems that it isn't simply physical tiredness that overcomes men just after they have

had an orgasm, although undoubtedly this is a factor. There is also a mental and emotional response. For a short while, men enter a euphoric, almost dangerously happy, fulfilled and vulnerable state. They are physically spent and their hormonal system is temporarily shut down. All their basic instincts, including by this time sexual impulses, are in abeyance and the feeling of relaxation is complete and overwhelming. If she chooses to, a woman could consider that his falling asleep is an indication of total trust.

Of course, there are no absolute rules and many men don't fall asleep and do like to talk after sex. Some light a cigarette, others switch on the radio. Naturally, it is usually in the early stages of a relationship that men make the most effort to please their partners after sex. Falling asleep

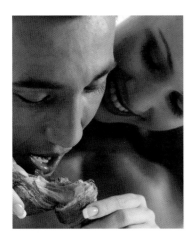

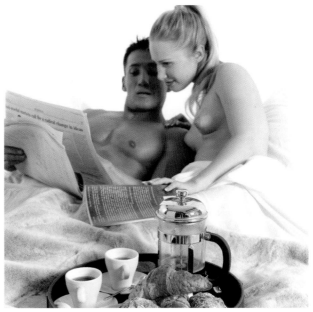

immediately is more typical of a long-term relationship because a man feels secure enough to do so. Women behave slightly differently. Some will fall asleep quickly or may not feel like talking, but most like cuddling up. Whatever happens, lying together in the "spoons" position or falling asleep in each other's arms can give you both a feeling of closeness, security and peace.

enjoying the afterglow

According to the Kama Sutra, lovemaking hasn't finished until the man has rubbed sandalwood ointment on to his partner's body. They should then eat sweetmeats and drink fresh juice, while enjoying the moonlight and an agreeable conversation. Finally, as the woman turns her face towards the moon, the man gives her a lesson in astronomy, pointing out the different planets.

Perhaps stargazing is not such a fabulous idea, but eating after sex is truly divine. You can have breakfast, lunch and dinner in bed and it's easy to prepare a delicious selection of fruits, chocolates, savoury nibbles and wine or champagne

beforehand to enjoy post-coitally. And if you have no veranda, there's no moon and it's freezing outside, how about taking a bath together? Put some lovely scented oil in the bath, create an atmosphere, perhaps put candles around the bathroom, and slide in. Make time in your busy lives for some special time together.

Many women are able to enjoy more than one orgasm and men may also want to go in for another session. All men require some recovery time – even very young, fit men usually need about 20 minutes before trying again. This time of lying together, talking and enjoying each other's bodies can sometimes lead to a surprise, especially if the woman starts licking her partner's penis, and, of course, repeating penetrative sex is not the only option.

ABOVE LEFT | Sharing something to eat after sex is a deliciously sensuous experience and may even refuel your energies for more.

ABOVE RIGHT | Making love, then enjoying a lazy breakfast in bed reading the weekend newspapers is one of life's greatest pleasures.

BELOW | Enjoy a long and indulgent bubble bath together, prolonging the intimacy of touch after you have made love.

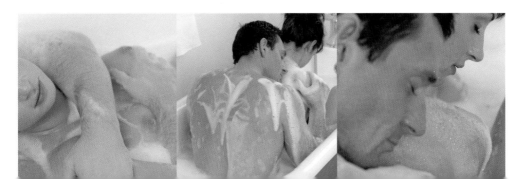

pillow talk

COMMUNICATION IS KEY even in the shortest relationships – it is important that you let the other person know what you are expecting. This is not just to avoid misunderstandings, but also in order to get what you want.

What are your sexual preferences? Are there things you really don't like your partner doing, but are unwilling to mention in case they feel criticized? Are there things you would love your partner to try, but are still too embarrassed to mention? Is there something slightly perverse that you would like to do during sex, but are afraid to broach it in case you seem a little weird?

Being intimate and speaking about your innermost feelings is generally difficult for both men and women. In an ideal world, we would be able to tell each other everything but, in reality, few people actually do, especially if there is a problem, until they have to deal with the subject. It takes time, sometimes years, to build up trust within a relationship and to discuss your innermost fantasies, fears and needs. Over this period, you can begin to know by verbal and body language what your lover enjoys or dislikes at certain times because you know them very well.

sexual communication

A good place for intimate chats is obviously the bedroom or lying cosily together on the sofa. The best way to tell your partner about your likes and dislikes is by affirmation – "I love it when you touch me there," or "It feels better this way." Direct criticism can be very intimidating and upsetting, so it is best avoided, but describing what you didn't like in previous sexual relationships may be constructive: "I felt embarrassed when my previous lover used to talk dirty when we were making love," or "The way my previous wife bit me each time she had an orgasm was really irritating." However, intimate disclosures about previous partners can

BELOW | Communication is the essence of a mutually satisfying sex life. It can be heartbreaking if you have a problem that can easily be resolved but you are afraid to discuss it with each other.

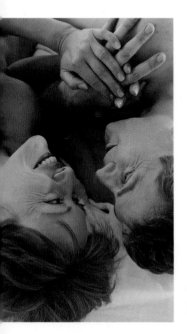

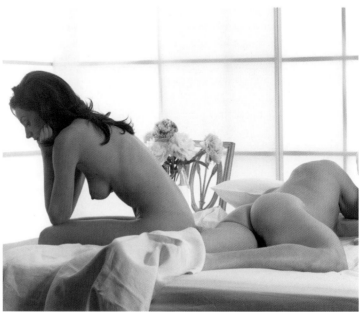

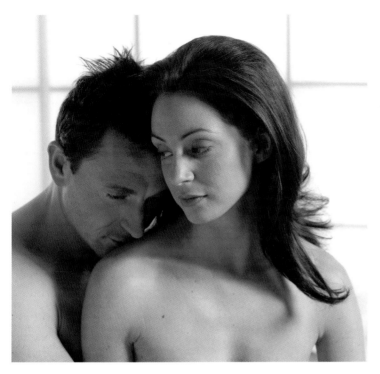

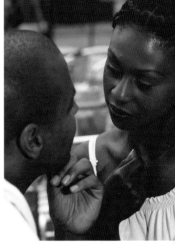

also upset current ones and a long list of differently skilled lovers is not recommended. Apart from anything else, it is likely to be interpreted as a comparative scale. You have to gauge your partner's response and act accordingly, remembering to build on the positive aspects of your relationship.

Theoretically, the longer you are with someone, the easier it should be to discuss your needs. However, all sexual relationships change over time and just because the sex was vigorous during the first year doesn't mean it will be during the tenth. Continuing communication and co-operation is vital, especially when you have to deal with problems. If left unresolved, problems can eat into the relationship, creating rifts between you. If the problem is shared, however, then she won't feel resentful or frustrated and he won't feel upset and to blame – or vice versa.

Some serious issues, such as bisexuality, might come out as a bolt from the blue at a later stage in a relationship, and that can be quite devastating

for the uninformed partner, if the subject has never been broached before. Besides the nature of the discovery, a major secret can seem like a betrayal. There are no instant solutions for the big sexual surprises, but it is important to be aware that professional support is available and if you are faced with something really challenging, you should seek advice to help you get to grips with the implications for the relationship. As always, it is far better to confront issues as they arise, rather than to let them fester.

If you are treating each other badly in general, then your sex life will probably be dire. There is no drug in the world that will cure a relationship problem like this as you get older. One of the most successful ways of keeping an intimate relationship flourishing is by being best friends. You may end up having sex only once a week or twice a month or much less frequently, but being respectful, loving and open with one another is the key. Honesty really is the best policy.

ABOVE | Sex is just an extension of a relationship. Communication is the key. So make sure you are clear about what you need and expect for yourself.

gay sex

RIGHT | Best friends can be lovers as well.

BELOW AND BELOW RIGHT | Giving and receiving pleasure and relishing each other's sexuality is at the heart of all relationships between couples, whatever their sex.

THIS BOOK IS written primarily from a heterosexual point of view, but what do you do if you find you are attracted to or seduced by a member of the same sex? It is worth noting that gay sex, both male and female, is not so very different from so-called straight sex – the relationships have many of the same problems, the partners have many of the same feelings and the sexual techniques are pretty similar. Society's attitude, however, is still quite mixed and this can impose additional pressures on gay partners.

coming out

Telling the family often poses a problem. Not everyone's family consists of middle-class liberals with a pansexual view of the world. In fact, it will probably take time for most parents to come to terms with the fact that their child is gay.

Although some families are truly homophobic, most will ultimately support their kids. The first reaction is often, "I'm never going to become a grandparent," then, "What about AIDS?" But

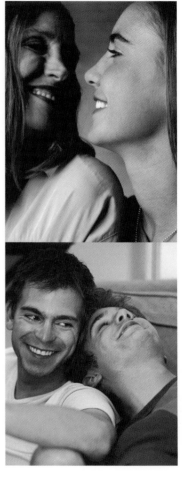

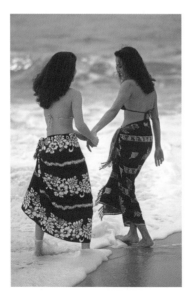

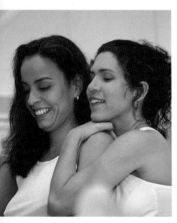

overall, the most common worry is, "Where are they going to meet someone who will help them have a stable and happy life?" If you can't manage to tell your family face to face, it's often a good idea to write to them. Reassure them that whatever your sexual preferences are you are still the same person they know and love. It's no big deal. There are support groups that can help families through this tricky stage.

Whether you are still at school, college or in the workplace, check the organization's policy on privacy before telling anyone – friend, teacher or fellow staff. In some instances, they may be legally obliged to tell someone else. Before you know it, a confidence could become a juicy story – people in groups are natural gossips, whether they mean to be or not.

Never come out when you are high or drunk – you may regret it the next day. Public announcements embarrass everybody. Outing someone else is, at the very least, bad manners and could cause grief and pain to a number of friends and relations. Great sensitivity is required for mature people coming out to their partners or children, as this is bound to be traumatic for all parties. Seeking advice before you approach the subject is recommended and again, there are lesbian and gay helplines with a wealth of experience in how to handle this delicate situation.

how to look after yourself

Whether you are gay or heterosexual, safer sex is the name of the game. You can acquire sexually transmitted infections (STIs) from kissing, petting and oral sex, as well as from intercourse. If you are into multiple partners, it's essential for your sake and theirs to use protection.

what gays do in bed

Gay or heterosexual, the body's erogenous zones are exactly the same and, in both cases, are not confined to the genitalia. Both gay women and men love to kiss, cuddle, massage, stroke, pet and kiss each other's erogenous zones, including nipples, arms, toes, fingers, ears, face, neck and genitalia. They masturbate each other and may indulge in fantasy, sometimes cross-dressing. Women may use strap-ons for vaginal or anal sex or insert fingers or hands. Men may have anal sex and non-penetrative sex. Gay men and women are just as likely or unlikely to indulge in S&M as heterosexual men and women. In other words, couples like to give pleasure to their partners, whatever their sex, and explore and enjoy their own sexuality.

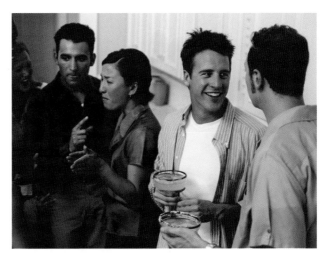

how do you know if you are gay?

The jury is still out on whether people are born with a genetic package that predetermines sexual preference or whether it's possible to be "turned into" a gay man or woman by your parenting and/or environment. The argument is still raging about nature and nurture:

"I first knew when I was a teenager and was more aroused by the men's underwear advertisements than the women's."

"I first became aware of being a gay women when I was kissed by the high-school heart-throb and realized that I was more interested in the art teacher."

"I'd never enjoyed sex with my husband and thought it was just one of those things. When we split up after the children had grown up and I met Joan, it was as if someone had switched on a light in my life."

"I kind of knew that I had gay tendencies as a boy, but my parents were so religious that it just wasn't acceptable. I had some therapy before I married and then was happily married for several years. My wife and kids have been through hell since I came out, but as the years go by, we are managing to support one another and rebuild our family life."

ABOVE | Gay relationships have much in common with heterosexual ones.

BELOW | Meeting other gay people is easier today with gay clubs and the Internet.

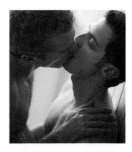

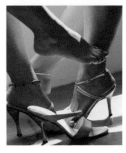

coitus

For really good sex you need to have a repertoire of different positions
to keep your lovemaking interesting, stimulating and truly satisfying.
Although more than 600 sexual postures have been recorded – some very
weird and wonderful – most of them in fact stem from six basic positions.

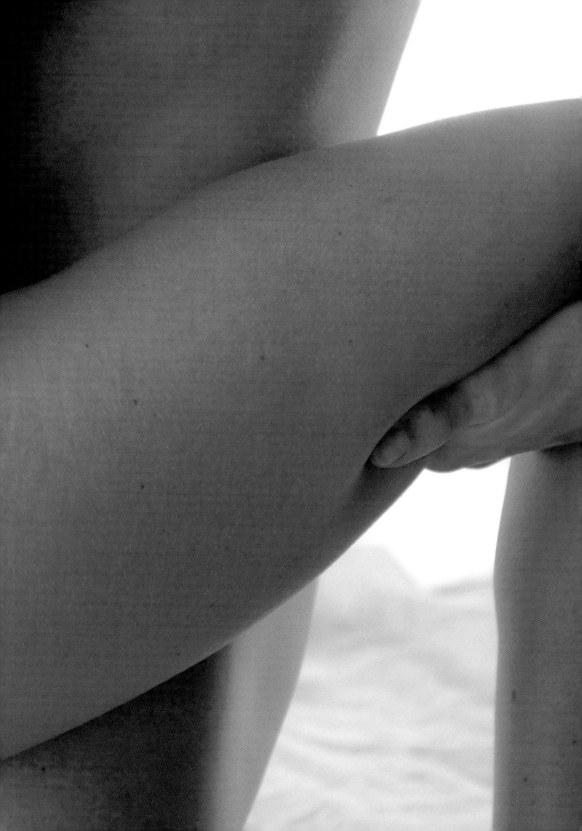

how to do it

EVERYONE HAS AN OPINION and preference on sexual positions. Some are spoons subscribers, while others are doggy devotees. The quest for the ultimate position is a little like letting a child loose in a chocolate factory. We all know there's plenty to choose from, starting with the well-tried and tested missionary position and progressing to something that any acrobat would be proud of. Some positions even look downright painful and others defy the imagination. However, regardless of the complicated twists and tangles your pals may boast of, there are really only six basic positions: man on top, woman on top, side by side (spoons), sitting or kneeling, rear entry (doggy) and standing. All the rest are, in effect, variations on these six.

It certainly makes for a more interesting sex life if you vary your positions and, although this doesn't need to be done with military precision, it can be great fun experimenting with something new. Some positions allow deeper penetration, while others let you stimulate different areas of each other's bodies during intercourse. There's a position for every type of passion. Each can be adapted to suit individual needs, regardless of height and weight differences, penis width and length, mobility, age and flexibility. All it takes is a little imagination, practice and enthusiasm (and of course, the magic ingredient, humour).

Physical and verbal communication with your partner is paramount. As you learn each other's likes and dislikes, you'll be able to anticipate when to change positions or lead where necessary. It's always a great turn-on if one of you suggests a new position, saying, "I've read about this one. Shall we give it a go?"

ringing the changes

Most of us are creatures of habit and usually opt for only two or three sexual positions because they are tried and tested favourites. However, familiarity is said to breed contempt and could lead to bedroom boredom. Trying new positions may seem strange at first, but really does add spice and adventure to your sex life.

This is not to suggest that you should swing from the chandeliers like an urban Tarzan. Know your limitations and don't attempt any positions that are too physically strenuous for you. The posture you choose must be comfortable for both you and your partner or you'll end up in a frustrating, unsatisfying and possibly painful tangle. If a new position doesn't quite work, don't worry. You may discover something amazing on the way that would reinvent this chapter.

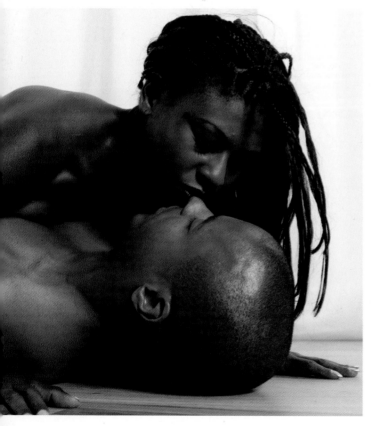

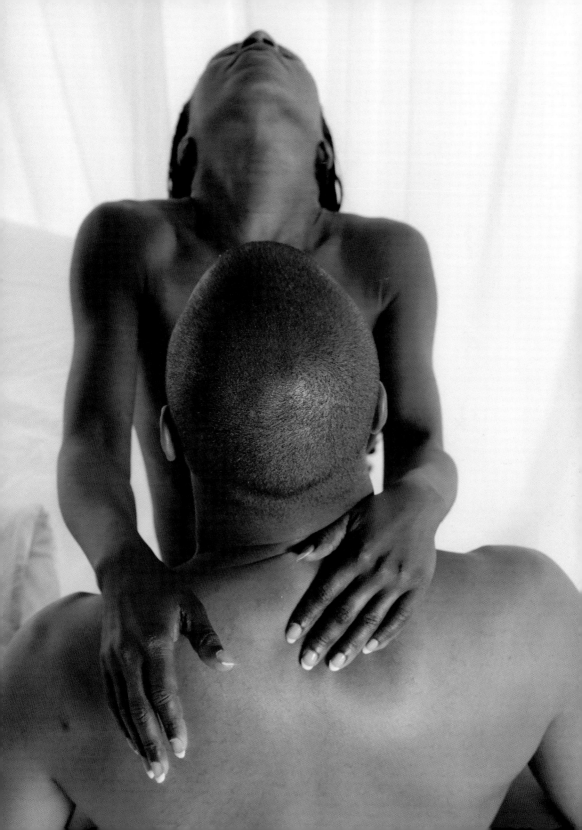

compatibility

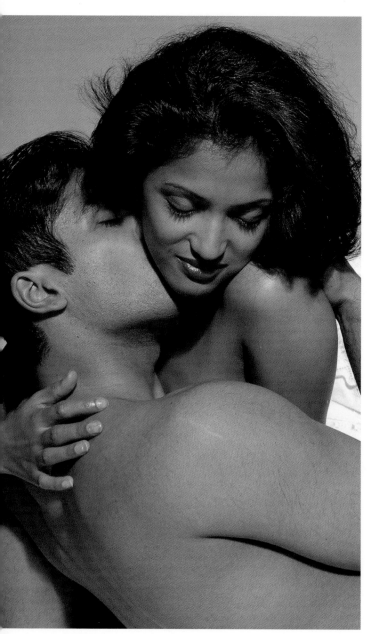

THERE ARE NO DEFINITE RULES about the positions you take or the things you do while making love, except one – that both of you should feel at ease with each other and physically and emotionally satisfied by the experience.

Often, at the beginning of a relationship, you need time to gauge what gives pleasure and feels good, which movements work harmoniously and what pace and rhythm feels right. Lovemaking tends to improve as you get to know one another's preferences and responses. You then begin to fall in tune with each other in much the same way that musicians or dancers do when they continually practise their art together.

What will increase your sexual compatibility is not an array of impressive techniques, nor a unique sexual position, but intimacy and tenderness, and the willingness to be honest, learn from, and be open to, each other.

The way you make love may change from one episode to another because the act of sexual intercourse should reflect the mood and feelings of the moment, rather than following a pre-conceived pattern. Passionate lovemaking may feel exhilarating on one occasion, yet on another, a vulnerable and tender approach will suit your needs better.

Well tried and tested formulas of lovemaking may need to be jettisoned if new lovers are to remain spontaneous with each other. What worked well in a past liaison may simply not be appropriate to a new sexual relationship. Everyone's timing, arousal levels and bodily responses are unique – unravelling those mysteries together is the key to a long and fulfilling relationship.

LEFT | Sometimes in a relationship intimacy and tenderness are more appropriate than passion.

sharing and caring

Sexual intercourse is not just about body positions and movement, or skills and techniques – it involves the heart, mind and emotional being of each person concerned. Love and intimacy, and a sense of comfort, appreciation and sharing, are the main ingredients necessary to ensure that coitus and nurture is going to satisfy both parties.

time to explore

With a new sexual relationship, allow plenty of time for sensuality, exploring your partner's body during foreplay, so that you get to know each other's physical responses. Being in tune with one another leads to compatible lovemaking.

During intercourse, tactile contact should not be confined to the genitals alone. For example, the female partner can use her breasts and hair to caress the man's chest as she sensually sways her body from side to side. Continue touching and kissing the whole body throughout lovemaking.

After making love, you can lie in each other's arms, bathed in a warm glow of contentment, rested, relaxed and nourished by the sexual experience. For some people, these are the happiest moments of all.

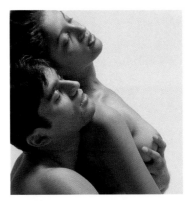

LEFT | Explore different positions to discover what suits both of you.

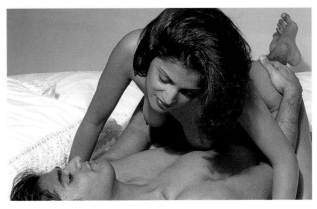

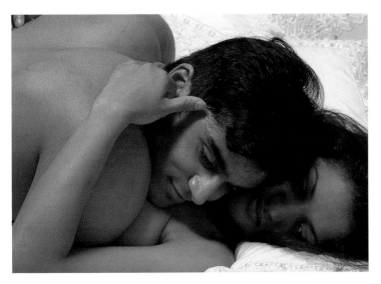

ABOVE | The woman-on-top position allows her to sway from side to side.

LEFT | Lying in each other's arms after making love is an important part of a sexual relationship.

the basic positions

THERE ARE A NUMBER of lovemaking positions in common practice that most couples feel comfortable with. These allow both the man and woman to express themselves sexually in different ways by taking more active or passive roles in the lovemaking, and thereby eliciting a variety of physical and emotional responses. An equal and balanced sexual partnership is capable of sharing the more dominant and submissive roles quite easily, allowing a natural transfer between the two, either within one episode of lovemaking, or on different occasions.

Exploration, experimentation and a sense of humour are important to keep a sexual relationship interesting and alive. Once you feel comfortable and secure with each other, it is worth trying something new to add variety, fun and excitement to your lovemaking.

BELOW | Cuddling up close to each other in bed after a passionate and varied lovemaking session is one of the sensations that most men and women enjoy.

Here, we sum up the basic lovemaking positions, and then on the following pages of this chapter, some of the more popular sexual positions assumed by couples in coitus will be discussed in greater detail. In other sections of this book you will find more adventurous positions that you can add to your lovemaking repertoire, as well as ideas on spontaneous and fun lovemaking.

man on top

The most commonly practised position for lovemaking, also known as the missionary position, is when the man assumes the more active role and moves on top of his partner. This allows face-to-face intimacy and full, front-of-the-body contact. The nature of this position means the man takes the more dominant role, while the female role is more submissive.

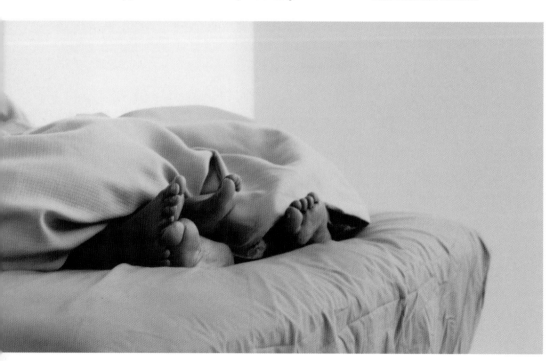

woman on top

The woman-on-top position enables the couple to swap the more active and passive roles and allows them to experience and express other aspects of their sexuality. The woman has more freedom to move and is better able to control the depth of the man's thrusts and the stimulation she may need to reach orgasm.

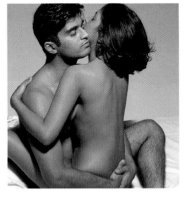

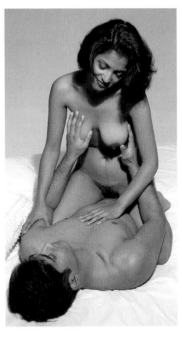

FAR LEFT | From embracing each other in this sitting position you can alter your lovemaking positions so that either partner can go on top.

LEFT | With the woman on top, the man can see and caress her breasts.

BELOW | In the man-on-top position the man has the more active role.

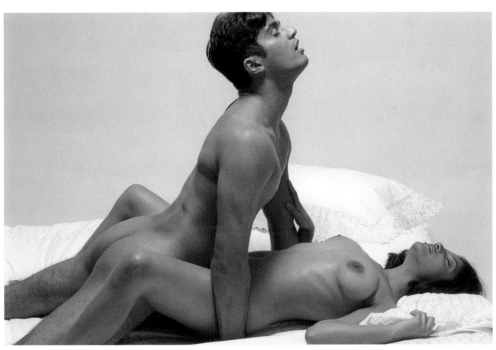

man on top

THIS WAS THE POSITION said to have been promoted by 19th-century missionaries as they travelled the world and discovered other cultures enjoying multi-positional and uninhibited sex. It was decided that the position of man dominant on top of woman was the only acceptable one and so attempts were made to impose it on anyone having sex.

Perhaps because of this history, the position has got rather a bad name. Images of bored women looking at their watches over their partners' shoulders or deciding on a new colour for the bedroom ceiling are all associated with the missionary position. It is also a position that people, particularly women, may resort to because

they are not very confident about their bodies. Their stomachs are flatter lying supine, and because it is a fairly standard position, there are no worries about being shown up for physical inflexibility, having your breasts dangling or worrying about showing a large bottom. Most people try this position for the first few times when having sex with a new partner, and when they feel more confident, move on to more challenging positions.

Having said all this, the missionary position is one of the most intimate; where your bodies converge and meld into each other, where you can kiss, caress and have your skins touching, and where you can have long, lingering sex.

BELOW | The missionary position is a very natural and easy position for sex, so it is a favourite for both a speedy romp and a prolonged session of love for couples of all ages.

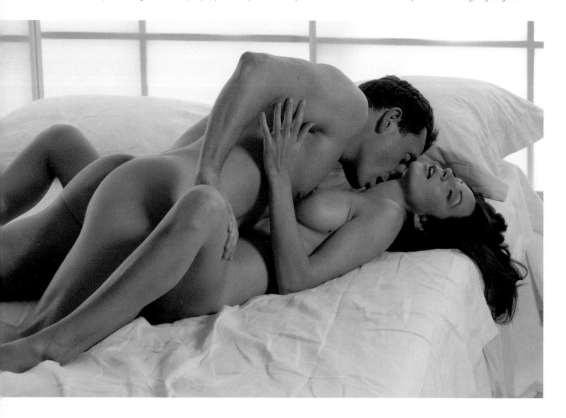

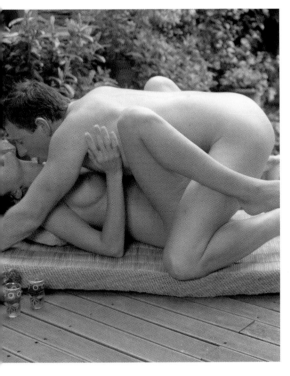
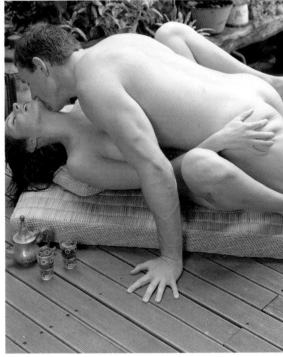

basic man on top

This is the classic man on top position. To begin with, his legs are usually positioned in between the woman's legs, which are both slightly splayed out. The woman can put her hands around her partner's neck and the man, resting on his elbows, can cup his hands around her head.

This is a great position for kissing and caressing each other, nibbling at each other's ears, whispering lovely things and then having long, slow sex. You can place your hands under each other's bottoms and rock to and fro, as this helps with clitoral arousal.

For the woman, once you are aroused, part your legs and let him in. At the same time, caress his testicles and the shaft of his penis before he enters you. Stroke his back and work your way down with your free hands to play with his anus.

For men, you are more able to control the rate of your thrust and, therefore, when you come in this position. Slow entry and almost total withdrawal of your penis will drive her mad: place the tip of the penis just inside the vagina and withdraw it, repeating this slowly or quickly. This creates a wonderful feeling and heightens sexual tension. However, be careful if you are highly aroused, as you may come too soon.

The main problem with this position is that it is not so good for clitoral stimulation, because the penis is often not at the best angle. If the woman arches her back, he can penetrate even deeper.

PLUS POINTS You can watch each other's faces, both as a guide to what excites your partner most and to arouse your own feelings still more.
It is a very versatile position that can be adapted to all kinds of places besides the bed or sofa.

MINUS POINTS A small, light woman can be quite squashed by a heavy partner, even if he takes most of his weight on his hands or elbows.
It is not very comfortable for either partner to make love in this position following a large meal.

ABOVE | Having sex *al fresco* is wonderfully liberating. However, do make sure that you have total privacy to avoid the risk of being overlooked or offending other people.

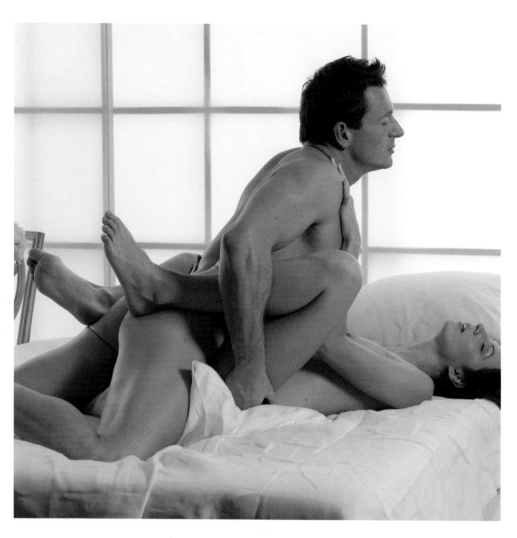

ABOVE | Man on top 1 and 2. Placing a pillow under the woman's bottom or back will increase contact between the clitoris and his pubic bone.

OPPOSITE | Man on top 3. Resting her feet on his shoulders makes penetration very deep. Both partners can still watch each other's faces.

man on top 1

The woman places a pillow under her bottom and bends her legs. The man can then kneel over her, holding her waist while he enters. The pillow helps to increase the contact between the clitoris and the man's pubic bone, so that it can be stimulated as the penis thrusts. Try different angles to get it perfect. This positions allows mostly for shallow penetration and you both need to be quite agile. The man can gently pull his partner's body towards him on each thrust. He can stroke her breasts and stomach and move off easily to stimulate her clitoris with his tongue. Since the woman is stretched right out in front of the man, he will be able to watch his penis thrusting in and out, which is visually very exciting.

PLUS POINTS This is good for a woman because her partner has more access to her breasts and clitoris.

MINUS POINTS This can be very tiring for a man, as he is holding himself and his partner up.

man on top 2

The woman wraps her legs around her partner's waist, with a pillow or two under her back if necessary. Her partner pulls her up so that he is holding her bottom. She can also stroke his back. The woman pulls the man inside her and can control the rhythm of the thrusts. Since this allows deeper penetration, her clitoris is more likely to be stimulated than if she were lying flat. The man enters his partner at a steep angle. If you can both manage it, lean forward for a kiss.

PLUS POINTS Because of the angle of penetration, a man who believes his penis is small will feel like a stud. The woman can stimulate herself at the same time, which both partners find a turn-on.

MINUS POINTS It can be tricky for the woman to get the rhythm right and for the man to let her.

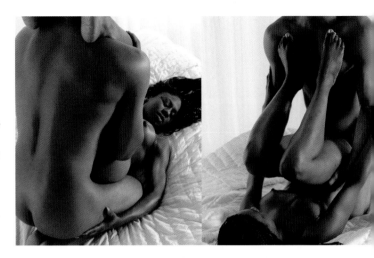

man on top 3

Here the woman pulls her knees up to her chest with one or both feet resting on her partner's shoulders. She can hold the man's hips for support and he can put his hands under her bottom. This is excellent for really deep penetration. If the woman then places her legs to one side, the side walls of her vagina will be massaged. She can also try pressing her hand on her belly to feel her partner's penis as it moves in and out. This is very arousing because you can watch each other's expressions and if the woman reaches down to masturbate herself, he will love watching this too. But some women will find the deepness of the thrusting too painful to tolerate for long.

PLUS POINTS Deep penetration makes this position extremely exciting for both partners – great for relatively quick sex.
He can watch his penis as it slides in and out and can also watch his partner masturbate herself, so it is visually a very stimulating position.

MINUS POINTS All men, but especially those with big penises, must avoid getting too carried away, as very deep thrusts can cause a woman considerable pain.

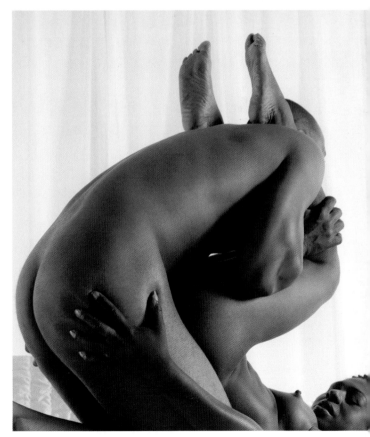

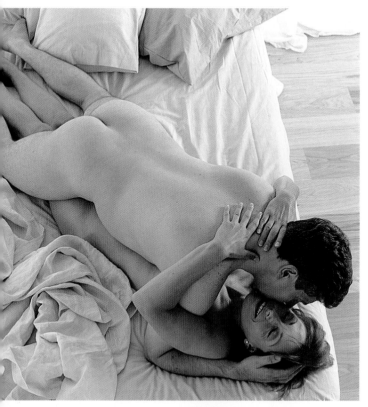

man on top 4

The man places his legs either side of the woman's and she squeezes her legs together, placing her hands around his head or neck.

This is a wonderful position for total body contact and slow sex with lots of kissing and caressing. If the woman keeps her thighs squeezed together after her partner has entered her, her vagina will be tighter and a stronger stimulation to her partner's penis. For the man there is only shallow penetration, so the penis can slip out if he's not careful. But it is also a very arousing and tantalizing position, so he has to be careful not to come too quickly.

PLUS POINTS As some concentration is essential to avoid the penis slipping out, sex is prolonged, slow and gentle, building inexorably to a spectacular climax.

It is ideal for women who worry about a slack vagina after childbirth as squeezing her thighs means that her partner's penis is also gently gripped – something he will find irresistible.

MINUS POINTS The eroticism of this position can be surprising, causing the man to come much more quickly than expected.

A small, light woman can feel crushed by her partner.

ABOVE | Man on top 4. It is precisely because this position is a little more difficult to maintain and the thrusts are shallow that the sensations are so powerful and intense.

RIGHT | Man on top 5. This position allows the woman to caress the head and face of her partner while he has access to her neck and breasts with his mouth.

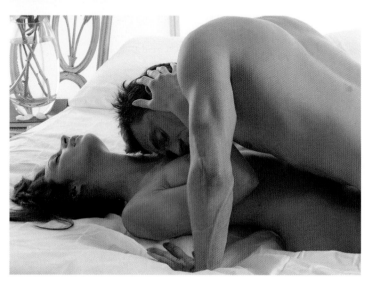

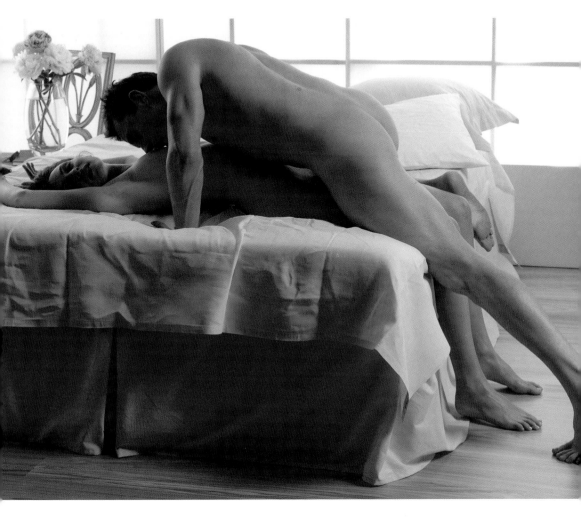

man on top 5

The woman dangles her legs over the edge of the bed, with the backs of her knees on the edge, and throws her arms back over her head. She may need pillows under her bottom on the bed in order to obtain a better angle for penetration. The man lies over her, supporting himself with his arms, with his feet on the floor. (A short man can put a couple of pillows under his feet.) The woman can suck her fingers and then masturbate herself – a great turn-on for both of you. This position is great for the man because he can see everything.

Although too far away to kiss, he can nuzzle and lick her nipples and both partners can watch each other's expressions as they come.

PLUS POINTS Watching his partner's arousal and abandonment to her passion is a turn-on for the man. He will have to be especially imaginative about ways to excite her, as his hands are occupied, taking his weight.

MINUS POINTS As the woman has limited control, she can feel dominated, but if she simply gives in to the moment she will just feel wonderfully indulged.

ABOVE | Man on top 5. With her arms flung over her head the woman can abandon herself totally to the attentions of her lover.

becoming a better male lover

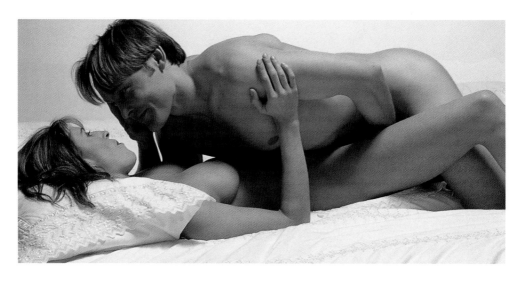

THE ADVANTAGE OF THE MAN-ON-TOP position for a man is that he has more command over his pelvic movements. His penis is at a comfortable angle to enter the woman's vagina, and he has better control over the depth of its thrusts, which enables him to regulate his pace and rhythm so that he is able to gain the maximum stimulation needed to reach orgasm.

A woman who, on other occasions, enjoys exploring and expressing the more active part of her erotic nature may also enjoy relaxing sexually into the more submissive role, and letting her man take charge. While this position obviously suits a man who prefers to be the active sexual partner, he should also be prepared to explore other postures if his partner so desires.

preparing for penetration

When sensual play progresses to intercourse it is a moment of physical and psychological transition for the man and woman. Both need to be ready in body and mind for this deeper level of intimacy and penetration, so it is important to stay in touch with your own and your partner's

responses. Don't rush into penetration if either of you is not quite ready for it. If both are fully aroused by the touches, kisses, words and embraces of foreplay, the woman's vulva will have swelled, and her vagina will be secreting its juices, in readiness to receive the penis; the man's penis will be erect and firm, and able to enter her. Emotionally, both should be open and available to each other, as they enter into coitus. To check that the woman is sufficiently lubricated to accept his penis, the man can stroke his fingers over her vulva and vaginal opening, or simply ask her if she is ready for penetration. She may indicate by words, sounds or touch that she wants him to enter her. He can then guide his penis into her vagina.

slow entry

In this position, the man is between the woman's legs as his penis begins to penetrate her vagina. She lies on her back, and opens her legs wide to give him room to enter her. Slow and careful manoeuvring will ensure the penis remains in the vagina and does not slip out, which can happen if

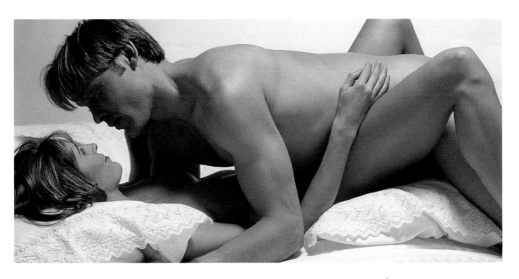

either tries to move too rapidly before both bodies have adjusted their fit to each other. Many women love a slow entry, when the tip of the penis enters and lingers teasingly just within the vaginal orifice. This can give her further time to relax, emotionally and physically, so that her vagina is flooded with the total desire to be filled. She can also reach down to caress his scrotum and the shaft of his penis, which is waiting to enter.

aiding mobility

For a woman, mobility is more difficult when making love in the man-on-top position. She may find it helpful if a pillow is placed beneath her buttocks to tilt her pelvis. This gives her more freedom of hip movement and takes the strain away from her lower back. By placing her feet firmly against the mattress, she can use her leg muscles to add leverage to her pelvic motions, to increase sensation for both of them, and to allow greater clitoral stimulation as it rubs against his pubic bone. The man should support his own weight with his arms and hands, keeping the trunk of his body slightly lifted above her.

ABOVE | The woman can place her hands on her lover's hips to help control his movements.

LEFT | Later the man can support his weight so that his partner has more freedom to move.

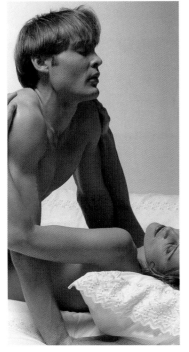

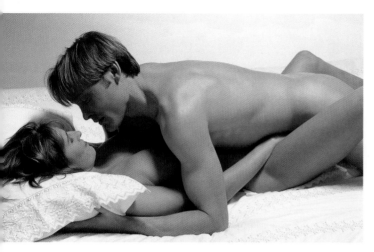

experiment with the woman-on-top positions which may slow the man down and give him greater control over his ejaculation.

intimacy in intercourse

The man should always remain aware of his partner's sexual responses, and ensure that the shared intimacy which inspired the lovemaking is not suddenly abandoned in the heat of arousal. Unfortunately, some men see penetration as a green light to go, and start thrusting away intent on an orgasm regardless of what is happening to their partners. In other scenarios, a man may be conscious of the woman's needs and start performing a series of mechanical manoeuvres aimed at giving her an orgasm so that he can go ahead and achieve his own. Neither type of behaviour is particularly desirable nor likely to please the woman, because intercourse is not a race or a gymnastic show, or a question of pushing the right buttons to gain an end result. It is all about two people meeting and merging, breathing and moving together, feeling and responding, and abandoning themselves equally to the sheer physical and emotional pleasure of the moment.

Fortunately, recent research shows that most sexually active men, while still considering female sexuality to be something of a mystery, believe that their partner's satisfaction is as important as their own. For many men, giving sexual joy to their women is the best part of making love. According to the studies, the majority of men believe that intimacy and affection during lovemaking are very important factors in a woman's sexual happiness.

penetration with care

Full penetration can create feelings of vulnerability as well as physical pleasure. These feelings need to be experienced and there is no need to rush ahead into immediate thrusting. It is important, too, that the man thrusts deeply only when his partner is physically and psychologically ready to receive him, otherwise it may cause her discomfort. Initially, she can place her hands on his hips to help control his pelvic movements until she is ready.

ABOVE | The man can begin thrusting with shallow actions, moving his pelvis slowly and gently back and forth, and allowing more time for attunement. On arousal, the first part of her vagina constricts, enabling it to grip the penis securely, adding to the pleasurable sensations of friction. However, if the man is in a state of high arousal, he needs to be careful not to overstimulate the erotically sensitive tip of his penis if he is prone to ejaculating too quickly.

making it comfortable

For the woman, the main disadvantages of the man-on-top position are the restrictions to her own pelvic movements and, unless her partner is particularly aware of his actions, the inadequacy of the clitoral stimulation – an important factor if she wishes to be aroused to orgasm.

Other situations can make this position an unsuitable choice. If a woman is suffering from a back condition, she may find that making love in this position will add to the strain. If her partner is much heavier than her, she may feel confined and burdened by the size difference.

A pregnant woman can feel anxious and uncomfortable about having any weight bearing down on her abdomen especially in the last trimester of the pregancy. Her breasts may feel particularly sensitive to pressure and, in the later stages of her pregnancy, this position may simply be impossible. In all of these cases, if the man is on top of his partner, he should take care not to put all his weight on her.

The man-on-top position puts the onus on the man to perform, and this may not suit him if he is tired or under stress. While he may desire physical intimacy with his partner, at a time like this it is usually preferable if the woman takes the more active role. Also, if the man is prone to premature ejaculation, the couple would do well to

sex with sensitivity

It is important to stay in touch on an emotional
level throughout intercourse. Slow down once in
a while, and look deeply into each other's eyes.
By allowing the intimacy you feel to be expressed,
silently or with words, your lovemaking will
become deeply satisfying.

Women need and prefer to feel emotionally
nourished as well as physically aroused during
the sexual act. Men can benefit too if they try to
get in touch with the side of their softer and more
vulnerable feelings.

focusing inwards

Some lovers like to keep their eyes open during
lovemaking, while others prefer to keep their eyes
closed. It is entirely optional. If your eyes are open,
you can take great pleasure in looking at your
partner's body and watching his or her arousal
and responses. Closing your eyes while making
love takes you into a different dimension of
sensual feeling because you are able to focus on
and enjoy the exquisite bodily sensations arising
within you.

To savour both experiences, switch from one
to the other, so that sometimes you have a total
awareness of your partner, and at other times you
have complete awareness of yourself.

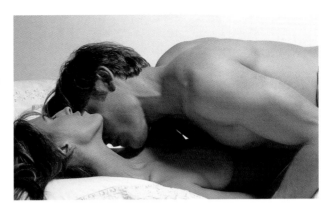

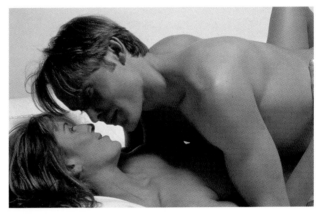

ABOVE AND LEFT | Alternate
between closing your eyes
and gazing into each
other's eyes.

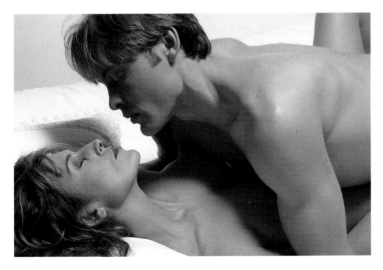

varying the movements

When lovers are sexually compatible, their rhythm and movement seem to flow from one beat to another without orchestrated effort. This harmony arises when a couple have allowed sufficient time in foreplay for full sexual arousal, or because they are familiar and comfortable with each other's bodies and share a deep sense of mutual trust.

To experience a whole range of pleasurable sexual sensations when the man is on top, it is important to change the position and angle of your bodies occasionally, and to vary your pelvic movements. The man should take care not to thrust his penis in and out of the vagina with a monotonous regularity of rhythm and motion. This can make the whole experience very unsatisfying for his partner, not only because she may be unable to receive the clitoral stimulation she needs, but also because the sex act itself can

begin to seem automatic and boring. When this happens, and unfortunately it sometimes occurs in even the best sexual partnerships, the woman may start thinking about something else altogether. She may mentally vacate her body, beginning to wish the whole episode was over.

Pelvic motions can be wild, passionate and thrusting, or they may be deliciously subtle, depending on the intensity of sexual energy at any given moment of lovemaking. The man obviously has more freedom of movement in this position, but both partners should try to reach a synchronicity and fluidity in their motions to avoid the "bump and grind" effect. You can try moving your hips from side to side to create a sexy wiggle, or circulate both pelvises simultaneously to produce some highly erotic sensations and to add a touch of variety to the more usual back-and-forth rocking motion.

If your movements do fall out of rhythm, don't hesitate to tell your partner you need to slow down for a while. Relax and breathe together and make eye contact so you regain harmony. You can remain like this for quite a long period of time, just moving your hips enough to ensure the penis receives sufficient stimulation to remain erect inside the vagina. Let the sexual feelings rise again, and focus on these inner sensations, letting them move you gradually into a new and easy flow of movement.

Enjoy the range of depth to which the penis can penetrate the vagina. Play teasingly between shallower and deeper thrusts. Shallow penetration can be very exciting to both sexes because it produces friction on the tip of the penis and stimulates the outer reaches of the vagina, both regions that are richly served with erotically charged nerve endings.

Deep penetration produces more powerful emotional responses, creating a profound sense of fulfilment and connection between the partners. So do add spice and vitality to your love life by enjoying and experimenting with varying thrusts, positions, pressures and angles to create maximum pleasure for you both. Let sex be adventurous and fun.

RIGHT | Angles of thrusting should be changed throughout intercourse to produce a variety of sensations, and to stimulate different areas of the vagina. The man can use his hand to lift and tilt the woman's pelvis in one direction, so that his penis strokes along the side of her vaginal wall.

RIGHT | Deep penetration can be achieved from a position in which the woman arches her back slightly so that her vagina is raised and open. The man can help by lifting and supporting her pelvis, while pulling her slightly towards him.

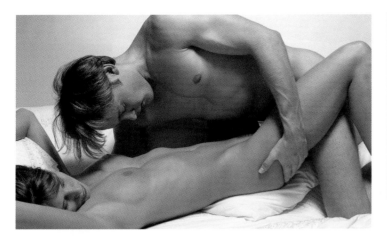

LEFT | Watching the motions of the penis thrusting in and out of the woman's vagina can be highly erotic for both partners. By lifting his body a little way from hers, they are able to enjoy this visual stimulation. To make it more arousing, vary the speed and depth of the penile thrusts. For the man, having the woman watch his actions can make him feel very potent.

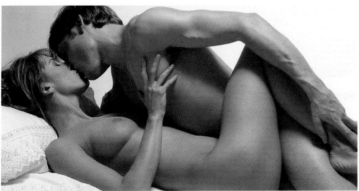

LEFT | In this position, the man shifts his weight to one side, using one arm for support, and inserts his penis into the vagina from a slight sideways angle. This allows the woman to use more of her body and she can caress his thigh with her leg and foot, while he, in turn, strokes them. Men also enjoy being touched and stroked during intercourse.

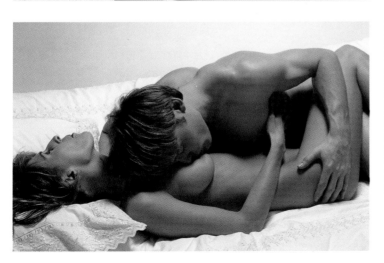

LEFT | Whole body sensuality should not finish just because intercourse has begun. This is important to a woman because every part of her body is sensitive to erotic stimulation, not just her genitals. While making love, the man should continue to kiss, lick and caress her body and not just concentrate on thrusting movements.

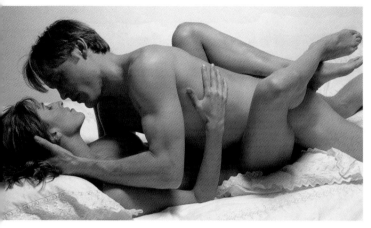

the woman's satisfaction

Even though the woman assumes a more passive role in lovemaking when her partner takes the on-top position, it is important that she receives the right kind of stimulation to achieve sexual satisfaction. What constitutes satisfaction will be different for each woman. For many it will mean being able to reach their full orgasmic potential, while for some it may be the need to feel as involved as their partners. Others would say that emotional and physical intimacy is the most important aspect of lovemaking, whether or not they reach orgasm.

Sexual performance is as much subject to mood and change as any other function in life. It

ABOVE | The woman can use her legs to pull the man closer and increase friction on her clitoris.

RIGHT | The side and rear entry position is particularly exciting for the woman.

BELOW | Running her fingers up and down her lover's spine will increase his pleasure as they lie close together.

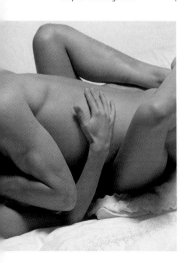

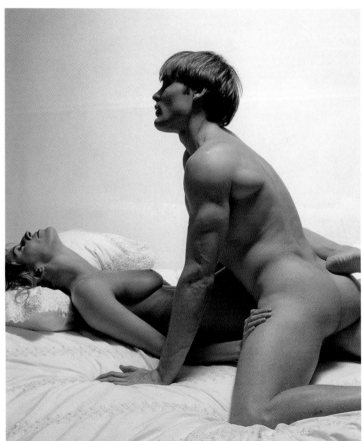

can be ecstatic, passionate and mutually orgasmic, or it may be comfortable and cosy – more like a cuddle. Most couples do take a realistic view of their sex lives, and do not expect to "feel the earth move" on every occasion. However, when a man is in the more dominant on-top position, he needs to exercise a certain amount of conscious control over his movements and arousal level. He may need to slow down from time to time, so the duration of lovemaking and the involvement of his partner provide fulfilment for them both.

How long it should last is a matter for the couple concerned, but the answer will probably lie in whether each person feels sexually and emotionally fulfilled during and after a session of lovemaking.

side and rear entry

This is an exciting lovemaking position, and one which adds to the woman's pleasure because of the pressure of his body against the back of her thigh and vulva. The man enters his partner partly from the side and partly from the rear of her body, so that her leg is drawn up and wrapped around his waist. He will need to support his weight with both hands.

pulling in tighter

While beneath her man, a woman may want to become more involved in the action. One way is for her to wrap her legs around the man's back, pulling him close in to her. This will bring their genitals in close contact, creating a pleasurable friction on the clitoris, especially when the pelvic motions are circular or rocking from side to side. It is not a position that can be prolonged, however, as the man's movements are somewhat restricted, and it may also become tiring for the woman.

pulling him close

Kissing and fondling should continue, no matter how intense the genital contact has become. The woman can stroke and caress her lover's back, running her fingers up and down his spine. She in her turn will enjoy the close embrace, touching, and kissing of her neck and face. This position,

where the man is pulled in close to the woman's body, is particularly helpful if the man's penis is short and unable to penetrate the vagina too deeply.

position for full penetration

With the woman's legs resting on the man's shoulders, the penis can penetrate the vagina deeply. This can be an exciting variation to add to lovemaking positions, but it is a vulnerable one for the female partner and not all women feel at ease with it. The action is almost all with the man and while this sense of helplessness can add its own dimension of excitement for the woman, she may not want to spend too long like this.

BELOW | Resting the woman's legs on top of the man's shoulders allows deeper penetration.

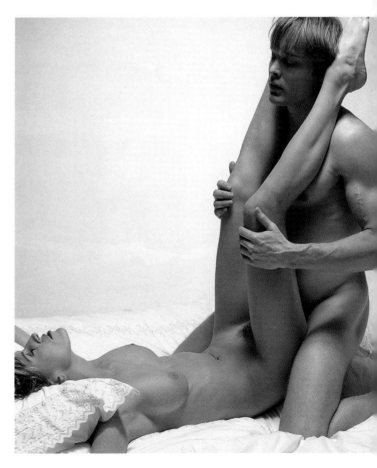

what turns men on?

Simon, 57, a teacher, divorced, father of three: What turns you on most about a woman? "The eyes and the voice." What do you enjoy most about lovemaking? "The sense of merging with another person." When do you experience your most powerful orgasms? "When I'm not too tired. It depends on how close and secure I feel with my partner."

Dean, aged 23, a student, single: What turns you on most about a woman? "Beauty and a feeling of warmth between me and the woman I'm attracted to." What do you enjoy most about lovemaking? "The closeness." When do you experience your most powerful orgasms? "When I'm in love. If it's a one-night stand it's more like a release."

Terry, 42, a postal worker, divorced. What turns you on the most about a woman? "The eyes, the smell, the breasts, her femininity." What do you enjoy most about lovemaking? "The closeness; the bonding, expressing our love." When do you experience your most powerful orgasms? "In a good relationship, sex is just more intense; or if I haven't had sex for a while. It's also a special mood, all openness, it is not something that can be planned."

Paul, 30, a decorator, with girlfriend: What turns you on most about a woman? "Everything, and all kinds of women!" What do you enjoy most about lovemaking? "The intimacy, the closeness, giving and receiving pleasure." When do you experience your most powerful orgasms? "With my current girlfriend."

What is more important is that both people continue to explore their potential for pleasure, allowing themselves to be more spontaneous yet constantly sensitive to each other's feelings, sensations and responses.

While the man remains on top of the women, he should ensure that she is able to adjust her pelvic movements to increase her sensual pleasure and that both her clitoris and vagina are receiving stimulation. This can be achieved by allowing continuing contact between his pubic bone and her clitoris, or he can add gentle pressure to her vulva with his hand, or stroke her clitoris sensitively with his fingers.

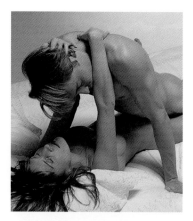

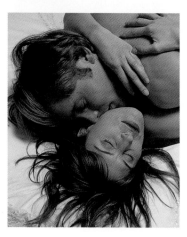

ABOVE RIGHT | Although this position does not allow the woman much pelvic movement, she can reach out to hold him tightly around the neck and shoulders and draw him closer to her. Some women like to scratch their partner's back as they become excited – he will enjoy this too, if it is not too rough.

RIGHT | While the man is in the more active position when he is on top of his partner, she can exert her power too by enfolding him in her arms so that he surrenders to her embrace.

increasing a woman's pleasure

Unlike in past decades, few women today would put up with a sexual encounter that only lasted a few minutes or was very unsatisfactory. On the other hand, anxiety about performance can lead some men to become too controlled, and that can also cause discomfort if the thrusting becomes prolonged and mechanical and out of tune with a woman's wishes.

Greater sexual awareness and openness have changed some basic patterns of male sexual behaviour. Only three decades ago, the famous American sex researcher Alfred Kinsey stated that, according to his studies, the majority of men interviewed considered it perfectly normal to ejaculate within the first two minutes of intercourse. Nowadays, most men are much better informed about a woman's sexual responses and her orgasmic capacity.

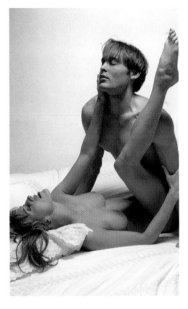

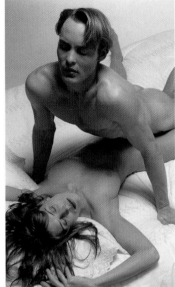

FAR LEFT | Lifting one leg only can be a more comfortable variation.

LEFT | If the woman's legs are straight and spread out wide, then her clitoris is in a good position to receive strong stimulation from the man's thrusting movements. He will need to support his own weight with his arms as he rocks his pelvis back and forth. A teasing side-to-side motion will rub and stimulate her whole vulva for even greater arousal.

lifting one leg

A more comfortable variation of the legs-raised position is for the man to lift one of his partner's legs over his shoulder. He is then able to thrust and move his body more easily, while also increasing the pressure on her thigh and vulva. However, the woman needs to be supple enough to stay relaxed and should be fully aroused as deep penetration is possible.

squeezing thighs

Here the woman's legs are positioned tightly between the man's as he squeezes her thighs with his. Although she has very little movement in this position, the extra pressure on her vulva is very arousing, while his penis fits tightly into her vagina. She can wiggle her hips around a little or contract her pelvic floor muscles for extra sensations.

BELOW | Here the man squeezes her thighs to increase the pressure.

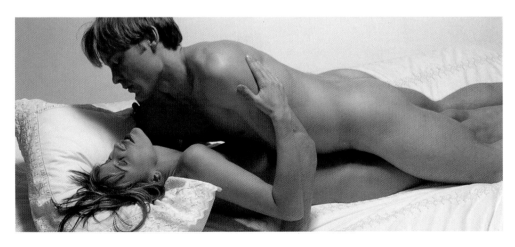

over the edge

Sooner or later, if the lovemaking is sufficiently abandoned, the couple will work their way all around the bed. It usually takes some time before two people become so attuned to each other's bodily responses that these movements are compatible and graceful, and do not cause them to interrupt the flow of their intercourse. Winding and unwinding the limbs, rolling over, changing the postures, swapping active and passive positions, all require skilful and nimble movements if they are to be executed with ease and fluidity. However, once a couple are comfortable with each other, they can let themselves go into passionate activity which can take them from one side of the bed to the other, and even over the edge.

locked in congress

Here, the woman is below the man, with her head just slightly hanging off the edge of the mattress.

She can hold the man very tightly to her body while she wraps her feet around his buttocks and thighs and locks him into her. This will inhibit his movement a little but the pressure of her feet will add extra pleasurable sensations, and they can just writhe, wriggle and rotate their hips for a while to create a whole variety of different stimulating motions.

exhilarating sex

The man or woman can end up in a position in which the head is completely off the mattress and is resting against the floor. This can cause an exhilarating rush of blood to the head, but should not be maintained for too long or the pressure can build up too strongly, especially if the person is approaching an orgasm. There is something very liberating, though, about being so abandoned in your lovemaking that you almost topple out of bed.

BELOW | The whole bed can become a sexual playground, even extending over the edge.

BELOW RIGHT | Exerting pressure on the man's buttocks will give him extra pleasure.

OPPOSITE | Whichever variation you choose, the man-on-top position gives plenty of opportunities for both of you to stimulate each other to achieve orgasm.

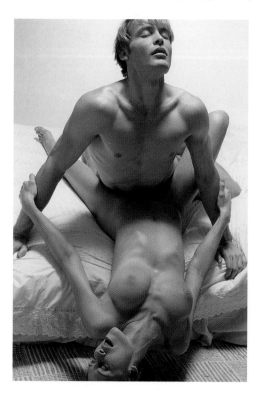

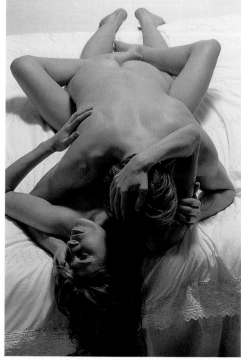

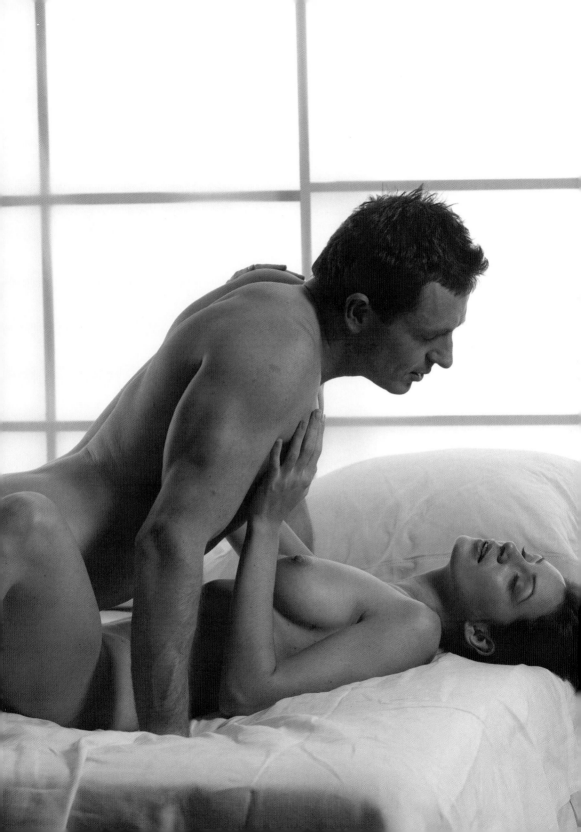

woman on top

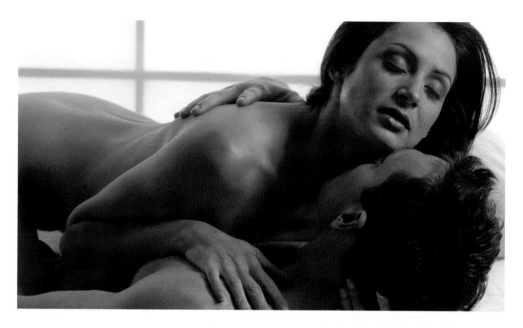

ABOVE | Being on top is an empowering position for women, which can be a real turn-on for him, especially if he is used to being the more dominant partner.

FAR RIGHT TOP | Woman on top 1. This position enables the woman to move freely, so stimulating whatever parts of her own body she likes at whatever pace best suits her, while simultaneously driving her partner into a frenzy of sheer sexual ecstasy.

THIS IS WHERE THE WOMAN dominates, and some of the most erotic positions are played out here. In these positions, the woman can regulate the depth of penetration of her partner's penis and decide on the rhythm of sex, and thus the stimulation needed to reach orgasm. The man can watch his penis thrusting in and out and admire his partner's breasts or bottom. For those men who tend to come quickly, your partner can slow the pace down and help you to control your orgasm.

basic woman on top

The woman climbs on to the man, facing him, with her legs pulled up slightly, so she has freedom of movement. Once he is aroused – and he probably will be already – she places his penis inside her before lying down on his chest. The man can caress his partner's bottom and help with the thrusting by pulling her up and down on to his penis. In this position there is plenty of intimate skin-on-skin contact.

PLUS POINTS There is no pressure for the man to "perform" and he can enjoy feeling especially loved. She has control of her own arousal, as well as his.

MINUS POINTS Some men dislike not being in control, although usually they can be persuaded.

woman on top 1

The woman straddles the man, facing him, but remains upright. Both partners have their hands free and can make good use of them. The woman can massage his chest, bend over to lick his nipples and upper body, rock back and forth, and go round and round with her hips. If she contracts her vaginal muscles around his penis, he will be in heaven as well. She can pause at the top of the penis as he comes out and touch the end of his member at the entrance to the vagina. She can touch her clitoris at the same time, if she can balance and her legs are strong enough. She can also lean back and grab his ankles for stability.

The man can caress his partner's breasts and body as she rises up and down. He can grab her around her hips and buttocks to help with the rhythm. And just watch her as she begins to come.

PLUS POINTS This position is both highly tactile and visually stimulating.
Penetration is very deep, so it is great for most men and for those women who particularly like that.
It's a fabulous way for a woman to indulge all her basic instincts and demonstrate her feelings for her lover.

MINUS POINTS It is quite a strain on the woman's thigh muscles and sense of balance.
Inhibited women or those who are sensitive about their bodies will probably not enjoy this position.

woman on top 2

In this position, the woman squats on top of her partner, facing him, and the man keeps his legs stretched out so that she doesn't fall off. The woman then guides his penis inside her. The man helps the thrusting movement, although he will not be able to do too much, by placing his hands under her bottom. It is up to the woman to set the pace and rhythm. This is a good position for deep penetration. However, the woman has complete control over the depth, so she can vary it as much as she likes.

To enhance the experience, the woman can pause at the top for a few seconds to give her man a tantalizing sense of anticipation. She can also pull both legs apart so that her partner can see his penis going in and out. He can fondle her breasts, caress her body and watch everything that is going on.

There are numerous variations for this position: she can pivot around slowly, kneel and sit on his groin with her legs crossed. Men must be careful, as it is more difficult for them to control their orgasm in this position. Maintaining a stiff erection is essential for maximum effect, as a floppy penis will slide out easily.

PLUS POINTS This is a very versatile position, so it is a good one for imaginative and creative lovers.

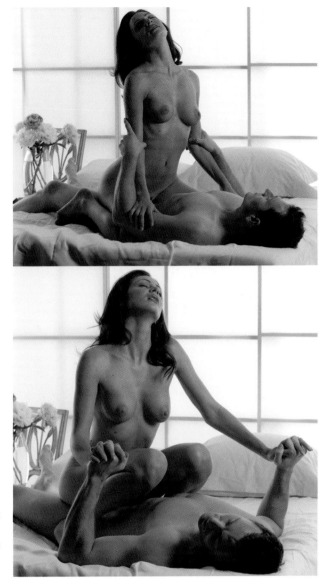

The woman is completely in control of all aspects of lovemaking – this is satisfying for her and hugely exciting for him.

MINUS POINTS She needs to be fit, as this position is quite tiring. It is also a strain on her knees.

ABOVE | Woman on top 2. When she is squatting on top, the man can support some of her weight by holding her hands, which will enable her to move more freely.

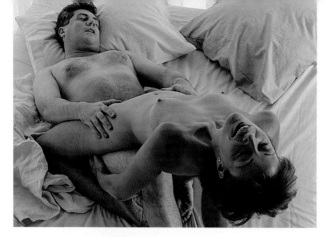

PLUS POINTS He can see his penis as it moves in and out and this is a real turn-on.

By leaning back and tensing her muscles, she is in a great position for his penis to stimulate her G spot.

MINUS POINTS She is unable to clearly watch her partner's arousal or see his face as he comes without changing her position to upright.

woman on top 4

The woman sits on top of the man, facing his feet with her bottom directly in line with his eyes, something most men relish. She can lean either forwards or slightly back. As well as watching her bottom bouncing up and down, the man can watch his penis thrusting in and out. For most men, this more than makes up for the fact that they can't see their partner's face and some women love to show off this normally concealed, even ignored part of their body.

If the woman leans back, she can stimulate her clitoris with one hand while resting on the other. However, she must take care to avoid hurting her partner's penis by sitting down roughly

spice of life

The last thing sex should be is a series of mechanical steps that follow instructions – even from this book. Just because you start your lovemaking in one position doesn't mean that you have to stay there until you both come. You can move and change position entirely, from woman on top to man on top, for example, as the mood takes you. You might like to start in a gentle, relaxed way, such as woman on top 3, and then, as feelings intensify, switch to a position where deeper penetration is easier. Equally, you might choose to change from woman on top 4 to a position where there is more skin contact and you can see each other's faces. Follow your instincts and have fun, but keep your partner in the loop by telling them which position's next.

TOP | Woman on top 3. Lovely if you are in the mood for some slow rhythms.

ABOVE | Woman on top 4. Some women love having their hair gently pulled or teased during sex.

woman on top 3

The man lies on the bed and pulls his knees up and the woman sits on top, with her legs bent and feet flat on the bed, or out behind her, facing him. Once she has guided his penis inside her, she can then lean back to support herself on his knees. This is quite hard work for both people and it may take some time to get a rhythm going.

on top of it or bending it the wrong way. If she sits up slightly, he can contribute to the thrusting with his hips and she can be still. If she leans forwards, then the man can massage her back and buttocks and, if she likes it, place his finger around or into her anus. (Remember to have the lubrication handy before you begin.) There are many erotic nerves in this area which will enhance the feeling of intensity in her vagina.

In return, the woman can fondle his testicles, or, if she is very supple, bend right over and lick them. She will need to lean forward to obtain the right angle, but again, should be careful with the angle of the man's penis, as it is bending away from the body so it could cause discomfort.

PLUS POINTS Men usually find this different viewpoint of their partner during sex very exciting.
The woman can adapt her position to stimulate different parts of her own and her partner's body, constantly changing levels of arousal and pleasure.

MINUS POINTS Some women dislike not being able to see their partner's face.
This position can be inhibiting for a woman as she will be taking care not to injure her partner as she moves.

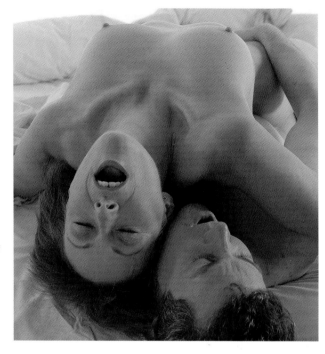

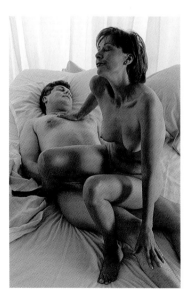

woman on top 5

Here the woman mounts the man's erect penis, facing him. She then pivots around, with his penis still inside her, until she is lying back on his chest. Her partner can then hold her by her bottom or hips to pull her back and forth. Pivoting can be tricky, as the penis can easily slip out, but once it is accomplished, this is a great position. The man can play with his partner's breasts in between thrusts and she can stimulate herself throughout.

PLUS POINTS This has great novelty value, as it is quite different from the usual woman-on-top positions.
There is lots of skin contact and the man can caress his partner's breasts and both can stimulate her clitoris.
With a little imagination, there are plenty of opportunities for exciting variations of this position.

MINUS POINTS The angle can make it difficult for the man to keep his penis in place.
Even a small woman can feel quite heavy in this position and some men find its restrictions a little suffocating.

ABOVE | Woman on top 5. This position would be perfect for couples who have a mirrored ceiling as they can watch themselves in action.

LEFT | Woman on top 5. Pivoting can be hard work, so the woman can pause on her way round. In a "side saddle" type position, the man can stimulate her breasts and either he or she can give clitoral stimulation.

becoming a better female lover

THE BEDROOM, OF ALL PLACES, should never be a battleground for power. So the question of who takes the dominant and submissive positions, or the active and passive sexual roles, should be a matter for lovers to decide after they have conducted a shared and joyful exploration into what feels natural, pleasurable, satisfying and sexually creative to them both. These days, most couples like to swap sexual positions and roles because it allows them to experience all the nuances of their sexual nature, which will have both feminine and masculine qualities, regardless of gender. This is how it should be because men and women today are breaking away from gender conditioning in every other aspect of their lives too.

Men do not always want to be "macho", and sometimes need to express the more sensitive side of their nature, while women are no longer content to be typecast purely in the "gentler sex" role. Since our sexuality is a profound expression of who we are, there should be enough scope within any sexual relationship for it to reflect the whole diversity of our inner selves.

Over the last three decades, women have enjoyed more sexual freedom than ever before. This may partly be due to the availability of efficient contraception, which has reduced their anxieties about unwanted pregnancy, and liberated them from the constraints of their biology to enjoy sex for reasons of pure intimacy and pleasure. In addition, women now know that

BELOW | It can be a relief to a man to be able to surrender himself into the more passive role, and totally relax while he receives her tender and nourishing caresses. She can kiss him gently all over his face, and tenderly stroke his head, while rotating her pelvis to maintain genital stimulation at the same time so that his whole body begins to melt into hers.

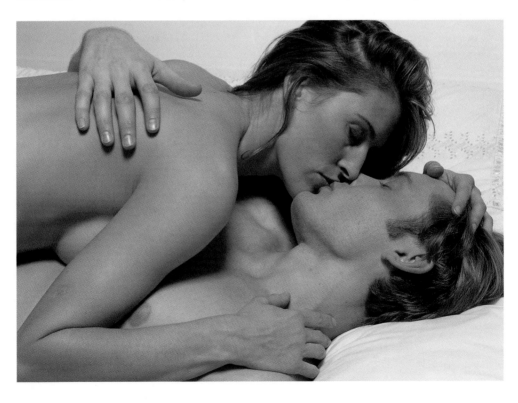

they have an equal, if not greater orgasmic capacity than their male partners. Gone are the days when a sexually ecstatic woman was considered to be an aberration of her sex.

Women want and expect to have a satisfying sex life, and to take charge of their bodies in order to do so. While it is largely true that for a woman the emotional, sensual and nurturing aspects of a relationship remain integral to her sexual happiness, she may also desire to reach the heights of physical pleasure during lovemaking for which her body is uniquely designed.

greater freedom and control

A woman is able to express her innate sensuality and eroticism to a greater degree in the woman-on-top sexual positions than when the man takes the active role. Most of the positions illustrated in this section not only allow a woman greater freedom of movement and to enjoy the pleasure

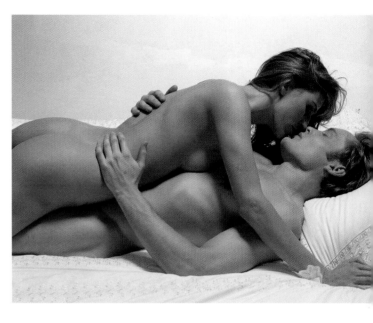

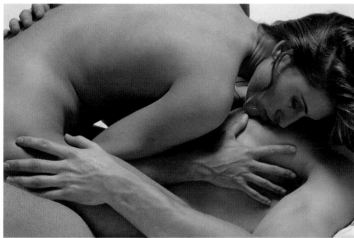

of taking her lover's penis inside her vagina, but also the choice of movements whereby her vulva and clitoris receive adequate friction too. Deep penetration is possible with many of these positions, particularly when she is squatting over her man, yet at the same time, she is better able to control the depth according to what feels comfortable.

For the man, having a partner on top and in charge of the movements can come as a great relief, especially if he is fatigued or would like some respite from the role of main performer. Not only is it erotically and visually arousing for him to watch his woman express her sexuality so powerfully, he can enjoy relaxing into the more passive side of his own sexual nature.

ABOVE | When the woman is making love to her partner from the on-top position, she can lean towards him for full sensual skin-to-skin contact, lowering her body to cover his. She can kiss and stroke him, while at the same time moving her pelvis from side to side or back and forth to rub her vulva against his pubic bone. If his thighs are between her legs, she can squeeze them gently between her own to create an extra teasing pressure.

LEFT | Many women enjoy the possibility of extending sensual play into lovemaking, and this position allows them to continue giving erotic stimulation to different parts of the man's body.

Couples can use the woman-on-top position for the whole duration of a lovemaking episode, or incorporate it into any number of other exciting sexual manoeuvres. A change of positions should be made gracefully, slowing down the pace of action if necessary so that both partners can adjust their limbs and posture to become comfortable. When the rhythm and motion of lovemaking is harmonious and fluid, a couple can constantly change positions without interrupting their intercourse. Sometimes, however, it may be necessary for the man to withdraw his penis from the vagina for some moments in order to avoid clumsy movements.

The woman-on-top position requires some caution from the woman as she lowers herself on to her lover's penis. Sudden, abrupt or speedy movements from her before he has found a comfortable fit can injure him by bending his penis at an acute angle. She needs to remain aware of his comfort too if she is abandoning herself to uninhibited movement.

clitoral stimulation

Many women complain that men either ignore the clitoris, concentrating too much on vaginal thrusting, or they zone in too much on the clitoris, to the exclusion of the rest of the body. This looks like a no-win situation for the man. Happily, there is a way he can give her the clitoral stimulation she needs, and without her feeling she is being tuned up like a car before a motor race.

It is important for the woman to continue receiving clitoral stimulation throughout intercourse and during orgasm. This can be achieved by positions, which either partner can take, that give the woman freedom of movement and allow her vulva to press against the man's pubic bone. During penetrative sex, the man or the woman can also press on, or sensually stimulate, her clitoris manually. Stroking of the vaginal lips and over the mons pubis will also stimulate the clitoris, and may be more arousing and enjoyable than pressure placed directly on to it. Remember, though, that the clitoris is a delicate organ with a high density of sensitive nerves, so frantic rubbing or excessive pressure can be irritating and even painful.

While a woman may desire and need clitoral stimulation to reach the peak of sexual arousal, she may not want to receive it to the exclusion of loving, tender touches and kisses bestowed on the rest of her body. This also applies to her breasts, which when stroked, kissed and licked during intercourse can take her into sexual bliss, yet she does not want them to be the sole centre of attention while the rest of her is ignored. Every part of a woman's body is erogenous, and she can be greatly turned on by the emotional depth of the lovemaking too.

BELOW | While the woman is moving up and down on the man's penis, she is able to control the depth of its penetration into her vagina. If he lifts up to lick, kiss or suck her nipples, he can take her to the edge of orgasmic ecstasy.

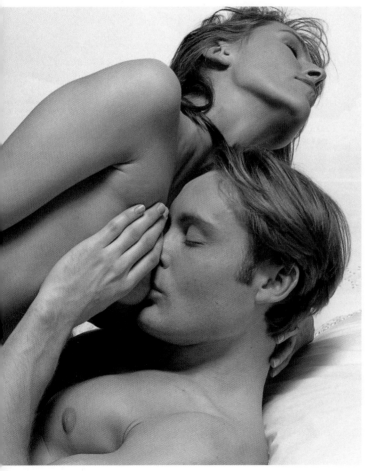

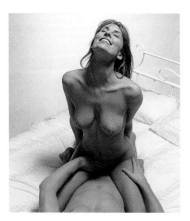

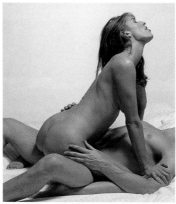

FAR LEFT | As the man lies back in this position, he can use his hands to stroke and caress his partner's whole body. He can also increase her arousal by stroking her vulva or rubbing her clitoris.

LEFT | Intense genital stimulation can be achieved once the woman lifts her body away from her partner and begins to gyrate her pelvis in varying motions to gain maximum vaginal and clitoral stimulation. While the contact between the lovers' bodies becomes less intimate, the arousal grows stronger.

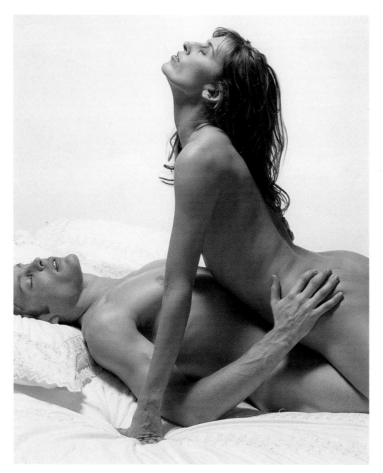

LEFT | To keep a sustained and arousing pressure on her clitoris, the woman can raise her back and push her vulva towards the man's pelvic bone, leaning into it without motion for several moments. She can heighten her pleasure by tightening her buttocks and thigh muscles, thereby constricting her vaginal muscles.

RIGHT | If she is supple
enough the woman can lean
right back. She is now in a
perfect position for her lover
to caress her belly and thighs,
before stroking and rubbing
her clitoris and labia.

ecstatic moments

Most women would probably say that they want
all the tender, erotic touching and caressing of
sensual play to continue after penetration, plus
the right amount of clitoral stimulation – and they
want their lovemaking to be exciting, yet relaxed
and spontaneous too.

They do not want to feel that they are
being programmed for an orgasm by excessive
mechanical stimulation, or that their total
sensuality is being neglected.

When a woman feels confident enough to
take the more active sexual role, she can really let
go into her orgasmic sexual energy. Suddenly her
whole body is free, and she can move, turn and
sway so that the waves of pleasure can rush
through every part of her. If she has a partner who
relishes in her ecstatic expression, the experience
can be intensely erotic for them both. If she is truly
uninhibited, she may even shout and scream,
moan, or even cry and laugh in turns, and all of

this can be very exciting to a man who is not
afraid to see powerful female sexual energy
unleashed. Or she may want to move in a very
soft and sensual way, stroking and kissing her
man, teasing him with playful and arousing
movements, and touching his heart deeply with
her gentle and nurturing femininity.

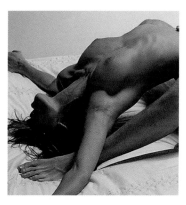

BELOW | Lowering herself back
gently, the woman can arch
her body as she leans against
her partner's raised thighs.
With the pressure of his penis
against the front wall of her
vagina, she can rock back and
forth with tiny movements.

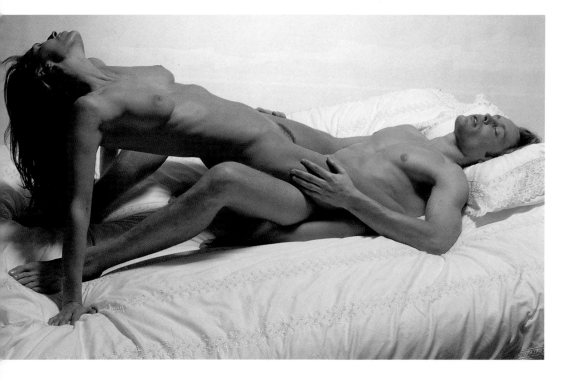

taking charge

One of the advantages for the woman when she assumes the on-top position is that she can take control of the movements to satisfy her needs in all the previously mentioned ways. Also, when a man is in the passive role, he is likely to be more attentive to her whole body, reaching out to touch and caress her because he is able to relinquish the tension of being the main performer. Yet at the same time, a woman needs to carry the same awareness that she expects from her man when he is the dominant sexual partner. Just like a woman, a man does not want to feel that his body is being used purely for sexual gratification, as if it is somehow separate from his whole person.

If both want to enjoy a prolonged session of lovemaking, she needs to be in tune with his sexual responses, so that the stimulation he is receiving does not propel him too quickly to his orgasm threshold. For a man, there is a certain point of no return, when he no longer has control over the process of ejaculation. The woman should remain alert to his signals, slowing down the pace of her movements, or even staying still, until the excitement level has subsided sufficiently to allow sexual activity to continue.

However, men who are prone to premature or early ejaculation can benefit from having their partner take the top position since it is likely to create less intense stimulation to the penis and can slow down the ejaculatory process.

sensate exercise

As the woman rides her man, she can begin to move slowly up and down on his penis, lowering herself so it penetrates deep into her vagina, and then raising herself so she is barely containing its tip. Closing her eyes, she should then try to merge herself entirely into each sensation, letting herself imagine what each subtle change of depth and movement must feel like for her partner. She can also ask him to describe those feelings to her. Gradually, those sensations will transfer themselves into her sexual consciousness.

If the woman becomes extremely sensitive to her man, she may actually begin to feel what he is experiencing, as if the sensations his penis are receiving are also occurring within her own body. It is an experiment certainly worth trying, for it can lead to a deepening of mutual sexual joy and understanding.

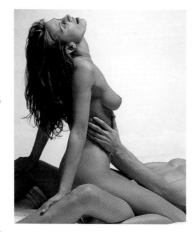

LEFT | The woman can brace her back, clasping the man's legs behind her and then breathe deeply. In this position, the penis will be exerting its pressure on to the front wall of her vagina to add increased stimulation to her G spot.

BELOW | Between the waves of high-energy activity and rapturous movement, it is always wonderful to rest awhile in a position that brings you both back to a sense of merging and melting with each other.

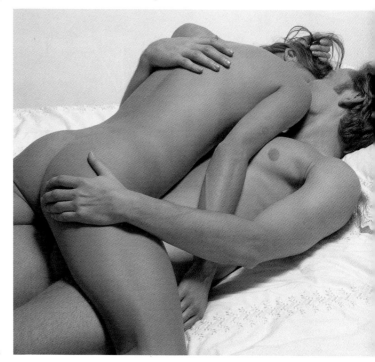

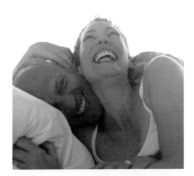

what turns women on?

Vanessa, 27, graphic artist, single. What turns you on most about a man? "His humour, his eyes, his sensuality." What do you enjoy most about lovemaking? "The tenderness and intimacy, lots of cuddling and kissing." When do you experience your strongest orgasms? "When I trust my lover completely with my vulnerability."

Renuka, 31, a personal assistant, married. What turns you on most about a man? "I was attracted to my husband because he was good looking and kind." What do you enjoy most about lovemaking? "When he takes control and is powerful and strong. It makes me feel very feminine." When do you experience your strongest orgasms? "When we are relaxed and I am not worrying about the children."

Deirdre, 42, psychologist, divorced. What turns you on most about a man? "His charisma, his looks, and his self-confidence." What do you enjoy most about lovemaking? "I enjoy mostly everything, especially if we can laugh and have fun." When do you experience your strongest orgasms? "When I am in love."

Carolyn, 22, married with one baby. What turns you on most about a man? "Physically, I would have to say his height, his build and his buttocks. Emotionally, I would pick his ability to communicate and love me." What do you enjoy most about lovemaking? "When it is slow and gentle yet very erotic." When do you experience your strongest orgasms? "When we are making love at the same rhythm and pace, and when we feel especially close with each other."

Freda, 35, artist, divorced. What turns you on most about a man? "Everything, I love them all." What do you enjoy most about lovemaking? "When it is hot, passionate and lusty." When do you experience your strongest orgasms? "When I feel free enough to scream and shout and generally let go."

feeling confident

There are some women who simply do not feel comfortable about taking the sexual initiative or adopting the superior position while making love. There can be all kinds of reasons for this and no one should feel forced into doing something which makes them feel ill at ease.

If it is simply embarrassment, it is worth gathering the confidence to give it a try, and almost certainly the male partner will love the new variation and the chance to lie back and enjoy. If, however, the man insists on always taking the dominant sexual role, this may be a symptom of a deeper problem within the relationship. No woman should allow herself to feel sexually repressed, and if she feels that she is, the couple may benefit from talking the issues over, or seeking advice from a counsellor.

A woman may be reluctant to assume the on-top position because of a sense of low self-esteem regarding her body. Perhaps she is shy to expose it so boldly to her partner, or maybe she feels overweight and too heavy to climb on top of her man. Most women make critical judgements about their bodies, but more often than not these views are not shared by their partners.

Feeling good about your body is more to do with your self-regard than your actual weight. You can be big and beautiful or thin and beautiful, if you are truly in touch with your inner beauty. However, if your concerns about your body image are actually interfering with your sexual relationship, and stopping you from expressing yourself to your full potential, then it is worth doing something about it.

increasing your sexual confidence

A balanced diet, containing lots of fruit, vegetables and grains, will give you vitality and energy and help you to stabilize your weight. Exercise will strengthen your muscles, giving you extra power for some of the more exciting sexual manoeuvres. Toning up your abdomen, buttocks and thighs will not only make you feel good, but add to your agility and suppleness, and ability to accomplish an exciting range of sexual positions. Working on your pelvic floor exercises will benefit your vaginal muscle control to the delight of you and your man, and may increase the intensity of your orgasm.

new angles of pleasure

In this position, the woman squats or kneels with her back to her partner. Although there is less intimacy, because they are not able to see each other's faces, it can be an exciting variation. The woman should lower herself carefully on to the penis so that it enters her vagina at a comfortable angle. Penetration can be deep with any of the woman-on-top squatting positions, so care should be taken to avoid thrusting movements that may cause the penis to jar the cervix. To maintain the squatting position, the woman will need to be supple in her hips and legs; kneeling astride the partner may be easier for her. The advantage of

this position is that the woman is free to stimulate her own clitoris, while the man surrenders to the pleasurable sensations of her movements.

sensuously slow motions

If the man is sitting up when the woman kneels or squats with her back to him, then much greater physical contact and intimacy can ensue. Her back and buttocks will be moving against and stroking the front of his body, and he will be able to caress her. Intimate contact on the back of her body will be pleasant for her as this area is largely neglected during more traditional sexual postures. He can also reach around to stroke her breasts, belly and thighs. Using her feet and legs for leverage in her movements up and down on the penis, she may enjoy savouring the sensual feeling and the slow motions of this position. In addition, she can continue to stimulate her own clitoris.

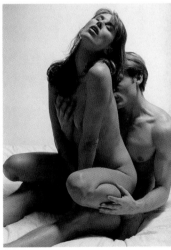

BELOW | More contact is possible when the man sits up and caresses her back, legs and breasts.

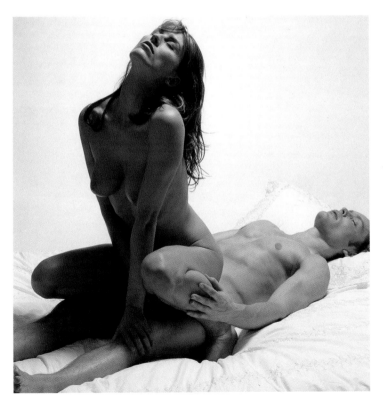

LEFT | The woman is totally in control, stimulating her clitoris.

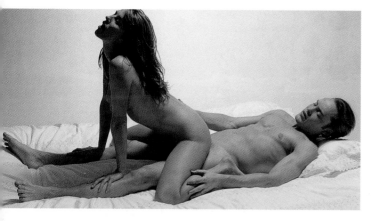

in particular may be very visually stimulated by looking at his partner's buttocks, especially if she is kneeling and leaning forward so they are on display. Gentle stimulation on her anal area with his fingers can also increase her sexual arousal, though for hygiene reasons the fingers should not then be transferred to her vagina until the hands are washed. The woman's movements can become quite active in this position, as she lifts and lowers herself on the penis, or she can tantalizingly raise herself so the lower end of her vagina clasps just the tip of the man's penis, to make small but deliciously sensual and erotically exciting motions.

heightened bodily contact

If the woman is light and supple enough, she can follow on from the previous position, to lean her body back to lie flat against her partner's trunk. This will bring them both back into a very intimate contact as the length of her upper body sinks into the front of his. In this position, the couple should take time to relax deeply and breathe together, allowing a sense of physical and emotional merging. The pressure of his penis inside her vagina will rest against its front wall, supplying an intense stimulation to her G-spot area. While there is little movement in this position, the woman can tighten her vaginal muscles around the penis to exert pleasurable contractions on to it. The open and exposed position of the woman's body means that both of them can touch and caress her breasts and vulva at the same time.

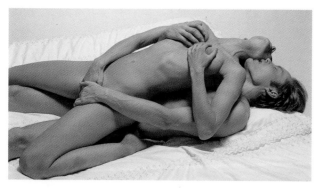

TOP | Most men enjoy the sight of a woman's buttocks on display.

ABOVE AND RIGHT | The woman can then lie back against her lover and both of them can caress her body.

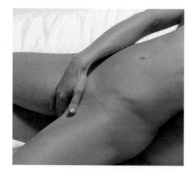

visual variations

While many women may be shy of exposing their buttocks and thighs so prominently to their partners, both sexes can find this variation of the woman-on-top position with her back towards the man a very exciting part of their love play. A man

stimulating strokes

When the woman has lowered the back of her body against her partner's chest and belly, as in the previously described position, she can also easily masturbate herself to reach a peak of arousal or orgasm while the man strokes and palpates her breasts and nipples. This can be tremendously exciting for the man as he feels the waves of pleasure running through her body vibrate against his skin, and as she surrenders to her involuntary contractions against the safe support of his body.

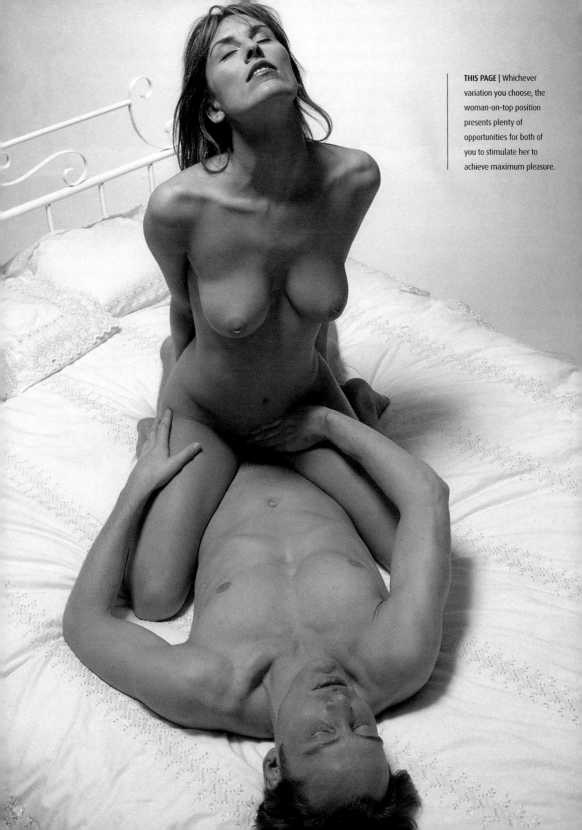

THIS PAGE | Whichever variation you choose, the woman-on-top position presents plenty of opportunities for both of you to stimulate her to achieve maximum pleasure.

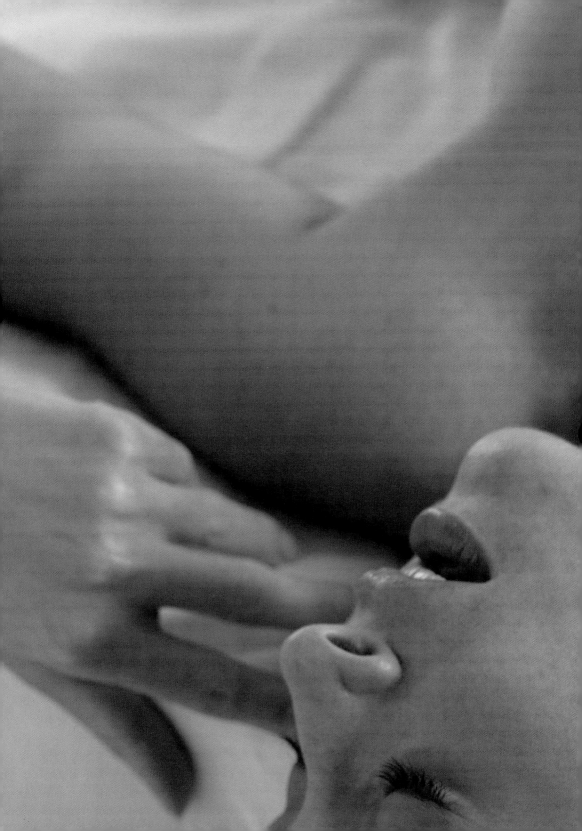

orgasm

Orgasms last seconds or minutes. They trigger divine sensations throughout the body, starting in the pelvis and genital area and sending overwhelming waves of delight rushing through you. They can make you feel relaxed, energized or exhausted, ecstatic, overjoyed or tearful, but always absolutely wonderful – and the even better news is that they are also good for you.

the big o

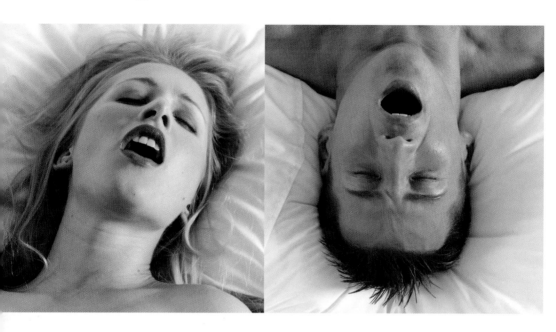

IT IS SOMETHING that fascinates us and that we aspire to – the ecstatic shiver that we feel at the end of making love. *La petite mort* (the little death), as the French call it, is the extreme pleasure. You can have orgasms by yourself through masturbation or together with your partner.

For a man, orgasm is a relatively simple process. He becomes aroused, is stimulated to the point of no return and ejaculates, although there are techniques, notably Tantrism, for achieving orgasm without ejaculation. For women, orgasm has always been more controversial and complicated. Sigmund Freud, for example, while not denying that there was such a thing as a clitoral orgasm, believed that the most satisfying orgasm for a woman was a vaginal one, experienced through penetration by the penis. But then, how much did Freud really know about how women feel and what they experience? Since it is estimated that only around 30 per cent of women can have orgasms through intercourse alone,

Freud's insistence has made many women, who need extra clitoral stimulation to reach a climax, feel like failures. More recently, sexologists have recognized that when women have orgasms, they are as a direct result of clitoral stimulation.

more than one way...

Your orgasm will unleash different sensations according to the different methods used to reach it: masturbation, oral sex or penetration. It is often said that orgasm through masturbation, for example, is more intense than orgasm with a partner, because we ourselves know the best means of delivery. Equally, many women say that they need to feel a penis, fingers or a dildo inside them during orgasm because it makes it a more body-intense experience.

There is no one way of having the ultimate orgasm. Some men need only look at a naked woman; some women, especially during ovulation, climax while fantasizing, or even by being involved in an intellectual discussion. Everyone is different and you must explore, by yourself or with your partner, the most satisfying and exciting methods of achieving your orgasms.

different strokes

There is evidence that both men and women can experience orgasm in other parts of their bodies, not simply around their genital and pelvic areas. People who have suffered nerve damage to their genital area develop orgasmic feelings in other areas of their bodies. Some women can have an orgasm only through nipple stimulation, some men only through fellatio. Women have reported orgasms while giving birth, and breast-feeding women may experience sexual sensations as suckling induces similar uterine contractions and nipple erections to those of orgasm.

all in the head?

Orgasms also have an important psychological dimension. The brain has been described as the most important erogenous zone in the entire body. Warm, loving and positive emotional and psychological feelings towards your partner and towards making love set you directly on the path to reaching orgasm.

However, many negative emotions, such as anger at your partner or even depression over your finances, can put a damper on reaching orgasm. If either partner is having problems attaining orgasm, forget it for a while. Do other things instead, such as lots of kissing and caressing. If you get the most important element of your relationship right, being best friends, your orgasms will flow from there. Communication on both sides is necessary for mutual delight.

BELOW LEFT AND RIGHT | What may bring a man to orgasm the quickest (rhythmic thrusting) is not necessarily the best method for achieving female orgasm. Sex is not always an intuitive practice but can be learned together.

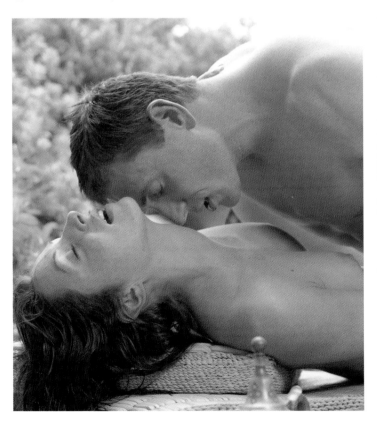

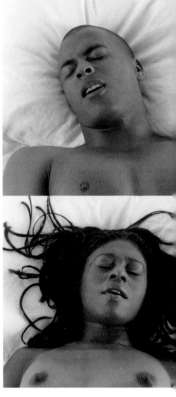

the science of orgasm

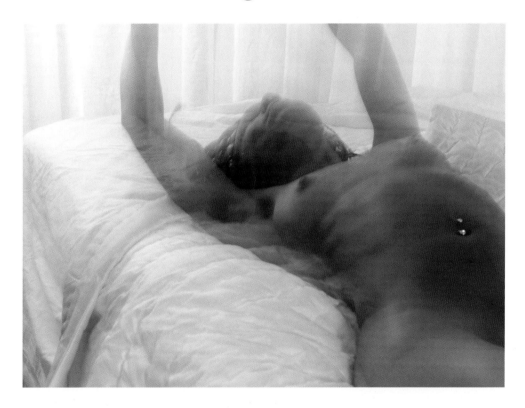

ABOVE | Orgasm is not essentially a shared experience. Most people disappear momentarily into their own worlds, which can lead to feelings of separation. A kiss and a cuddle can easily rectify this when you come back down to earth.

WHAT ACTUALLY HAPPENS during orgasm is different for each gender. However, while individual male and female responses and intensity may vary, the science of the process is the same for all men and for all women.

women

When a woman's clitoris is stimulated and she becomes aroused – the excitement phase – blood rushes to the pelvic area and her vagina becomes moist. The vagina expands and lengthens, the clitoris and breasts swell and the nipples become erect. In the plateau phase, the vaginal lips puff up further, parts of the vagina wall swell with blood and the opening to the vagina narrows. The woman's heartbeat increases, her muscles stiffen

and a pink flush may appear over her body. At this point the clitoris sometimes disappears; if the woman's partner is in the middle of stimulation, this can be a little disconcerting. Just before orgasm, the inner labia (lips) change colour.

At orgasm, the third phase, the muscular tension and engorgement of blood vessels reach a peak. When the orgasm happens, feelings of warmth and delight emanate from the body. The vaginal walls contract rhythmically for a few seconds and tension is released. The number and intensity of the contractions vary. Stimulation of the G spot can induce female ejaculation of a liquid similar to male prostate fluid. The muscles of the uterus also contract, pulling up the sperm to help them find their way to the right place.

In the fourth phase, resolution, the genitals return to normal. This phase can sometimes last for up to half an hour.

men

The blissful sensations of orgasm come, in part, from the seminal fluid exploding into the urinary passage deep in the prostate gland. Most men experience orgasm as sensation and ejaculation.

When a man becomes aroused, his penis stiffens, his heart rate increases and his muscles tighten. The most obvious sign of the build-up towards orgasm is in the penis and testicles: the veins start to bulge, the colour of the glans (head) becomes darker and the testicles rise up towards the body. Once the penis is standing at its biggest, the ridge around the head becomes extra sensitive and the man has reached the point of no return. He will then orgasm, in up to eight contractions, at around one-second intervals.

enhancing orgasm

Women are capable of having multiple orgasms, but some don't realize that they can just keep on going. Multiple orgasms come in a series of waves, one after the other.

Sequential orgasms are slightly different and come on and off after a few minutes. For both, you simply have to keep stimulating the clitoris. If it is painful to do so after orgasm, which it quite often

is, try stroking the vulva area or other parts of the body, or more penetration instead. Many women have difficulty reaching orgasm through penetration alone and need extra stimulation of the clitoris by finger or a vibrator. Try pushing your clitoris against the penis or pubic bone.

Some men say that having their testicles stroked at orgasm heightens the sensation; others love it when their nipples are sucked. The nearest a man will ever get to a multiple orgasm, though, will probably be when he's a teenager and can ejaculate several times in a row. If a man has a second orgasm within a couple of hours, the sensations can be much more intense. There is no proven medical explanation for this but one reason may be that his senses have been heightened by his first orgasm.

For men, extended sexual pleasure has to be mastered. The longer the foreplay, the more intense the orgasm. The ancient art of Tantric sex teaches men how to peak and plateau without going to orgasm immediately. It also teaches men to orgasm without ejaculation and, by moving the energy away from the penis and testicles, to have a whole body orgasm. In the meantime, try the squeeze technique. Just before orgasm, place your thumb on one side of the base of the penis and the tips of your index and middle fingers on the other side, then squeeze. This stops the blood flowing to the penis and slows everything down.

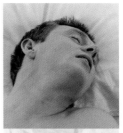
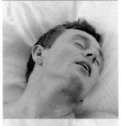
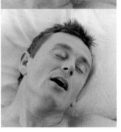

ABOVE AND BELOW LEFT |
Some people are concerned about what they look like and how they behave during orgasm. But the best orgasms are those where you throw inhibition to the wind and succumb to ecstasy.

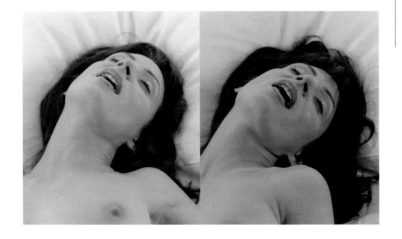

find the spot

THERE HAVE BEEN MANY CLAIMS for the miraculous orgasms that are possible from the stimulation of various areas of the body and many publications have been sold extolling their virtues, although there is no clinical proof that any of them exist.

G spot

This sensitive area, discovered by a Dr Grafenberg, is supposedly located in women on the roof of the vagina, about 5cm/2in up on the outer wall, on the tissue that surrounds the urethra. Many women say that the orgasms from G spot stimulation are really spectacular, while others report only discomfort. To stimulate this patch, insert a finger into an aroused vagina (it may be easier if you squat down). You can buy vibrators specially made for G spot stimulation. It is said to be easier to have multiple orgasms with G spot stimulation and you may experience a full body sensation. You may feel that you need to pass water when you touch this spot, so watch out – and empty your bladder first.

The male G spot is his prostate gland which, when stimulated, can produce the most wonderful orgasms, sometimes even if his penis isn't being touched. The nerve pathway from the penis to the brain runs through the rectum and a nerve centre is located beneath the prostate, so the sensations are powerful. A lubricated finger inserted into his anus – avoid long fingernails – will find the walnut-sized prostate gland about 5cm/2in up, towards the belly button. Caress this and his orgasm will be intensified.

AFE zone and U spot

The AFE (anterior fornix erotic) zone is on the opposite wall of the vagina to the G spot. It is bigger, easier to access and more sensitive than

BELOW AND RIGHT | There seems to be a spot for every letter of the alphabet, with new discoveries every day. However, they all appear to be located around the same area as the G spot, the good news being that if you miss the G spot you've a host of other potential targets.

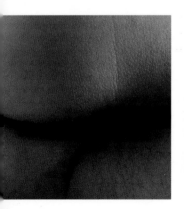

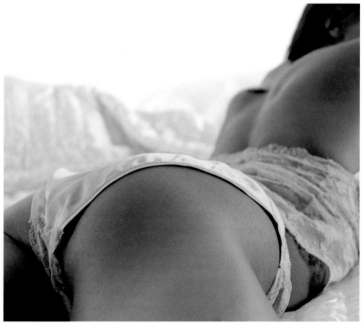

the G spot. Apart from manual stimulation, the woman can mount the man and work his penis to find the spot. Another recently hyped erotic zone is the U spot, a tiny area of external tissue above the opening of the urethra and right below the clitoris. Any stimulation here needs to be very gentle as a urinary tract infection will put a stop to any fun. The fact is that this whole area has so many nerve endings that all of it is an erogenous zone, so you can make up your own special spots.

simultaneous orgasm

This is said to be the ultimate goal of lovemaking. If it happens, then simultaneous orgasm is fantastic. However, not many couples manage it, so don't let yourself be disappointed. in fact, there are reasons why it may not be such a good idea. What about watching your partner orgasm? Isn't that the most erotic thing in the world? And if both partners are concentrating on their own orgasm, there can be a sense of dislocation in which both feel momentarily separated from the other.

faking it

It's not only women who fake orgasms. An increasing number of men are doing it too, as a result of pressure, expectation and lack of confidence. If a partner fails to orgasm, it is not a good idea to insist that you help them have one. You may be projecting your own fears on to them and seeking reassurance that you are a good lover. Just let it be for a little while. If a relationship falls apart, it is more likely to be for other emotional reasons than from difficulties in obtaining orgasm.

problems with orgasm

Anorgasmia is the inability of women to achieve orgasm, even with stimulation. It may have a physical cause, including illnesses, such as advanced diabetes, or if you are on certain medication, have hormone deficiencies or anorexia. It is also caused by a rare condition called vaginismus, an involuntary spasm of the muscles surrounding the vaginal opening. The spasm makes it very difficult, or even impossible, for a penis to enter. If you think you have a

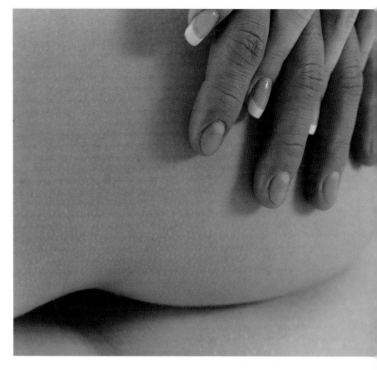

physical problem, check with your gynaecologist. For the majority of women who can't orgasm, it is generally for a psychological reason. A number of cultural, social or relationship issues may be involved – anxiety, control issues within a relationship, past sexual abuse, or a fear of being penetrated. It can also have roots in your religious or moral upbringing. Remember, too, that reaching orgasm may just take time at the beginning of a relationship, especially if a woman is extra anxious to make everything work out well.

Men sometimes suffer from the reverse problem – premature ejaculation. This, too, may have physical causes and you should check with your doctor if it is a recurring problem. This is also true of repeated failure to maintain an erection. However, more often than not, both these problems are occasional and can be resolved with patience, understanding and a little imagination within the context of a loving relationship. Anxiety often plays a major causal role.

ABOVE | No spot is a magic button and orgasms don't happen to schedules, so don't neglect loving caresses as well as powerful stimulation or you may create anxiety and defeat your purpose.

BELOW | Explore every nook and cranny of your bodies to find your pleasure spots.

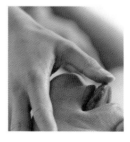

orgasmic variety

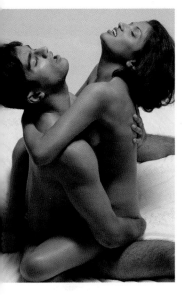

It is not necessary to have penetrative sex in order to have an orgasm. It can be attained from self-masturbation, mutual masturbation and oral sex. Sometimes, during intercourse, a couple may choose to switch to oral sex to complete the orgasmic experience. A man who is concerned that he might not sustain his erection, or that he might ejaculate too soon, may even perform cunnilingus so that his partner has an orgasm before he enters her. So orgasm is very versatile and can be adapted to the mood of the individual or the lovers concerned.

the body's response in orgasm

Studies conducted into human sexual behaviour by American researchers William Masters and Virginia Johnson in the 1950s revealed for the first time that men and women follow a very similar physiological pattern before, during and after orgasm. They discovered that the sexual response of men and women is divided into four phases: the arousal or excitement phase, the plateau phase, orgasm or climax, and the resolution or recovery phase.

ABOVE | Both the man and the woman can feel as if they are melting and merging and letting go into something that is greater than themselves. For some moments the individual ego is dissolved, and for this reason orgasm has often been described as a potentially transforming experience.

RIGHT | During orgasm, both sexes experience rhythmic contractions in the sex organs and pelvic floor muscles, followed by a release of tension which creates a surge of pleasurable sensations spreading through the body.

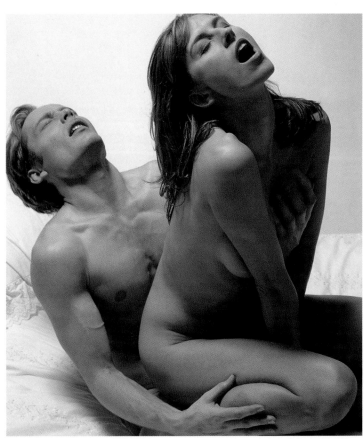

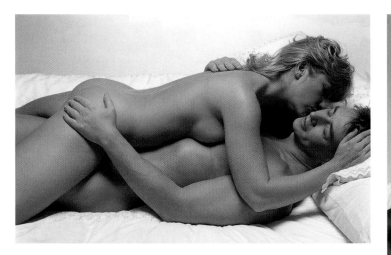

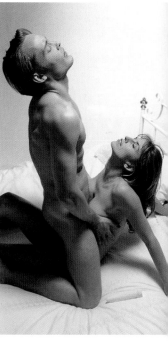

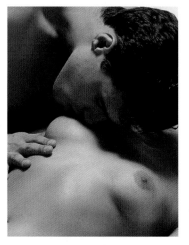

penis, and its sustained stimulation during intercourse may be necessary if she is to achieve orgasm. They also noted other distinct parallels between the male and female physiological responses, such as the build-up of neuro-muscular tension, the increase in heart rate and blood pressure, the quickening of breathing, and, if it occurs, a reddening or flushing that can spread over the skin.

varying orgasm

There are times when a man may choose not to ejaculate into his partner's vagina. Maybe penetrative sex is unwise because of a current infection, or there is a risk of pregnancy, or perhaps the couple want to add a little variety to their repertoire. In such cases the man can reach his orgasm threshold and then ejaculate on to his partner's belly, or even between the warm soft mounds of her breasts. (It goes without saying that he should only do this with her consent.)

self-discovery

Quite often, self-masturbation is recommended as an exercise for people who are experiencing difficulty in obtaining an orgasm with a sexual partner. By bringing yourself to orgasm, you can learn exactly what kind of stimulation you enjoy.

However, they also discovered that the sexes differ in many respects. For example, the plateau phase in males can be much shorter than in females, with the result that the man may ejaculate before the woman has had an orgasm, unless he makes an effort to prolong this phase. In contrast, the resolution phase can be much shorter in females compared with men, enabling many women to achieve several orgasms during a single lovemaking session.

In addition, Masters and Johnson showed that the woman's clitoris is as erotogenic as the man's

ABOVE LEFT | Become more sensual and relaxed with each other so your bodies begin to resonate together. Try different positions for making love to see which ones can bring you to greater heights of arousal.

ABOVE | Ejaculating between his lover's breasts is a possible variation.

LEFT | The man can caress his partner as she masturbates.

male physical response

Orgasm is triggered in the man when the muscular tension in his body and nerve stimulation of the sex organs has reached the orgasm peak in what has been termed "the point of no return". Just before the man ejaculates, rhythmic contractions of muscles around the prostate gland, the seminal vesicles, and the epididymides, push seminal fluids and sperm into the base of the urethra – the urethral bulb – where they mix together.

At this stage, the man's testicles are fully elevated and the opening between his urethra and bladder closes. At ejaculation, intense rhythmic contractions of the urethral bulb and spasms of the pelvic floor muscles pump the semen through the penis, where it spurts out at the tip. These ejaculatory contractions follow each other in rapid succession. Initially they can be very powerful, though they progressively decrease in strength. At the same time the man experiences the intensely pleasurable sensations of orgasm.

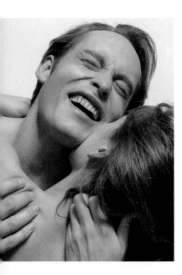

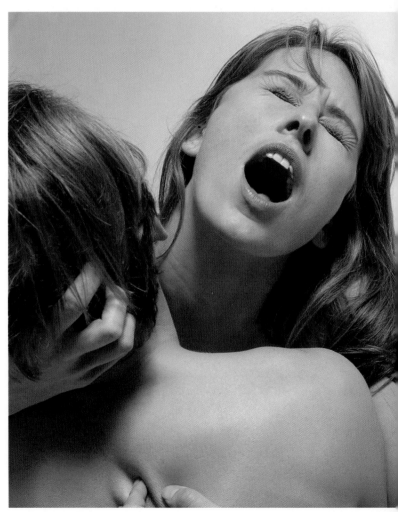

ABOVE | Some men experience sexual contractions only in their genital area, while others feel them throughout the body. During these moments of orgasm, a man may shout, and his face may contort for a few ecstatic moments as a result of muscular spasms.

RIGHT | During orgasm, the woman loses voluntary control over her muscles, so her face may spasm, and even her fingers and toes can curl.

female physical response

Women do not always have an orgasm, even though they may have attained a high level of arousal during the excitement and plateau stage, and there can be a number of reasons for this. Some women may not reach orgasm at all during lovemaking, or during a particular episode of sexual activity, but this does not necessarily detract from the pleasure they have experienced during the other stages of intercourse, and they may feel sexually fulfilled just the same. In addition, a woman can be more easily distracted by her thoughts or concerns at this stage, in which case even the effort of trying to reach an orgasm can be counter-productive.

Most women do not reach orgasm through vaginal friction alone, and need more direct clitoral stimulation during intercourse, either by skilfully applied pressure from the man's pubic bone, by her own movements, or by additional oral or manual stimulation.

When the conditions are right for the woman to have an orgasm, she may begin to feel it as an intense sensation of warmth spreading from her clitoris throughout her body, and a throbbing sensation in her vagina and the muscles in her pelvic region.

When this tension reaches its peak, it gives way to powerful rhythmic contractions which can occur in the lower portion of the vagina, the uterus, and around the anus. For many women, these waves of sensation can pulsate through their whole body. The first contractions are the strongest, but they may be followed by a series of milder pulsations – rather like the aftershocks that often follow an earthquake.

These involuntary contractions work as a pump to release the vaso-congested genital area, so if a woman has almost reached the point of climax, but orgasm is interrupted, for whatever reason, this pent-up feeling of tension in her genitals can make her feel physically very uncomfortable and emotionally let down. She must either wait for this physiological feeling to subside by itself, or for her partner to bring her to orgasm – by oral or manual stimulation if he has already ejaculated.

resolution

Resolution is the final phase of the sexual cycle of response, as defined by Masters and Johnson. Here, for both the man and the woman, the body now returns to its normal pre-arousal state. In a man, the immediate stage after ejaculation is termed the refractory period, and it is impossible for him to resume sexual activity at this time. The length of time the phase lasts varies greatly from one man to another, but in most cases it increases with age.

Most men feel depleted after orgasm and need a period of time to recover, often wanting to withdraw into themselves, or go to sleep. However, a post-orgasmic woman can often remain in a state of sexual excitement after climaxing and may want the lovemaking to continue. As explained, a woman is often capable of going on to achieve more orgasms.

This fundamental difference in the male and female response in the moments immediately after making love can create real problems in a relationship. If after-sex behaviour is disrupting the harmony of your love life, it is really worthwhile talking about the issue with each other. It is best to try to understand your partner's needs and point of view, rather than becoming angry or defensive.

BELOW | If the man is able to delay his own orgasm the woman may be able to have one climax after another.

BOTTOM | During the resolution phase, a couple can lie together in each other's arms, simply enjoying their close physical presence and the intimacy of the moment.

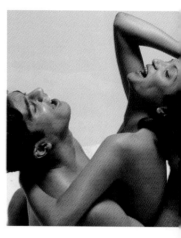

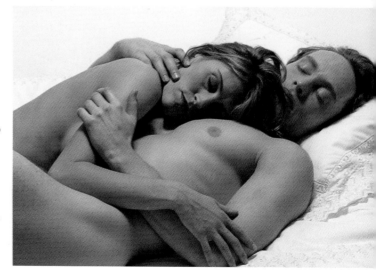

multiple orgasms

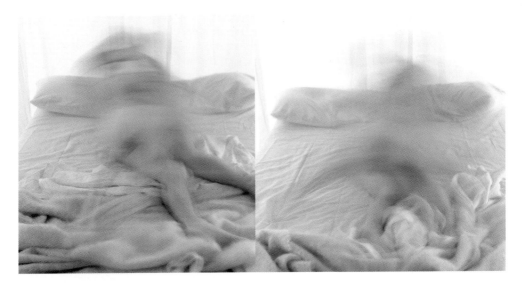

ABOVE AND BELOW | Lack of genital geography can make orgasm during penetrative sex elusive for some women. CAT can bring this into focus and is actually fun for both partners.

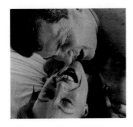

MANY WOMEN HAVE INFREQUENT ORGASMS or no orgasms at all and, over the years, this can take its toll on a relationship. This doesn't necessarily mean that they are not having good sex, but the dynamics of a woman's arousal are quite complex and it doesn't help that the design and position of the clitoris make stimulation somewhat hit or miss. The Coital Alignment Technique (CAT) and the Extended Sexual Orgasm technique (ESO) are two methods that have been designed to overcome some of these difficulties.

coital alignment technique

CAT is a position that has been adapted from the missionary position to greatly increase the likelihood of a woman reaching orgasm during penetrative sex. It is ideal for women who have difficulties achieving orgasm during penetration, although it helps only if these difficulties are technical ones and not psychological.

The clitoris of most women is approximately 2–3cm/¾–1¼in away from the vaginal opening, so clitoral stimulation during penetration is often sporadic, indirect or totally absent. The difference with CAT is that the man penetrates his partner from a more acute angle, so that his thrusting penis stimulates her clitoris.

Start in the normal missionary position with the man on top, between his partner's spread legs, which she gently bends from the knees. As he enters her, he should lift himself forwards, further up her body, so that his thrusts make contact with her clitoris, keeping his upper body relaxed by leaning either to the left or right to rest part of his weight on the bed. The woman can wrap her legs around her partner's legs, keeping her pelvis stretched so that her ankles lie around the vicinity of his calves.

Another option is for the woman to keep her legs closed while her partner places his legs on the outside of hers. Try both ways to see which one suits you better. The latter may be more beneficial to women with a very sensitive clitoris which does not respond well to direct contact. From here, the couple should begin a light rocking motion back and forth, keeping in rhythm with each other. He should grind and rotate or make figures-of-eight with his pelvis from time to time, as many women respond well to the stimulation of a circular motion around their clitoris.

extended sexual orgasm

ESO was developed by psychiatrist Alan Brauer and psychotherapist Donna Brauer and is designed to help women to extend their orgasms to up to 30 minutes in duration. The woman should begin by training both her mind and body, cleansing herself of any negative barriers or fears she may have about sex by focusing on the enjoyment of sex with her partner. What this means is that she should begin with a couple of weeks of daily pelvic floor (PC) muscle workouts and a regular masturbation programme concentrating on learning precisely the types of stimulation she finds the most effective.

ESO is done with the woman lying on her back and her partner between her legs, either kneeling or sitting. As he could be there for anything up to half an hour, he should choose a comfortable position. The man begins by applying lubrication to her entire genital area, massaging everywhere except the clitoris. When the woman begins to move her body to the rhythm of the massage, he should begin slow, rhythmic clitoral stimulation, while she flexes her PC muscles and takes deep breaths. When the first set of orgasmic contractions commences, he should shift stimulation from the clitoris to the vaginal walls, by inserting a couple of fingers, but keeping the rhythm steady and slow. Once she achieves her first orgasm, he should wait for it to subside slightly, but not so long that the contractions stop. He must then continue massaging the vaginal walls slowly and rhythmically and if she feels the contractions subsiding, move back to the clitoris, maintaining the momentum. This should trigger further contractions and so he should move back to the vaginal wall massage, continuing this back and forth movement until the contractions become continuous. Finally, he stimulates both areas at the same time, resulting in wave after wave of continual orgasms.

go again, and again…

For some women it is possible to have more than one orgasm. Some claim that the second or third is less intense, whereas others claim that intensity builds with each one. The techniques for achieving multiple orgasms in women are similar to those described in ESO, where stimulation after the first orgasm continues. Many women find that their clitorises are hypersensitive to touch after orgasm, so instead of stimulating the clitoris directly, her partner should stimulate the surrounding areas until feelings of arousal return.

For men, the multiple orgasm is more difficult to achieve, as many enter a refractory period after ejaculation, which usually means a light snooze. It is believed that men who can separate orgasm and ejaculation are able to experience multiple orgasmic sensations. This is one of the tenets of Tantric and Taoist sex.

In order to achieve this separation, men need to develop strong PC muscles with Kegel exercises. When the man gets to the point of orgasm, he should stop all stimulation and contract his PC muscles, then relax all the muscles of the pelvis and bottom area. He should then resume stimulation and repeat the whole process, before finally squeezing the PC muscles tightly at the point of orgasm. The man should then experience the pleasurable sensations of orgasm without releasing any semen. Anyone with a prostate problem should consult a doctor before trying this.

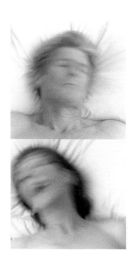

ABOVE AND BELOW |
Practising what is known as semen retention, by contracting the PC muscle, enables a man not only to prolong lovemaking and so stimulate his partner to orgasm, but also to have multiple orgasms himself.

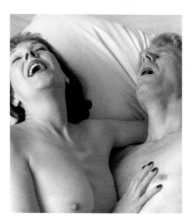

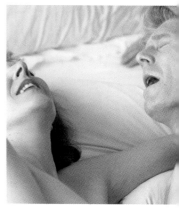

self-pleasuring

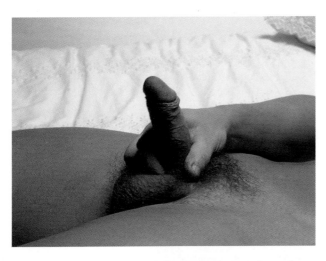

ABOVE | Experiment with different strokes, pressures and speeds of movement, sliding your hand up and down the whole shaft of the penis, from the base to above the ridge of its head, or focus more on applying pressure to the erotically sensitive frenulum.

RIGHT | Stroke around your vaginal lips and clitoral area, sometimes letting your fingers caress the outer edges of the vagina itself, or slipping into it. As you approach orgasm, increase the pressure and speed of your strokes.

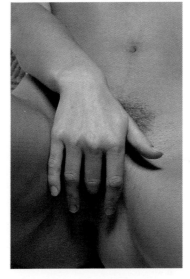

NOWADAYS, MASTURBATION IS REGARDED by most sex experts as a normal and even beneficial sexual activity for health reasons. However, until quite recent times, masturbation was a taboo subject. It was considered immoral, termed a "sin", and many young people were warned that it would make them mad, blind or infertile, or ruin their chances of sexual happiness in marriage, in order to stop them doing it.

Attitudes to masturbation began to alter in the late 1940s and early 1950s, when the Kinsey reports on male and female sexuality stated that, according to their studies, 94 per cent of American men and 40 per cent of American women masturbated to orgasm. More recent research suggests that, while the figure for male masturbation remains the same, female masturbation is now considerably higher, though still less than for men.

Masturbation, which is the self-stimulation of one's own genitals for sexual pleasure and orgasm, is clearly, then, a normal part of human sexual activity. In fact, the Kinsey report concluded that the only harmful side-effects of masturbation were the anxiety and guilt it might evoke in those who practised it.

Masturbation is now seen more as a valuable way for males and females, young and old, to learn more about their bodies, and to enjoy their sexual and orgasmic responses. It can be a useful way to release sexual tension, but more importantly, it gives men and women the chance to enjoy sexual pleasure and body sensuality, regardless of whether or not they are currently in a relationship.

These days, masturbation is one of the basic tools used in sex therapy, and clients are often encouraged to masturbate in the privacy of their homes as one of the key methods of discovering and encouraging their sexual and orgasmic responses and of overcoming their anxieties, guilt or other problems surrounding sexual issues.

art of self-pleasuring

Masturbation is often carried out in a speedy and rather unsensual fashion, with the aim of achieving a climax in the fastest way possible. This method has its uses, especially if the aim is to obtain a quick release from sexual tension. However, to turn it into the art of self-pleasuring, you should learn to make love to yourself in a wholly sensual way.

Try to create some time for yourself that is dedicated to self-pleasuring. Ensure that you have complete privacy and that you won't be interrupted. Warm your bedroom and light some candles, if it is dark, to create a sensual ambience. Play some music that will help you feel sexy, and then lie naked on your bed. Begin to stroke and caress your whole body, including your genital area, but do not at this point focus specifically on it. If you have an imaginative mind, allow your fantasies to unfold, but also remain totally involved in the physical sensations happening in your body.

self-pleasuring for men

Most men, when they masturbate, concentrate the stimulation solely on the penis. Instead, try to let your hands also stroke your chest, belly, thighs, scrotum, perineum and buttocks, sweeping them over your penis as they move from one part of your body to another. If you choose, fantasize that your dream woman is stroking your body, or indulge yourself in whatever imagery works as a powerful aphrodisiac for you.

Uncircumcised men should draw back the foreskin to expose the glans while masturbating. The most erogenously responsive area is usually around the frenulum, on the underside of the shaft, just beneath the head of the penis. Experiment with pressures and strokes, speeds and rhythms, delighting in all the different sensations that you can create.

As your sexual feelings rise, let yourself go, breathing deeply and moving your body, thrusting your pelvis, and making sounds to express your growing excitement. If you feel you are approaching ejaculation, slow down to prolong your self-pleasuring, then build up the tempo towards climax again.

For a truly sensual experience, try to let this pleasuring last for 15 minutes, or even longer, before you climax. As you approach an orgasm,

abandon yourself totally to the sensations. Then rest awhile, touching your body and relaxing.

self-pleasuring for women

Women tend to be more naturally sensual in the way they masturbate, and also quite inventive in their style of touching and stimulation. First, though, why not take a bath enhanced by the aroma of aphrodisiac essential oils, such as ylang-ylang, sandalwood, jasmine, rose, basil, patchouli and black pepper. Choose up to three of these oils, mixing a maximum of seven drops.

When you have dried yourself and used moisturizer on your skin, lie on the bed and allow your erotic fantasies to take over. Touch and stroke your body, including your genital area, thighs, breasts and nipples. As you become mentally and physically aroused, apply different pressures and strokes of your hands and fingers to your pubic and genital area. You can begin by gently arousing the whole area with a circular motion, placing the heel of your hand on your pubic bone and resting your fingers against your vulva.

As you become aroused, part your vaginal lips with your fingers, and stroke all over the inner folds, around the opening of your vagina, and the area surrounding your clitoris. You may want to pull back the hood of the clitoris to apply pressure on it directly, but if this kind of stimulation feels too intense, rub the skin above and beside it instead.

Experiment with different strokes, vibrations, pressures, and rhythms, finding out exactly which sequence of movements is the most erotic for you. Increase the pressure and speed of your touches as your arousal builds, and then, as you approach your climax, maintain a more regular tempo, sustaining pressure on your clitoris throughout your orgasm. Let yourself go into the orgasmic contractions, allowing them to pulsate through your whole body. Moan, sigh or cry out, and move your pelvis to enhance the powerful sensations of your orgasmic release.

For even more arousing sensations, men and women can apply a water-soluble lubrication to their genital area while masturbating. However, avoid oil-based products such as petroleum jelly.

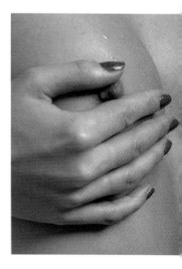

BELOW | Many women touch and caress their whole bodies while they are masturbating. Try stroking and caressing your most erogenous zones, such as your breasts and nipples, to experience a new intensity of sexual arousal.

men and masturbation

IN THE PAST, standard dictionaries defined masturbation as "self-abuse". Today, it is more accurately defined as "self-pleasuring". Around 95 per cent of men masturbate, a statistic that has probably not changed over the years. Sex experts believe that masturbation is an integral part of a healthy lifestyle. It is a sexual practice that is now recognized as both normal and beneficial.

BELOW | The shower is a popular venue as it offers privacy and no need to clean up after oneself.

Men are inclined to masturbate more frequently than women. Some men masturbate two or more times a day and some a few times per month. It's possible that men masturbate more than women because, biologically, they need to "clean the tubes" more often, removing old semen so it can be replaced with new. Whatever the reason, masturbation forms an integral part of the average male's routine, whether he is conscious of this or not.

light relief

All too often, masturbation is done with only the end point in mind, the orgasm. It is tempting to creep between the sheets, sit on the toilet or have a quick pull elsewhere to relieve sexual tension. This is fine, but in order to get more from your orgasm, it's worth taking time and practising the art of masturbation to prolong the delicious sensations that lead up to climax. This will result in a more intense orgasm, as well as training for those long-distance sessions with your partner.

Like sex, masturbation can be divided into two categories, the "quickie" and the long, drawn-out sensual session. Instead of concentrating solely on the penis when masturbating, try to explore other areas such as your nipples, chest, thighs, perineum and buttocks. If you have never tried stimulating your anus, give it a go. No one can see you.

Masturbation is a great opportunity to let your imagination run wild. Different people have different fantasies and the content of yours is personal and not something you should feel ashamed or embarrassed about. Everyone has fantasies and they may be the absolute pinnacle of depravity. Often what gets your rocks off in your head would have the totally opposite effect in reality.

There is no right or wrong way to masturbate. Some men prefer a strong gripping movement, others prefer a lighter touch. Many men prefer to confine stimulation to the head or glans alone. This may involve a pulling action, which stimulates just the head and frenulum area. Other men incorporate

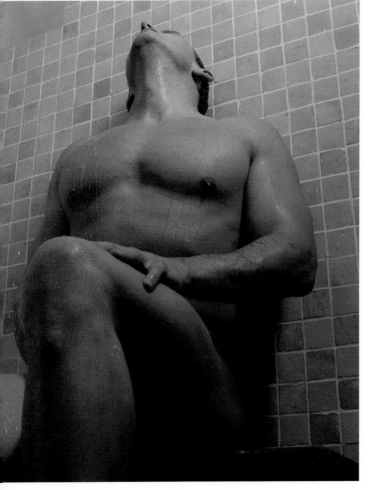

the shaft into their technique. Whatever works for you wins. The idea of this book is not to teach correct technique, but to encourage a little extra variety and new discovery.

The techniques described here have been tried and tested. They are merely a guide, however, as teaching a man to masturbate is comparable to preaching to the converted. It is interesting that masturbation is still one of the hardest topics to discuss in a relationship, so leaving this chapter open on your girlfriend's pillow may be helpful.

calligraphy grip

Hold your penis in the same way that you would a pen, with your thumb nearest you and your forefinger furthest away. Stroke your penis up and down in this way, stimulating your frenulum and glans. If you want more contact, simply wrap the rest of your fingers around to form a fist and use your thumb at the top to stimulate the head.

turn and twist

Grip the top of the head like a water tap and twist as you would if turning a tap on or off. This may be better with some lubrication and stimulation of the shaft with your other hand.

the mattress massage

This involves lying on the mattress and rubbing your penis up and down the fabric. You can spice this up with cushions strategically placed along your penis to increase the pressure and friction.

prayer pumper

Put your hands tightly together as if in prayer. Add some lubrication and then insert your penis into the groove formed at the joining of your wrists. Using your pelvis, thrust into your hands, adjusting the depth of your penetration.

san francisco shuffle

Hold your penis in a similar way to the calligraphy grip, using either a fist or your thumb and forefinger. Stroke up and instead of going back down, go over the top of the head, maintaining contact, and down the other side, so that the top

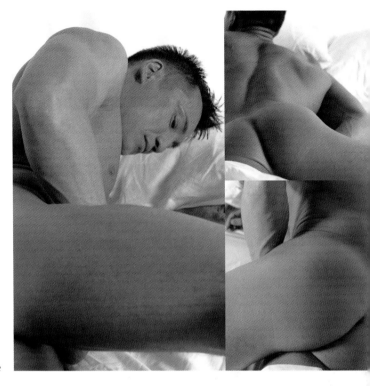

of your hand is closest to your stomach and your thumb is pointing away from your body. Then reverse the direction.

dressing up

For this one, all you need to do is experiment with different fabrics and textures by placing socks, gloves and other garments over your penis. Different fabrics will provide a variety of sensations; just be sure to get permission from your girlfriend before using her gloves.

Fabrics have different textures that will stimulate your nerve endings in different ways. The cool chill of silk for example, will induce a sensation similar to water, whereas the harder, rougher and warmer feel of leather, combined with its distinctive smell, is a completely different sensory experience. Experimentation is the key here and soon you will become more aware of what fabrics and textures turn you on.

ABOVE | There are as many positions and places for masturbation as there are men on the planet.

BELOW | The television is a great source of stimulating material to inspire a session of self-pleasuring.

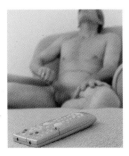

women and masturbation

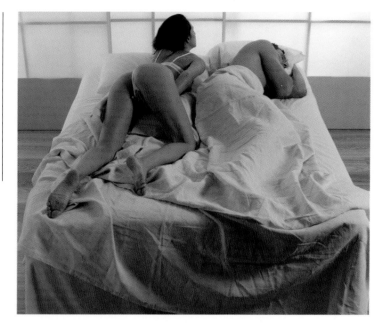

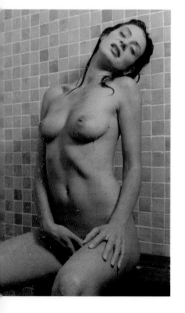

FOR YEARS IT WAS SEEN as dirty and depraved to pleasure yourself, especially if you happened to be a woman. It was not until 1972 that the American Medical Association declared masturbation a normal sexual activity.

Although today some women find it hard to approach the subject of masturbation, the truth is that the majority of women are doing it. Recent statistics show that 82 per cent of women masturbate, a statistic that is increasing with time. Are more women masturbating now? Probably not, they are just more inclined to admit to it.

For many women, masturbation is the only means of getting sexual fulfilment and orgasm and it is thought that a woman is three times as likely to orgasm through masturbation than through penetrative sex. A huge number of women find it difficult or even impossible to climax with a partner through penetrative sex alone and need clitoral stimulation.

cliterati

Emily Dubberley, journalist and sexpert on masturbation says of the orgasm, "It's like one of those water balloons that just slips through your fingers when you try to get hold of it, or a bar of soap in the bath. Try to grab on to it too hard and it just flies away." Because there wasn't enough masturbation material for women on the Internet, she founded cliterati.co.uk, so if you are not feeling imaginative enough to think of something yourself, look up the site for some raunchy inspiration.

setting the scene

Most men can masturbate almost any time, anywhere, with pleasing results, but for women it is often more complex. Masturbation is a fine art that involves all the senses to set the mood.

It's often worth doing some preparation beforehand to get you in the right frame of mind. Solitude is a must. Turn off your pager, unhook the phone and feed the dog, making sure that you give yourself a window of distraction-free time, unless you are excited by rushing and perhaps the possibility of being discovered.

There is no set place that leads to a more orgasmic experience. Wherever you feel comfortable is ideal, but it's sometimes fun to seek variety and try different positions, from lying on your front in bed, standing in the shower or jumping into the back seat of your car. Any literature or visual aids should be ready to hand.

techniques

There is no correct or incorrect technique – the important first step is to explore your body and find out what goes where in your pleasure zone. It's also important to experiment with touch and caress to find out what you like and what does it for you, as preferences vary greatly from woman to woman.

Many women like to fantasize as they play with themselves. If you are a fantasizer, this is an opportunity to let your mind wander into the impossible, sordid or even dangerous. It doesn't matter, your mind is totally secure and you should never feel guilty about what turns you on. Fantasy and reality are two different worlds.

Using lubrication can often help to get things moving a bit more smoothly. You can use water-based lubricants, which are usually odourless and tasteless, or even your own saliva. Some women produce more love juices than others and feel that lubrication is not necessary. Either way, it evokes a different sensation and experience, so experiment.

crossed clitoris caress

Using your third and fourth finger, caress your clitoris and the surrounding areas in a cross-like movement, moving from north to south and then east to west, with your clitoris as the central point. Change the direction and pressure until you discover your most sensitive spots.

passion pinching

Gently squeeze your clitoris between your thumb and forefinger or middle finger and lift it slightly, squeezing at the same time. Roll it between your

fingers, starting slowly and then picking up momentum. Again, experiment with different paces and pressures. For women with super-sensitive clitorises direct contact may be too intense. If this is the case with you, try to keep the clitoris covered with a layer of the inner labia, avoiding direct stimulation.

circular cyclone

This is an old favourite that, once perfected, will guarantee orgasm. Place your forefinger and middle finger just over the top of your clitoris and rub in a circular motion over your clitoris, varying the size and frequency of the circles. Because you are stimulating just above the clitoris, you can use a bit more pressure.

figure of eight

Another favourite that is fairly self-explanatory. The top of the eight concentrates on the clitoris and the bottom incorporates the vulva and labia. Use a smaller circle for the clitoris and larger, more sweeping circles for the bottom circle. Use forefinger and middle finger or whichever two fingers feel more comfortable.

tri-digit fidget

This one uses three fingers. Use your fourth finger and forefinger to hold back the inner and outer labia folds, leaving your middle finger free to concentrate on clitoral stimulation. With your free hand you could use a vibrator.

victory roll

With your middle finger and forefinger in a V shape, rub up and down your vulva with the clitoris in the middle. This stimulates the sides of your clitoris and the inner labia. By varying the width of the V, you can experiment with the different sensations.

tapping

Spread your labia to fully expose the clitoris. With your index finger, lightly tap the tip of your clitoris. This is not for everyone and some may find this sensation too much, but it adds variety and spice in combination with other techniques.

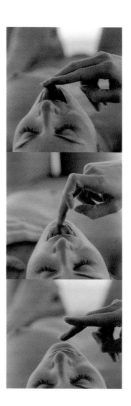

ABOVE AND BELOW | If you do not have any lubricant handy, use your saliva to lubricate yourself when masturbating.

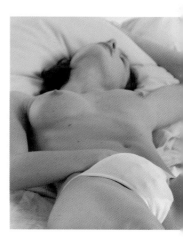

doing it together

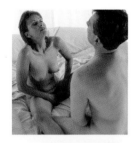

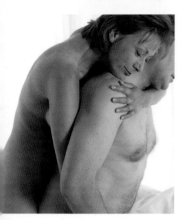

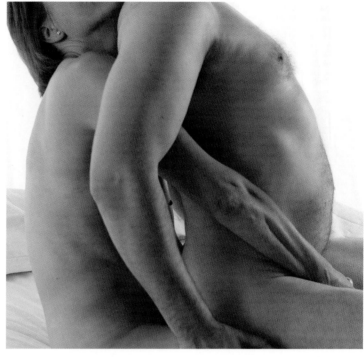

TOP | Watching each other masturbating can be a learning experience.

ABOVE AND ABOVE RIGHT | Sharing the experience of masturbation is simply another form of intimacy, which can be deeply erotic and exciting. It does not replace the pleasures of penetrative sex, but actually enhances them.

OPPOSITE | Body shapes can fit together in many different ways.

MUTUAL MASTURBATION ENHANCES the sensuality of foreplay by increasing arousal for either partner prior to penetration and intercourse, and it is a sure way to get the love juices flowing. It may also be enjoyed as a complete and totally fulfilling sexual act in itself through which lovers can attain orgasm even without penetrative sex. It is a delightful way to initiate a second round of lovemaking when both people are sufficiently rested from the first bout, and it can be used to lovingly assist a partner to complete sexual satisfaction if the other person has climaxed first or is unable to continue lovemaking.

An important skill in the art of lovemaking is to learn how to masturbate your partner properly. To do it well is to know which touches bring maximum pleasure and to share in your lover's delight.

Many couples, particularly the young, use masturbation as a way of exploring and enjoying each other's bodies before committing themselves to a full sexual relationship. It provides a safe means of exploring and becoming familiar with each other's sexual responses as well as enjoying sexual satisfaction without the implications and responsibilities involved in full penetrative intercourse.

Some people find masturbation acceptable but would only allow intercourse within the context of a committed relationship or marriage. Others may wisely consider the consequences of pregnancy or sexually transmitted infections and prefer to abstain from a full sexual relationship, using masturbation as an alternative until these issues have been safely resolved.

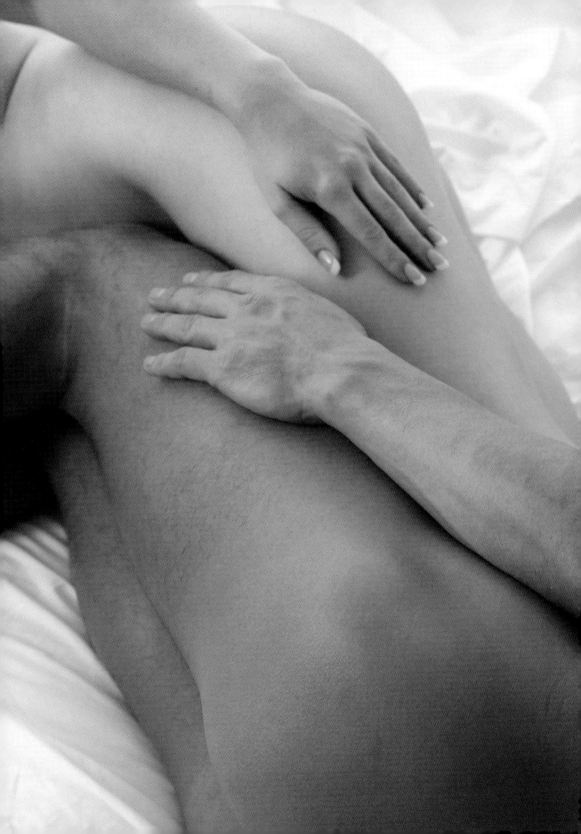

satisfying your partner

Mutual masturbation should remain an integral part of any couple's range of lovemaking techniques, for it continues to provide an erotic enhancement throughout a sexual relationship. Arousing and satisfying your partner by skilful masturbation without asking for anything in return, except the joy gained from his or her pleasure, can be a very erotic experience.

If your libido is at a low ebb, perhaps as a result of tiredness or stress and you are not in the mood for making love, while your partner is, masturbating your lover can be a perfect way to answer both of your needs. If you have a back injury which makes movement difficult, or you are heavily pregnant, then again mutual masturbation can provide an extremely sensual alternative to full sexual intercourse. In addition to masturbating each other, either of you can indulge in the pleasure of self-masturbation with the other partner closely involved in the process. This can be a very erotic experience, as you watch your partner self-pleasure his or her body next to yours. You participate with touches and caresses to increase the arousal and you can even join in the sighs, moans and changing patterns of breath as if the sensations are being transferred into your body too.

You can take it in turns to masturbate each other, or you may do it simultaneously while standing, kneeling or lying next to your partner so that your bodies begin to vibrate together with the mounting tension of your sexual excitement.

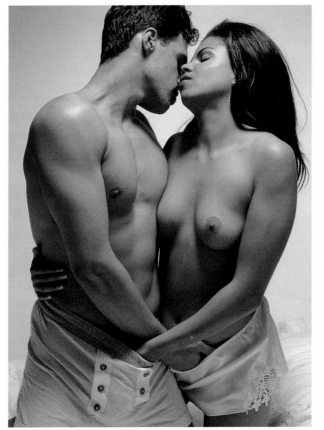

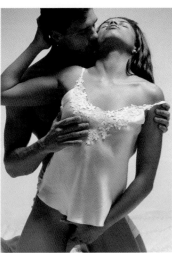

ABOVE | Watching your partner self-masturbate is very erotic.

LEFT | Masturbating mutually as you undress adds extra spice.

Many lovers feel that the orgasms they experience through masturbation provide a quite different sensation than those resulting from intercourse. The masturbatory orgasm is sometimes described as being more physically intense than an intercourse orgasm, probably because it ensues from a sustained and specific stimulation applied to the most erotically sensitive areas of the genitals, and possibly because if you are on the receiving end, you can lie back and surrender yourself totally and quite selfishly into its powerful sensations.

For some women, careful and loving masturbation combined with oral stimulation from the partner are the only way in which they can achieve orgasmic satisfaction while making love. It may not, however, bring the same deeply nourishing and fulfilling sense of emotional bonding and fulfilment which is more likely to occur when a couple climax during the act of penetrative sex.

Sexuality, however, is multi-dimensional – a kaleidoscope of physical and emotional experiences – and mutual masturbation is there to be enjoyed as one of its many exquisite hues.

quick-release sex

Mutual masturbation can provide fast erotic arousal whether it is part of a whole lovemaking session or a separate episode from intercourse. By masturbating each other to orgasm, both of you can receive a satisfying release of sexual tension. Mutual masturbation while still partly clothed can be particularly exciting because it can recall memories of early sexual experimentation, and also because the friction of material against the genitals can be an additional form of stimulation.

caresses and fantasies

You can masturbate yourself to orgasm while your partner holds you close to his body, and touches and caresses your breasts and kisses your face and neck. You can let your own sexual fantasies run free in your mind, or he can even whisper his sexual fantasies to you while you are turning yourself on. Again, this type of masturbation can become even more enticing if you are wearing a silky textured item of clothing, like a camisole, which will rub sensuously against your nipples and skin.

BELOW | You can masturbate each other at the same time. If you are attuned to each other's responses, it may even be possible to reach a simultaneous orgasm, or if not, take it in turns to satisfy one another sexually. Or you may only want to take the arousal level so far with your masturbatory motions before progressing towards other forms of lovemaking. Lie close to each other to have skin-to-skin contact, but position yourselves comfortably so that you can easily touch and stroke each other's genitals.

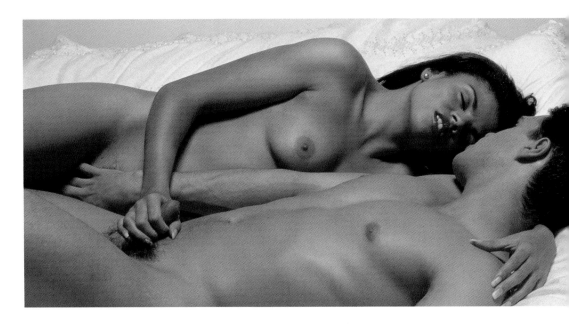

the right touch

Most people perfect their masturbation skills on themselves. So it makes sense that the person who can best show you how to apply just the right erotic touch in masturbation is your partner. Only he or she knows the rhythm and pace of the strokes which can be guaranteed to take them to the heights of arousal and on towards a mind-blowing orgasm. However, that does not exclude the other partner being able to add something entirely new and extremely exciting of their own invention to this type of sexual arousal – so stay open to the possibility of experiencing some hitherto unknown peaks of pleasure.

Men and women masturbate themselves in quite different ways. Generally, a man will focus his attention almost entirely on his penis, though he may possibly include some self-arousing caresses to his scrotum, or finger-pressure on his anus. He is also likely to simulate the action of intercourse by creating the same type of pumping friction on the shaft of his penis, only this time by hand. He almost certainly prefers to use a firm grip of the hand, and may apply increasingly vigorous strokes until the moment of ejaculation.

A woman's way of masturbating herself is likely to be more sensual and slow, and involve more of her body, for she may caress her breasts and rub her nipples, and stroke her belly and thighs as if she is making love to herself. She is unlikely to concentrate her manual stimulation solely on her clitoris, but will move her fingers all around it and over her vaginal lips, separating them carefully to stroke over their folds and occasionally inserting the tips of her fingers to stroke around the lower part of her vagina. She may also rub and vibrate the pubic bone area above her clitoris, and tug gently on her pubic hair to stimulate the highly erotogenic nerve endings at the base of the hair follicles.

A woman is likely to start her self-masturbation in a slow, gentle and languid manner, varying the motions of her strokes, and building up speed and pressure only as she approaches her climax. She is more likely to lavish her attentions on her vulva, and less inclined to try to recreate the actions of intercourse, though some women insert a dildo or sex toy into the vagina during self-masturbation to increase the stimulation.

BELOW LEFT | The best way to learn how she likes to be touched and stimulated in order to attain an orgasm through masturbation is to watch her do it to herself. She can show you exactly what she enjoys, because she has explored the best means of self-arousal.

BELOW RIGHT | Look also at how her whole body responds to her self-stimulation. Watch how her facial expressions change as she registers the waves of pleasure rising within her. Notice too how she also caresses other parts of her body.

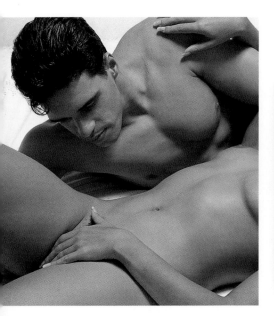

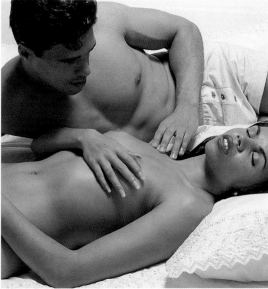

observing each other

Knowing about the different methods employed by men and women during self-pleasuring will help you and your partner to become more sensitive to each other's sexual needs. If you can overcome your shyness, you can watch each other masturbate. If you are observing your partner masturbate, notice everything he or she is doing, which parts of the hands are used, what motions are employed and how the strokes vary at different stages of arousal.

Watch your lover's facial expressions and listen to the changing patterns of breath and the sounds he or she makes, for these will all give you cues to your partner's physical response and arousal patterns during masturbation.

If you are masturbating yourself, tell your partner exactly what you are doing and why a certain stroke or pressure is giving you pleasure. Describe the sensations as well as you can so your partner can begin to absorb all the nuances of those physical feelings into his or her own sexual consciousness. Then, when he or she touches your genitals in a certain way, the physical pleasure you are receiving can also be transmitted

to, and consequently experienced by, your partner. Note, especially, what your partner does as he or she approaches orgasm. Does the friction and stimulation speed up, and does the pressure of palm and fingers increase? What happens on the point of ejaculation and orgasm, and immediately afterwards? In all of these things, your partner is your perfect teacher, but see below for more guidance on masturbation techniques specific to either sex.

make it like music

Mutual masturbation, like oral sex, is a way of getting right down to your partner's genitals. Learn to love them completely so your touches convey your reverence, awe and pleasure for these most intimate parts of your lover's body. Become as familiar with them as you would with any other part of the body.

Use your hands and fingers to play on and stroke over your partner's genitals as you would if you were making beautiful music on a classical instrument. Learn to perfect your rhythm and pace, recognize when to be subtle and when to go for the "grande finale".

BELOW | Mutual masturbation can be enjoyed when both of you simultaneously pleasure yourselves. One way to do this is to lie comfortably next to each other in a top-to-tail position. Continue tactile contact with each other by resting a hand or arm over the other's body then focus totally into giving yourself pleasure, doing all the things that bring you sexual joy, but at the same time feeling the warmth of your partner close by.

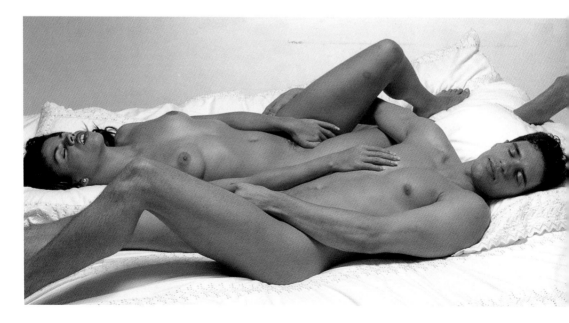

BELOW | Let the man tell you exactly how he enjoys to be stimulated during masturbation. Lay your hand over his to find out how he begins to arouse himself, what strokes he may like to receive on his scrotum, and other parts of his body. If your relationship is open enough, he may like to describe to you the sexual fantasies he uses while masturbating.

masturbating the male partner

If you are going to engage yourself fully and wholeheartedly into masturbating your male partner you will want to be comfortable yourself. You can lie beside him, sit or kneel between his legs, or straddle across his body so that you are facing his genitals. Remember that most men prefer the feeling of a firm grip on the shaft of the penis, so it makes sense to use your strongest and most agile hand. You can, however, swap the action over to the other hand if you are going in for a longer bout of masturbation.

You can hold the base of the penis with your more passive hand to keep it steady, and then clasp your active hand around the top end, settling it just below the coronal ridge. (If your partner is uncircumcised, draw the foreskin gently backwards to expose the head of the penis, but do not overstimulate the tip itself as it may be overly sensitive – unless of course, your partner insists otherwise.)

You can circle the penis with your thumb and index finger to form a ring around it, using this part of your hand as the main tool of stimulation. Alternatively, you can stroke your clasped hand up and down the shaft of the penis from its base to just above the ridge of the glans.

The focal point of stimulation is the erogenously sensitive coronal ridge and the frenulum on the underside, but all-over stroking of the shaft is also pleasurable. You can also roll his penis between your hands, against your thigh and belly, or very erotically between your breasts, although you may need to complete with hand movements to actually bring him to orgasm.

You can start off slowly and sensually, increasing pressure and speed as your strokes progress. Follow what your partner has shown you, varying between short and long, slow and rapid strokes. Build up a rhythm and pace that suits your partner and is in tune with his responses, increasing the tempo as his arousal heightens.

If you both want to prolong the moment of his orgasm, you can slow down teasingly and temporarily just before the ejaculatory process begins, and then start the action all over again. If you do this several times, he may feel as if he is going to burst with increasing sensation and his orgasm, when you allow it to happen, is likely to be very intense.

Learn to recognize the signs that your partner is about to climax so you can speed up your strokes, but stop or slow down once he has started to ejaculate. Continued stimulation at this point may not be welcome as the tip of the penis becomes extremely sensitive and further rubbing can even be painful.

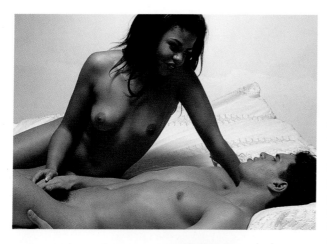

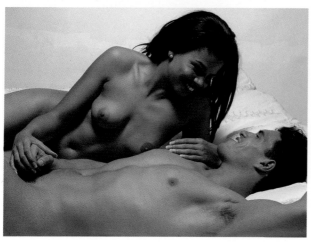

His pleasure may be increased during masturbation if you also caress his thighs and belly, stroke and palpate his testicles, apply finger pressure onto his perineum, or press or stroke around his anus. Try it and check out his responses.

use firm pressure

A mistake that women often make when masturbating their partner is to use only light pressure because they are afraid of hurting him. Most men, however, prefer a firm strong grip on the penis, and fairly vigorous strokes. He may have particular preferences on how he likes the pace of masturbation to progress; whether he likes to start off slowly and then speed up, or enjoys to tease himself towards an orgasm by taking the heat off just before the ejaculatory process begins and then resume his strokes. He can also show you exactly where the most erogenously sensitive parts of his penis are and which areas respond most to your touch. By clasping your hand over his while he masturbates, you can learn exactly what brings him the most pleasure.

masturbating the female partner

Start by stroking, gently rotating and vibrating the flat of one hand over the whole of her vulva, applying some pressure from its heel onto her pubic bone. You should aim to get her love juices to flow, so remember to caress her whole body, giving loving attention, especially, to her breasts.

Do not zone in right away on her clitoris, and then rub away madly. If you do, you will irritate her, and make this delicate organ feel bruised and sore. Also, remember that she needs to be well lubricated when you are stimulating her clitoral area. Use your finger to gently spread some of her vaginal juices around and over her clitoris. You can also use a little saliva or a drop of KY jelly as a lubricant, but most exciting would be to moisten her with your tongue.

Softly but deftly explore her vulva with your fingers, parting its lips gently and stroking the tip of a finger all around them, and then rub your finger back and forth just above the clitoris. Your middle finger, pointing downwards, is the one long enough to easily stroke over her clitoris, while its tip can gently massage inside her vagina.

Give to her the pleasure she is able to create for herself, applying your strokes with the motions, pressures, and rhythms you have seen her use. Let her guide you with her pelvic movements, and her sighs of delight. Build up your pressure slowly and remember, if she climaxes, to sustain it for the duration of her orgasmic contractions. If the rhythm is wrong or pressure is reduced during these precious moments, you can interrupt the full intensity of her orgasm.

BELOW | Lay your hand gently over hers as she continues to touch, rub and vibrate her fingers against her vulva and clitoris. Try to imagine that your hand is hers, but let hers lead yours in movement and rhythm. Notice how she not only stimulates the clitoris directly, but also strokes her fingers over its surrounding areas and caresses her labia and vagina.

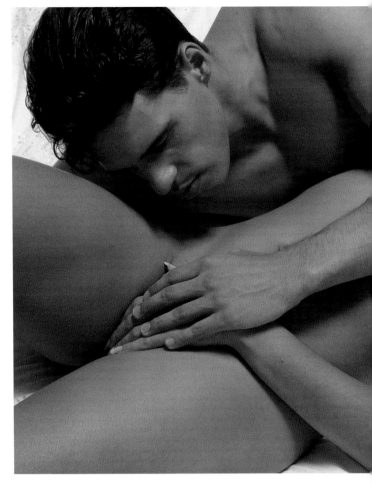

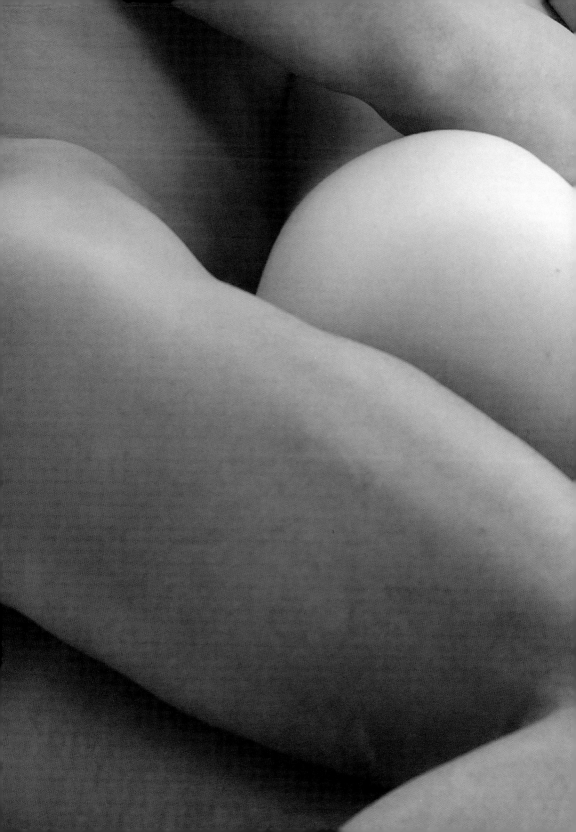

adventurous positions

As a couple achieve greater sexual harmony by becoming more in tune with their partner's body and sexual responses, they will want to push back the boundaries of sexual expression and explore new routes to erotic rapture. This is an age-old quest, and past masters of the sexual arts devoted lifetimes to discovering numerous postures and positions that offer men and women new experiences of sexual intensity and orgasmic joy. But other, much simpler forms of sexuality can also provide powerfully new erotic experiences, such as allowing your partner to share your innermost sexual fantasies, or even acting them out yourself. Finding ways to enhance the full range of the skin's exquisite sensitivity, or just yielding to the animal passion of the moment, can take you to different states of sexual bliss. Whichever route you choose, you will soon discover that the sensual body is an unbounded playground of sexual delights.

adventurous lovemaking

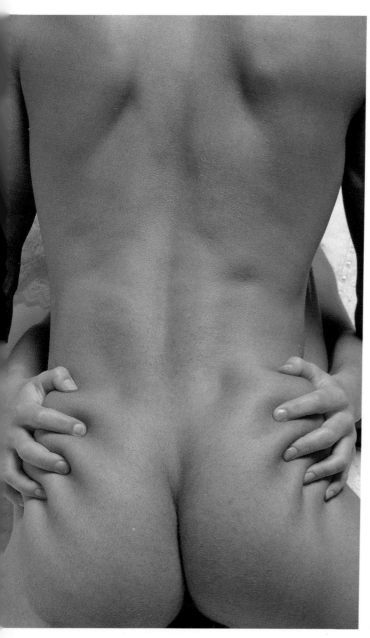

THERE IS NOTHING NEW ABOUT adventurous sexual positions, despite the plethora of advice that is currently in vogue. Sexual imagery is often found on ancient Roman and Greek pottery and detailed texts and manuscripts on the best ways to achieve sexual happiness, and explicit descriptions on sexual positions and practices have appeared in many ancient cultures, including India, China and the Middle East. Some of these texts dealt with the pursuit of sensual and erotic pleasure, others were medically informed scripts to help couples achieve sexual health and happiness, and some referred to sexo-yogic practices through which men and women could attain a higher spiritual state of consciousness.

The Kama Sutra of Vatsyayana, which was written in India in about the fourth century AD, is one of the most famous of the texts giving frank and exact advice on how to achieve sexual fulfilment. The first English version of the Kama Sutra was translated from Sanskrit by the Victorian explorer Sir Richard Burton in 1883, and privately printed for The Kama Sastra Society of London and Benares. At that time, this organization was devoted to the acquisition and translation of important and historical texts dedicated to the subject of erotic love.

It was not until 1964, however, that the text was widely published in the West, when its forthright descriptions of the sexual behaviour of the Indian bourgeoisie of an earlier era caused a considerable stir among the public. In particular, its ample detail of a variety of erotic practices and sexual positions really excited the readers' imaginations. The publication of the Kama Sutra during the 1960s was one of the many events of that decade that heralded a more open attitude to sexuality.

LEFT | Find the positions that give you both most pleasure.

The work is based on the principle of kama, or desire, which is the celebration of the physical senses and the longing for love. In a spiritual context, this can be perceived as the human yearning to be united with the Divine.

It is the section on sexual union, however, which has spanned the divide of culture and history to become meaningful and relevant to modern readers. *The Kama Sutra* does not shrink from an explicit discussion on sexuality, even though it embraces the social mores of its time, some of which may seem alien to the contemporary reader.

It talks candidly about every aspect of erotic behaviour, including how to touch and caress, the art of kissing, biting and scratching, varying sexual positions, themes of domination and submission, and oral and even anal sex. This is not a text book for the inhibited, or for puritans, or those who are content with the missionary position for sex.

It encourages its readers to explore every aspect of their sexuality, from their bestial instincts to their more sensitive and tender expressions of sexual love. It impresses upon men the importance of satisfying a woman sexually, speaks of woman-on-top positions, and comments that the use of certain types of sexual behaviour should "…generate love, friendship, and respect in the hearts of women".

exploring variety

To describe lovemaking positions with the kind of practical detail that appears in this section of the book necessitates adopting a somewhat clinical approach to the subject, and this has the unfortunate tendency of divorcing sexual activity from its wider context of affection, intimacy, tenderness and passion. By discussing movements, angles of penetration and the various techniques of arousal for either partner, it inevitably risks reducing the wonder of making love to that of a how-to guide perhaps more in keeping with a gymnastics or keep-fit manual.

No one can tell two people what is the correct way for them to have intercourse – lovemaking is their own personal act of creativity and an expression of their emotional, psychological and physical make-up. How a couple want to make love, or what they require from a sexual relationship, depends on the needs of the individual or the relationship. Those needs can change from day to day, year to year or from one partnership to another. Telling someone how best to achieve an orgasm cannot possibly address the complex emotions which are also integral to every person's sexuality, or even touch on the shared vulnerability and love which is surely the essence of a truly fulfilling sexual relationship.

Yet in even the most loving partnerships, certain patterns can set in which make the sexual relationship repetitive and eventually boring. Exploration and variety can be as much an enhancement to a sexual relationship as any other aspect of a creative life. Then there are simple physical facts about sexuality that people may simply not know or fully understand because it is often difficult or embarrassing to talk about the nitty-gritty details of sexual performance.

So, for instance, a man could regard himself as an experienced lover, yet despite his Olympian efforts in bed, still fail to satisfy his partner sexually because the positions he favours do not provide the stimulation she needs to achieve an orgasm. The woman, herself, may not understand exactly why she has been unable to reach her peak of arousal, for she may be attracted to her partner and even enjoy those same positions for all the other emotional feelings they provoke.

Examples of this are the various positions shown here where the woman's legs are vertical and resting on the man's shoulders. This position can be exciting for them both, because the man feels powerful and potent, while the woman may enjoy the sensation of surrendering her body to his thrusts. Yet this position precludes the possibility of her receiving direct clitoral stimulation, and is unlikely to lead her to orgasm, so it is not an ideal one to continue for any length of time. Knowing about the subtle variations of position gives partners a greater range of choices and also more understanding of how to fulfil their own and each other's overall sexual and emotional needs.

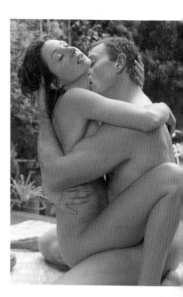

ABOVE | Orgasm has often been described as a potentially transforming experience and it can be even more intense and exhilarating if your lovemaking is in an unusual place.

sitting positions

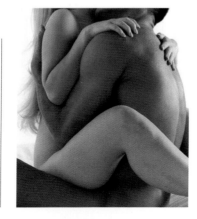

RIGHT | Sex in a sitting position is very loving and reassuring as there is plenty of skin contact and lots of opportunities for cuddling, kissing and caressing.

BELOW | Sitting position 1. Leaning back from each other allows greater freedom of movement and also provides exciting visual impact.

THIS SET OF POSITIONS is very intimate, allowing for lots of kissing and caressing. The movements are limited, but there is no need to rush so you can spend time perfecting them. They allow the woman to rock back and forth and thus to stimulate her clitoris. Why not try placing the chair in front of a mirror, so that you can watch yourselves? Some people find this very erotic.

basic sitting position

The man is sitting up with the woman on top – her legs wrapped around him. Initially, if the woman sits slightly away from the man, she can stroke his penis and he can stimulate her clitoris and caress her breasts. When he enters, they can rock their way to an orgasm.

PLUS POINTS This is a very easy way to introduce an element of variety. Circular movements work well. It is a really intimate position, a little like giving each other an extra special hug.

MINUS POINTS With so much body contact, unless you're outdoors you can become very sweaty on a hot day.

sitting position 1

The woman sits on the man's thighs, as he leans back. She puts her arms behind her, leaning back to support herself. Timing is of the essence here, as the woman raises her body up and down and her partner joins in with smaller thrusts. You can tease each other by looking, because you can't touch – unless you sit up slightly and take each other's hands. And you can both see the penis as it goes in and out.

PLUS POINTS Visual stimulation scores highly in this position for both partners. The hands-off effect is really tantalizing.

MINUS POINTS It can take some practice – not exactly a hardship – to get the timing synchronized.

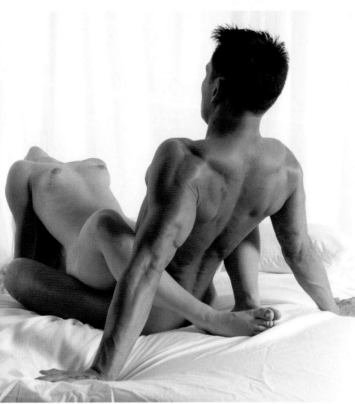

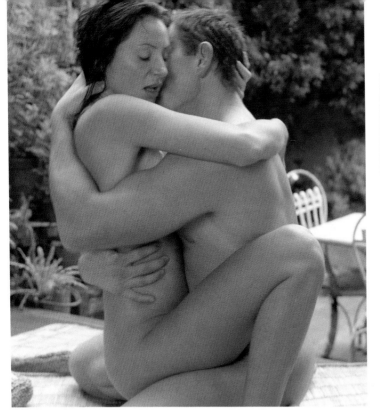

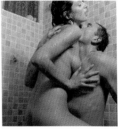

LEFT | Sitting position 2. Enjoy sitting out in the garden on a balmy evening, as long as you're not overlooked.

ABOVE | Sitting position 2. If you have a strong seat in the shower, use it.

BELOW | Sitting position 2. Chairs are great for this position. Rock back and forth, but be careful not to tip over.

sitting position 2

The woman is more in control in this one. If she places her feet flat, she can easily push herself up and down. Rotating the hips and making circular motions are excellent for clitoral stimulation. If you are on the floor raise yourself up with your legs and pause momentarily, then go down on to his tip and come up again before he has entered you.

The man can thrust upward at the same time, but it may take a while to get the timing right together. Since penetration will be quite shallow, experiment with the angles. He can also explore her upper body with his tongue. This is a lovely position for hugging, kissing and full body contact.

PLUS POINTS Great for women who like to be in charge. This is a good position for varying the location – from the garden to the office, on a chair or on the floor.

MINUS POINTS This position is slightly difficult for short women, but placing the feet on the rungs of the chair can solve the problem.

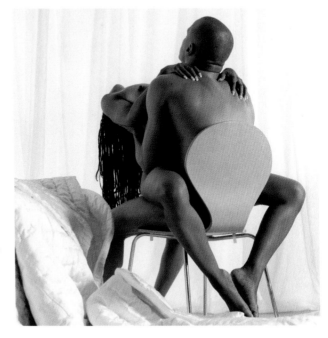

sitting position 3

In this position, the woman squats on her lover's thighs as he kneels and supports her buttocks and back with his hands. The position itself does not allow for a great deal of movement, and is more often used in between other manoeuvres, or when the couple need to find a more restful connection during intercourse. Yet it can create a very profound feeling of intimacy and bonding between both people, allowing them to have close eye and body contact. Holding each other, and breathing together, can be emotionally fulfilling. It can also transform the excitement and passion of lovemaking into a more meditative quality of deep merging and union of mind, body and spirit.

BELOW | Sitting position 3. In this position the man's knees are together.

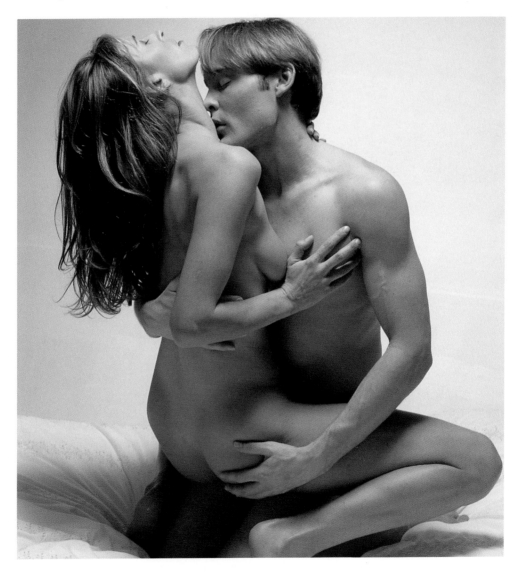

PLUS POINTS The man can take a more active role in this position.

MINUS POINTS The woman cannot maintain this position for long.

synchronized sexuality

While making love in the sitting position, more movement can be attained if the couple separate their bodies, leaning back and supporting their own weight on their arms and hands. The woman can use the strength in her leg muscles to lever herself up and down on the shaft of the penis, and the man can thrust into her. Movements should synchronize, or be made by one or the other partner. The more separated position of the bodies also enables the man to stimulate the woman's clitoris with his fingers.

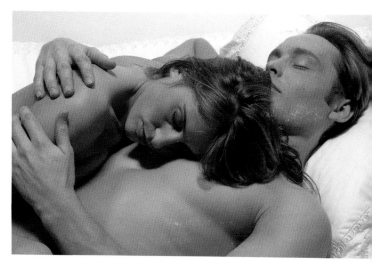

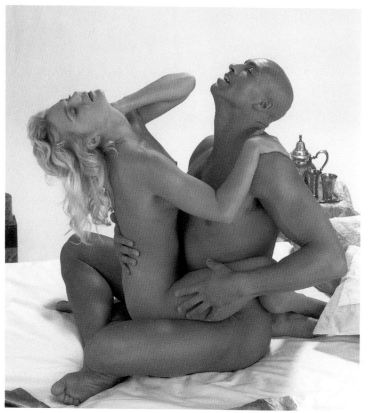

ABOVE | Harmonious lovemaking can draw the man and woman into a deep sense of joyful union, from which arises a profound feeling of peace and inner integration. Wrapped in each other's arms, they may want to just lie quietly together in a state of blissful repose.

LEFT | Here the woman is sitting in her partner's lap, with her legs wrapped around his back, and gently moves her pelvis as she enters into the state of sexual ecstasy.

meditative sex

The sitting position for lovemaking is popular for its particular ability to enhance a meditative sexual mood. It can be used while the couple remain on the bed, or chairs or the edge of the bed can be utilized to make it more comfortable for posture and movements. The following examples show the many diverse ways to adapt this particularly sensual and relaxed form of making love.

When making love on a chair, the vertical posture of both partners enables them to relax deeply and bond emotionally and physically. They can embrace each other closely so their bodies are in intimate contact. This position is not chosen for vigorous movement, but more for slow, sensual and tender sex. As the man holds his partner tight to his body, he can lovingly kiss her neck.

Making love whilst seated can also become very still and meditative, and the couple can sometimes just hold each other closely, harmonizing their breathing and even allowing their bodies to rock and sway gently together, but

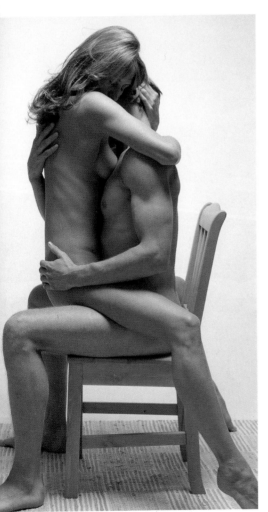

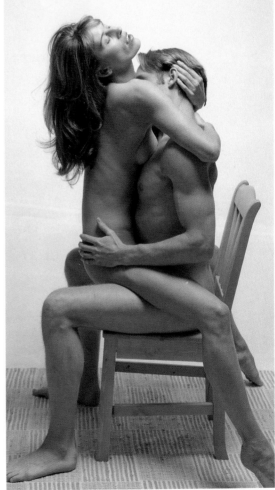

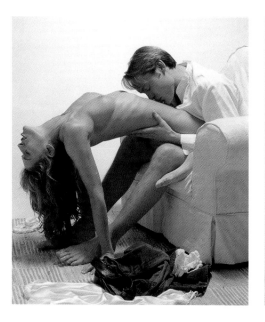

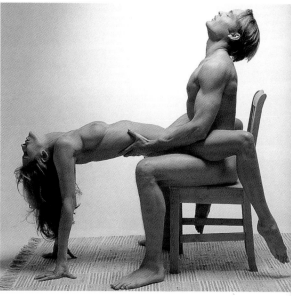

without excitement. During these quieter moments of lovemaking, if the man's penis becomes softer, the woman can tighten her thighs or her pelvic and vaginal muscles to create just enough pressure and friction to keep it erect. Intimacy here is much more important than excitement.

changing angles

If she is supple and confident enough the woman can slowly lean backwards so that her hands reach to the floor behind her while she is secured by her partner's hold. The angle of her pelvis will enable the erect penis inside her to put sustained pressure on the front wall of her vagina and G spot. The exposure of her body and genitals will be sexually exhilarating to them both visually and physically.

The bow-shape of the woman's body as she leans back against the support of her partner's thighs while kneeling astride him in an armchair, will, like the previous position, open and expand her lungs, diaphragm and abdomen so that she can breathe deeply. This will help her whole body to become charged with vibrant sexual energy.

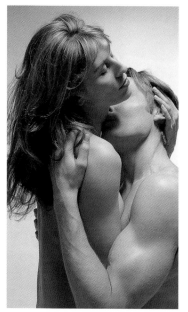

These positions are quite physically challenging so you may not be able to stay in them for very long, but they will add excitement to your lovemaking.

ABOVE LEFT | In an armchair the woman can wiggle her hips so that her vulva rubs against her partner's body. The man can lean forwards to kiss and lick her belly, which will increase the intensity of her sensations.

ABOVE | If the woman can relax into this position, the effort will be worthwhile.

LEFT | If both partners are sitting vertically, the man can caress his lover's neck.

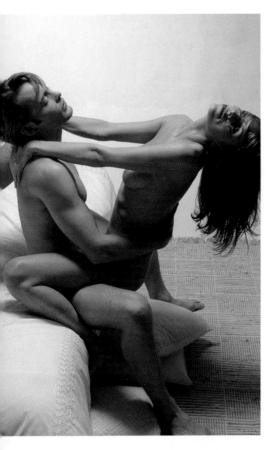

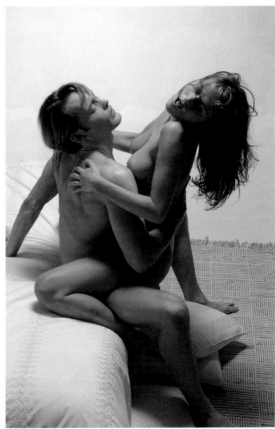

ABOVE AND RIGHT | The man
uses his feet and hands to
balance himself and his
partner even when she is
fully aroused.

taking it further

The sitting posture of lovemaking can be one of a
whole variety of positions which a couple adopt
during a period of coitus to express the wide range
of shifting emotional and physical sensations that
sweeps through them. By using the edge of the
bed for a sexual sitting position, the couple can
become more active and passionate than in other
sitting situations which are more conducive to
meditative lovemaking. Here, the man can
balance himself with his feet and hands while the
woman is astride his lap, enabling her to move
more freely without fear of toppling them both
over. Perching on the edge of the bed while
making love in the sitting position will enable the
man to place his feet firmly on the floor so that

the couple have better support and balance if
their movements become more abandoned. The
woman can grip the man's shoulders firmly, and
while leaning her body away from her partner,
can gyrate her pelvis vigorously back and forth to
create strong sensations of friction.

Pressing one hand against the mattress for
additional support, the man can clasp his partner
close to him with his other hand, while rocking
his hips back and forth. He should co-ordinate his
thrusts to move simultaneously with the woman's
motions, which are made by her levering herself
up and down from flexed knees. When the
woman lets go fully into her sexual energy, she
may also begin to toss her head and neck from
side to side.

easing down

This sexual position follows on naturally from when the woman is sitting astride her partner's lap in the sitting position on the bed. She can then slowly and gently relax back, using her partner's grip to ease herself down gracefully, even while his penis is still erect inside her. Then, with some careful manoeuvring, she can bring the leg that was lying across his thigh to rest beneath it.

If the man lies back on the bed after his partner has done so, the couple's position falls into a cross-shape, and they can engage in a very relaxed form of lovemaking which will, at the same time, keep them both in a high state of arousal. By moving their hips around, they will receive adequate friction to keep them both stimulated, but they will also be able to rest before resuming a more active position.

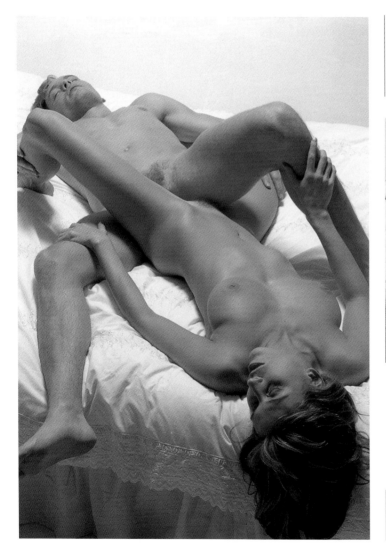

LEFT | In this comfortable position, the woman can move her hips from side to side to stimulate her clitoris.

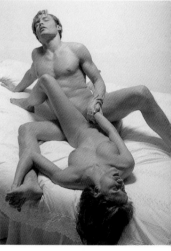

BELOW | When they are ready to change positions again, the man sits up and then pulls his partner upwards and they can continue with other movements.

kneeling positions

BELOW | The man controls both rhythm and depth of penetration. The woman can create even greater pleasure by clenching the muscles of her buttocks and vagina to squeeze his penis – a delicious sensation for both partners.

THESE POSITIONS ALLOW the man to control thrusting in and out of his partner. While they are close and intimate because you are facing each other, they are physically harder for both partners and need determination and knowledge of each other's movements. You have to be reasonably agile for these positions, with good knees, so make sure you have plenty of pillows around.

basic kneeling position

The man kneels on the bed leaning over the woman, as she lies flat. He places his hands under her bottom to lift her on to him. Her legs are bent, with her feet flat on the bed, and her back is arched. He has a full view of her body and, with plenty of eye contact, this is the perfect opportunity for talking dirty and discussing fantasies.

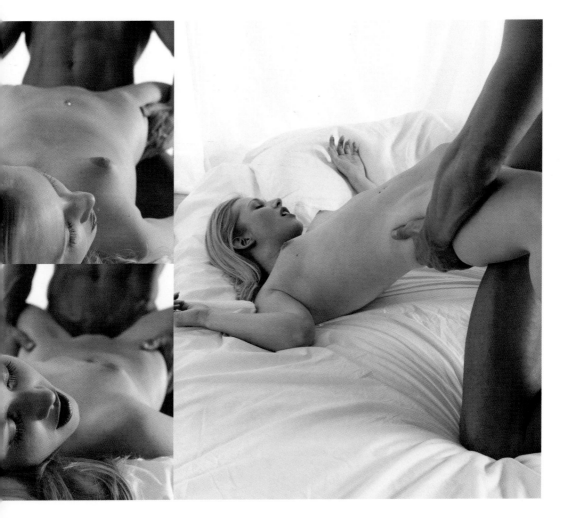

PLUS POINTS Penetration can be as deep or shallow as you like, as it is easy to vary depth and pace.

MINUS POINTS The man may find it difficult to support his partner's weight and penetrate her without shunting her across the bed.

kneeling position 1

The man sits on his heels on the bed. He lifts the woman on to him as she pushes herself up with one hand behind her on the bed, and the other holding on to his neck. He holds her buttocks with one hand and her back with the other, supporting her. This is quite a tiring and athletic pose, and would probably be best for quick sex. Again, there is plenty of opportunity for eye contact.

PLUS POINTS Deep penetration and clitoral stimulation mean both partners are rapidly aroused, so this is a great position for those times when you just can't wait. You can do this almost anywhere private, not just the bedroom – and a comfortable floor offers extra support.

MINUS POINTS He needs to be quite strong, but it helps if she takes some of her own weight on her hand.

kneeling position 2

The woman sits on a chair. The man kneels in front of her, holding her waist, and the woman's legs are wrapped around his waist. (There may be a problem with getting the heights right on this one, so choose a chair or footstool that is the right height and come forward slightly on the chair.)

This is a very sexy pose if you manage to do it right. The woman can lean backwards to facilitate entry, holding on to the man's neck. The man can put his hand on the chair to help steady his partner and can also reach his partner's breasts and clitoris to stimulate them.

PLUS POINTS This is a perfect position for making love quickly with your clothes on.
Penetration is deep – deeper if she places a leg over one of his shoulders.

MINUS POINTS Hard on his knees, but great for her.

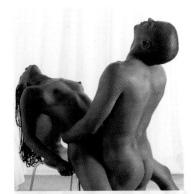

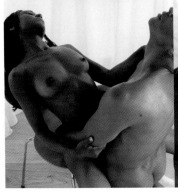

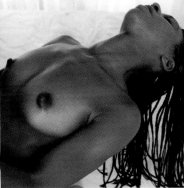

LEFT AND BELOW | Kneeling position 2. The woman's legs can wrap around his body, or stay firmly on the floor if the chair is not too stable.

kneeling position 3

The man kneels back on his heels on the bed with the woman kneeling on top with her knees on either side of his. It may be easier if she raises one leg, placing her foot flat on the bed. She has her arms around his neck and his arms are around her waist. The man should thrust up and down. This is very intimate and erotic and you can stay in this position for a long time. This is a terrific position for fondling the woman's breasts, rubbing the man's back and stroking his neck, nibbling each other's ears and a long, delicious kiss.

PLUS POINTS Unlike most kneeling positions, this is a good position for prolonged sex, although it's also great for a quickie, as penetration is very deep.

MINUS POINTS Cramp in the leg muscles can bring proceedings to an abrupt halt.

mix and match

Kneeling positions are wonderfully adaptable and you can move very easily from one to another – from a gentle, relaxed pose, such as kneeling position 3, to a more urgent and physically demanding one, such as kneeling position 1. Moving from most kneeling positions to rear entry or man on top are other options.

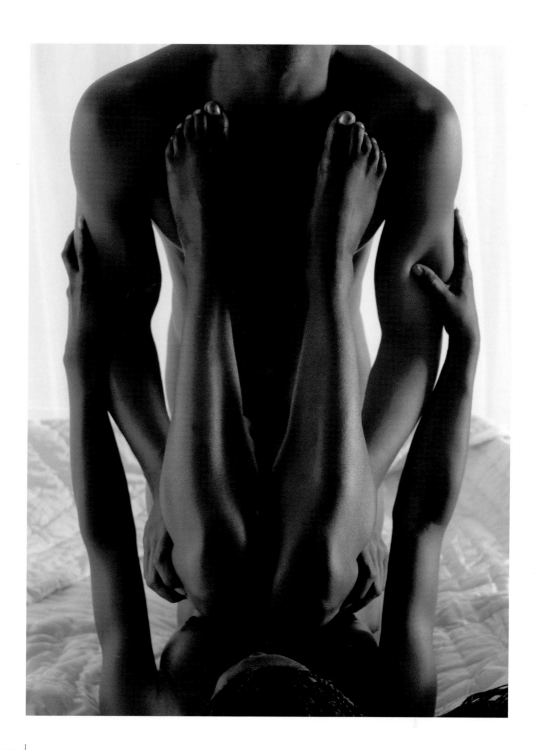

kneeling position 4

The man kneels back on his heels with the woman's legs wrapped around his neck or up on his chest. She lies back on some pillows. The man can lean forward and caress her breasts and nipples. If the woman has her legs wrapped around his neck, this is perfect for deep thrusting as they will be wide open and her partner has a great view of the penetration and can play with her clitoris. If her feet are resting on his chest, this will make her vagina feel tighter, as if gently gripping his penis.

PLUS POINTS If you are both quite fit and strong with well-toned muscles, this position is intensely thrilling. This is great for women who really relish feelings of passionate sexual abandonment.

MINUS POINTS This can strain the woman's back and demands muscular strength from the man.

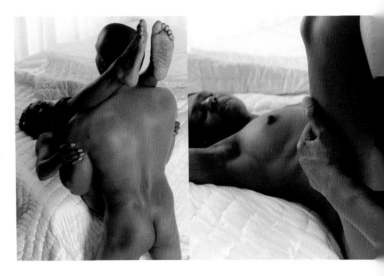

bed versus floor

Whatever the position, you don't have to limit your location to the bedroom, but kneeling positions are favourites for sex on the floor in other rooms. This is often for the purely practical reason that the floor offers greater resistance than the softer, springier bed, so you are more stable and less likely to topple over – a real risk with some of the more demanding and vigorous positions. The disadvantage is the same thing, the hardness of the surface. It's not always noticeable at the time, but afterwards you may find aching knees and, in several positions a sore spine, a high price to pay. Even thick carpet provides only limited protection and can, in any case, cause painful friction burns. It takes only a few seconds to grab some pillows or cushions. It's even better if you fetch a quilt from the bedroom. Not only does this provide some comfortable padding, you can wrap yourselves in it afterwards for cosy, post-coital intimacy.

kneeling position 5

The man kneels on the floor, and the woman lies down on the bed or a couch or sofa. She puts her legs up against his chest, making sure she is right at the edge of the bed. The man holds the woman's buttocks and pulls them towards him as he gently enters her. It is essential that there is a carpet or quilt on the floor to protect the man's knees.

Here, the man has the opportunity for deep penetration and both partners can watch his penis thrusting in and out. He also has a great view of her breasts and can lean forward to massage and fondle them if he is agile. All the woman has to do is lie there, watch his face as he builds up to orgasm, and enjoy.

PLUS POINTS This is great for those who love the sensation of deep, powerful thrusting.
Sex in this position can be fast and urgent or prolonged and intimate, depending on your mood.
It is highly arousing visually.

MINUS POINTS This is not ideal for women who like to be in at least partial control of the action.
As with all positions where penetration is very deep, it is important that the man is sensitive to the possibility of causing his partner discomfort.

OPPOSITE | Kneeling position 4. Simply by moving her feet from his chest to behind his head creates all sorts of utterly delicious sensations.

ABOVE | Kneeling position 5. She wriggles right to the edge of the bed, but he must hold on tight, otherwise you may both end up in an untidy heap on the floor.

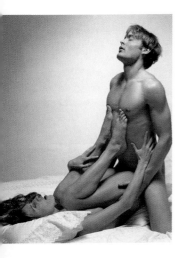

kneeling position 6

This position offers a fun and unusual opportunity for role-reversal. Here, the man lies on his back with his knees drawn up and his legs raised so that he is assuming a position viewed more typically as a female one. The woman lowers herself on to his penis carefully, making sure its angle is right and that she does not bend it awkwardly by moving too quickly. She squats, so the backs of her thighs rest against the backs of his, but she supports her weight on her feet, and uses her legs as leverage to move up and down, or she can wiggle her hips from side to side. Only a supple man will be able to maintain this position for long, but it will certainly help him to understand a woman's perspective of the submissive role.

The woman's body becomes even more compact if she draws her knees towards her breasts and places the soles of her feet on to the man's chest. This position provides little clitoral stimulation as her vulva is lifted away from her partner and her movements are limited. However, she may find the powerful surge of her partner's thrusts very thrilling and be content to submit to a passive role. While the man can enjoy feelings of power and strength as he makes love to his partner like this, he needs to be careful not to penetrate her so deeply or vigorously that he is hurting her cervix. If, in this position, he stops thrusting for a while and leans his body back a little, he can apply an exciting pressure from his erect penis to the woman's G spot.

ABOVE | Total surrender: For deep vaginal penetration, the woman can draw her legs right back into her body, and bend her knees to rest the heels of her feet against his shoulders. The man can then lean into her, pushing her legs even further back, while thrusting his pelvis freely. Again, the woman is able to move very little in this position, but can enjoy surrendering to the thrusting sensations. For easier penetration into the vagina, he can raise her hips by placing a pillow beneath her buttocks.

RIGHT | Kneeling position 6. Here it is the man who lies back on the bed with the woman on top.

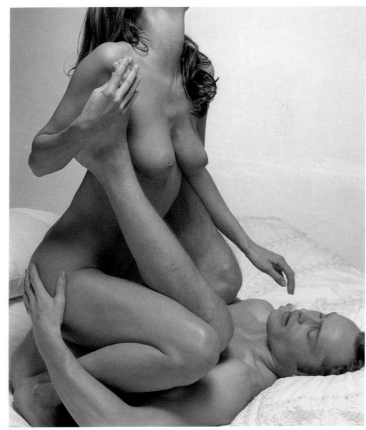

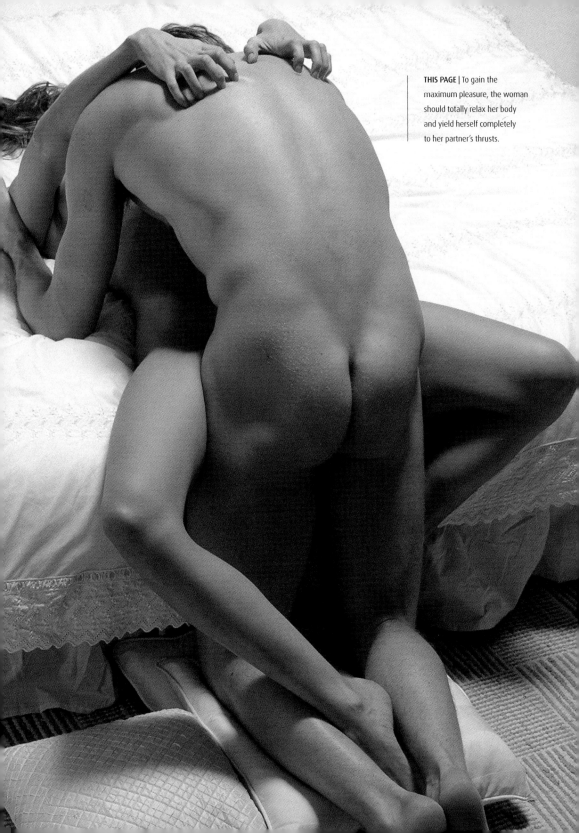

THIS PAGE | To gain the maximum pleasure, the woman should totally relax her body and yield herself completely to her partner's thrusts.

side by side

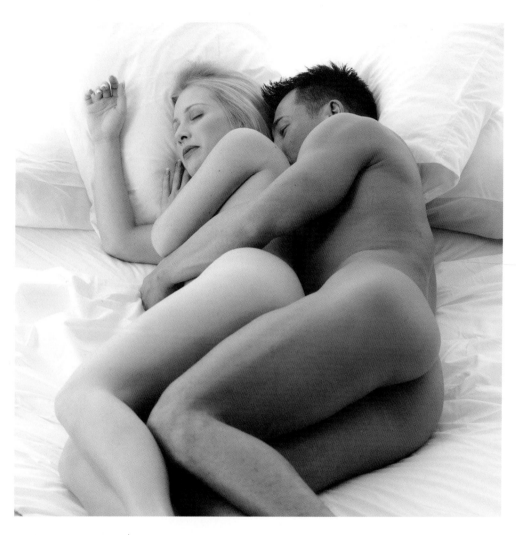

ABOVE | The basic side-by-side position is the most comforting, and so restful that it is easy to fall asleep afterwards without moving.

THIS IS CONSIDERED the least active of the sexual positions. It is perfect to do first thing in the morning when you just want some meditative and relaxing sex, on a lazy, hot afternoon or late at night when you're feeling romantic but sleepy. It is wonderfully cosy and very intimate, with lots of cuddling and caressing. It is good for tired people

and those who aren't very agile. It is difficult for heavily pregnant women to find a comfortable sexual position that is not painful with deep thrusting, so this is a good one for them. It allows for hours of stop-and-go sex, and you can just fall asleep afterwards in exactly the same position, still connected if you are lucky.

basic side by side

Neither of you has to do a lot of work here, but there are infinite possibilities for touching, as your hands are free. The man snuggles up behind his partner as she draws up her knees towards her waist and he slots in behind her. This is pure skin-on-skin contact. He can kiss his partner's shoulders and neck and nibble her ears, while reaching around to cup her breasts. He can also reach down and stimulate her clitoris or alternatively, if there is some lubrication handy, place his finger around or into her anus.

The woman can reach back and massage his testicles or slowly masturbate him between sessions. She can also suck or nibble at his fingers. By lifting her leg over his, she can massage his thigh with the inner surface of hers – a surprisingly sensual sensation.

PLUS POINTS Good for a first-thing wake-up call as morning breath can be avoided.
This position still works if he has only a partial erection.
Great for whispering dirty things to each other.

MINUS POINTS This can be tricky for partners of very different height. The woman will need to bend her knees quite far and arch her back for the man to enter her. Not great for those who like to watch each other's faces.

side by side 1

From the basic side by side position, the man leans back. The woman places her leg over his and leans to a different angle. The man should grip the woman's hips when he enters her. This allows for deeper penetration than the basic position and involves a little more energy. It can feel slightly impersonal as you don't have much body contact apart from the genitals.

PLUS POINTS Women often find the sensation of being gripped firmly as penetration deepens very erotic.
Men often find that feeling their partner's bottom pressed tightly against them is highly stimulating.

MINUS POINTS As you're further apart than the basic position, it is difficult to whisper in each other's ears.

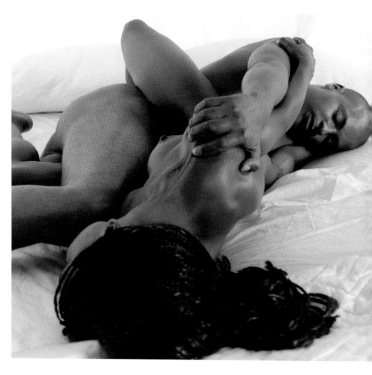

side by side 2

This is a great position for slow sex, but it requires agility and there is some choreography to learn. The woman lies in front of the man in spoons with his penis inside her. Slowly, both partners should lean away from each other with their legs stretched out straight, until their heads are at opposite ends of the bed. They then grab each other's hands or shoulders to prevent themselves coming apart. This position requires both verbal and non-verbal communication and co-ordination in slow movements.

PLUS POINTS Quite different from most other positions, this is good when you want some variety.
The man can watch and play with his partner's bottom, which is erotic for both him and her.

MINUS POINTS Not so great for the unsupple and unco-ordinated, but still worth trying if you share a sense of humour.

ABOVE | Side by side 2. This is also known as position X because of the shape.

BELOW | Side by side 1. Lean away from each other to vary the angles.

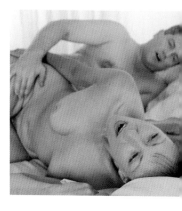

standing positions

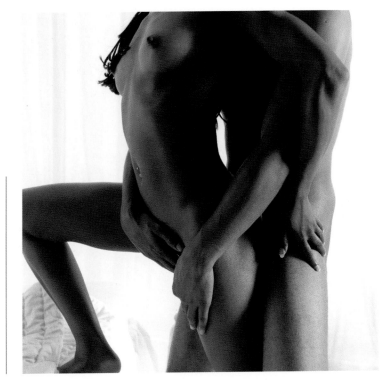

RIGHT | Standing position 3. Unfortunately, standing positions are often neglected in the bedroom in favour of more supine poses, but they may offer considerable scope for variation.

BELOW | Even in the basic standing position, it is easier for the man to enter his partner – and to stay there – if he lifts one of her thighs, supporting it with his hand.

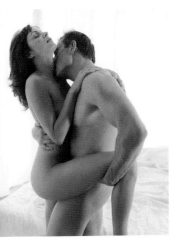

STANDING POSITIONS WORK better if you are both of a similar size, although you can always use the first one or two steps on the staircase to get the height correct. These positions engender very intimate embraces, because you have total body contact and can kiss and caress each other constantly. However, penetration is not very deep.

basic standing position

This is one you see regularly in movies, whether it's in the shower, up against a garden wall, or against a door. It's fantastic for passionate, spur-of-the-moment sex in a place you never expected it to happen. If you're in the shower, before you even start penetration, lather up your hands with soap and wash each other all over, leaving the

pubic area until last, but then rinse thoroughly, as it may sting if used for lubrication. Then the man gently pins his partner up against the wall and enters her, grabbing her by the bottom. She can put her arms either up against the wall for balance or around his neck. He can suck her nipples and breasts and she can massage all down his spine.

PLUS POINTS Spontaneous sex is incredibly erotic, not least because it somehow seems a little naughty. There's plenty of scope for touching, caressing, nibbling, nuzzling, licking and every kind of body contact.

MINUS POINTS Falling over, especially if you are in a slippery shower, is always a risk.
Make sure the shower you are in is structurally stable.

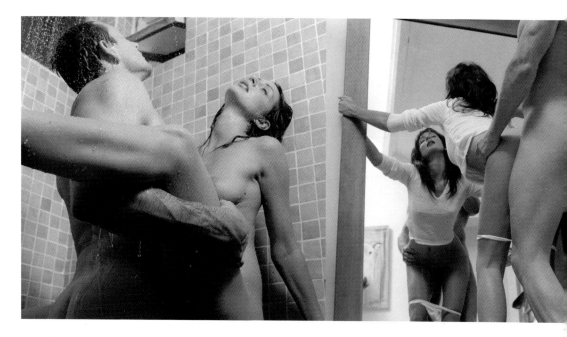

standing position 1

The woman stands with one leg over her partner's forearm or shoulder if she can manage it. A strong grip is needed to keep a balance, so it will be best if the woman has her back up against the wall. This position gives the woman deeper penetration than the previous one, with plenty of opportunity for kissing, licking and general nuzzling.

PLUS POINTS This is a great opportunity for any woman who practises yoga or even went to ballet classes as a child to surprise and delight her partner.

MINUS POINTS Only for the supple – otherwise pulled muscles and/or falling over may occur.

standing position 2

Stand in front of a mirror, so you both have a view of what's going on. The man enters his partner from behind, holding on to her hips. The thrusting will be shallow, so you both might have to lean slightly forward in order to keep the penis inside. The man can nuzzle into his partner's neck and there's plenty of skin contact.

PLUS POINTS An irresistible temptation to talk dirty as well as to watch yourselves.

MINUS POINTS It is quite difficult for the man to prevent his penis from slipping out, so there is not much scope for vigorous movement.

standing position 3

This is another rear entry position. Both stand by the bed (just in case you fall over) with the man holding his partner's thigh, so her leg is lifted and foot resting on the bed – her knee being bent will allow deeper penetration. He lowers himself slightly and enters her from the rear. With one hand free he will be able to offer some clitoral stimulation as well.

PLUS POINTS Because this is more stable than other upright positions the woman has more opportunity to match her partner's thrusts.
He has a hand free for extra caressing.

MINUS POINTS While he can caress her body, she will be unable to reach much of his.

ABOVE LEFT | Standing position 1. Only for the supple.

ABOVE RIGHT | Standing room only for position 2.

dangerous liaisons

Astonishingly, thousands of people each year are, apparently, admitted to A&E (the Emergency Room) with injuries sustained while attempting unusual sexual positions. When trying out exciting new positions with your partner, remember to keep within your limitations and although alcohol may remove inhibitions, it doesn't make you any more flexible, more supple or any younger.

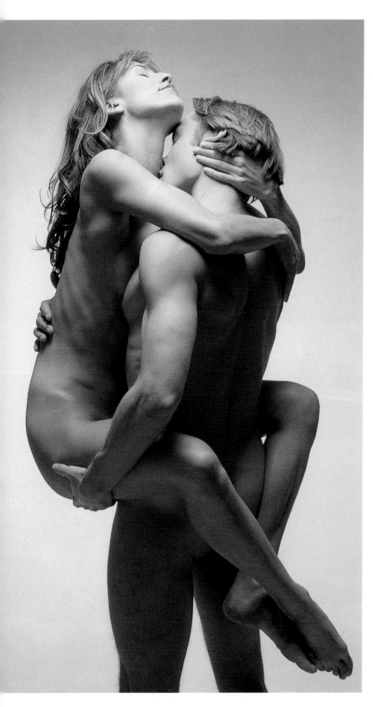

standing position 4

Among the many positions of intercourse suggested by *The Kama Sutra* is the one it calls the "supported congress". This is a standing position in which the lovers support themselves, either against each other, or propped up against a wall. The woman will need to be lighter than her partner if he is to pick her up and hold her securely. She can swing her legs up around his waist and clasp him around the shoulders and neck, while he supports her buttocks and back with his hands.

PLUS POINTS Use it to add variation and adventure to your other lovemaking manoeuvres, rather than as the sole position for intercourse.

MINUS POINTS While this is fun and sensual, it can also become awkward and tiring, especially for the man.

standing position 5

To make the standing lovemaking position a little more acrobatic and adventurous, the woman can lower herself slowly down towards the floor, supporting her upper body with her hands against the ground, while her partner secures her lower back and waist with a firm and secure hold. He can then move her pelvis gently to and fro to create the thrusting sensations. The man should then carefully assist the woman in raising herself upwards, taking care she does not strain her back, or, alternatively, he can slowly and gently sink down on his knees until it is possible to lay her whole back safely against the floor.

PLUS POINTS This is an exciting and unusual sexual position but should only be attempted by those lovers who are supple and fit.

MINUS POINTS This position cannot be maintained for too long before either partner becomes tired.

LEFT | Standing position 4. This position is for the athletic couple, and used only as part of making love otherwise he will get tired.

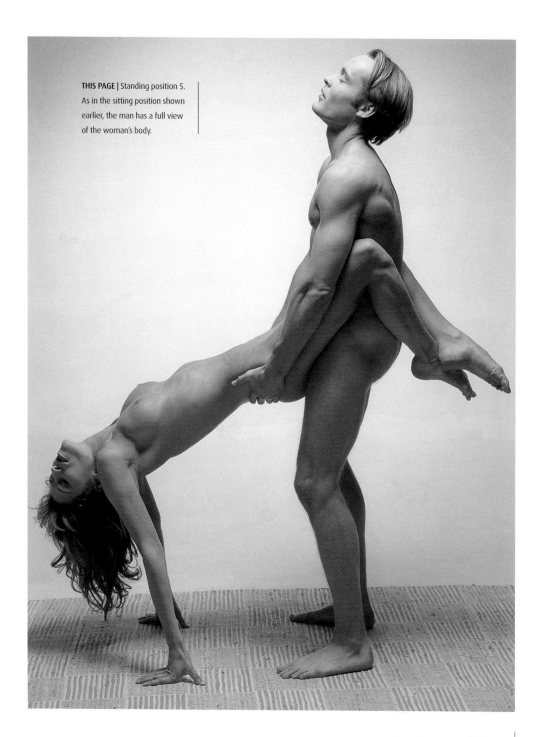

THIS PAGE | Standing position 5. As in the sitting position shown earlier, the man has a full view of the woman's body.

rear entry

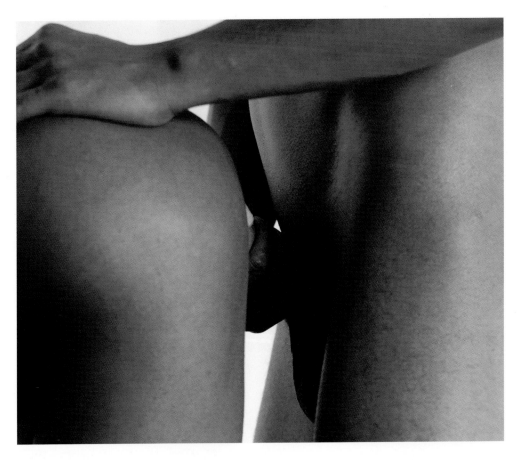

ABOVE | For a quickie, rear entry can be a tremendous thrill, but go gently as penetration can be deep.

ENTRY FROM BEHIND IS FANTASTIC for deep, penetrative sex. The penis is naturally angled to maximize impact for clitoral stimulation, although the woman may still need a little manual assistance, and the man's testicles rub and bounce against the vulva with each stroke, creating a most sensuous feeling for both partners.

Psychologically, some women find these positions difficult, as they have little control over the depth of penetration or the rhythm of the thrusts. A few find the position exceptionally unappealing, as it makes them feel almost like a depersonalized sex object. Rear entry positions can also be uncomfortable, with deep, heavy thrusting, as the penis goes in very deep and hits the cervix. Men should be careful and experiment to see what works without causing discomfort.

In spite of these provisos, these positions can be breathtakingly exciting for both partners, as, with limited visual stimulation, they concentrate physical sensation intensely. Consequently, the pitch of excitement increases very rapidly and orgasm tends to be an even more mind-blowing explosion than usual.

basic position

Sometimes known as "doggy" style, this can be extremely erotic. If you are both on the floor, make sure the carpet is soft, or kneel on cushions.

The woman kneels on the floor or bed on all fours with her arms straight or resting on her forearms. The man kneels behind her, holding her hips or waist. Then he enters her. Men who are shorter than their partners may need to kneel on cushions. Going up on one knee will help raise the level of the penis.

As the woman is being penetrated, she can touch her own clitoris or reach back and stroke the man's testicles. He will love this. He can lean over and fondle her breasts or stimulate her anus with firm finger pressure. (Many women enjoy the sensation of pressure just in front of the anus.). When doing this, he may be able to feel his penis through the wall between anus and vagina. You can use a small vibrator rather than a finger to do this if you prefer, but don't put the vibrator into the vagina until you've washed it.

Linger with the tip of the penis at the opening of the vagina, doing several smaller thrusts before going in hard and deep. If there is sufficient control to do this several times, she'll find this breathtaking and almost unbearably exciting. The natural curve of the vagina fits with the curve of the penis, so deep thrusting is possible.

This is a favourite position during pregnancy, as the "bump" doesn't get in the way. Take care not to cause discomfort with deep penetration, although sex in pregnancy is generally not dangerous.

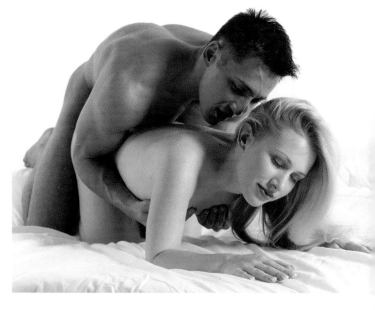

PLUS POINTS Many women love the slightly naughty feeling of being "taken" in this position.

This is great for an intense passionate romp, as both partners are aroused very quickly.

If he kneels up, the man can see his penis moving in and out and has a tantalizing view of his partner's body.

MINUS POINTS Penetration is so deep, it can cause discomfort to the woman.

The woman cannot see her partner's face.

ABOVE | The doggy position can suit your internal shape well, giving opportunities for using the hands as well as deep thrusting. Be sure to use extra-strong condoms here, as the strain may be more than they can normally stand up to.

LEFT | Most men find the sight of their partner's bottom an inspiration for imaginative sex and exciting positions.

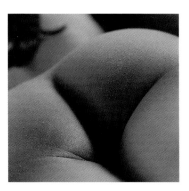

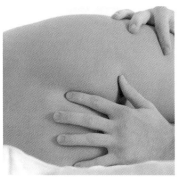

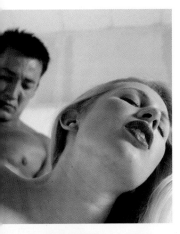

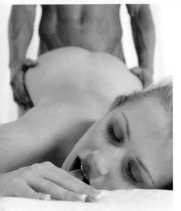

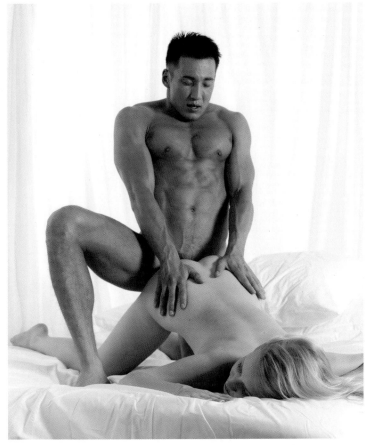

let him know how you feel, as
he cannot see your face.

ABOVE RIGHT | Rear entry 1.
With one of the man's knees
raised, penetration will be
even deeper, so he should
take it easy and be guided by
his partner's verbal and
physical responses.

OPPOSITE | Rear entry 2. Use
pillows to raise yourself up
enough to get the right angle.

rear entry 1

This is like the doggy position, but the woman,
while keeping her bottom in the air, puts her head
on the bed. The man is behind her on one knee,
holding her shoulders or waist. This allows for
even deeper penetration than the traditional
doggy style. She can hook her legs over his,
pulling him into her, and the couple can thrust
simultaneously with a little practice.

PLUS POINTS This takes the weight off her arms so the
woman finds it more relaxing.

MINUS POINTS It can cause headaches or a stiff neck if
the woman is positioned awkwardly.

rear entry 2

Here, the woman lies down flat, legs spread out,
and the man kneels behind her and then lies on
top of her. She needs to raise her bottom high
enough, perhaps with a pillow underneath her.
Penetration will be shallow. However, this position
is very comforting and close, with plenty of body
contact and the opportunity for the man to kiss
and nuzzle the woman's neck and lick her ear lobes.

PLUS POINTS He can whisper dirty things in her ear.
Friction over her buttocks can be a real turn-on for her.

MINUS POINTS As penetration is shallow, there is a risk
of the penis slipping out.

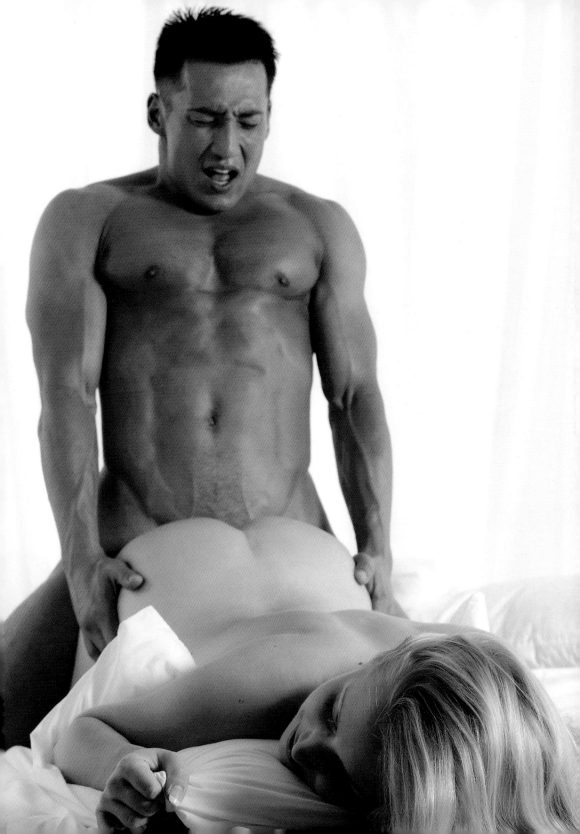

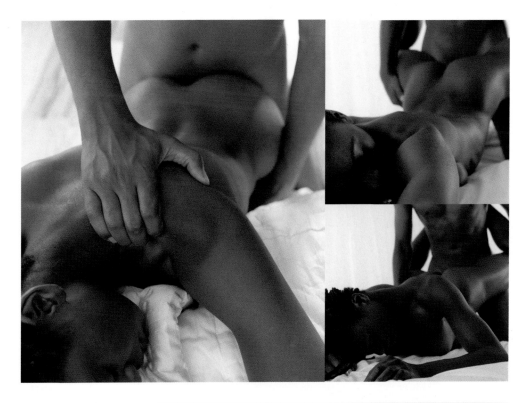

ABOVE | Rear entry 3. This is a variation on the wheelbarrow, with the man kneeling so that most of the woman's weight is taken by the bed.

the thrust debate

Deep penetration can be equally enjoyable for men and women. It can stimulate the female G spot if the correct angle is achieved and men like the sensation of the tip of their penis coming into contact with their partner's cervix.

It's good psychologically too. It makes him feel like a well-endowed stud and it makes her feel that she is so irresistible that he can't control his surging desire for her.

However, shallow penetration can be equally gratifying for both parties. For the woman, the opening of the vagina is rich in nerve endings and for the man, shallow penetration provides constant stimulation of the frenulum and head of the penis, which can be squeezed and stimulated by the muscles at the vaginal opening.

Many couples enjoy shallow penetration that involves rocking together back and forth: it is highly stimulating at the same time as being very relaxing, close and loving.

Partners soon find out what level of thrusting and penetration they prefer and consequently use positions that best suit them. Equally, they will choose a position for deep or shallow penetration depending on their particular mood or sense of sexual urgency. If deep penetration is your thing, plenty of lubrication heightens the experience, especially as many women don't secrete enough naturally.

rear entry 3

This is only for the fit and athletic. The man stands behind his partner and holds her straight legs while she bends forward and supports herself on her hands on the bed or the floor. You will both be more stable on the floor.

This position has a passing similarity to a wheelbarrow race on a children's sports day – with some very obvious differences. You don't have to run your partner around the room – unless you want to, of course – but you do need to have strong arms and she needs to be fairly light.

Once lifted up by the thighs, pull her on to your penis slowly while she supports herself. Neither of you will be able to do anything else with your hands. Unless you are an athlete, this will be a quick one, with vigorous thrusting. If you get into trouble, the woman can rest her legs on the bed or floor. You will have a wonderful view of your partner's bottom and back. There's not a lot the woman can do except enjoy. Lots of laughs are guaranteed.

PLUS POINTS This is great when you are in a really raunchy mood and want to feel like porn stars. Perfecting the technique is fairly tricky, but enormous fun for couples who love to laugh together.

MINUS POINTS This does have to be a quickie, as her arms will begin to hurt quite soon and the blood will rush to her head.

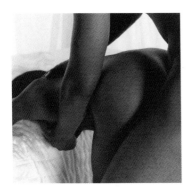

ABOVE | It may be easier for the woman to lean on the bed in this position.

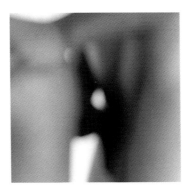

LEFT | Rear entry 3. The man may need some assistance to guide himself in.

BELOW | Rear entry 3. The wheelbarrow may be too strenuous to keep up for a long time. Have a rest and change of angle by both kneeling down, if you can manage it without collapsing in fits of giggles.

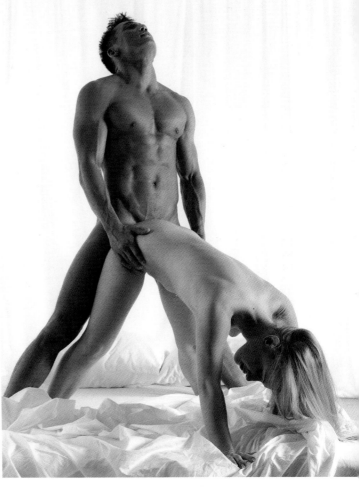

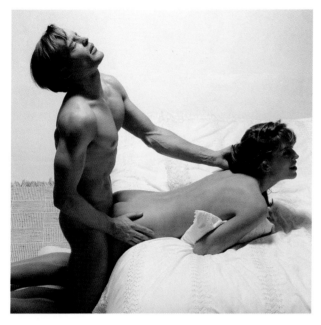

rear entry 4

If the woman kneels on the floor and lays the upper half of her body across the bed, she can position herself comfortably for rear-entry sex, especially if she pads her chest with a pillow. The man then kneels behind her, so the floor gives him some solid support for his movements. If the woman enjoys making love in the "doggy position", she may be aroused by the slightly dominating aspect of her partner and by her own more submissive stance. Although they are not face to face, the man can be very intimate with her body, and can stroke her hair, back, and buttocks easily. He can also lift her away from the bed slightly to fondle her breasts, caress her belly, or to stimulate her vulva and clitoris with his fingers while making thrusting movements.

rear entry 5

An armchair lends itself very well to rear-entry lovemaking, if the furniture is deep enough to

ABOVE | Rear entry 4. Strategically placed pillows are useful in this position.

RIGHT | Rear entry 5. A deep armchair is ideal for a change of venue.

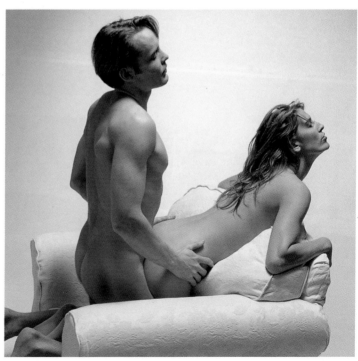

take both partners on its seat. She can lean her body against the padded support of the back of the chair and avoid any feeling of collapsing forward under the pressure of his thrusts. The man can then kneel behind her and, as she leans forward, enter her vagina from the rear position. He can use his hands to stroke and caress her erogenous zones.

rear entry 6

This is another creative and fun way of enjoying rear-entry sex in the comfort of the armchair. The woman starts by kneeling astride her partner's lap but with her back turned to him, and then she carefully guides his penis into her vagina. Once the penis is fully erect, she can then lean forward slowly and support herself by placing her hands on the floor.

The man's movements are restricted, but he can lift her hips up and down with his hands to create more friction, and the woman can also wiggle sexily from side to side to increase the arousal for them both.

rear entry 7

Anatomically, it is obviously not possible for the "doggy position" to be reversed for penetrative sex. The couple, however, can enjoy other thrilling sexual sensations by having the man take the usual female position for rear-entry sex. First of all, he can be aroused by assuming the more submissive stance, while experiencing the sensual feel of his partner's breasts and belly moving against his back. He can wiggle his hips to rub himself against the edge of the bed, while the woman can use her hands to squeeze and pat his buttocks, or stroke and fondle his testicles or the erotically sensitive tip of his penis.

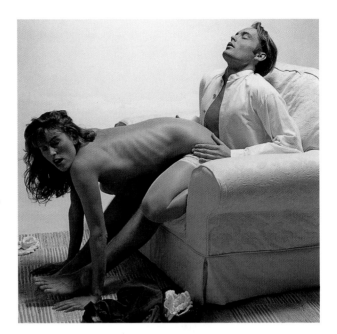

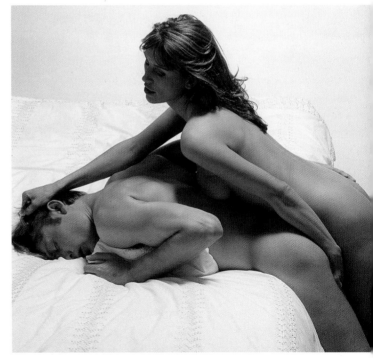

ABOVE RIGHT | Rear entry 6. Another way to use the same armchair.

RIGHT | Rear entry 7. The woman cannot penetrate her partner, but she can arouse him in this position.

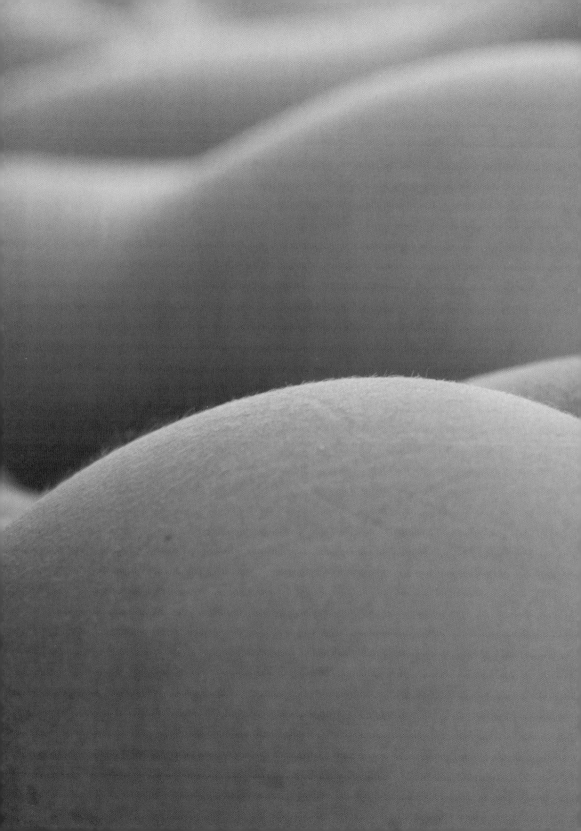

x-factors

There is more to a sensational sex life than vaginal sex, delicious and important though that is. Both oral and anal sex can bring some spice to a relationship, creating unique sensations of extreme pleasure – both when giving and when receiving.

please your partner

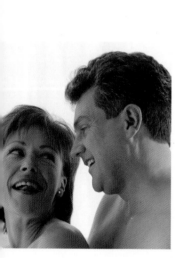

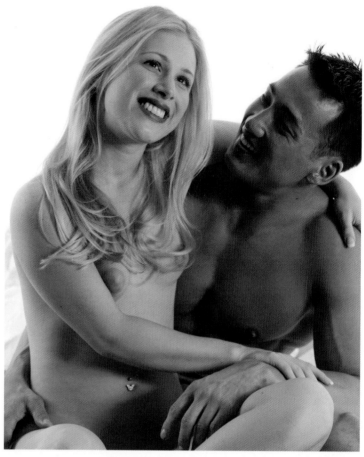

ABOVE LEFT AND RIGHT | The time to discuss more adventurous sexual activities is when you are feeling close, so that you can explore the ideas freely together without anyone feeling that he or she is being humiliatingly criticized or put down.

IN THE LAST FEW DECADES there has been a definite trend towards demystifying sex and dispensing with sexual taboos and many sexual barriers have been broken down by increased information and greater liberation. Masturbation is now considered normal practice, although some women are still only just beginning to feel comfortable admitting to self-pleasure. It's much the same with anal and oral sex. Pleasing your partner with your mouth –

or vice versa – is as natural as doing it any other way. In fact, with the added bonus of that most mobile organ, the tongue, the erotic potential might even be increased.

Sex is all about pleasure and intimacy. If you find pleasure from anal penetration or oral sex, then where's the problem? Equally, if you're not keen, there's no reason why you should feel obliged to include them in your sexual repertoire.

talking about it

Reading about positive aspects of what, in the immediate past, was regarded as a sexual taboo, might well create a desire in you to try it out for yourself. But even the most liberated people sometimes find it tricky to discuss their innermost sexual thoughts with their partner. How, then, do you go further still and raise adventurous topics such as fellatio, cunnilingus and anal penetration?

Perhaps you and your partner already have a great sex life, but you feel there is always time and space to try something new. Whatever your reasons, it may be hard to put them into words for fear that you may offend your lover by making him or her feel inadequate or threatened. You may also be concerned that they may regard you as a little perverted for bringing up the possibility of

more risqué sexual options. The likelihood, though, is that they won't feel anything except excitement at the prospect of jazzing things up.

So where to begin? A straightforward request is probably too blunt and might provoke a straightforward negative reply that closes off that prospect forever. Instead, be a little more subtle and sensitive. If you'd like to explore anal sex, for example, you could take his or her hand during foreplay and gently guide it to your anus. If he or she pulls back in fright or horror, then just smile and explain that you have never done it before and thought it might be fun to give it a try. Don't make a big deal of it and he or she probably won't either. In fact your partner will probably be keen to please you and as curious to try something new as you are, so why not mull it over together?

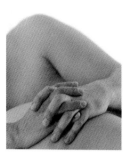

ABOVE AND BELOW | By discussing issues such as oral and anal sex beforehand, you are less likely to hurt each other's feelings and overstep each other's boundaries.

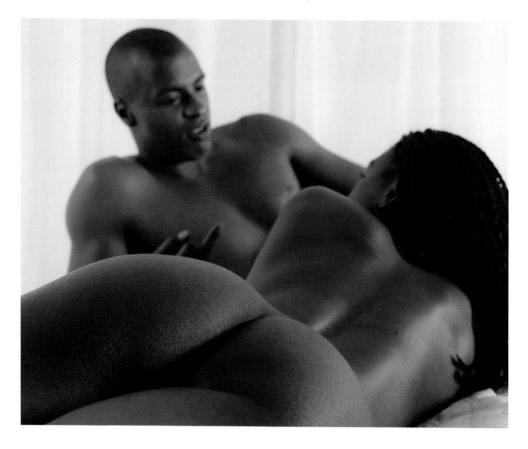

oral sex

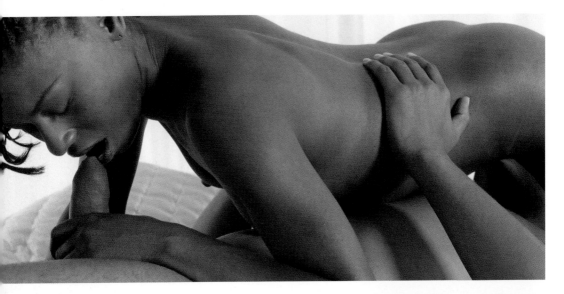

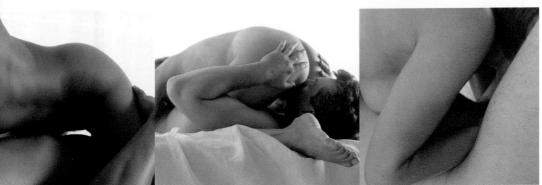

ABOVE | Whatever position you choose, the tongue is an extraordinarily flexible organ and can be made hard or soft. Try it on your hand to vary your technique and then practise on your partner.

THE ACT OF ORAL SEX is an extremely intimate and trusting one in which you invariably find yourself opening up to your partner and allowing them access to your most sensitive and private places. When you think about it subjectively, it is actually quite a bizarre ritual. Licking, sucking, tasting and pleasuring your partner is a very emotional experience that requires commitment, not only to your partner but also to the task in hand. All too many people think of oral sex as a prelude to penetrative sex. In actual fact, it is really a quite separate act. The techniques used for explosive oral sex are extremely different from those of penetrative sex. By refining the art, you can get a greater understanding of your partner's sexual preferences. It is an exciting journey of exploration into your partner's hot spots – a journey that is equally, if not more, exciting for them.

For many people, the difference between being an average and an exceptional lover lies here. Skilful fellatio and cunnilingus – giving good head, providing a great blow-job or going down with the best of them – whatever you call it, is worthy of an award. There is nothing more sensual and pleasurable than lying back and being orally stimulated by a genital genius.

You must remember that tastes – literally and metaphorically – differ tremendously in this department. What may be a great oral sex technique on one individual may be totally inappropriate for another. In order to be a great oral aficionado, the secret is timing, listening and responding. Once again, it's all to do with communication. Take time to do oral sex, and do it sometimes without penetration in mind. Listen to your partner's moans, groans and body movements to work out what is working for them and what isn't. Respond according to what is working and *keep doing it.*

Make it apparent to your partner that you are enjoying yourself too. Oral sex is not something you just do to someone else; you are participating and sharing in the activity and relishing the intimacy, the effects you are having and, in fact, the entire experience. (If you're not, perhaps you shouldn't be doing it at all.) Some people worry that the active partner in oral sex is not getting their "fair share". Sexual pleasure and orgasm are not like a bank balance – you don't have to keep in credit all the time.

soixante-neuf

The 69 is tricky. Many people find it hard to concentrate on stimulating as well as being simultaneously stimulated. It can be difficult for the man to hit the woman's spot in this position, as his chin is stimulating her clitoris. Similarly, it is the less sensitive top side of the penis that receives most stimulation in this position. Height differences can cause problems too, making one partner curl and the other stretch.

So why do it? Well apart from the fact that it is a real giggle, it can also be quite effective. The sight of each other's most private places up so

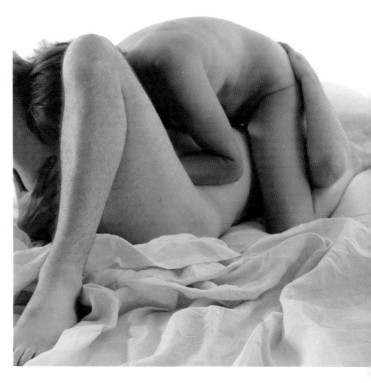

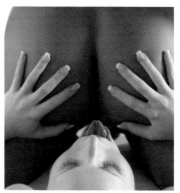

close can prove to be an astonishingly erotic experience. If the woman goes on top, she is more in control and her partner can stimulate her dangling breasts. The man can massage her buttocks – most men find their partners' bottoms arousing – or just concentrate on her genital area.

ABOVE | Soixante-neuf is an expression of ultimate togetherness and complete trust in each other.

LEFT | Rimming is the term used to describe licking around the anus. It is a highly pleasurable experience but as always the area must be scrupulously clean. If rimming a casual partner a dental dam of clear film (plastic wrap) is a good barrier method to prevent contracting sexually transmitted infections.

fellatio

PUTTING YOUR MOUTH around a man's penis requires trust on both sides – you assume that he's washed and that he won't choke you, and he assumes that no biting will be involved, something men commonly have nightmares about. The secret to giving good head is, without a doubt, enthusiasm, but most men agree that the mere idea of a blow-job is a massive turn-on. If you don't want to do it, then simply refrain – a half-hearted effort will disappoint him and make you resentful and there are lots of other delicious things to do. However, if you are willing, it's unfair for him to expect you to do so if he's not prepared to return the compliment himself every once in a while.

BELOW | Fellatio works from any direction. Straddle your partner's chest, for example. He won't be able to see what you are doing, but can enjoy the rear view.

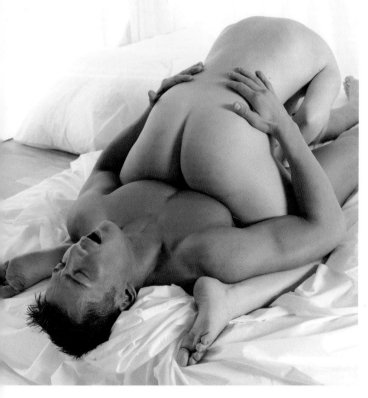

where to begin

The best blow-jobs are those given as a luxurious, time-consuming package. Rather than heading straight for the penis, it's often nice to incorporate an element of anticipation. Lie him flat on his back and begin either at his feet, working up, or at his chest, working down. The secret here is to ignore time and to immerse yourself in both his body and his needs. Sucking toes, licking nipples, massaging his inner thighs and flicking a tongue around his belly button are just some of the delights you can provide for him, but stay away from the genital area to begin with. He will read the road you are following, so as you start to home in towards his groin, he will be almost literally bursting with excitement. Once down there, you can tease him by licking around the outline of his penis on his belly, allowing your breath to pass over it or brushing your lips suggestively over the head of his penis before using direct stimulation.

technique

From this point there are a variety of techniques that you can use. Different men like to be stimulated in different ways, so why not try them all and see which ones he likes the most? You can discuss what his likes and dislikes are or simply read his body. If he's groaning and grinding, then you are on to a winner. If he is quieter or pulling away from you, try something else.

Position yourself so that you are comfortable. Most women like to be between their partner's legs, with him lying back. This positions the tongue so it can easily stimulate the front of the penis, the most sensitive area, and also allows your partner to look down and watch you in action, which will excite him even more.

Use a lot of saliva to lubricate the lower part of the shaft, which you can stimulate with your hands. Wrap your lips over your teeth. The merest hint of anything sharp near a man's penis will have him leaping away from you in fear.

Get your tongue working. Little flicks of the tongue around the head and over the frenulum are very stimulating. Roll your tongue both quickly and slowly around the head and, if you can, use the thin layer of skin that joins your tongue to your mouth to stimulate the frenulum.

The term "blow-job" is really a misnomer, as you don't actually need to blow. As you go up and down the penis, you can create an airtight seal with your lips. This means that as you move up the penis, a vacuum will naturally suck so you don't have to. Use quite a firm grip with your mouth and twist your head around at the same time for added stimulation. Use your tongue too, applying extra pressure or using a quick flicking action.

The head of the penis is often more sensitive in uncircumcised men. You can place the tip of your tongue underneath the foreskin and run circles around the head, or you can pull the foreskin back with your hands by wrapping them around the shaft, just above the base, and pulling down to the base. This exposure heightens sensitivity and will make it more exciting for him.

A good blow-job is a partnership of both the mouth and the hands. While your mouth concentrates mainly on the top end of his penis, your hands can be working on the lower shaft. The

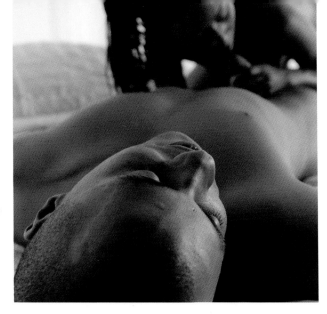

most successful technique is to synchronize your movements, allowing your hands to follow the pumping action of your mouth.

spicing it up

Experimentation with different tastes and textures can spice up a blow-job even more. Try sucking on a mint beforehand. The added ingredient of menthol in your saliva will provide a different sensation on your partner's penis. Sucking ice cubes or licking

ABOVE | Don't neglect his testicles and perineum while you are giving him a blow-job. It will enhance his experience if you gently stroke these areas with your free hand.

BELOW | Sitting or lying down, make sure you are both comfortable before you begin.

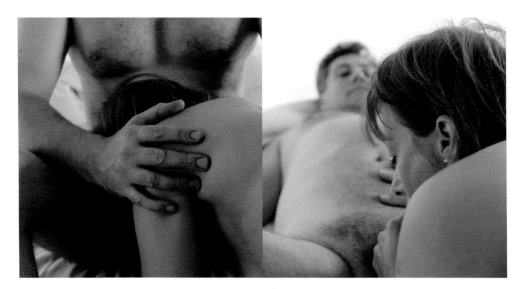

BELOW | In the chair – he sits in the armchair and she kneels on the floor in front of him. This is liable to make him feel like an emperor.

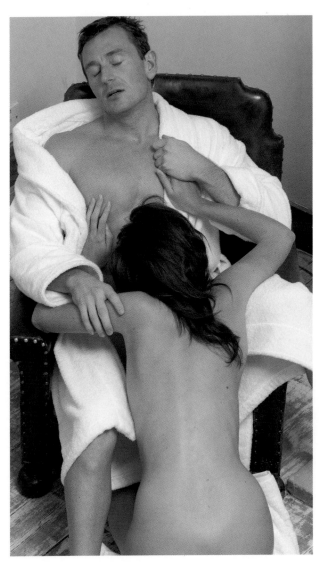

ice cream and then drinking hot drinks also adds variety in the form of hot and cold sensations, but beware of extremes. Your favourite spreads, such as chocolate or jam, can also make it a tastier experience for you and you can have lots of fun with the application.

Some men like to have their prostate or anus stimulated during oral sex and many of them say that orgasm is greatly heightened when the prostate is stimulated at the same time. Using a little lubrication, massage around the area for a while to relax him before gradually slipping in one finger. Once inside, very gently massage the area towards his belly button, taking care not to scratch with your fingernail. Licking around the anus, known as rimming, is also a source of pleasure for some men.

Another technique worth trying is called "flicking". Don't panic – despite the name it's actually a pleasurable experience for him if done properly. During a blow-job, slide the shaft out of your mouth and then flick his penis gently against your cheek or neck a few times; you get a breather and he gets a different sensation.

blow-job basics

edging This is a great move if your mouth needs a bit of a breather. Hold his penis in one hand and place your lips at the bottom end of the shaft on the top side. Use your lips as if you were kissing and create a light suction, then move your mouth and head steadily up and down the shaft, increasing and decreasing the pace. You can use your other free hand to caress the head or glans of his penis at the same time.

rolling This produces a wonderful sensation as it concentrates on the head of the penis, the most sensitive area. Place your mouth over the head of the penis so that it is completely in your mouth. Use your tongue to stroke all around the edges of the head in a circular motion, quickening and lessening the pace and changing direction every now and again. When your tongue passes over the frenulum at the front of the head (facing you) use the bit of skin that attaches your tongue to the bottom of your mouth to stimulate it. You can also

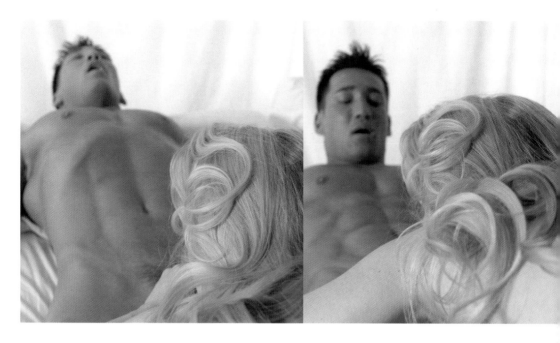

use your tongue to massage the tip, as if you were licking an ice cream.

balling Men's balls are very sensitive and you can give a lot of pleasure by playing with them. Just before a man comes, his balls contract and move up towards to the body to prepare for ejaculation: by gently gripping them at the top and pulling down (gently, gently) you can hold off his orgasm. Putting both his balls in your mouth and sucking them and massaging them with your tongue can produce a wonderful sensation.

pumping Placing your mouth over his penis, form a tight vacuum with your lips, making sure that they cover your teeth to prevent scratching him. Then, using a slight sucking action, move your head up and down the shaft. Keeping your neck relaxed and taking a breath when you get to the top, and breathing out through your nose as you move down the shaft, will help you take more of him in your mouth and prevent you from gagging. Use either one or two hands to follow your mouth up and down the shaft, gripping it as you would a tennis racket. You can have quite a firm grip, the firmer the better.

humming As you are sucking him, try humming or moaning at the same time, as the vibrations from your voice box will penetrate through to his penis and make it more stimulating.

the swallow debate

The pros and cons of swallowing semen are individual to each woman. Some women don't like the idea of it, others wouldn't consider spitting and see swallowing as the ultimate finale. Men's preferences vary almost as much.

Knowing when a man is about to ejaculate can be quite tricky. Things to look for – apart from an obvious screaming announcement – are a tightening of the muscles and increased rate of breathing. His facial expression, if you can see it, is often a giveaway, too.

If you don't want to swallow, you can either withdraw and finish him off with your hand, or you can spit, but do it discreetly, or it will put you both off. Another alternative is to ask him to come on your breasts, which is known as a pearl necklace, or face. Semen is, after all, very good for the condition of your skin.

ABOVE | Decide before you begin giving him a blow-job whether you want to swallow or not. If you don't want to swallow, try not to be too obvious about it; excessive spitting and face-pulling is likely to spoil the whole experience for him.

when to abstain from oral sex

The chapter on Sexual Health explains the risks involved in HIV/AIDS transmission during oral-genital sex practices. If you are unsure about your own or your partner's health, or know little about each other's sexual history, then fellatio should be performed only when using a condom or, in the case of cunnilingus, a dental dam.

You should not participate in oral sex if you have an active cold sore around your mouth, or a genital herpes sore, or any other kind of infection or sexually transmitted disease, until it has been treated and cleared up. Oral sex is not advisable during a menstrual period because of the risk of blood-transmitted infections.

BELOW | Work your way slowly and sensuously down his body towards his genitals, bringing the whole surface of his skin alive with your breath, lips, tongue and touches. Linger over his belly, kissing teasingly around the pubic area, and moving inch by inch closer to his genitals.

concerns and objections

Many couples feel that oral sex is an integral and natural feature of their sex lives and, for some, is the best part of it. Oral sex has always been an option in sexual relationships and is recorded in ancient texts such as *The Kama Sutra*.

However, at different times in history, and in different cultures, it has been considered deviant behaviour. In the early part of the last century a request for oral sex could be considered grounds for divorce. In some states of America it was outlawed. Research now shows that the majority of sexually active people have participated in oral sex at some point in their lives, though statistics indicate that more men than women enjoy it. This may have something to do with the fact that men are not always so skilled in performing oral sex to their women's satisfaction.

Women, too, can have deep anxieties about the smell, taste and appearance of their vaginal area. They may be against the idea of putting the penis into their mouths for fear of choking, or repulsed by the idea of swallowing seminal fluids if the man ejaculates.

Oral sex is a normal, healthy activity in an intimate relationship. However, if you do not want to engage in it, you should not consider yourself lacking or abnormal in any way. It is a very personal choice. You should never try to pressurize your partner, or be forced against your will into performing or receiving oral sex, or any other sexual activity, if either one of you objects, even if you participate in it on some occasions but are just not in the mood right now.

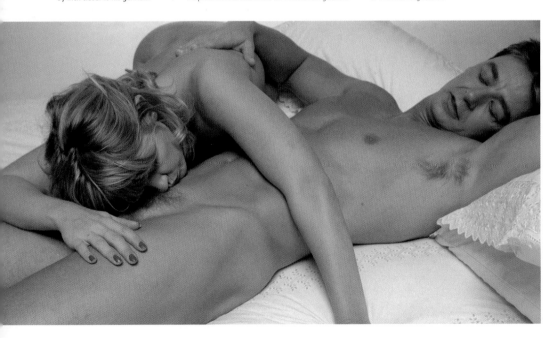

It is an extremely intimate activity, and should only be performed with total mutual consent. A partner's refusal to participate in oral sex may be rooted in deep moral or religious convictions and is not necessarily a rejection of the other person. Everyone has their own sexual boundaries, and while many loving couples feel secure enough to abandon all or most of their sexual inhibitions, some individuals may need to set rules.

Discuss these issues honestly with each other because understanding and accepting each other's truths is an important part of a loving and intimate relationship. Some men have a fear of being bitten during oral sex and some women have a fear of being choked. Some people, particularly women, can only participate in oral sex activities if they are deeply in love and feel the relationship is a committed one. They may come to enjoy oral-genital contact once the sexual relationship has become established and secure. Patience can often be rewarded.

Some of the objections people have to oral sex may be based more on fears, misconceptions and misinformation, such as that it is "dirty" or harmful, or they may have anxieties about the genitals being ugly, or smelling or tasting unpleasant. Such anxieties can usually be alleviated with gentle understanding, exploration and support. Reading sex manuals like this one or speaking to a psycho-sexual counsellor can also help to alleviate unnecessarily inhibiting anxieties or phobias.

smelling and tasting good

As a woman, probably your biggest concern about receiving oral sex is whether those intimate parts of you are going to taste and smell good to your man. Make sure you have had a bath or shower beforehand and do not use too much scent. Normally, your natural, special, musky, and earthy sexual scent and taste will be very appealing to him. Those men who are squeamish about vaginal secretions and smells will probably avoid oral sex altogether, or move on quickly. The taste and smell of your sexual secretions can be affected, however, if you have eaten lots of spicy or garlic-flavoured food.

The secretions sometimes become more acrid or metallic tasting just before a menstrual period. Try sexual honesty, and ask your partner to let you know if the taste suddenly changes and he would rather abstain. If you notice a strong smell or discharge from your vagina, you may have an infection. In that case, put oral sex on hold and seek a medical check-up.

The normal amount of seminal fluid in each ejaculation is about a teaspoonful, and for those who are weight conscious, it contains about five calories and is mainly protein. It has the consistency of raw egg white and tastes a little salty. Except in the case of infection or sexually transmitted disease (in which case oral sex should be avoided), there is no evidence to prove that swallowing semen is harmful in any way to a woman, providing she is a willing participant in the act.

BELOW LEFT | When you are ready, take his penis into your mouth, to whatever depth you feel most comfortable with. You can suck on his penis or vibrate your tongue over the shaft.

BELOW | Many men love the sensation of having their scrotum gently stimulated by loving licks and kisses. Move his penis gently to one side and explore the whole area with your tongue, while stroking his thighs and buttocks and perineal region with your other hand.

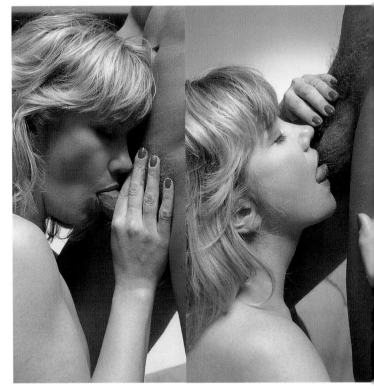

cunnilingus

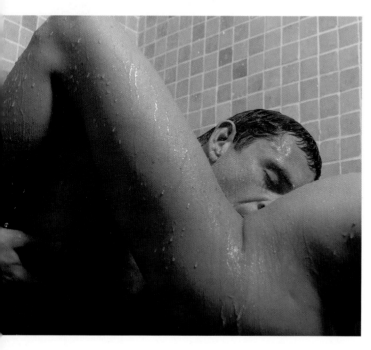

are those in which both your bodies are pointing in the same direction, but as long as your tongue can reach her vagina, then any position will do.

Begin by kissing and sucking around the vulva, luxuriating in everything, excluding the clitoris. The clitoris is highly sensitive and needs plenty of forewarning before it is touched. Heading straight there can cause discomfort and, at times, even pain. Gently spread your partner's outer labia with your fingers and kiss and suck her inner labia in the same way that you would if you were kissing her passionately on the mouth. When you notice her starting to respond, glide your tongue between the folds of the inner labia. If her response is a sharp jerk or she pushes away from you, stay away from there for a while, concentrating, instead, on the outer edges and massaging her pubic mound with your hand.

Once your partner is sufficiently relaxed and turned on, you can expose the clitoral shaft which runs down from the top of the labia to the clitoral head, underneath the inner labia. You may find it helps to spread the labia with two hands to make the skin taut, exposing the shaft. This area of densely packed nerve endings is extremely sensitive and a soft tongue, hard tongue approach usually works best. Try to stimulate it first with your tongue relaxed and soft and if she begins grinding towards you, you can increase the pressure by tensing and firming your tongue muscles. Remember to keep your tongue well lubricated with saliva.

How you stimulate the clitoris is very individual to the woman. Some like a soft sucking or caressing action, while others prefer a harder and sharper flicking action, either up and down or sideways.

If the clitoris enlarges, then she likes what you are doing; if it shrinks, then stop. However, remember that just before orgasm, the clitoris often retracts and seemingly disappears, so it is important to read other signs from her as well.

ABOVE AND OPPOSITE | Whatever the position for cunnilingus, it must be comfortable for both partners. Then he can lavish time and attention on her, while she can abandon herself to pure sensation.

THE WHOLE ISSUE of oral stimulation for women – going down – is one that sends spasms of fear through many men. How a woman wishes to be stimulated is so individual that it takes a lot of time and communication to get it just right. It is difficult to gauge exactly how to stimulate the clitoris without some help from your partner and even then it can be tricky, as many women know how to stimulate themselves but often find it difficult to explain and teach. As your relationship progresses and you begin to read each other's bodies, cunnilingus gets better and easier; practice does, after all, make perfect.

where to begin

Performing cunnilingus, as with fellatio, is a luxuriously time-consuming act. Bear in mind that you may be doing it for a while and make sure that you are both comfortable. The best positions

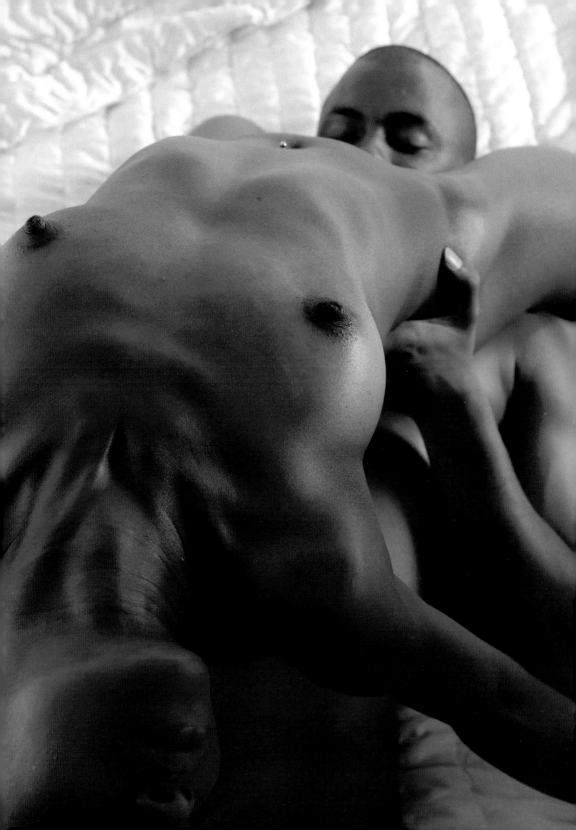

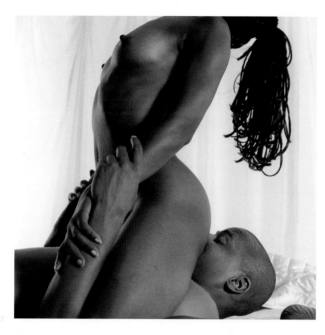

spicing it up

In the same way as with fellatio, drinking hot and cold drinks before oral sex can lead to different sensations for your partner, but do be aware that the clitoral head is hypersensitive and may not necessarily respond well to extremes. Occasionally the head can become irritated, which will certainly cool down the proceedings.

Incorporating a vibrator can add to the experience; place it under your tongue, so the vibrations transmit through you.

To really extend playtime, bring her to the brink of orgasm and then stop for a good half a minute, do the same but stop for less time, and so on. Some women may not appreciate this, so it's best to discuss it first.

keep the rhythm going

Just before your partner is about to come, make sure you don't change a thing. Whatever you're doing is working, so just hold your ground and

ABOVE | For many men, cunnilingus with their partner sitting on their face is the realization of their dreams.

RIGHT | You need to be sensitive to your partner's responses. As she becomes increasingly aroused, you can put on the pressure and move your tongue more rapidly – but don't try to force the pace.

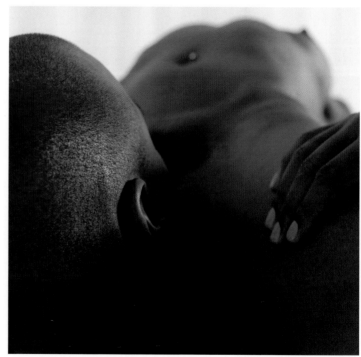

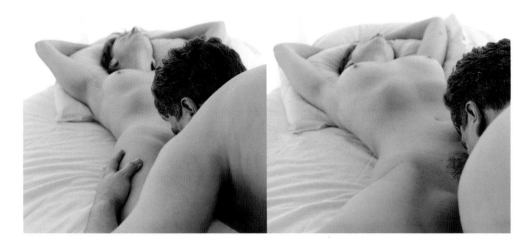

prepare for the tsunami. When she comes, don't necessarily stop unless she asks you to, but lighten the touch slightly and perhaps take the emphasis away from the clitoris. Continuing stimulation can increase the orgasm and some women even report multiple orgasms from good oral sex.

licking the clitoris

Imagine you're drawing small circles on and around her clitoris with your tongue. The smaller circles will concentrate on the tip and larger ones will deal with the base. Alternate the speed and direction of the circles, as some women respond better if the circles rotate in a specific direction.

Draw figures-of-eight over her clitoris with your tongue. This may be too much stimulation for some women but for others it will work wonders. Experiment with the speed and frequency.

Use your tongue to either flick the clitoris up and down with a short pause between each flick, or from left to right, aiming just underneath the base of the head. Vary the pressure of the flicks along with their frequency.

the bridge

Remember doing the bridge in the gym, when you raise your arched body up, supporting yourself only with your feet and hands? Well this is a variation for the more supple lover. He sits while

the woman positions herself face up with her knees hooked over his shoulders and her head between his knees or legs. From here she arches her back and uses her hands to support herself, raising her genitals closer to his face.

the edge

She lies down on the bed, on her front or back, with her bottom over the edge of the bed. He kneels on the floor between her legs and uses his hands on her bottom or pelvis to support her. She hooks her legs over his shoulders and he can raise her up or lower her down with his hands.

the triangle

She positions herself face down on the bed or floor with her bottom in the air and her legs straight and spread, similar to a triangle. He then sits so that the tops of her thighs are supported by his shoulders with his legs straight out on either side of her head.

face sitting

The man lies on his back while the woman crouches or kneels over his face, facing in either direction. This is great for women as they can control the pressure by either easing off or grinding down, but be careful not to suffocate him in the throes of passion.

ABOVE | There are no hard and fast rules for cunnilingus. Try to keep in tune with your partner so you can both get the most out of the experience.

anal sex

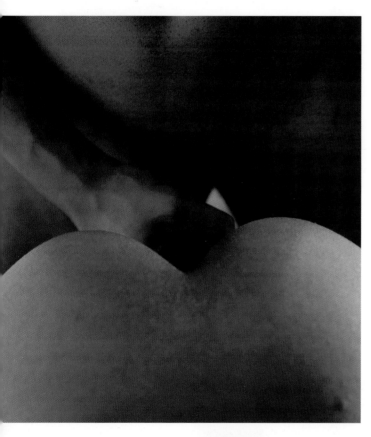

THOSE WHO PRACTISE anal sex insist that it can be one of the most stimulating experiences in the sexual repertoire. They claim that because the area concerned is jam-packed with sensitive nerve endings, when stimulated they produce a more intense and dramatic orgasm. Some people have tried it and found it a painful experience not worth repeating. Others see their anus as a one-way passage and find the mere thought of incorporating it in sex play plain disgusting and unnatural. The fact is that the anus is composed of two anal sphincters – rings of muscle – that are designed to control only outgoing matter. With training however, they can learn to facilitate a two-way traffic.

demystifying anal sex

Although no one should ever be forced to take part in any kind of sexual act that they are not comfortable with, it is worth mentioning that many people, both men and women, find anal sex a hugely enjoyable experience.

So why the taboo? There are several reasons, the most obvious of which is that, just like masturbation, people rarely admitted to the practice in the past. Secondly, when the AIDS virus became so prevalent in the western world in the 1980s, anal sex came to be seen as a gay practice that increased the risk of HIV and AIDS.

However, today people have a greater understanding of these viruses and so are less cautious about practising anal sex. Although it is true that unprotected anal sex can increase the risk of HIV and AIDS – the thin membrane in the rectum can easily be torn – with proper safety precautions (which should be used in all sexual adventures with new partners, be they anal or vaginal), the risk of contracting these viruses is minimal. The key word here is simply precautions. It is possible to buy harder-wearing condoms that are specifically designed for anal penetration or penetration where there is extra strain.

ABOVE | Absolute trust in your partner is the key to relaxation – essential for practising anal sex.

RIGHT | Couples who practise anal sex agree that it has added a new dimension of pleasure to their sex lives.

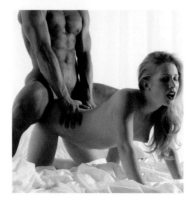

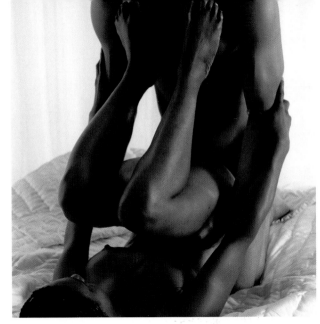

the gay factor

Anal sex is not an exclusively homosexual practice. In fact, only about half the gay population practises it. We already know that the male prostate gland is an area of great erotic potential that, when stimulated by a man or a woman, enhances sexual sensation and orgasm. The prostate gland, however, can only be accessed through the anus, so should it be ignored just because of inhibitions? If this is so, then we could be missing out on a whole array of potential sexual experiences purely because of the implied connotations.

In fact for men, practising anal sex on a woman is a tighter and more intense experience. For women, if it is done correctly and carefully, the vaginal and rectal walls can swell during arousal, stimulating the G spot and providing sensations that they could not get from vaginal penetration. Men receiving anal sex from a woman with the help of a strap-on, finger or vibrator can have their prostate stimulated at the same time as their penis.

the hygiene factor

This is another reason for the taboo. There's always the chance that a bit of faeces will still be in the rectum when it is penetrated, although most of the time it is stored in the colon until defecation. To combat this problem, you should empty your bowels before anal sex and not just when you need to go. If this is still not satisfactory, then you can buy an enema kit from the chemist and clear the system out in the bathroom beforehand. This may seem somewhat over the top, but performing anal sex does call for a little preparation.

getting down to it

The secret of successful and satisfying anal sex is trust and communication. Before you even think about doing it for the first time, you should be absolutely certain that your partner is someone you can trust. Discussing it beforehand is also important and if you can't do this, forget about it. Without these two essential ingredients you can only end up hurting, and possibly damaging yourself or your partner.

relax and do it

The difference between anal pain and pleasure is relaxation. When you are tense, your natural reaction is to clench your buttocks, so it's important that the environment and pre-anal play is relaxing and complementary. A massage, soft lighting, a warm bath and soothing music can all help in setting the right scene.

When practising anal sex for the first time, the key is to use plenty of lubrication and take it very slowly. Initially, you will probably find the sphincter tightens up, making entry seem impossible. Get your partner to use more lubrication and gently massage the area for a while before even contemplating putting anything up there. Stimulate each other's genitals at the same time, as nervousness can lead to loss of arousal. If this happens, it's best to stop and try again later.

For the first few times it is advisable just to insert a clean, manicured finger, slowly and gently. By doing this, the rectum learns to relax and not to "clam up" every time anything goes near it. Gentle massage with the inserted finger, bending slightly towards the coccyx (tailbone), following the natural curve of the rectum, can also help you to relax. It's a good idea if the receiver inserts his or her own finger up the anus to get a better understanding of how it all works.

ABOVE | Men enjoy the tighter feeling of anal penetration. For a woman, the stimulation of the G spot is exciting.

BELOW | Gentle, lubricated massage is the way to start.

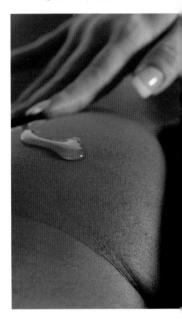

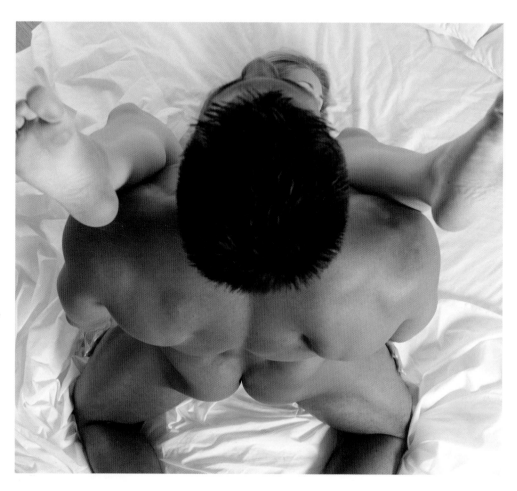

ABOVE | Once anal sex has become part of a couple's sensual repertoire, they can experiment with confidence to explore a whole range of different positions.

Entry is usually the most difficult part and must always be done slowly and with care. It's often better if the receiver lowers herself or himself on to the partner's well-lubricated penis or dildo with the partner applying constant pressure and a guiding hand. (Unlike the vagina, there is no natural lubrication in the anus.) Remember, though, that both entry *and* exit must be done slowly. A quick exit can cause a lot of pain and even damage. Remember, slow equals safe.

Once in, thrusting should be minimal to start with. Keep applying the lubrication and check frequently that your partner is all right. If there is any discomfort, stop for a while, with the penis or dildo still inside, and calm things down by stimulating the genitals or by giving a soothing massage. If the discomfort continues, it's best to stop altogether and try again another time. Remember that before entering the vagina after the anus, you must wash your penis to prevent any potential infection.

strap-on fun

Some men like their female partner to wear a strap-on anal dildo to stimulate their prostate. Others feel it has some stigma attached. Once tried, lots of straight couples enjoy the delights of anal sex and it becomes a regular part of their lives.

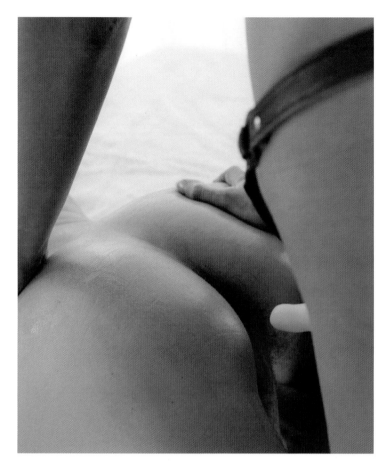

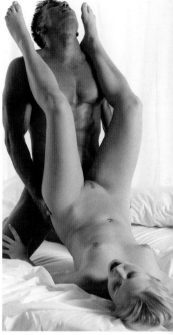

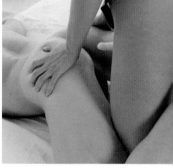

anal sex and the law

The term sodomy refers not only to anal sex but also to "lewd and lascivious behaviour". Many countries and US states use sodomy laws as a means of preventing homosexual behaviour regardless of whether penetrative sex is present or not. However, sodomy laws affect gays and straights alike.

In Massachusetts, for instance, sodomy is illegal. Anyone convicted faces a maximum sentence of 20 years plus another eight for "lewd and lascivious behaviour".

Countries that have sodomy laws include Jamaica, USA, Morocco, Saudi Arabia, India, Mauritius, Trinidad and Tobago, Malaysia, Tunisia and the Seychelles. Countries where sodomy is punishable by death include Afghanistan, Pakistan, Yemen, Iran, Saudi Arabia, Mauritania and Sudan.

In the UK there is no sodomy law at present, and the legal status of gay couples has been strengthened with the introduction of civil partnerships.

TOP RIGHT | There are as many positions for anal sex as there are for vaginal rear entry.

ABOVE LEFT AND RIGHT | Being penetrated by a woman may be disconcerting to begin with, but many find that seeing their partner with a strap-on is highly erotic.

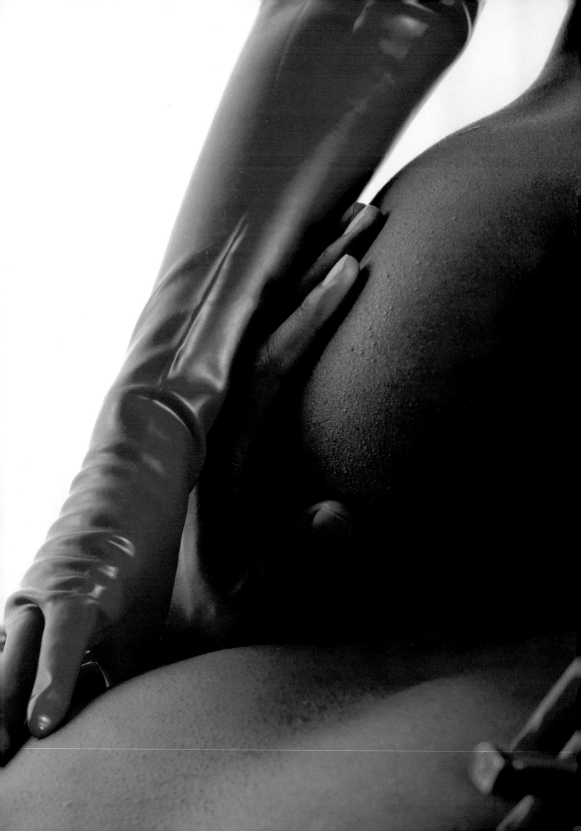

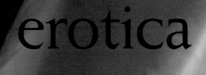

erotica

There comes a time in many couples' lives when sex can become rather routine and occasionally you might need a little stimulation from outside. Incorporating pornography, reading erotic literature together or shopping for sex toys can add that extra zing to your lovemaking, especially if you both have a good sense of humour.

the senses and sensuality

BELOW | What used to be called "sex aids" now come in all shapes and sizes. Artists and designers are turning their skills to making sex toys more approachable and more aesthetically pleasing.

THIS CHAPTER IS A JOURNEY through the more advanced and esoteric practices of sex. It covers sexual acts that push the boundaries out just that little further. You don't have to be a leather-masked, latex-wearing, whip-wielding dominatrix to appreciate this chapter. Erotica is more to do with stimulating the senses, all five of them, removing the emphasis from actual penetration and

technique. To that end, this chapter could be seen as the most sensual of them all – a delicious exploration of the darker side to sex.

Although sado-masochism (S&M), body manipulation and whipping are touched on in these pages, this chapter is more about the sensuality of using different media in your sex play. Wearing leather in bed can be very arousing,

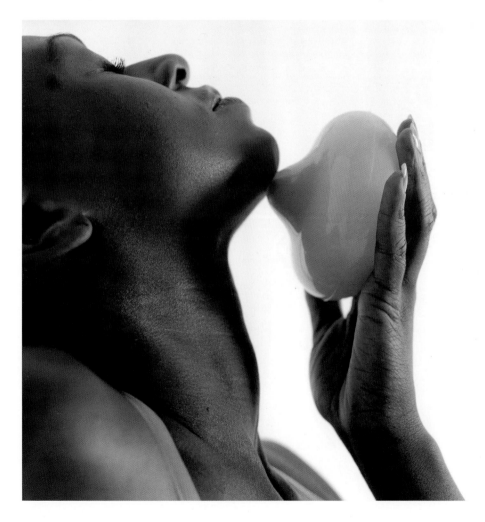

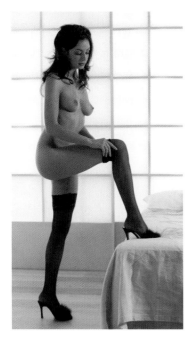

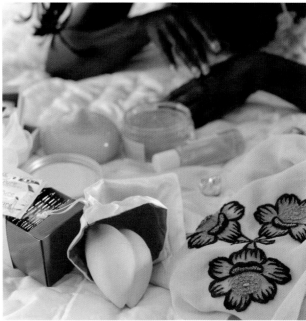

for example, purely because of its sexy connotations and the texture of it against your skin. It does not necessarily mean that you are about to embark on some sinister role play with your partner, involving nipple clamps, whips and chains. It could be quite the opposite.

sensuality

There are plenty of ways to introduce the sensual touch to your sex life. For instance, silk scarves, with their cool soft slippery texture, are sexy when used to tie up your partner. The emphasis is not so much on the tying up, but on the sensuousness of the material against your skin. This form of tying up allows you to luxuriate in your partner while he or she lies back and enjoys the sensations.

Try to incorporate much more sensuality into your sex play by concentrating on your five senses:

touch Be aware of the pressure you use when caressing your lover, use just your fingertips and then the pads of your fingers when stroking each other. Use different textures on your skin: feathers, silk, satin, velvet, rubber, a soft brush.

sound Choose music to go with your mood. Jazz is always mellow and helps you relax, or you may be a Beethoven or Mozart type of person who likes a good crescendo. Brazilian, Cuban and other World music is very sensual and can strongly influence the way you move and groove together.

sight Create your own magic space with lighting, candles or dimmers. Use fairy lights around a mirror or tea lights along a mantelpiece. Soft lighting is conducive to relaxation and the flickering flames can be hypnotic.

smell Rub musk or vanilla scented oil into your body, sprinkle rose petals on your bed, use scented candles, burn incense, or have your favourite flowers in full bloom.

taste The best taste is the taste of sex – that musty, musky, heavy, natural perfume that attracts us to one another. However, you might also enjoy some delicious titbits to tempt each other with. Choose different flavours and sensations: the satin of melting chocolate, the juiciness of ripe mangoes, the saltiness of caviar, the softness of yogurt or cream, the coldness of ice cream.

ABOVE LEFT | Stockings and high heels may be a cliché, but they are still a turn-on.

ABOVE RIGHT | Sex accessories are abundant. There is a huge variety of places that will help you to stock up.

sharing sexual fantasies

SEXUAL FANTASIES ARE COMMON to many people and provide a rich resource of aphrodisiac material which contributes towards their heightened sexual arousal, either during masturbation or intercourse. These fantasies can be extremely diverse, even bizarre by real-life standards, but very erotically imaginative. Whether the content of someone's sexual fantasy is lurid or mild, it is deeply personal to that individual's sexual psyche and private world of erotic imagery. Some people have a consistent theme to their fantasies, other people change the material, adding new detail, new scenarios and different characters to their fertile sexual imagery. Studies show, however, that there are certain common patterns of imagination prevalent in people's fantasies, such as themes of domination, submission, being forced into sex against their will, making love to a stranger, an ex-lover or a favourite film star, or being watched while having intercourse.

BELOW | Being tied to the bed is a common fantasy for both partners.

varying kinds of fantasy

Sex researchers believe that for many people fantasies are formed in substance from their earliest associations with sexual feelings, while others are constantly updating their erotic imagery to reflect the changing circumstances of their lives. Fantasies based on primal experiences can explain why, for some people, themes such as spanking or other punishment from an authority figure can feature so strongly.

In another circumstance, a fantasy involving forced sexual compliance, such as a rape scene, may be just a creative way of permitting intense feelings of sexual arousal without having the burden of guilt. In the imagination, that person has no control over what is happening and therefore carries no responsibility for the ensuing erotic feelings.

It is important to realize, however, that fantasies involving forced sex, however descriptive on an imaginative level, will bear little relation to an individual's real-life behaviour or desires, and so do not necessarily indicate that a person has masochistic tendencies. The fantasizer is always in control of events within the fantasy, because he or she is the creator of those images and can carefully manipulate them to bring about the desired result: increased sexual response and orgasm. This scenario is totally different from a real-life event, during which they would have absolutely no control over aggressive behaviour resulting in forced sex,

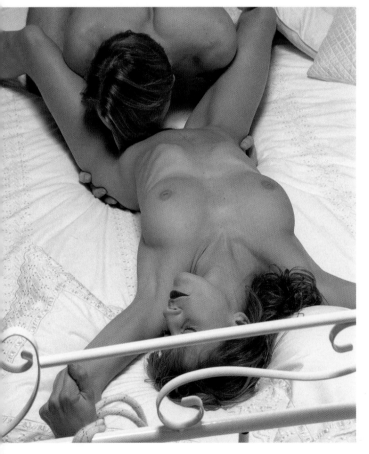

from which they would derive no sexual pleasure at all. Many people love their sexual fantasy world, using these mental images to enhance and enrich their sex lives and sexual responses. Their fantasies seem to have a life of their own, emerging and existing within a vivid arena of sexual imagination.

Some people, however, may feel guilt and anxiety associated with them, fearing that the extraordinary content of their mentally created eroticism reflects a deep inner psychological disturbance. This anxiety may be compounded when the fantasies contain material which is strongly in contrast to their normal moral values and sexual behaviour.

Members of both sexes may have sexual fantasies, although some people do not have them at all, and cannot see any value in this mental erotic resource. Such couples may regard fantasy as a mental distraction which will prevent a truly spontaneous interaction between the lovers – a flight into cerebral sex.

Most sex experts agree that sexual fantasizing is normal behaviour, and can be an important and useful way for people to explore their capacity for sexual arousal and response, either during masturbation or lovemaking. Sex therapy can help, however, if sexual fantasizing has become disturbing to an individual, or is having a serious adverse effect on a sexual relationship.

BELOW | Stockings, high heels and leather all have their followers. A silk blindfold makes the experience even more exciting.

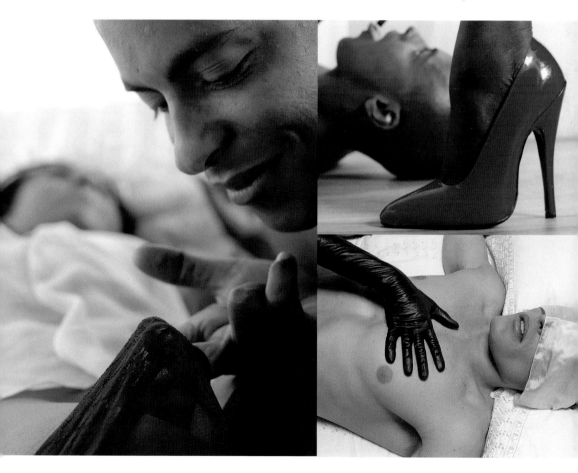

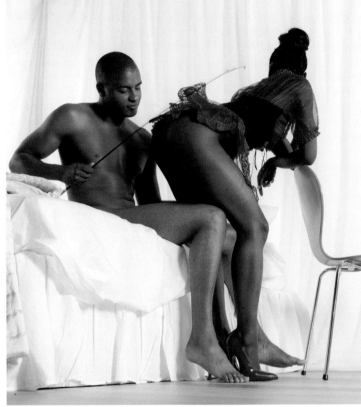

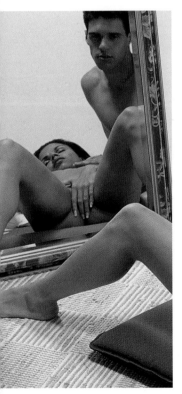

to share or not to share

Many people who enjoy using sexual fantasy to induce sexual arousal or orgasm would never consider revealing the content of these mental images to anyone else, not even a partner. For them, the fantasies must and do stay within the realm of privacy. They may feel that once a fantasy has been verbalized or shared it loses much of its power and impact.

Other couples discuss their fantasies with each other, and even describe them openly during lovemaking to increase mutual sexual excitement. Some people even feel safe enough within their relationship to act out their fantasies with each other. Not every person is able to understand or tolerate the erotic imagery that may be part of a partner's sexual consciousness. You need to know

and trust your partner's ability to handle this information before revealing your fantasies, or discretion may be a wiser course of action. Your partner may be less than thrilled to know that during lovemaking you have been fantasizing about having sex with your favourite film star.

If fantasy is not part of your partner's sexual agenda, then he or she may have no comprehension of your need for it and may even regard it as a personal rejection. In that case, it may be better just to enjoy your fantasies as your own private creation.

This section explores some of the sexual fantasies which can be shared and played out between couples. Some of them are mild and teasing and generally involve a playful content which would probably be viewed as unthreatening and fun by both partners. Other fantasy games, such as domination and bondage, or even cross-dressing, would need to be revealed or acted on only when a relationship is strong enough to withstand their impact. No one should ever try to impose a private sexual fantasy on another person, or coerce them into acting it out against their will. However, as a loving couple, if you can enjoy sharing each other's fantasy world in a context of trust and mutual exploration, then your erotic imagination can add a new and exciting dimension to your love-life.

mirror fantasies

Some people like to use mirrors when they make love because the thrill of watching themselves in different sexual positions increases the excitement of intercourse. It adds a voyeuristic element to their lovemaking because they can actually see themselves making love, as well as watching their partner's body from a different vantage point.

When a mirror is strategically placed, the couple can see the more erotic and intimate parts of the body in action, such as the vulva, the scrotum, and particularly the buttocks and anus, and they can even witness the process of penetration and thrusting. It can seem as if you are watching yourself and your lover acting the part in a blue-movie, which is an added turn-on to those couples who enjoy watching pornographic films.

Another fantasy that can arise through the use of a mirror is a sense that other people are copulating alongside you while you are making love. This can provide a safer and less emotionally damaging way of acting out a group orgy sexual fantasy rather than doing it for real. Some couples are blatant about their mirror fantasies, and have one permanently fixed to the bedroom ceiling.

BELOW | As the man, you are able to see your partner's breasts in the mirror as you fondle them from this rear position.

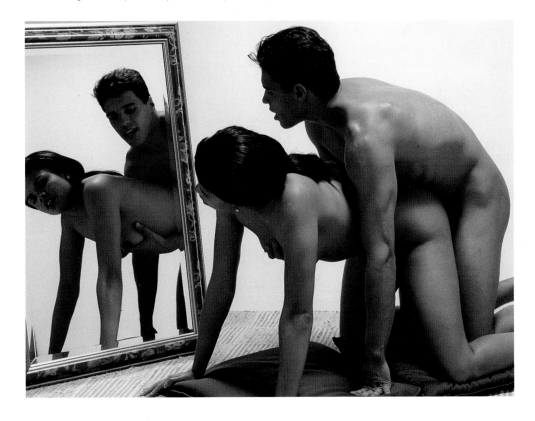

striptease fantasy

IT HAS BEEN SAID, in a tongue-in-cheek way of course, that inside every woman there is a stripper trying to get out. Even among the most reserved, the idea of doing a strip-tease can hold a certain allure. It may even provide material for a sexual fantasy.

If you do a strip-tease then you must be the one who is in charge of your sexual exhibitionism, and during it your partner is in your control and at your command. He can watch and relish the sight of you, but he must not touch you unless you so desire. The tease is the main point of the exercise so you are allowed to arouse and play with him,

promising hints of your naked body, but you alone must decide when and how to take off your clothes, and how much he can touch you.

Perform your exotic dance for your own pleasure as well as his. You are celebrating your own eroticism, and what is more, you are enjoying showing it off.

One of the more fascinating aspects of performing strip-tease is that it allows you to counteract an aspect of your gender conditioning. While women are often portrayed as objects of desire, society also expects them to behave in a

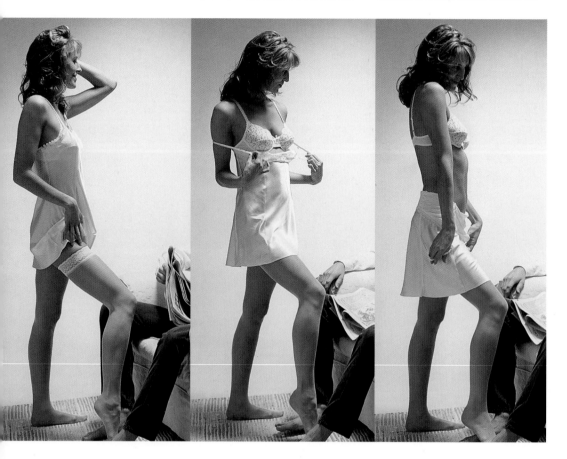

demure and chaste manner. Stripping for your lover helps you to challenge that restraint, and you can flaunt your body in such as way that you are making a statement about your own sexuality.

If it is your fantasy to do a strip-tease, then pluck up the courage to do it for your lover. It could be one of his fantasies too, but he may have been too shy to ask you to do it. Visual arousal is an important part of male sexuality, and he is sure to enjoy the invitation to become your captive audience. Devise your own dance routine, and if you need to build up some confidence, practise your steps in front of a mirror when you are alone. The illustrations and further suggestions shown here should provide you with some inspiring ideas on how to turn your strip-tease into an art.

build the suspense

One of the more fun ways of acting out your strip-tease is to perform for your partner when he is least suspecting it. Or you can set a date for it to build up his eager anticipation. Put on some of your prettiest or sexiest lingerie, but make sure you have a few layers of clothing on top so you can take your time peeling them off, keeping him in suspense.

White underwear is a particularly good choice – the combination of snow-white innocence and your sexy routine will add extra appeal and excitement to the strip-tease. Also, wear pretty stockings which you can roll sexily down your legs, or you can add a suspender or garter belt to the strip-tease outfit.

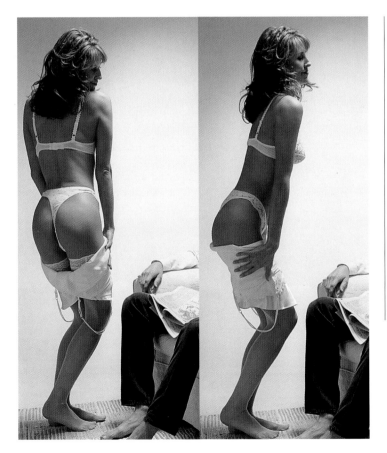

FROM LEFT TO RIGHT | Once you have got his interest, begin your strip routine. To the sound of raunchy music, start to move and sway in front of him. Tease your petticoat straps on and off of your shoulders, tossing your hair with each seductive turn. Gradually expose your chest and belly, posing in such a way that you accentuate your curves. At this stage, the man should look but not touch. Very slowly reveal your buttocks. You can tantalize him further by letting your petticoat slip a little, then re-adjusting it. Sway your hips seductively, then turn a little to the side.

the art of strip-tease

Good strip-tease should be an art, a dance and a performance, so it is worth preparing properly to do it. If you have practised a few routines on your own, you should, by now, have built up your confidence. The two most important props for your show are the right music and sexy underwear. You might like to use additional items like a feather boa which you can trail all over your skin, and which you can use to reveal a glimpse of your body.

The music you choose should be sexy, or slow and sensual, depending on your dance routine. Or select songs which hold romantic memories for you and your partner. Whatever music you pick, it should have just the right rhythm to put you into an arousing and playful mood.

If you want to make strip-tease a regular part of your fantasy play to enjoy with your lover, it is worth investing in several sets of lingerie. Select different colours and styles, and save them for these occasions as well as for your most romantic nights. You need a bra and panties of matching colours and soft fabrics. Silk and lace items always look wonderful. You might like to wear a suspender belt, or choose stockings which cling to your legs. You then need a sexy petticoat, or a slinky dress, so that you are fully covered when you first appear. The fun of strip-tease comes from peeling off the layers piece by piece. You can go for the vamp look, dressed all in black, and even wear high-heeled shoes. Red is exotic and brazen, while white is pure and innocent.

BELOW | Give him your leg to hold and have him peel the stocking right off your foot while you sexily stroke over your own leg, thigh and buttocks. Self-caressing is an alluring aspect of strip-tease.

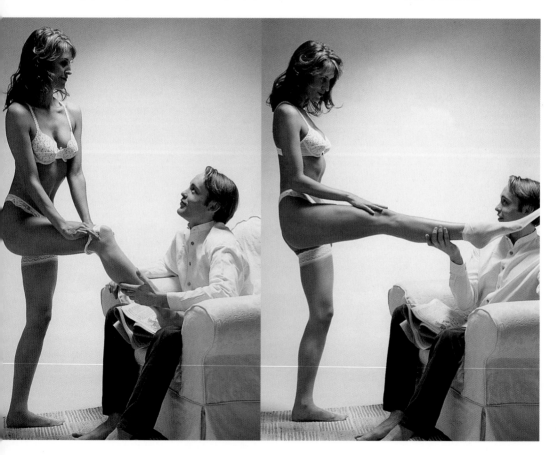

The correct actions during the strip-tease are very important if you are to create the right alluring effect. They should be slow and sexy but slightly exaggerated. Your aim is to pose and move your body as erotically as possible. Lots of pelvic gyrations will excite him and you.

However, you should let your dance be an expression of your own inner sexuality. Do what feels good to you and what turns you on. Find that sex queen part in yourself and act it out to the full.

While you tease your partner and peel away your clothes, stroke and caress your own body as if you are making love to yourself. You can run your hands sensuously over your breasts, along your inner thighs, and in between your legs. Although the aim of the strip-tease is to excite and tantalize your partner, it should be done for your pleasure too. Love your body and have fun showing it off, and let your liberated eroticism turn you on too. Enjoy the thrill of your sexual power.

involve your partner

Everything in strip-tease should be done slowly with a constant "Will I? Won't I?" tease. You can roll your stockings down your legs – one at a time – either by yourself, or involve your partner in the action. Before, he had simply been a spectator, but now he gets a chance to touch. However, you must stay in control, and allow him to touch you only to help you undress – part of the fun of strip-tease is that he knows that you always have the upper hand.

BELOW | When you are just wearing your panties and bra, take lots of time to remove them. Stand close enough that he can begin to touch and caress you, and even let him tug at your panties with his teeth.

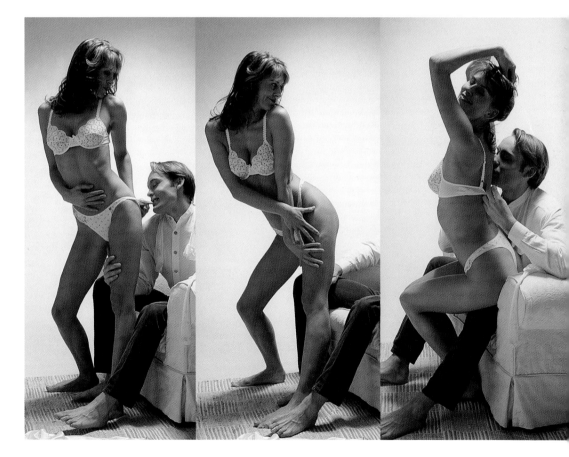

unsnap the strap

You can enlist his help to undo your bra fastener, especially if undoing it yourself would prove too awkward. Perch saucily on his lap with your back to him and stay in your performance mode, gyrating your pelvis subtly on his knee. If you have long hair, sweep it sexily away from your shoulders and back to expose more bare flesh to him, and if he wants to, let him plant little kisses on your skin. It is too soon to let the bra slip off, so once he has undone it, cup it to your breasts with your hands. The point is to keep him wanting more.

caress your breasts

Let the rounded swell of your breasts begin to show, but don't expose your nipples yet. Turn to face your partner, and incline towards him so your breasts come close to his body. Gently palpate your breasts with your hands as if caressing them, and let the bra material stroke across their skin. Don't let your partner touch your breasts yet – at this point you are using visual stimulation to arouse him – but you can move your leg closer to him so he can stroke your thighs. Gradually let your bra slide down from your breasts, to expose the edge of your nipples.

panty time

Now comes the really sexy part, as you start to peel off your panties. Keep the movement going in your body as you turn from side to side and back and forth, sometimes leaning your hips or

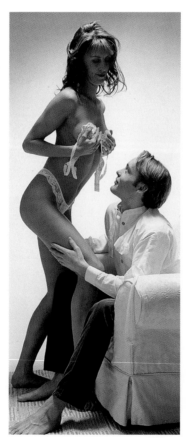

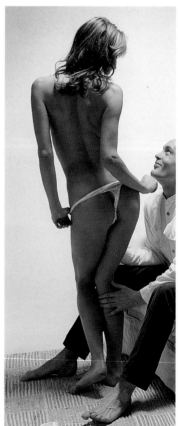

buttocks within reach of his touch. Begin to edge your panties very slowly downwards. Turn around sometimes to give him a glimpse of your pubic hair, but change angles constantly so he gets an all-round view of this very erotic part of your body.

move in close

Still holding on to your panties, languidly roll them over the curve of your buttocks so they rest on the top of your thighs. At this point, your whole body is almost entirely naked. Make the most of these last tantalizing moments of your strip-tease, but moving very close to your partner and dancing erotically in front of him. Let different parts of your body brush and rub against him, and then allow him to reach out and caress you a little more.

fun finale

Find an easy way to roll your panties down your legs so you remove them completely from your body. If necessary, you can rest one foot on the chair for easy manoeuvring. Then use your panties as part of your dance. Stroke them softly over your skin, between your legs, against your partner's face, and hook them around his neck to pull him playfully towards you. The strip-tease is over, what you do next with all that smouldering sexual excitement is up to you.

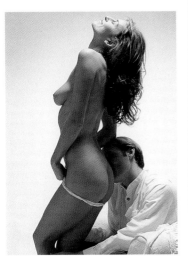

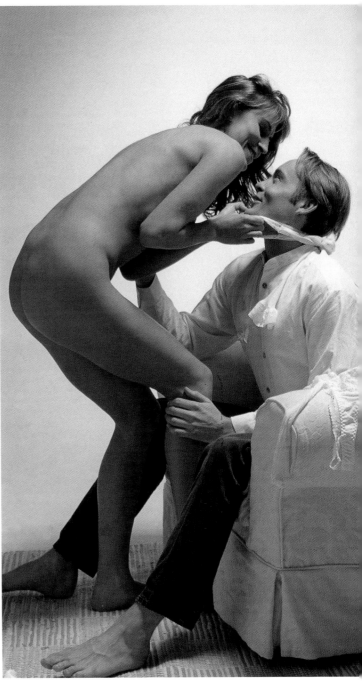

sex games

RIGHT | You don't have to take dressing up very seriously – it's usually more fun if you don't – but it can be a good way to discover all kinds of feelings and desires you didn't even know you had.

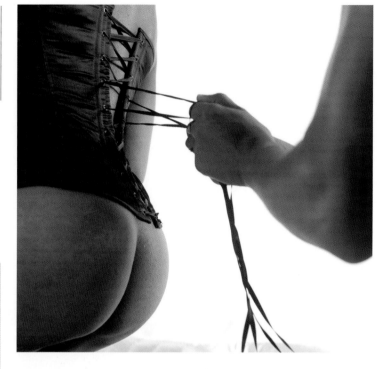

party games

dice games Get two dice. Write down one sexual position for each number on the first dice. Then write down six places for the second dice (the car, the broom closet, the stairs and so on). Roll the two dice together and obey dutifully.

truth or dare Take it in turns between either answering a personal question (truth) or performing some naughty act (dare) – great after a couple of glasses of wine.

spin the bottle This is a game for an adult party. Each of you should write a list of sexual forfeits. Spin an empty wine bottle, and the person it points at must undertake the next forfeit.

LET'S FACE IT, repeated sex with the same person can get rather, well, repetitive. A common complaint is, "Our sex lives have become boring. What can we do to spice things up?"

play time

Sex is meant to be fun. When you recognize that glint in your partner's eye, you will know that it's time to go and have a bit of adult play time. There are lots of games that you and your partner can share to enliven the average bedroom and not all of them have to involve his wearing your underwear. You can play naked scrabble, hide and seek in the garden, have dinner in the nude when the kids are away at camp – and cook it wearing nothing but an apron. The list is endless, and the main goal? To have a laugh and enjoy each other.

dressing up

Nurses, doctors, chambermaids and dominatrices: these are all well known in the repertoire of role-plays that many people enjoy. Less obvious scenarios include the bored housewife and the plumber, starring in a porn movie, a visit from a high-class call girl and even pretending to be complete strangers.

Dressing up and role-play are not just for drama students; you can re-create your bedroom as a dungeon of depravity, a hospital of hedonism or even Lara Croft's lair. It's an opportunity to put those fantasies into reality. You can buy outfits or make your own. Your boyfriend's a fire fighter? Wear his uniform; it's bound to keep him smiling the next day at work. Your girlfriend is a doctor? It's what white coats were made for.

board games

Dust off those board games you play only at Christmas. Although there are games that you can buy that involve an element of stripping or sex play, you can just as easily reinvent the rules of the old favourites. Instead of paying the fine when you have to "go directly to jail", change the cards for your own set, with whatever your desire dictates as the forfeits.

strangers

The following ideas allow you to act out your desires. Surprise your partner on your anniversary by secretly booking a hotel room. Tell him or her to meet you at a specific time in a restaurant nearby but make sure he or she understands that this is a blind date and that you have never met before.

Arrive at the restaurant and introduce yourself. Order wine and sumptuous food, and flirt in the manner that you did before you met one another. As the evening progresses, become more provocative. Tell him or her that you are wearing no underwear or that you have a partner but would be interested in playing away from home on this occasion. As the meal comes to a close, ask them if they would be up for a one-night stand of no-strings-attached unadulterated sex.

As you leave, do not tell them where you are going, but arrive at the hotel and accept the booking under pseudonyms such as Mr and Mrs Smith. Then, staying in character, play the ultimate sexual host or hostess, asking what they want you

to do to them. If you can stay in character then this is guaranteed to release the naughty side to both your natures and result in some pretty hot and exciting sex.

midnight feast

Have some oysters and champagne hidden in the refrigerator, making sure your partner doesn't see them when he or she comes home. Have a normal evening, with a light meal, and then say that you want an early night because you have a headache. Make sure you set an alarm or stay awake while your partner sleeps so that at midnight you can quietly get up and set the scene in the bedroom with candles and soft music. Retrieve the champagne and oysters and bring them into the bedroom. Start the music and gently wake your partner. Eat and drink together and enjoy a night of passion. This is best done on a Friday or Saturday night so you can catch up on the sleep you will inevitably lose.

teaser

This is a great oral sex game to get you and your partner literally bursting with anticipation and sexual energy. Begin by lying him or her back on the bed and explain that they are not to move, and if they do then they will be punished. Massage their whole body from their chest, arms, legs and down to their toes, avoiding the genitals. Then start to kiss and caress the chest, sucking on his or her nipples and massaging with your hands. Work your way down slowly, paying attention to every crack and crevice of their body, and begin to work your way towards their genitals.

If they move, "punish" them by beginning all over again from the top. Give them oral pleasure, beginning lazily at first, every now and again stopping and moving to another part of the body. Make the breaks less and less frequent but every time they twitch or groan, begin from the chest again. This will build up so much sexual tension that they will soon learn and become stiff and still with anticipation. The final orgasm will be monumental and will have them eating out of the palm of your hand for days to come.

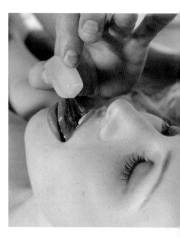

ABOVE | The sensation of an ice cube against your skin excites nerve endings in a way that hands and fingers can't.

BELOW | Removing your sight with a blindfold may heighten other senses.

BELOW LEFT | If you are sharing a croissant you must have made it as far as the morning after.

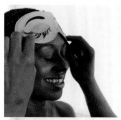

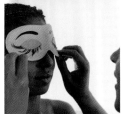

dressing up fantasies

WHILE MOST OF US PRESENT a particular personality to the outside world, with which we predominantly identify ourselves, within us all there are many other character traits which weave together to create the rich tapestry of our human psyches. At best, the varying shades of our personalities can mingle with each other and become integrated, each part having an opportunity to express itself at an appropriate time.

BELOW | If your sexual fantasy is to be assertive, try leather, rubber or chain mail.

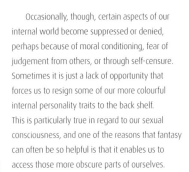

Occasionally, though, certain aspects of our internal world become suppressed or denied, perhaps because of moral conditioning, fear of judgement from others, or through self-censure. Sometimes it is just a lack of opportunity that forces us to resign some of our more colourful internal personality traits to the back shelf. This is particularly true in regard to our sexual consciousness, and one of the reasons that fantasy can often be so helpful is that it enables us to access those more obscure parts of ourselves.

In a close and loving relationship, where two people trust each other and are willing to share each other's fantasies without condemnation, there is a tremendous opportunity to play-act roles which allow them to express and have fun with some of their sexual identities. One way to do this is by dressing up, thereby allowing your hidden sexual fantasies to emerge in full regalia.

You can even dress up to be theatrical, turning your bedroom into a fantasy land where you act out heroes and heroines from the movies, the stage, literature – or even those from your imagination. You can turn yourselves into Heathcliff and Cathy, or Romeo and Juliet for the night. Or perhaps one or the other of you has a favourite film star – so why not be Humphrey Bogart, or Marilyn Monroe, or whoever else you admire, and play-act the part for the night for your favourite audience? Or, if you trust each other, dress up to manifest your sexual secrets and fantasies. Raid your wardrobe, or scour the sales for items of clothing which will help you to fulfil your complete sexual personality.

the temptress

So you have a respectable job, your life is well-organized, you may be a mother and have a secure long-term relationship. Or you have strong feelings about sexual equality, support the feminist movement, and hate to see women portrayed as sexual objects. There is, however, a part of you (it

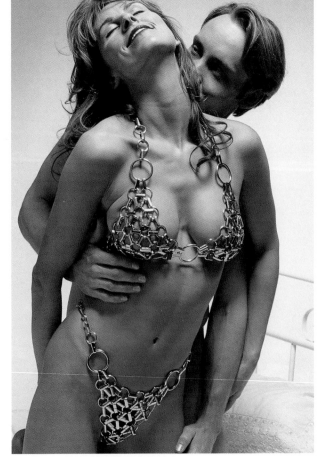

may be a very small part!) that has an on-going fantasy about being a scarlet woman, a femme fatale, a bordello queen, or a temptress.

If you give yourself permission to allow that side of your nature to come out once in a while, it does not mean to say that your whole value system and way of life is about to change. Dressing up and play-acting your sex queen or brazen woman fantasy in the safety of your bedroom and together with your partner will just be an exciting and fun way to express a certain side of yourself. You may feel enriched by it too, because an important aspect of who you are can claim its place in your life.

Look for the kind of outrageous outfit or underwear you would never normally wear. It should be pure showbiz or downright sexy. If you want to be a James Bond girl or an Amazon Queen, leather, latex, rubber or chain mail will give you the tough, sexually assertive look to help you play out your fantasy role.

You have succeeded in winning over the man and now he is putty in your hands. Wrap him up in your feather boa and pull him close to the warmth of your skin and into the soft curves of your body. Now that you have him in your arms, you are going to lavish attention on him. How about planting kisses from those full red lips of yours all over his face.

Pose yourself to look alluring, and make the most of your feminine curves. For extra effect, drape your feather boa around your body. Learn to pout seductively. Let everything you do signal a hint of promise and pleasure. Then pat the bed beside you expectantly and invite him to join you. How can he refuse?

fantasy femme fatale

Is there a temptress or a femme fatale inside you waiting to express herself? Do you have a fantasy about being a Mata Hari, a high-class courtesan, or an expensive mistress? Enjoy playing your role. Go for the glamour look, and keep it totally feminine. Choose passionate red, lace and feathers, and lots of make-up. Go all out to seduce your man.

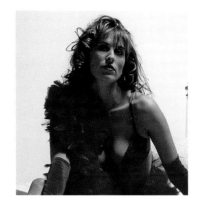

LEFT | A feather boa is a very effective accessory.

BELOW | Long gloves complete the temptress look.

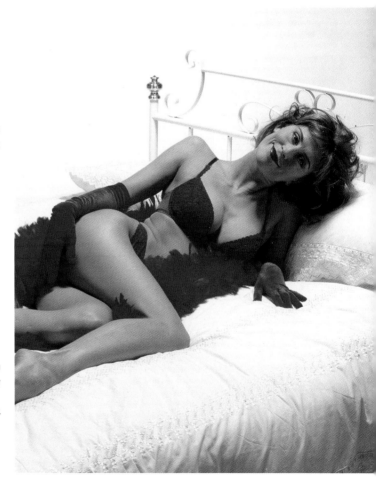

cross-dressing

BELOW | Not all women are
disturbed by a man's cross-
dressing fantasy. She can be
happy to join in, selecting
items of her clothing for him
to wear, or taking him out
shopping to choose his
female underwear.

NOBODY KNOWS FOR SURE how many men enjoy
cross-dressing or even fantasize about it. The
subject is still fairly taboo in our society, although
transvestite issues are now being discussed more
openly. However, research shows that many men
do cross-dress and become sexually aroused by
wearing, or thinking about wearing, women's
clothes, and especially women's underwear.

The reason why this is one of the most secret
fantasies of all is that many men, who clearly
identify themselves as heterosexuals and who
only want to make love to female partners, are
afraid of the ridicule and condemnation that cross-
dressing invariably causes.

Studies conducted on men who cross-dress
show that over 75 per cent of them are married

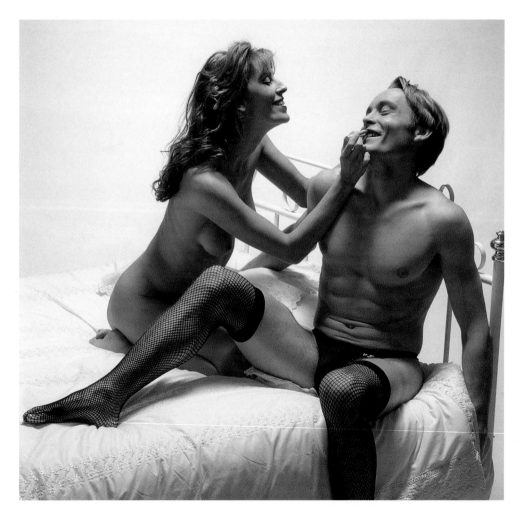

and have children. Their sexual orientation is towards the opposite sex, and they clearly identify their gender as male.

There are various reasons why a man may fantasize about cross-dressing. It may be due to curiosity and the desire to discover how it feels to "be like a woman"; soft, feminine or exotic underwear may appeal to him, or he may even need to wear female underwear or other clothing to become sexually aroused. In the latter case, this can be termed as a transvestite fetish, as the man is reliant on these objects to become sexually fulfilled.

Having fantasies, or wearing female clothing, is not necessarily a problem in itself, unless the man feels confused or unhappy about his sexual identity, is plagued with guilt about it, or his female partner feels distressed, offended and threatened by his transvestite tendencies. (Some sex counsellors specialize in cross-dressing, transvestite, or transsexual issues and are able to help the individuals concerned to talk through any problems that may result.)

Many wives and girlfriends who discover their partners are cross-dressers find it almost impossible to accept or even understand their behaviour. They may fear that their partners have homosexual tendencies, are effeminate, or they may regard the behaviour as a perversion.

Some female partners, though, are happy to comply with this aspect of the man's personality, and even enjoy dressing him up, putting make-up on him, or choosing his specialized items of clothing. It is their secret, and it becomes part of their sexual agenda – an important feature of their relationship, even if it is something that is hidden from others.

Perhaps your dressing-up fantasies might include cross-dressing. This could be a response to the man's real desire to sometimes wear women's clothing, or it might just be a one-off game to act out the opposite-sex gender role. If this is acceptable to both people involved, and you feel your relationship is strong enough to withstand the implications, cross-dressing can become a shared fantasy game involving you both.

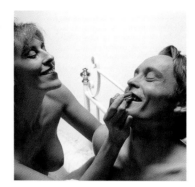

LEFT | He may just want to wear women's panties or stockings, but he might also want to dress up completely as a female and play-act the role of a woman for a while. You can put lipstick, and eye make-up on him, and even lend him some of your jewellery.

coming to terms with cross-dressing

Melanie, 42 years, has been married to Tom, also 42, for 14 years: "We had been married for about nine years before I discovered that Tom liked to wear women's underwear. I found out because I walked into the bedroom one afternoon and found him wearing a pair of my best knickers – a black, silky pair that I kept for special occasions. I don't know who looked more shocked – Tom, for being found out, or me.

"We had a terrible scene about it, during which he confessed that he often fantasized about wearing women's clothing, and that he did sometimes dress up as a woman, whenever he was alone in the house. I went a bit hysterical, and I said some awful things to him, accusing him of all kinds of perverted behaviour. He said he had always felt guilty about this trait, and he was obviously very distressed about me knowing about it.

"On my side, I felt he had turned into a stranger in a second, that he was no longer the man I knew, and I even wondered if he was actually a real man at all. Our relationship went through a very rocky patch, but somehow we managed to keep talking it through because the bottom line was that we really loved each other, and we had a good relationship. We were lucky because we met some people who knew a great deal more about cross-dressing than us and we were able to get advice from them.

"Slowly, Tom felt less guilty, and I came to accept this side of his sexuality. I became less suspicious and judgmental about the whole thing. In the end we even started to use his cross-dressing as an occasional 'extra' in our sexual relationship. When he feels the need, and I am ready for it, I dress and make him up. We don't discuss this with our friends, but it has become our special secret and we even make it fun."

Tom's response
"All I want to add to what Melanie has said is that none of this ever had anything to do with how I felt about her because I have always really loved her. At the end of the day, it was a relief that she knew. I am very lucky to have someone like Melanie who could eventually accept and understand this part of me."

skin teasing

SOME PEOPLE ARE VERY TURNED ON by the idea of skin teasing, where they are stroked all over the body with the lightest of touches and using all kinds of textures which can result in an almost unbearable intensity. At the other extreme, so long as both partners are willing, lovers can find it stimulating to act out fantasies that involve bondage and domination.

RIGHT | Experiment with the feeling of silk, velvet or chiffon.

BELOW | Barely any weight at all, a feather boa feels like a breeze whispering over the skin – watch the goose bumps come and go!

the lightest touch

It is not a fantasy for the ticklish, but if the idea of a session of skin excitation appeals to either of you, then gather around you all kinds of sensual materials so that you can enjoy a variety of tactile sensations. Find out from each other if either of you has a particular tactile fetish – perhaps you love the feeling of feathers, or of soft, luxurious silk on your skin, or even the firmer texture of leather or rubber being stroked against the surface of your body.

Even more exciting is to use different materials and different touches, perhaps even blowing or licking the body all over, or trailing your fingers very lightly over the most sensitive parts of the skin. Erotic touches on the skin involve brushing its surface, with almost no pressure, so they enliven the skin's most peripheral sensory nerves. All the hair follicles that cover the skin are packed with nerve endings that are stimulated by these erotic caresses. Sometimes your whole body is left tingling and quivering to the point that you are tempted to beg your partner to stop. Yet the pleasure is in being taken right to the height of skin sensation.

There are several ways to enjoy this fantasy game. You might want to try all the different kinds of skin stimulation in one session, so that you experience a whole variety of touches and textures. You can enjoy the caress of any material including leather, silk, satin, chiffon and feathers. Or you might make it a totally feathery event, tantalizing the skin with delicate caresses from a whole variety of exotic plumes. Perhaps you prefer to be excited by the warmth of your partner's touch. Your skin can be stroked all over with the light brush of fingertips, the sensual moistness of the tongue, or the caressing breeze of the breath. If you are being skin teased, try to relax as much as you can into the intensity of your skin responses. While the touch is exquisitely light, your sensory nerves will be in a state of high

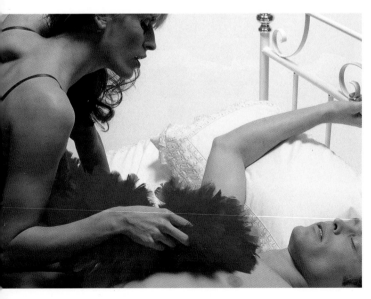

excitation. If you tense up it will become too ticklish, but if you surrender to the tantalizing touches, it can become an extremely pleasurable sensation.

feel of leather

If your partner is turned on by the idea of black leather, find a pair of erotic-looking soft leather gloves to wear and begin to stroke very lightly but slowly over his whole body. Blindfold him loosely with a silk scarf so he doesn't know where your touches will go, or exactly what you are planning to do, and this will add to his excitement. Stroke all over his face so he can take in the smell of the leather, and then draw one hand after the other lightly on the surface of his skin down over his body to the tips of his toes.

caress of silk

The soft caress of a silky scarf will create a contrasting skin sensation compared to the feel of leather. Its light sensual texture will barely put any pressure on the skin at all. This will heighten the nerve sensation, drawing your partner's feeling senses out to the very surface of his body. Silk can produce a wonderful sense of luxurious caress, particularly when trailed over areas of highly

sensitive skin. Velvet or chiffon are also texturally sensual materials.

featherlight touches

The ruffling of downy feathers against the skin will tickle and tease it pleasantly. Feathers are even softer than silk, so light they can fly away. For the tantalizing effect of many feathers stroking the skin, loosely bunch up an ostrich feathered boa, and rub it back and forth gently across his chest. Then you can loosen it and trail its length all over his body, asking your partner to turn over at some point, so it can caress the back of his body.

plumes of pleasure

Lots of people fantasize about having their skin teased lovingly by peacock feathers. The rich colours and beautiful designs in the peacock's plumage give them a very exotic appearance. Then the fan-shaped top of the feather and its delicate quill make it a perfect tool for exciting the skin if it is stroked very lightly all over the body. Give your partner a feathery thrill, running the peacock feather over the surface of her skin with almost imperceptible pressure. It will make her whole body tingle and shiver with pleasure.

BELOW LEFT AND RIGHT |
Sweep a delicate feather over all her erogenous pleasure zones. Run it around her nipples, under her arms, along the side of her neck, and over her belly, groin and thighs. When she turns over, skim the feather over the soles of her feet and on the very sensitive spot at the back of the knees, and then circulate it over her buttocks.

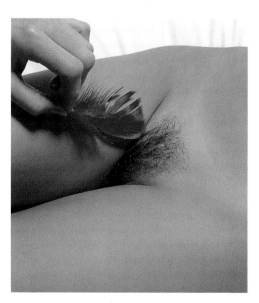
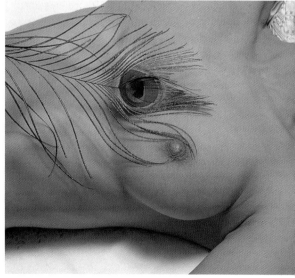

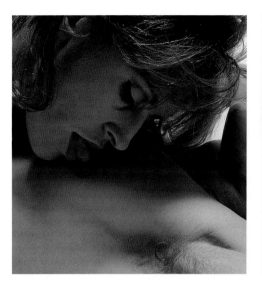

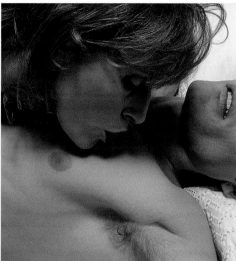

ABOVE | Vary the pressure of
your tongue from soft to hard.

ABOVE RIGHT | The warmth of
your breath against the damp
of the skin is very sensual.

tongue teasing

Bathe the whole body with the warm, moist
sensations of your tongue, flicking it and licking
lightly over the surface of the skin. This is a very
erotic form of skin teasing, inciting sensual and
sexual feelings to fever pitch. Languidly roll your
tongue around and around the surface of the lips
and the rims of the ears. Then dart it back and
forth over the nipples and further down, circle it
around the navel. Let your tongue travel down
lightly over the genitals, but try not to over-excite
your partner here. Continue running your tongue
over the whole of the body, to keep him or her on
the sensory edge.

sensual breath

When the skin has been moistened by the tongue,
blow gently over the wet areas. Brush the whole
body with sweeps of your breath, sometimes
caressing the skin like a gentle breeze, and
sometimes blowing a little stronger in circular
motions so it seems as if you are creating a mini-
whirlwind on the surface of their body. Breathe on
their nipples for a special effect.

He or she can lie back and surrender to the
gentle touch of your fingers running softly over
their face. There should be no pressure at all in

stroke play

Patsy, aged 33: "When we were little, my
sister and I used to spend hours tickling
each other and I loved that very light
touch on my skin. I had special places
where it felt particularly pleasurable,
like my back, my underarms, and most
especially my feet.

"In all of my relationships since
becoming an adult, I have always wanted
a boyfriend to touch and tease me in that
way. I just want to lie there, and be lightly
stroked all over – the more subtle it is, the
more exciting I find it. It is not always
sexual, but it is immensely physically
pleasurable.

"Now, finally, I have a boyfriend who
loves it too, so we spend quite a bit of our
physical time just teasing, tickling and
stroking each other's skin with all kinds
of things. We always take it in turns, so
one of us can just give in to enjoying the
pleasure of all those lovely skin sensations.
To me it feels like luxury and my dream
come true. Sometimes I enjoy it as much
as making love."

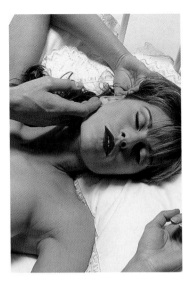

your hands, just a feathery motion that will awaken the most peripheral of their skin's sensory nerves. Let the feeling in your fingers be tender, and move them flowing down over the face, tracing the contours of the features. Run your fingertips delicately over the edge of the eyelashes and over the lips.

linger lovingly

Use the back of your fingers, your fingertips, and even the edge of your nails to heighten the skin's senses. Linger sensually over the most sensitive places where the skin is particularly soft and defenceless to tease and excite it. Stroke over the belly and along the sides of the rib-cage and then slide your fingers along the inside of the thighs with these teasing and pleasing touches which bring the warmth of your skin to the surface of your partner's body.

LEFT | Try to see how light you can make the touch of your fingers.

BELOW | Use the back of your fingers as well as your fingertips.

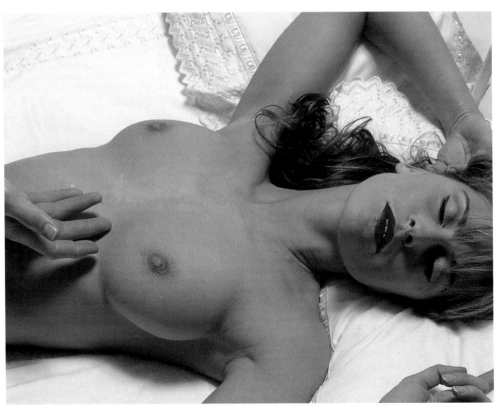

bondage, s&m and spanking

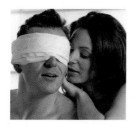

ABOVE | Tissue paper is a soft alternative with no hint of danger involved.

BELOW | When tying each other up, it is worth investing in some handcuffs or other restraints, such as this self-sticking bondage tape, to avoid ending up struggling with tight knots that simply won't come undone.

MENTION BONDAGE to most people and images of sinister black masks, chains, long whips and complicated harnesses spring to mind. Although there is definitely a culture of people who love all that, there is also a lighter side to the scene that a larger proportion of people indulge in.

Bondage can be described as any sexual act that involves the restraint, humiliation or even pain of a partner. In spite of the potential harm it can do, it is important to add that bondage is a consensual act, in which both parties agree exactly on what they are about to do to one another. Take away the word "consensual" and it becomes a criminal offence. It's a fine but definite line.

light bondage

This can include a little light bottom spanking or having your arms and feet tied to the bedposts, bed head or even the banisters, using handcuffs (often covered in fake fur), stockings, ribbon, silk scarves or your work tie. To save yourselves

considerable embarrassment later, before you start, make sure you know exactly where you have put the key if you are using locking handcuffs. Whatever you use, it can be fairly tight, or looser just to simulate restraint.

The person who is being restricted is often referred to as the "bottom", and the person inflicting the restraint as the "top". There are some who enjoy both roles and they are known as "switches". For the top, the pleasure in bondage is found in feelings of power and control. For the bottom, it is more about submission and victimization. In light bondage, the thrill is mainly a psychological one coupled with the fact that, when restrained, you no longer have to worry about reciprocating pleasure. You can concentrate exclusively on your own sensations, without any feelings of guilt about my turn/your turn. Some women who have difficulty achieving orgasm with penetrative sex, find that a little light bondage resolves the problem.

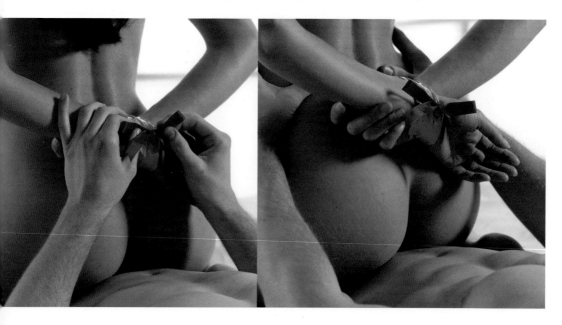

heavy bondage

This has a huge following and people who are into it form tight group connections. Orgasm takes second place to the infliction and receipt of pain. Many claim that when receiving extreme pain of this kind they are transported into a meditative state.

Bondage practitioners are very serious about their craft and it is not something that the experts take lightly. There are special codes, etiquette and release words that are used to prevent serious harm from being done. Anyone contemplating getting into heavy bondage must read about it first and learn how it all works. A lot of literature and advice is available.

sado-masochism

Like all forms of bondage, S&M is a game of role-playing in which the "sadist" inflicts the pain and the "masochist" receives it. It often involves whipping or body piercing, but extreme S&Ms have been known to brand the bottom with hot irons to enforce loyalty.

Research has shown that before climax the brain releases feel-good hormones called endorphins, which help the body to tolerate pain. After climax the top must stop, as the body becomes less tolerant of pain. S&Ms usually use a release word to prevent serious damage. "Stop" and "You're hurting me" are, apparently, no good, as the bottom will often shout these words when they don't actually want the top to stop or slow down, and use them as part of the game. Instead, the word "red" often means stop and "yellow" means ease off a little.

submission and domination

SubDom, as it is known, is similar in practice to S&M. However, where practitioners of S&M concentrate on the infliction of pain, SubDom is more about relinquishing control. It is more of a mental game that involves a lot of trust and discussion for both parties to get satisfaction and enjoyment. The dominator will remove all control from the Sub (or bottom) in the form of slavery by commanding the bottom where to sit, when to speak and how to behave.

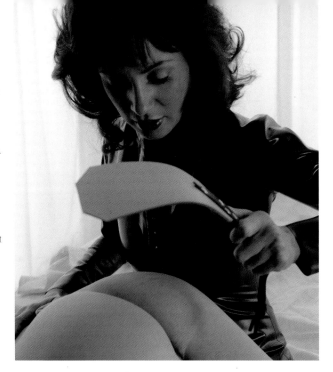

Most people either like to be a bit dominant or a bit submissive during sex, often switching roles depending on their mood. If you are playing the dominant role then you can command your partner where to lick you, what position to get into, how to touch you, where and for how long. Try switching roles so that you each get a chance to "play teacher" and each get a chance to be "dutiful student".

paddles and spanking

Spanking is used in bondage but also by "vanilla" sex practitioners, people who simply enjoy the odd thump on the rump.

Most people who spank each other for a bit of a laugh don't consider themselves as "real" bondage and discipline practitioners, so don't really need to organize a release word as such before they begin. But remember to keep within each of your boundaries to prevent either of you from getting unintentionally hurt. In the heat of the moment you may forget your own strength. Begin slowly and gently with a light slap or two and then, if you want, increase the pressure in response to your partner. Keep it light-hearted and fun, and make sure you give as good as you get.

ABOVE | If you want something kinkier than a hand, go with a wide paddle, as this produces more of a dull thud than a whip's sting.

BELOW | A little light-hearted bondage can be fun. These pink accessories are soft and gentle on the skin.

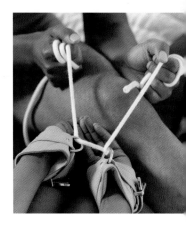

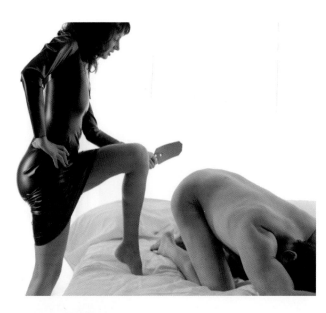

dominance and bondage

Domination and bondage are common themes in sexual fantasies. Images of being tied up, spanked, or even "forced" (albeit erotically) into having sex are typical fantasies which can run through some people's minds while having intercourse. More often than not, these day-dreams remain in the mind as a private fantasy and are never actually acted out in reality.

A lot of people would never even discuss these fantasies with their partners, either because they feel too shy, or just because they want to keep them in their own private world. However, for many, the fantasy of being the dominant or submissive partner in a sexual scenario, or being restrained while being slowly teased into an orgasm, is an imaginative way to become erotically aroused. Some couples even like to play out their sexual fantasies together in the bedroom,

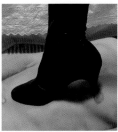

TOP | Dressing in leather may be attractive to some couples.

ABOVE | Some men have a fetish about women in high heels.

playing power games

Jonathan, aged 33, a salesman has lived with his girlfriend, Anja, for five years. "It was Anja who first suggested that we should introduce some domination and submission games into our sex life. She said that in her last relationship, her boyfriend would sometimes tie her arms and legs to the bed posts, and then make love to her, and that she found it to be incredibly sexually arousing. I was more than happy to give it a go because I had always wanted to do something like this myself, but my last girlfriend would have never agreed to it. Now, once in a while, we take it in turns to be tied up. Sometimes I do it to her, and she just goes wild, especially if I am giving her oral sex. She says that this kind of sex game gives her the most intense orgasms. It's the same for me, because there is something incredibly erotic about having to absolutely surrender and be helpless while she is making love to me. She does everything very slowly, and takes me almost to the point of an orgasm, then cools it down, and then starts again. In the end, I feel like I am going to explode – and I usually do."

Clara, aged 27, a landscape designer, has shared a home with her fiancé for two years. "Jack and I enjoy all kinds of sex games, and we are pretty hot on the ones with domination themes. He is the dominator, and I get turned on by the submissive role. We do all kinds of things, and I am sure people who know us would be quite shocked about what we get up to on some weekends because we look so normal. I trust him completely because I know he loves me and he would never do anything that would actually hurt me. I have my code word, and if I say it, he always stops. We also make love in all the more normal ways too because we don't want this to be our only sexual theme. The interesting thing is that it is only in our sexual relationship that Jack's domination fantasy comes out. In every other aspect of our relationship, we are absolutely on equal terms."

switching between the dominant and submissive roles from time to time, or settling into a particular routine depending on which excites them most. Bondage, discipline, or dressing up in leather and other fetishist gear may be a big turn on for some people but abhorrent to others.

The major rule of these sex games is that both partners are happy and willing to give them a go. No one should ever pressure his or her partner into this kind of fantasy sex play, nor should anyone submit to it just to please a demanding partner.

However, if you both enjoy a little rough play or dressing up in your sex life, and the idea of taking your eroticism right to the edge excites you, then there is no reason at all why you should not add these saucy alternatives to your sexual repertoire.

rules of the game

Some people fear that their tough love sex play could mean that they are bordering on sado-masochism. There is no need to worry unless you are actually hurting your partner or you feel you are receiving real pain and abuse. What we are discussing here is pretending to use domination and force and playing with these concepts because you find them sexually arousing and enriching to your sex life. So where do you draw the line?

First of all, these fantasy games must always be by mutual consent. Then make some rules and stick by them. Only act out domination and submission games when you are in a relationship you trust, and you know your partner well enough to be sure he or she would never hurt you, or ever force you into something you do not want to do.

BELOW | Both men and women enjoy being tied up and having their skin teased with different textures.

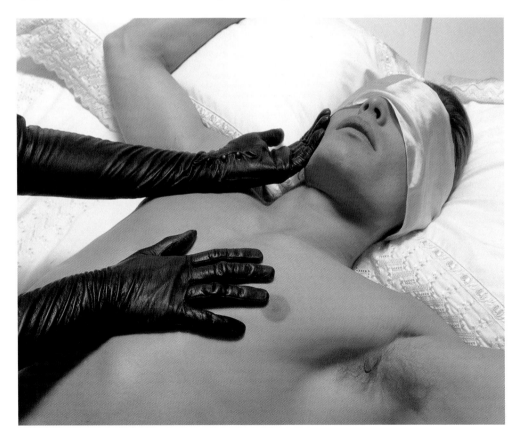

BELOW | Master and slave: Some men can be very aroused by playing a submissive role in a sex game, especially as a release of tension if they otherwise hold powerful positions. Some couples enjoy a "master and slave" game, where the woman dresses up to play a dominating role and disciplines her partner.

If spanking the buttocks is part of your play, then only take it so far as you find it fun and exciting.

Don't cause real pain, cause bruises or break the skin. You can pretend you are humiliating your partner, but you should know the boundaries between play and offence. Don't say things you may regret later or which will emotionally scar your partner. Talk over exactly what kind of fantasy behaviour turns you on, what your limits are, and what you do and do not want to happen, and then stick within these guidelines.

Make sure you have a signal or code word which you both recognize as the sign to stop the game immediately. The moment one or the other of you says this word or gives the sign, you must stop!

If being tied to the bedpost while your partner makes slow, tantalizing love to you or gives you orgasmic oral sex (research shows that restraint is probably the most popular fantasy) interests you and you plan to act it out, then make sure he or she does not tie the knots too tight, and that they can be undone immediately if you request it, or whenever necessary.

You can restrain the wrists and ankles, but you must never tie anything around the neck, and

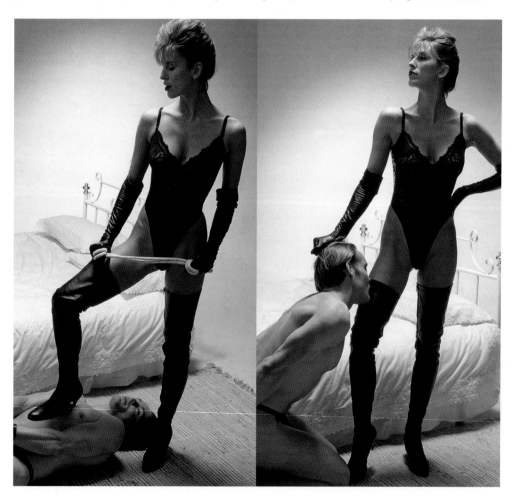

covering the mouth can also be dangerous. If your partner is restrained, do not leave him or her alone – even for a short time. You need to be conscious and present during the whole time your partner is tied up. Some people may fantasize about restraint, and even desire to act it out, but are simply too afraid to be tied up. Respect that anxiety and just pretend he or she is tied up. One way is for that person to grip the headboard so the arms are spread-eagled, and the legs are splayed out wide in the posture of restraint.

getting the gear

Fetishist tools may be in order for these games, and you can get these from a good sex shop, on the internet or by mail order. Black outfits are a popular choice for bondage and domination games. Thigh-high boots, lace-up corsets, armbands, and elbow-length gloves in leather, latex or rubber are the normal gear that turn people on. Men are more visually stimulated than their partners by these outfits, but women can enjoy dressing up to arouse their men. (Some women might find the whole idea chauvinistic and absurd!)

Soft ropes, silk scarves or strips of cotton material can all be used for restraint, but make sure that nothing you use will burn or chafe the skin. If you want to use more serious-looking equipment, there are sexy handcuffs available which both of you can undo, if necessary. Don't use real handcuffs which are too threatening and may be difficult to release.

Restraint, or being softly tied to the bedpost, and having your lover slowly, tantalizingly and deliberately turn you on while you pretend to be helpless can be extremely arousing. The added thrill is the restriction on movement which can take your excitement right to its peak. He should pay attention to every part of your body. If he licks and kisses your breasts and nipples while you are tied like this, you may feel as if you are going to explode with erotic sensation. He should deliberately do everything slowly, taking his time, to keep you dangling at this almost excruciating pitch of excitement.

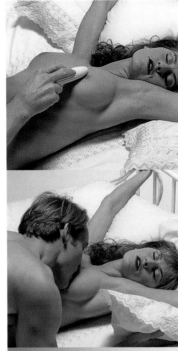

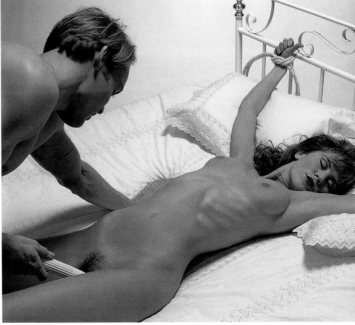

LEFT AND BELOW | You can caress each part of her body while she lies helpless.

Slow, erotic oral sex while being restrained can be an amazing sexual experience. Again, he should take his time, doing everything in a teasing and super-sensual way. If he is sensitive to your responses, he will know just when to slow down to delay your moment of orgasm, so that you beg him to go ahead.

Good vibrations: Another variation to add to your fantasy play is for him to use a vibrator to bring you to orgasm. After kissing and stroking every part of your body, and waiting till you have reached a peak of arousal, he can vibrate it against your vulva.

Demand his obedience: Stay haughty and proud as he grovels at your feet. Let him adore you from his lowly position. He must touch, kiss or caress you in any way you command, but you must appear to be above feeling excited by his attentions. Complain and make him do more. The fun is in acting as if you have total control and can demand complete obedience from him.

Assert your sexuality: If you think he has been "bad" or is showing too much will of his own, you can rough him around a little. Or you can display your assertive sexuality, pulling him to your body and holding his body tight to yours. You can even make love to him, but you must stay in charge.

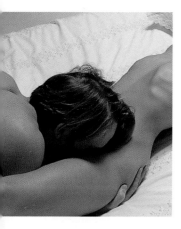

ABOVE AND RIGHT | Oral sex can be especially sensual for the woman while she is being restrained.

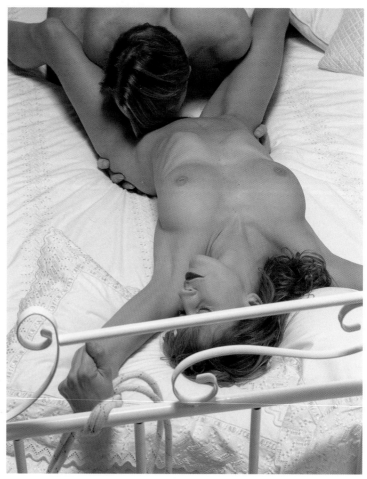

OPPOSITE | Sometimes it is the woman's turn to assert herself.

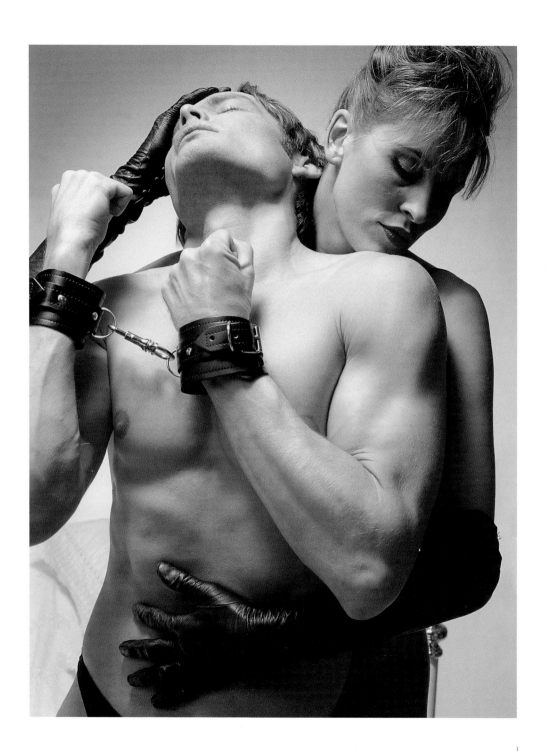

fun and fetish

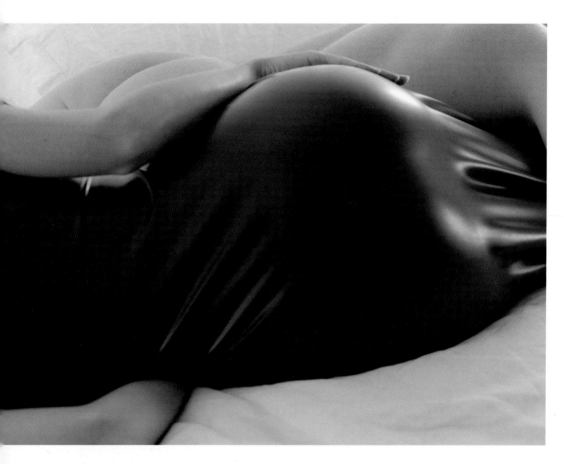

ABOVE | The feel of rubber and PVC against the skin can be a huge turn-on and some claim it makes them more sexually confident. Putting rubber and PVC garments on can be slightly less appealing – use plenty of talc to smooth your skin before you try.

OPPOSITE TOP LEFT | Piercing can be very erotic.

MOST PEOPLE LIKE TO PLAY around with fetishes – for example, getting their partner to keep her (or his) heels on while they make love. It's a titillating romp rather than a necessity. A stricter definition of a fetish, however, is a tangible object or an action that needs to be repeated over and over for sexual gratification. For example, we've already discussed talking dirty, which some people enjoy now and again. A talking dirty fetish, however, would mean that the person would not be sexually aroused unless the dirty talk is used in all sexual acts.

Fetishes are fine if both partners have the same one, but if they don't, then the relationship can break down and external guidance may be necessary. However, it's worth remembering that a person with a fetish usually loves his or her fetish immensely and is unwilling to part with it. It's usually better if the partner of someone with a fetish learns to accept the sexual foible, rather than trying to repress it. This assumes, of course, that the fetish is morally acceptable and legal. For example, an exhibitionist who gets sexual pleasure only or mainly from exposing his genitals

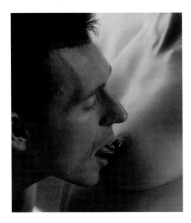

Cutting, piercing or branding may be permanent or temporary. Elaborate S&M piercing fetishes can involve piercing many needles shallowly through the skin with a variety of strings attached so that the strings can be pulled or weights hung from them. This is advanced S&M that is beyond the scope of this book. It requires trust and knowledge. There is a lot of literature on this type of sex play and anyone who wants to have a go at it needs to get informed advice.

watersports

Body fluid fetishes include a whole area of "dirty games" where body fluids are shared. This might be simply sharing sweat, saliva or other excretions, or sometimes involves urinating on your partner.

Some games involve exchanging blood, or body fluid bonding. Couples who try this have usually taken the precaution of being tested for disease before they begin – precautions should be taken so you are not putting yourself at risk.

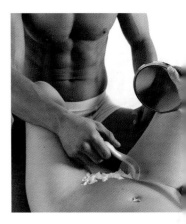

ABOVE | Try the infamous Brazilian wax, or get your partner to shave you.

BELOW | Tantalize him with a pair of spiked heels and rubber accessories.

to strangers should not be allowed to continue this fetish and must face both the legal and moral consequences of his actions.

Common fetishes include leather, fur, latex, stilettos, handcuffs and feet (shrimping), but some go as far as exhaust pipes or mud wallowing. Cross-dressing is a popular fetish. Some women go so far as to wear a fake penis ("packing"). There are many theories about why people find cross-dressing stimulating. One idea is that men and women feel more relaxed when they are able to express the other gender side to their personality. Some men find transvestism erotic. In most cases these men are straight but merely find eroticism in wearing female clothing. Many of these men are afraid to share this fetish with their partner for fear of rejection and of being thought of as less of a man.

body modification

Tattooing and piercing are fairly common nowadays, with a huge number of people decorating their bodies in some way. Doing it for sexual gratification highlights the difference between high-street trend and sexual fetish.

Piercing, tattooing, cutting, branding and body sculpting through corsetry are all forms of body modification. For some, having an absolute stranger wield a long needle and clamp around their nether regions is just not a problem. It's seen as a means of enhancing sexual sensation and a way of getting more sensation from a localized area.

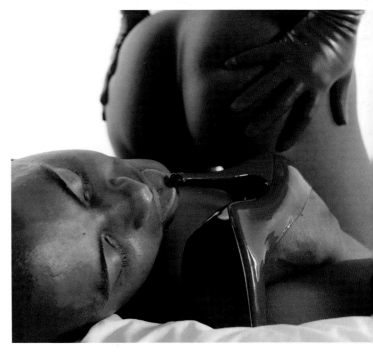

fantasy

VERY LITTLE HAS BEEN documented about male and female fantasy, probably because people guard their fantasies fiercely. Regardless of how liberated and open they may be or how close their friends are, people rarely discuss fantasy in the same way they may discuss, say, oral sex.

Nancy Friday was one of the first authors to bring women's erotic fantasies into the limelight in her bestseller *My Secret Garden* (1973). Until then, it was widely assumed that women did not have sexual fantasies, although most women must have known that they did. It has always

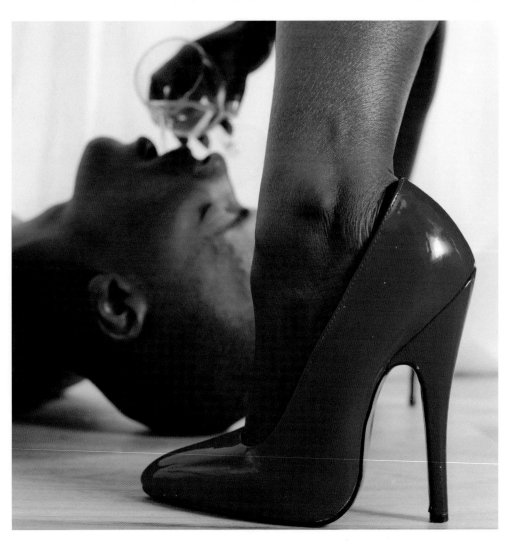

been accepted that men fantasize and whole industries have been built up to enable men to fulfil these with props and costumes.

Many people are embarrassed by the content of their fantasies. They may be extremely depraved and subversive; they may involve illegal acts that make most people angry or disturbed when they hear about them happening in real life. It is for this reason that many people become embarrassed and sometimes a bit disgusted by what they dream about during masturbation or lovemaking. Many people also worry that they fantasize about weird and wonderful scenarios while making love to their partner. This can lead to feelings of intense guilt and doubt. It is worth remembering that it is human instinct to be drawn precisely to those things that are forbidden.

Hardly surprisingly, men and women fantasize about different things. In general, men's fantasies tend to be impersonal, often involving several partners and complete strangers. Other common themes include watching others, especially two women, making love and watching their partner or another woman masturbate. Women's fantasies tend to be more about intimate, one-to-one relationships. Popular themes involve sex with a celebrity, sex with another woman and being dominated or dominating. Both men and women fantasize about having sex in public.

brain stimulation

Fantasy is one of the most important components in lovemaking. As humans we have very complex brains and mental capacities so it is often not enough merely to stimulate our genitals. We have to be in the correct mood and mind-set before we are relaxed enough to let our bodies go. Sometimes your fantasies are simple enough to enact: having sex in a smart hotel or on the kitchen table; being wooed in a romantic candlelit room. Others that involve a cast of thousands may be more difficult to arrange.

Many people fantasize about sex with a film or popstar. Try thinking about your fantasy figure while having sex with your partner. What they don't know won't hurt them. Just be sure not to scream

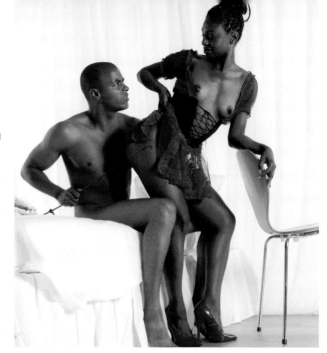

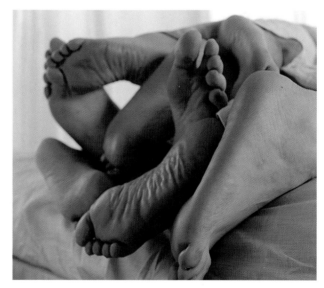

out the wrong name during a moment of heightened excitement. Keep your fantasies as a private store of erotic movies that you can switch on whenever you like. Remember that your brain is the biggest and most sensitive sex organ in your body and where the mind leads, the body will follow.

TOP AND ABOVE | It could be dressing up and role-playing, or having more than one partner in bed – whatever turns you on, as long as your accomplices are willing.

toys toys toys

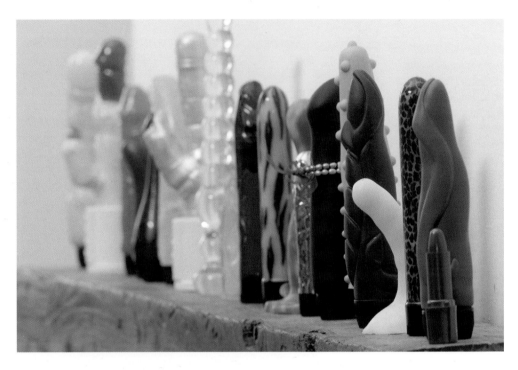

is a wide range of sex toys
available and a new style of
sex shop which caters for
women and is less seedy than
the stereotypical sex shop.

BELOW | A classic rabbit vibrator
has a clitoral stimulator.

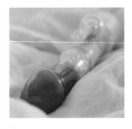

SEX TOYS ARE COMING out of the bedside drawer
and on to the coffee table. Vibrators and other sex
toys have become *de rigueur* as the face of sexual
awareness has changed. There are so many toys
to choose from, in all sorts of shapes, colours and
sizes. Design and aesthetics are as important as
function and nowadays sex toys are becoming
desirable designer items.

And they're not just for women. There are as
many gizmos and gadgets for men, from anal love
balls to penis rings. We are becoming more open
to the idea of incorporating toys into sex play. Sex
toys have the advantage of spicing it up between
the sheets, whether you are a man or a woman
together or going solo.

The whole purpose of sex toys is fun, but you
may need to be careful about how you introduce
the idea to your partner. Many men feel that they

are being criticized as inadequate lovers if their
partner buys a vibrator. Equally, a woman might
wonder about her partner's sexuality if he
suddenly starts using anal love balls.

Sex toys are great incorporated into foreplay.
They are exciting to use on each other and many
can be used to arouse both men and women. A
small, flexible vibrator with rubber nodules, for
example, is just as great for stimulating the
prostate as it is for hitting the G spot. Most
vibrators are better for external stimulation than
for penetration and feel fabulous on all kinds of
erogenous zones, such as the insides of the thighs
and the nipples, as well as the genitals.

Reassure your partner that you don't prefer the
toys to them. It's just a different and fun variation.
Sometimes you like oral sex, sometimes
penetration and sometimes playing with toys.

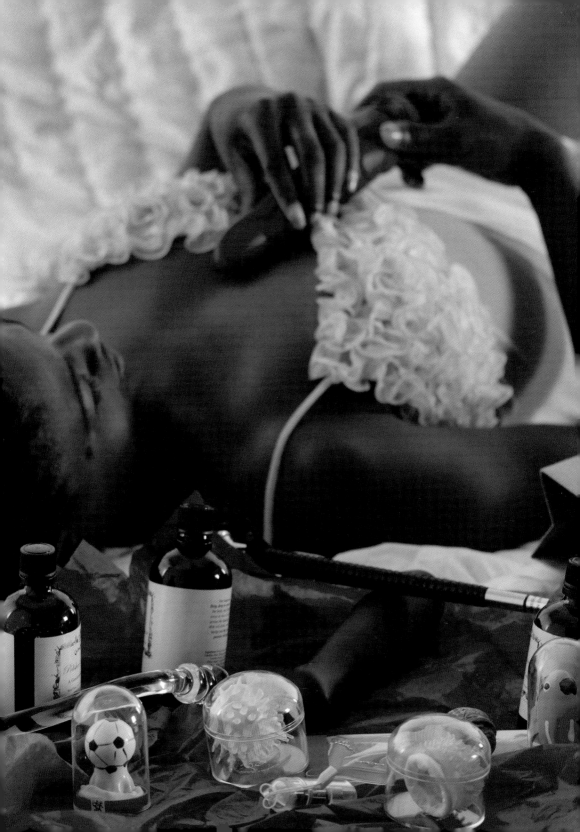

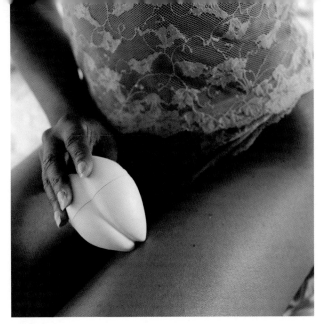

incorporate it into lovemaking or masturbation. Some women find the vibrator more effective than the hand, tongue or penis.

When using a vibrator, experiment with the different sensations it can produce. It may feel strange to begin with, but persevere. It can be used for massaging the clitoris, penis, testicles or anus, and not necessarily for penetration.

Vibrators can be made out of plastic or, more recently, soft elastomers, resins and silicon, and the most popular size is about 10cm/4in. The softer ones are better suited for penetration and are also quieter, as the softness absorbs the sound. The more rigid plastic variety may be better for more direct stimulation. As with any aspect of sex, it's important to keep it clean. Always wash and dry your vibrator after use. Remember to keep a supply of batteries handy, as there are few things worse than a pre-orgasmic power failure.

ABOVE | Designer toys are a far cry from the usual pink plastic fare. This vibrating "seed pod" is made from a soft, warm-to-the-touch elastomer material.

BELOW | These love balls are coated ball bearings which can be inserted into the vagina. Great for exercising your pelvic floor muscles, they come in a variety of weights and sizes.

bring on the toys

It's easy to confuse a vibrator with a dildo, so what is the difference? Well, the vibrator vibrates and the dildo doesn't. Vibrators are used more for genital massage and are not necessarily phallic in shape. Dildos are shaped like penises and are designed more for anal or vaginal penetrative use.

vibrators

Not just for women, many men use vibrators to stimulate their penises and report similar sensations to those of women. The advantage of the vibrator for women is that those who need constant clitoral stimulation to achieve orgasm can

the rabbit

One of the most popular and most expensive vibrators, the rabbit first hit the big time after *Sex and the City*'s Charlotte fell in love with her rabbit. It has the standard vibrating shaft and the added bonus of the "ears", providing a clitoris tickler at the front. Some also have an anal probe at the back. It's guaranteed to make you hopping horny.

the mojo

Designed by Marc Newson in silicon, this nipple-shaped five-speed toy concentrates less on vaginal penetration and more on clitoral stimulation. It's good for hitting the spot, but some women miss the vaginal penetration aspect.

dildos

Like vibrators, dildos are made in a variety of different shapes, sizes, colours and textures, and are associated with penetration. They are usually phallic in shape, but this can vary from a lifelike penis (often complete with testicles) to a simple cylindrical structure. Dildos have a history that stretches back 30,000 years, so if you're feeling embarrassed about buying one, remember you are by no means the first.

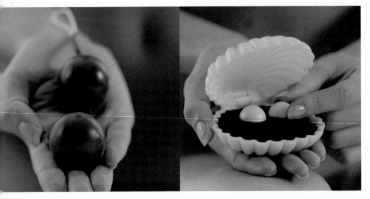

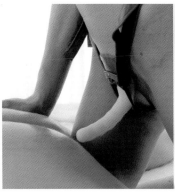
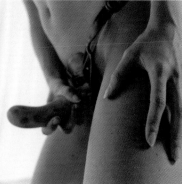

As well as being fun, dildos also have certain health benefits for women. Regular use of a dildo can help to strengthen the vaginal walls by exercising the muscles. They can also help to control the effects of vaginismus, a condition in which the vaginal muscles become tense and spasmodic, making penetration painful.

Dildos are often made from porous material that can accumulate infected semen or blood and vaginal discharge. If the dildo is shared, so is infection. If you want to share a dildo, protect it with a condom.

When buying a dildo intended for anal penetration, make sure that it has a flared end to prevent it disappearing up the rectum. You will thus prevent an embarrassing emergency trip to the local hospital. If you use a dildo for anal penetration, be sure to use a condom and dispose of it once you are finished, as the anus harbours many bacteria that could cause infection if the dildo is then used for vaginal penetration.

harnesses

Used in conjunction with dildos for strap-on sex, harnesses allow the wearer to ignore gender boundaries so that the woman can anally penetrate her partner or he can double penetrate her (vaginal and anal penetration at the same time). If he has erectile problems, he could also opt for the synthetic version to do the job. There is also an option that allows the woman wearing a dildo to have one inside her own body at the same

time. Strap-ons allow women to know what it is like to be the penetrator and the male to be the penetratee. Their use enables couples to role-play and has unlimited possibilities. They can be used by anyone – gay, straight, male or female.

love balls

These are two weighted balls of about 3cm/1¼in in diameter which are placed inside the vagina. The weights rock and jiggle together as you move around, so the balls move around. The advantage of them is that they help you with your pelvic floor exercises. They are also fairly discreet and can be worn anywhere. Some women love them, while others can't feel a thing.

lubrication

The production of love juice is not necessarily directly related to how aroused you are. In fact, it is hormone-controlled and its presence or absence can depend on a host of things from certain times in the menstrual cycle, effects of childbirth and hysterectomy to the drying effects of alcohol and marijuana. There is nothing worse than having to stop a steamy session because of drying up.

Some of the properties in commercial sexual lubricants kill sperm, so avoid these if you are trying to have a baby. Lubrication is an essential component in anal play, as the anus and surrounding area produce no natural lubrication. Be sure to use water-based lubricants if you are using sex toys or condoms.

ABOVE LEFT | Strap-on sex toys can be made in any colour and shape to order, for anal sex or for woman-on-woman vaginal penetration.

BELOW | Vibrators come in all shapes and sizes – a ring must be one of the most discreet.

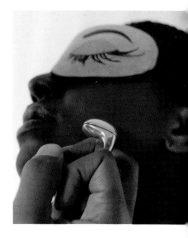

erotica and pornography

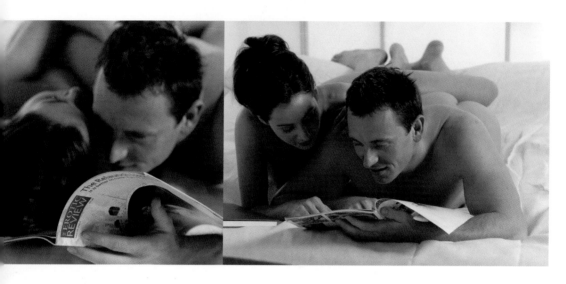

ABOVE AND ABOVE RIGHT |
Erotica is often more exciting
than straightforward porn, but
the range of sexy literature
and magazines covers the
entire spectrum. Reading it
together – or to each other –
can be a great turn-on.

*I KNELT DOWN in front of him again. His cock,
already thickly inflated, sprang up. I moved my
hand over his balls, back up to their base near the
anus. His cock stood up again, more violently. I
held it in my other hand, squeezed it, began
slowly pulling it up and down. The soapy water I
was lathered with provided perfect lubrication. My
hands were filled with a warm, living, magical
substance. I felt it beating like the heart of a bird, I
helped it ride to its deliverance. Up, down, always
the same movement, always the same rhythm,
and the moans above my head. And I was
moaning too, with the water from the shower
sticking to my dress like a tight silken glove, with
the world stopped at the level of my eyes, of his
belly, at the sound of the water tickling over us
and of his cock sliding under my fingers, at the
warm and tender and hard thing between my
hands, at the smell of the soap, of the soaking
flesh and of the sperm mounting under my palm.*

Taken from *The Butcher* by Alina Reyes, this is
a perfect example of contemporary erotica.
Reading it is like drinking a glass of single malt
whisky or fine wine – it makes you feel really good

all over. In addition, it stimulates the erogenous
zone that straightforward pornography simply
cannot reach – the brain.

Erotic literature can be a great aid to sex.
It can provide the warm-up act before your lover
comes on stage or can be part of the programme
together in bed. The choice is vast, whether books,
poetry, films or magazines. It gives you access to
your fantasies and often provides brilliant material
to act out in the reality and privacy of your bedroom.

Most people think of porn films and dirty
magazines when they think of literature associated
with sex. Getting away from the hard stuff, there is
a wonderful variety of sensual and erotic films that
are guaranteed to get you in the mood. You may
be inspired by a raunchy sex scene in an elevator,
or the idea of being blindfolded, lightly tied up and
fed delicious morsels on the kitchen floor.

At the other end of the scale, the gritty porn
film and dirty magazines can be appealing
because of their explicitness and lack of subtlety.
Many people watch porn and read dirty magazines
as masturbation tools or as extra stimulation in sex
play. Both men and women find it exciting to view

something that appears so naughty. It helps to vent fantasies that are active in people's minds but which would perhaps never be brought into reality. To this end it is by no means wrong or subversive to use porn, providing of course that it is legal.

make your own movie

Many people think that porn movies are generally smutty, badly acted and could be done better, so why not give it a go yourself? All you need is a camcorder and a bit of imagination.

Start by sitting down with your partner and discussing the "theme" of your movie. Don't make a script as all the best porn movies rarely have a good script anyway, but just get a general idea of how events will run together. Some ideas could be: the doctor's visit; the prostitute visiting his or her client; an alien sent from outer space to learn more about human procreation; the electrician coming to fix the television.

Set the scene, get any props that you might want, and dress up appropriately for your roles. Position the camera so that you have a good view of the room and, most importantly, the bed. Finally hit record and begin.

Making your own porn film is not only hilarious fun, but also watching it afterwards together can be an extremely erotic experience. Seeing yourselves making love from a different angle gives you a whole new perspective. Alternatively, if you don't have a camcorder then you could create your own kinky photo shoot – just be careful about where you get the pictures developed.

ABOVE | Sharing a pornographic book may end up as a joint exercise in humour or it might give you some interesting ideas.

erotic poetry

The choice of erotic poetry is vast, but sometimes the classics are the best, like DH. Lawrence's poem from *Women in Love*. Here is a taster of the first few lines, best sampled while resting under a ripe fig tree, accompanied by your partner, a good bottle of wine and the sun on your skin…

The proper way to eat a fig, in society,
Is to split it in four, holding it by the stump,
And open it, so that it is a glittering, rosy,
moist, honied, heavy-petalled four-
petalled flower.

Then you throw away the skin

Which is just like a four-sepalled calyx,
After you have taken off the blossom
with your lips.

But the vulgar way
Is just to put your mouth to the crack, and
take out the flesh in one bite.

Every fruit has its secret.
The fig is a very secretive fruit.
As you see it standing growing, you feel at
once it is symbolic:
And it seems male.
But when you come to know it better, you
agree with the Romans, it is female.

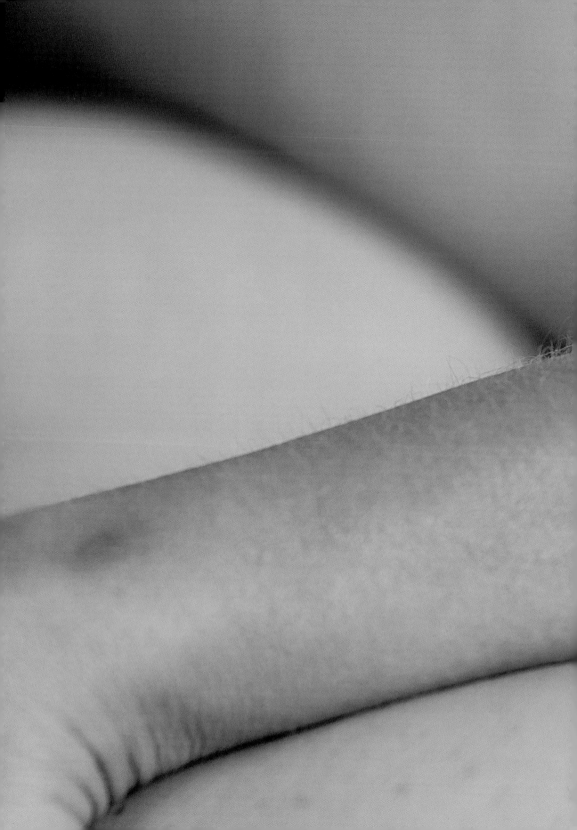

shaking it up

Many long-term relationships experience occasional periods of over-
familiarity and predictability. Add some spice and fire to your relationship
with some fun and exciting new ideas, allowing you to rediscover both
your own and your partner's desire.

spontaneous sex

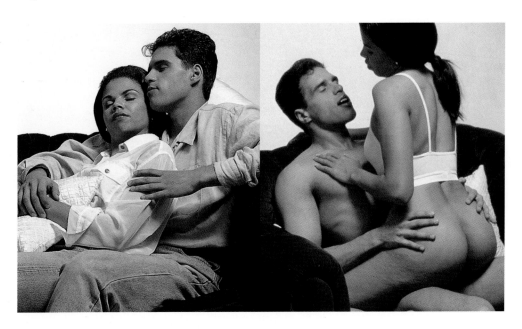

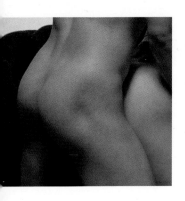

SPONTANEOUS SEX REFERS TO the proverbial "quickie". It is the stuff of best-selling airport novels, full of erotic heaving, panting and writhing bodies, bodice-ripping sex scenes and exotic or, at least, unusual locations. It is not slow and sensual, or particularly intimate, but it is hot and passionate and deliciously primitive. When spontaneous sex happens it is the meeting of the "wild" man and the "wild" woman – there are no formalities to play out and clothes are cast aside along with inhibitions.

Does spontaneous sex have any place in a loving and intimate sexual relationship? Yes, it certainly does, if the two people concerned are equally eager for the action. It is sexual appetite at its most voracious, a hunger immediately satisfied by two consenting partners.

Spontaneous sex can be extremely exciting and exhilarating, affirming a mutual physical attraction and enlivening any sexual relationship with its raw and untamed content.

It can happen anywhere, and when least expected, because by its nature it does not run to a schedule. The one thing you must guarantee, though, is complete privacy, with absolutely no one else in sight, because neither the law, nor your family, nor your neighbours will applaud you if you are caught in the act.

Spontaneous sex rarely happens in the bedroom, it is much more likely to occur in the kitchen, the living room, the bathroom or on the stairs. It may be even more licentious – forbidden moments in the office basement, on a bed of soft grass, against an inviting tree, or on a windswept beach at night.

The wonderful thing about this kind of sex is that it can recapture the excitement and spontaneity of your early days of romance, when your sex hormones were rampant and the two of you could hardly wait a second longer to make love. A "quickie" is the pep pill which can put the zest back into your sexual relationship.

change of mood

Sexual arousal can happen when you least expect it. You may be planning simply to relax with your partner after a tiring day at work and watch a little television before going to bed to sleep. The two of you snuggle up for a cosy but quiet evening, then suddenly the mood changes, and your bodies become electrified just from their closeness to each other.

A sense of urgency rises. You don't even feel you have time to go to the bedroom. Most of your clothes are hastily removed, either by yourself or your partner. You do not even have to take all your clothes off. Now you can make better use of that comfortable old sofa. As the woman, you can climb astride your partner's lap and mount him immediately. This sponteneity will be very exciting for your partner.

Both of you can let go into a passionate session of lovemaking, using the sofa to its best advantage. The back of the chair is a good place to sit if your partner wants to perform cunnilingus on you. The heat of the moment will increase the arousal and excitement for both of you and you can let go into waves of pleasure. You can also use a dining chair and the woman can keep her feet on the floor and hold on to the chair for support if necessary.

Making love in the rear entry or doggie position, with the male partner entering the vagina from behind, will add to the primal intensity of your spontaneous sexual happening. You can lean your weight on to the back of the settee, and while he is thrusting, he can also stimulate your clitoris with his fingers. This position gives both lovers the opportunity to thrust against each other, and is good for vigorous, passionate sex.

RIGHT | The back of a chair is good place to sit for the man to perform cunnilingus.

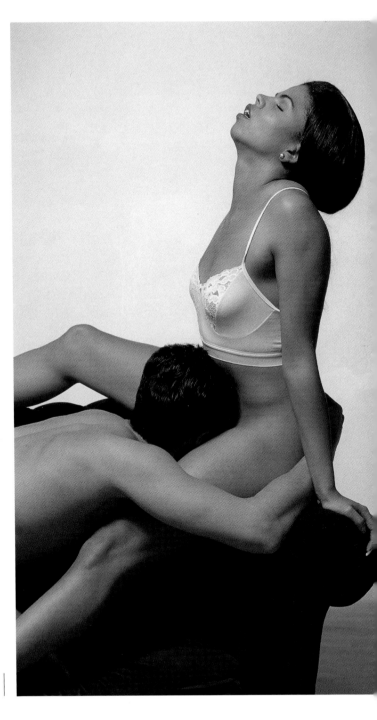

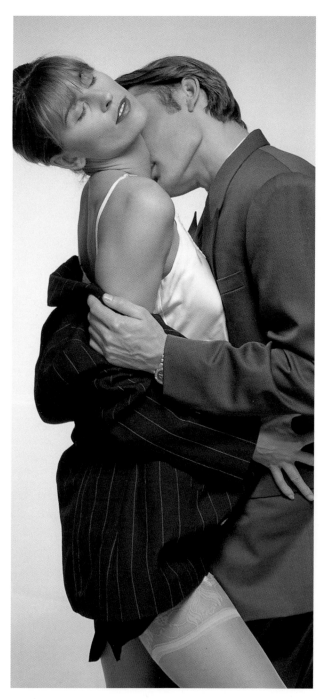

standing up

Standing up is a classic but awkward position for the "quickie" way of having intercourse. It usually implies fast and furious passionate sex, with no preliminaries, but it is hot and impetuous and therefore usually very exciting.

If you do it standing up, it is best to have something to lean on, such as a wall or a tree, and it definitely works better if the partners are a similar height and weight. The main problem is that the penis can very easily slip out of the vagina, and the vertical position makes it difficult for deep thrusting. However, the impulsiveness and thrill of the situation usually indicate that the man is so aroused he is likely to ejaculate very quickly.

This is not an uncommon position for young lovers to take when first exploring their sexuality, perhaps because they cannot take their partner home and so have to resort to more furtive methods of sexual contact. It may also be a natural follow-on from a heavy-petting session. However, in these situations, penetration does not necessarily take place, but the female may close her thighs around the penis, allowing it to rub against her genitals. In this way, both people can gain a quick release from their sexual excitement and tension.

standing sex

You can't wait to make it to the bedroom so, pressed against the wall, you make love to each other in the standing position. Your partner will be able to penetrate you deeper if he elevates you slightly, and you curl one leg around him. He must take care not to push you too hard against the wall while he is thrusting.

Sometimes, full spontaneous sex may be out of the question, especially if you are in a business situation, but if you and your partner meet up somewhere at work or a work function, you may not be able to resist a surreptitious petting session behind closed doors. There is something especially exciting about this kind of erotic and sometimes secret encounter because it will be in strict contrast to your professional persona.

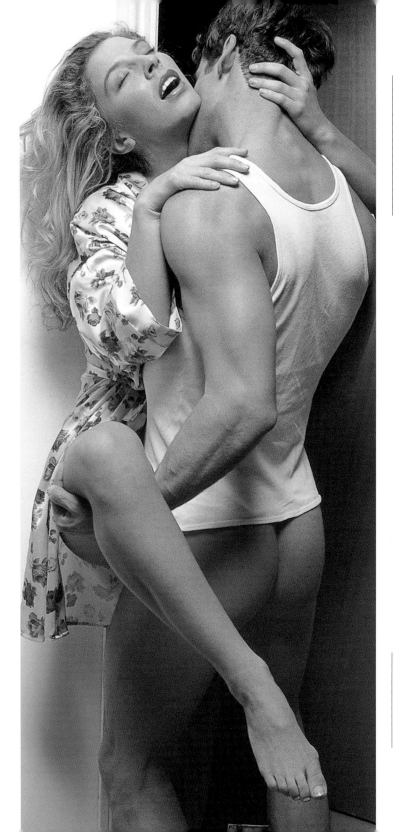

OPPOSITE | You may find yourself at a work function and the urge to have spontaneous sex or a heavy petting session overcomes you and your partner. These passionate embraces can fulfil sexual fantasies and keep the excitement in a long-term relationship.

LEFT | A "quickie" out of the bedroom can lead to a prolonged night of intense passion, or you might find yourselves returning from a night out and unable to wait until you get to the bedroom.

RIGHT | The kitchen table is a good place for torrid quick sex – even if you don't have time to clear it. You don't even have to wait to take all your clothes off.

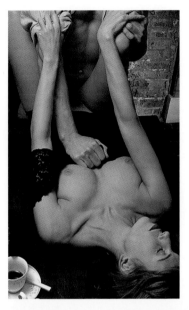

passion and lust

Passion is the spice of life – it's sexuality in Technicolor. It fascinates and frightens us a bit, because under its spell we temporarily lose our minds, while our emotions and bodies take over. Lust is a sign of a healthy libido racing along in top gear, and life would be pretty boring without it.

The main thing about sexual passion is the intensity and the speed with which it can come and go. While in the throes of a passionate love affair, all other areas of life pale by comparison. What else would drive politicians, amongst others, to risk careers, marriages and reputations which they have spent years building up?

Passion is the source of inspiration for a thousand books, films, songs and poems. It seems as if we need to have passion in our lives, even if we are not the ones actually experiencing it. Passion and lust inevitably burn themselves out, but in a stable relationship they can leave in their

RIGHT | This could be an extremely lustful episode of spontaneous lovemaking. You have torn off each other's clothes and she is laying face down across the table. You can enter her from the rear position, and make love to her passionately, but take care not to press her too hard against the surface of the table.

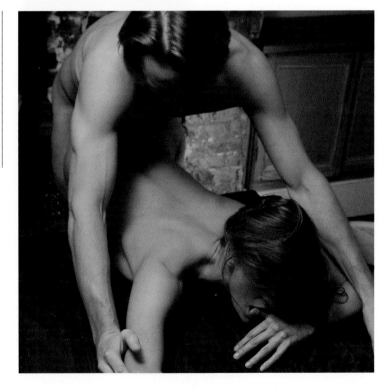

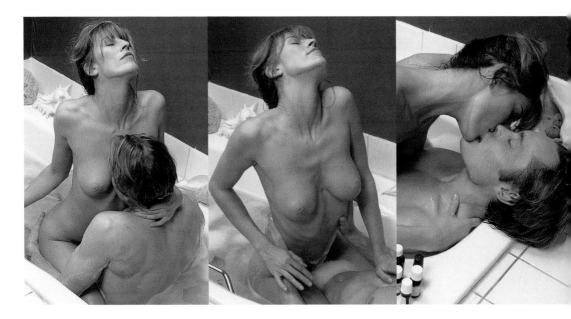

place the warm glow of intimacy and
companionship. Sexual love can grow instead,
and a physical relationship can become more
harmonious and compatible, integrating itself
within the context of everything else that is
meaningful in life.

Yet even within the most contented
relationships there is often a secret yearning for
the flame of passion to be lit again. We miss the
excitement, and the thrill of the unpredictable
and uncontrollable experience of overwhelming
physical and emotional sensation. Most of us
would become exhausted if we lived in a state
of passion all the time. However, it is a lucky
relationship which can retain its elements, for if a
couple can relive those moments of passion and
lust and magical chemistry which drew them
together in the first place, the mantle of
complacency and boredom which can descend on
any relationship would have difficulty taking hold.

So spontaneous, wild and lustful sex has a
therapeutic place within a relationship. When the
mood takes you, you can be creative with it. Let
go into it, and allow your erotic fantasies to come
true immediately. Don't worry about the time of

the day, or what part of the house you are in – let
your mutual passion surface unbridled, and use
whatever props you have around you, such as the
chairs, stairs or bathtub, to their best advantage.

sharing a bath

You may have shared your bath together to simply
wash away the cares of the day, but suddenly,
unfettered by clothes and warmed by the water,
your passion for your partner rises. Don't bother
to get out and dry yourselves to head for the
bedroom. Just use the sensual setting and go with
your feelings. Climb on top of your partner and kiss
him, bringing the whole of your body in contact
with his.

Making love in a bathtub of soothing warm
water, especially if scented with aromatic oils,
can be a wonderfully erotic experience. Let your
spontaneous urges take over. You will need to
straddle across his lap, but you can use the bath
rail for levering your body up and down while he
kisses and caresses you all over. You can even go
for the bodice-ripping "take me – I'm yours"
scenario if the urge takes over. Neither of you
should hold back; let lust command you.

ABOVE | Sharing a bath and
making love is an erotic and
sensual experience that you
can share with your partner.

out of the bedroom

BELOW | The steamy atmosphere and sensuous effects of hot water on bare skin heighten the pleasure of making love in the shower.

WHEN YOU HAVE BEEN TOGETHER for a long time, it can be difficult to keep the flames of passion burning brightly, especially if – whether out of habit or because you have children – the only place you have sex is your bedroom. As well as location, give a thought to timing and recall those days when you first met and couldn't keep your hands off each other. If you think about it, making love after a demanding day at work, cooking dinner and clearing up afterwards, then helping the kids with their homework, will almost certainly be less exciting and, frankly, more of a duty for both of you than rampant sex in the garden shed in the middle of an afternoon's weeding.

One of the most popular alternatives to the bedroom is the bathroom. As there is usually a lock on the door, even if the kids are at home, you are assured of some privacy. Sex in the shower or the bath is extremely sensual, as the hot water stimulates all your touch receptors, making your skin more sensitive. It is also very refreshing and revitalizing. Don't just go for the main event – relish the eroticism of lovingly soaping and rinsing every part of each other's bodies. Concentrating on giving your partner an invigorating body brush will not only produce its own rewards, but will also remind you why your lover's body is so special.

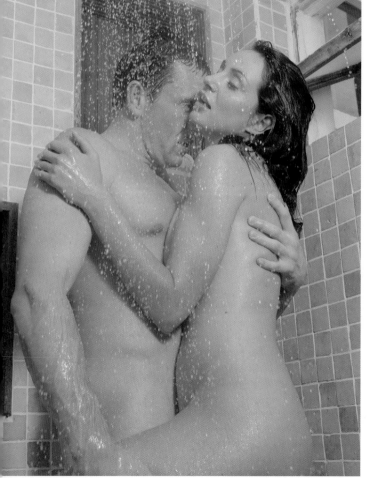

alternative venues

Chairs and sofas are also great places for making love and performing oral sex. Try sitting in your favourite chair in the front room with the curtains and windows open to add an extra notch of excitement and danger. Rocking chairs and recliners are fantastic, as the gentle motion gives a little extra movement to allow deeper penetration.

Cellars and attics are fun because of their secret atmosphere, although a little forethought about cushions and blankets might be a good idea. These places can become your own erotic dens and, if role-play is your thing, then there are unlimited scenarios, from dominatrix dungeons to caveman dwellings.

Stairs are fantastic settings for sex because the different levels allow you to experiment with positions that may otherwise not be possible. The vertical 69 is a challenge to the fittest. The woman sits on the second or third step while her partner kneels on a higher step, so her head is between his legs. Then – very carefully – he manoeuvres his

a change of scene

Try some of the following to spice up your sex life.

• Book into a motel for the afternoon – as Mr and Mrs Smith if you're not paying with a credit card.

• Hire a cabin cruiser for the weekend and enjoy the sensation of rocking on the water.

• Get away from it all with a tent or camper van (trailer) and make love under the stars.

• Splash out on a chauffeur-driven limousine, but make sure that it has privacy screens.

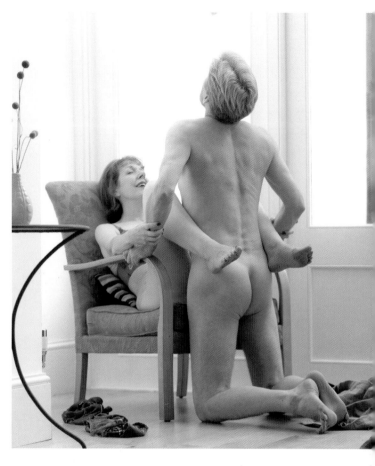

body so that he is head first down the stairs, supporting his weight with his hands on the floor at the bottom of the staircase, with his knees a few steps higher. Underneath him, the woman may need to move slightly or change the step she is on. Both partners' mouths are in contact with the other's genitals.

An easier position is for the man to kneel on the stairs, with the woman sitting one step above, facing him. She can then sit back and hold on to the banisters, while he grasps her by the hips. For additional spice, he can handcuff or tie her wrists to the banisters with a silk scarf and torment her with his hands, tongue and penis.

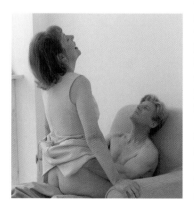

The kitchen, too, offers tasty possibilities. If the woman lies flat on the table and the man stands beside it, supporting her legs straight up in the air, the angle of penetration is intense. If she keeps her legs together, the tightness of her vagina will be immensely exciting for both partners. And, since you are already there, you can explore the possibilities of sensual and sexy foods – whether as an hors d'oeuvre or as a dessert.

There are couples who reckon that making love leaning against or with the woman sitting on an operating washing machine is one of life's truly erotic experiences. The vibration, especially if you time your "cycle" to the final spin, is said to be out of this world.

ABOVE AND LEFT | Chairs and sofas offer comfort as well as scope for some interesting and exciting positions. "Putting your feet up for half an hour" will never have the same meaning again.

the quickie

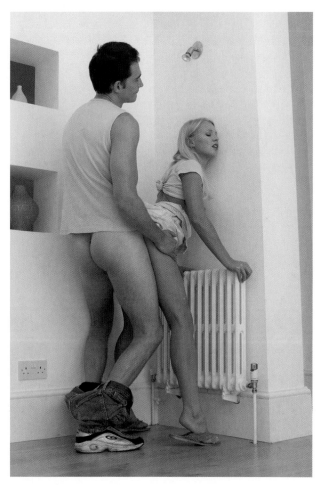

Quickie sex is a wonderfully erotic and lustful way of adding diversity to your love life. Although it cannot and should not replace the long sensual hours of foreplay and lovemaking that are essential in all loving and respectful relationships, it has a place, reaffirming each other's sexuality and reassuring your partner that you still find them the sexiest and most desirable person on the planet. Variety is not described as the spice of life without good reason.

mother of invention

Quick sex is often creative and inventive, two essential ingredients in lovemaking. Creeping up behind your partner while he or she clears the dishes in the kitchen in response to a completely overwhelming lustful urge is both delightful and flattering. There are no limits to when you can do it, whether sneaking off early from a party or a frantic session before you leave for work. It's up to you and your infectious desire.

The bedroom is usually the place where your loving, united encounters take place, so having a quick romp there may undermine the emotional importance of this room. The bathroom, on the other hand, is ideal. Steal in when your partner is having a shower and wordlessly show your intentions by kissing passionately under the hot jets.

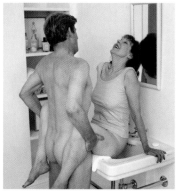

ABOVE | Sometimes, the less glamorous the venue, the more exciting the sex.

RIGHT | Surprising your partner in the bathroom can have, well, surprising results.

RETAINING YOUR SENSE OF SPONTANEITY is one of the keys to a successful long-term relationship. It is all too easy to slip into a habitual pattern without noticing, especially when you have family responsibilities, a demanding job and a busy life. Seizing the moment and surprising each other with unplanned flurries of passion keeps excitement and desire alive, adding spice and maintaining the longevity of the relationship.

Sometimes the best places are those that seem to be totally unsexy and mundane, such as against a radiator in the front hall. It's almost guaranteed that you will both smile each time you pass that particular radiator in the future. Shamelessly grabbing your partner as soon as they walk through the front door for a passionate encounter on the hall floor is an unmistakable demonstration of your feelings – and who cares if dinner is half an hour late?

The living room is also a great place to have quick, spontaneous sex. While your partner is watching television, why not surprise her with a sexy striptease to distract her? Suddenly blast some music from the stereo as you rip your clothes off in front of her in time to the beat. It's bound to have her in stitches, and laughter is a wonderful aphrodisiac. Alternatively, while he is relaxing in his favourite chair, why not silently hitch up your skirt and sit on his lap, either facing him or facing away, gently moving and rotating your hips until he becomes aroused? It certainly beats making coffee during the advertisement breaks.

timing

If quickie sex is what you have in mind, you do need to choose your moment wisely or the whole idea could backfire. You must also be open and sensitive to your partner's response. Selecting the final five minutes of a nail-biting match on television to give him a blow-job or suggesting steamy bathroom sex when she is in the middle of shaving her legs would be inappropriate. Your partner will either end up "submitting" and feeling exploited and irritable or else push you away and you will feel rejected, unloved and unimportant. Neither of these is conducive to promoting harmony and closeness in your relationship. Quickie sex is, after all, just as much about mutual pleasure as is prolonged, sensual lovemaking – just different. Although being ambushed for a quickie is a great turn-on, sometimes your partner may simply not feel like it and, if they are still unwilling after a little gentle persuasion and encouragement, then it's probably best to postpone the idea until another, rather more suitable moment.

the sky's the limit

Quickie sex does add an element of surprise and keeps your relationship exciting, fun and light-hearted. Just breaking the pattern of day-to-day life can ratchet up the libido for days afterwards.

Nor does quickie sex have to be restricted to the home. If you're feeling reckless – and you really are going to be quick – what about the back seat of the car in a carwash? Try stopping a hotel freight elevator between floors – but watch out for surveillance cameras, there may be penalties for being found out. Airline security permitting, you could go for membership of the Mile High Club. The balcony of a holiday hotel can offer the frisson of exhibitionism without any of the danger, if only the top half of you can be seen. The list is as endless as your imagination – just make sure that you don't get caught *in flagrante*.

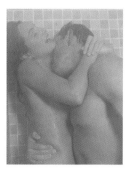

ABOVE AND BELOW | The occasional quickie helps keep the magic alive and can be a timely reminder of exactly how much you love and desire each other.

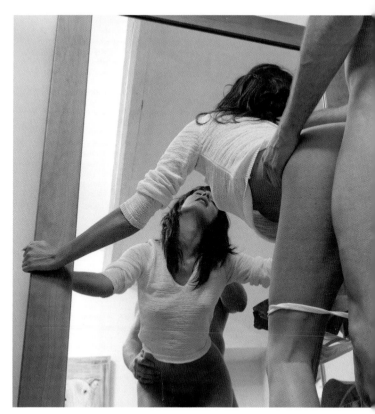

al fresco

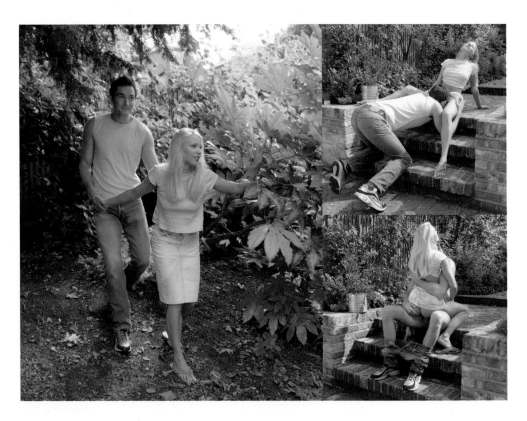

ABOVE | Fresh air and sunshine are natural aphrodisiacs. Whether you are walking in the woods or sitting in your own garden, why not follow your instincts and let nature take its course?

RELEASING YOUR SEXUAL ACTIVITIES from the confines of the four walls of your home and bringing them out into the open air can be a liberating experience. Enjoying each other in the outdoors puts you in touch with nature and makes the experience seem somehow more wholesome, purposeful and natural.

dangerous games

A word of caution here: having sex in public areas is illegal for reasons of public decency and it is vital not to cause offence. This is especially important to bear in mind if you are travelling abroad as some countries have harsh legal penalties. Equally, while some people find the risk – however slight – of being observed a positive turn-on, this can have precisely the opposite effect on others. As with all sexual activities, coercing an unwilling partner to have *al fresco* sex will sacrifice long-term fulfilment for short-term satisfaction.

There is something about the smell and feel of fresh air that ignites a basic passion in all of us. A long walk on a wintry day, with the wind literally taking the breath from your lungs, instils a sense of vitality, one of the most important ingredients of great sex. The proximity of lush vegetation, in the thick of a tall impressive wood or shaded by bushes and plants of nature's choosing, evokes fundamental animal desires and stirs our visceral energy. Even just strolling with your partner through a meadow, into a wood, along the beach or even to the local park is a wonderful prelude to get you both in the mood, whether you have sex outdoors or not.

basic instinct

The key to having great sex outside is to let nature be your guide and to go with whatever feels right. If the urge is suddenly to whip up your partner's skirt while you kneel before her and give her pleasure, it's doubtful she will complain. Open-air sex heightens the senses and intensifies feelings so that many people feel extra close and united. Being outdoors certainly gives an added dimension to the tried and tested positions that you enjoy in the privacy of your bedroom. Even the staid missionary position seems racy when you are outside. Sitting up, entwined in each other is also great, as you can do this with comparative ease. If you need to be quick, there is no need to remove all of your clothes, especially if the woman is wearing a flowing skirt.

The best place to have *al fresco* sex is in your own garden providing that it has suitably tall surrounding vegetation or a wall to prevent your being spotted by the neighbours. You can either spread out some blankets and pillows and,

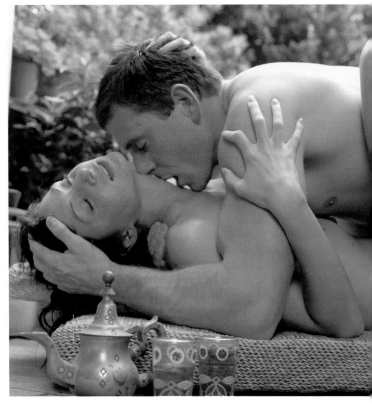

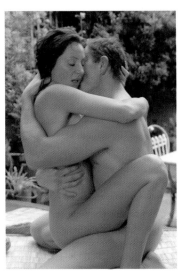

perhaps, some outdoor lights and candles if it is dark, or just go with the moment and get down and dirty in the mud. A garden hammock is a challenge worth taking on. It requires superb co-ordination, but can be done. A swinging garden seat provides a similar momentum with rather less risk of overturning.

Alternatively, if you live in the countryside, then research the area and work out where most people tend to walk and, more importantly, where they don't. Woods are always good, as there are many clearings and concealing bushes to choose from. Places that are harder to get to are usually better. A few things to consider are, how far away you are from a public footpath, where the nearest road is and whether there are any houses nearby. You don't want to end up making love in someone else's back garden.

ABOVE | A quiet cup of tea in the garden could turn into an intense and romantic lovemaking experience.

LEFT | Outdoor sex heightens the senses – touch most of all – and creates a powerful feeling of unity.

trying something new

BELOW | Nothing ventured, nothing gained. If sex is becoming more like a routine chore than a frenzy of ecstasy, you have the solution almost literally in your own hands. Try something that you have wondered about, but never done before, whether it is rimming, or using a vibrator. Suggest something you enjoyed with a previous partner, but have never done with your current one – you don't have to mention where the idea came from. Think back to the things you used to do together, but now no longer seem to have time for. Stretch your imagination and push the boundaries a little.

TRULY GREAT SEX is usually that which is totally uninhibited, where no holds are barred and where each partner feels completely at ease with their loved one. For many couples, perhaps the majority, this is not the case, even though they may have known their partner for many years, watched their body shape change and feel comfortable and safe in their presence. As time goes on, it gets harder to change, and couples reach a sexual stalemate where they have met their limits. In order to progress, a new level of intimacy must be achieved.

masturbating together
Most people view masturbation as an uninhibited self-pleasuring practice that they have done for many years in private. The idea of masturbating in front of someone else, regardless of how much you may love and trust them, can be daunting.

A good place to begin is to lie between your partner's legs, so they can embrace you, but you do not have the sensation of being watched. Get used to the idea of touching yourself in front of them without worrying about whether you orgasm or not, just to let them see how you like to

touch yourself. Once you are fully comfortable doing this, you can both try masturbating at the same time in front of each other and work on trying to orgasm simultaneously. It is worth noting that watching their partner masturbate is one of the top five male fantasies.

pushing the boundaries
It is precisely because couples feel safe and comfortable together that sex can actually become boring. For some couples, simply letting go of a few inhibitions – and almost everyone has some – can be enough to restore the magic. Try positions and activities that you haven't previously explored, even a little light S&M or anal stimulation.

Don't confront your partner as if this as a challenge or grit your teeth and systematically work through the entire Kama Sutra. However, if you would like to try, say, rimming – licking and kissing the anus – you could both test the water by gently licking and sucking each other's genitals, while stroking and massaging the anal area with your hands. Mirror each other, so that one copies the other. If one chooses to lead, then he or she massages their partner's anus in the way they would like him or her to massage them. The other partner can reciprocate by following this lead – or not, if they don't like it. This is a great way of communicating to each other how you like to be touched in new and sensitive areas.

crossing the line
Trying different positions may not be enough for some highly adventurous couples who feel that they need a more extreme stimulus to enliven a dull sex life and want to push the limits still further. A good place to start is the Internet, as there are plenty of websites catering for all manner of sexual tastes from swingers' clubs to voyeurism. This will give you the opportunity to discover the options, discuss them and form an opinion about whether you both really want to try something

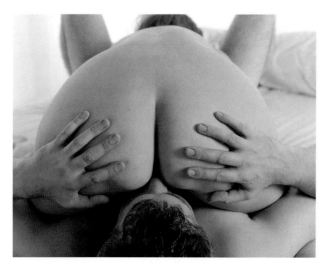

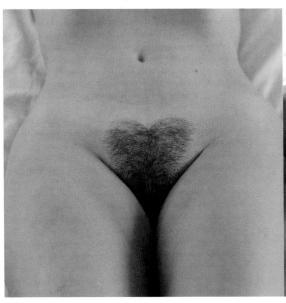

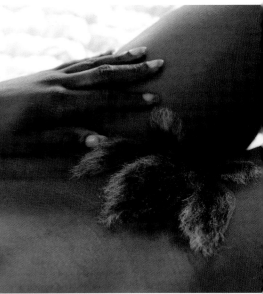

that, perhaps up till now, has just been a fantasy. A trip to a sex shop together would be another way to explore other possibilities, such as bondage and restraint fetishes.

It is important to discuss any activity that might be described as beyond the usual boundaries, especially if it involves other people. The reality of seeing your lover giving pleasure to a third party may be very different from the idea of it and could harm or even ruin a long-term relationship. If you both agree – and it must be both – to proceed with some more off-beat sexual thrills, set some limits about what is and isn't allowed and do some more research to make sure that you will be as safe as possible. If one of you is keen, but the other lukewarm or totally unenthusiastic, keep the idea at fantasy level and watch some blue movies or read porn magazines or raunchy books that will indulge this aspect of your libido.

a bit of fun

Never forget that laughter is a great aphrodisiac and that one reason couples reach a sexual stalemate is that life – and sex – has become boringly predictable and serious.

You might choose to give your partner a surprise the next time he or she sees you naked. There is a whole variety of things that you can do to your pubic hair that will guarantee that they will be equally amused and aroused. Many women wax or shave their pubic hair to keep it trim and tidy, but a variation on this is to shave it into fun patterns or even dye it for the total makeover. The amount of hair you have will determine how much you can do, but as it is pretty much already in a heart shape, it doesn't require too much skill or artistic flair to trim it and sculpt it into that shape, perfect for a Valentine's Day treat. Other shapes could be a star or a cross, or even a chessboard. A beard trimmer is an excellent tool for all genital artists, as it is often thinner and more precise than your average razor.

A merkin is basically a pubic wig or hairpiece, held in place with a special glue. They have been used throughout history for a variety of reasons, including health problems and "public decency", but today people use them for titillating fun. They vary in shape and colour, from fig leaves and flowers to national flags, and are guaranteed to raise more than a smile.

ABOVE LEFT | Heart-shaped pubic hair – the perfect private joke.

ABOVE | A fig-leaf merkin for playing Adam and Eve – watch out for the snake.

BELOW | Masturbating with your partner is deeply intimate.

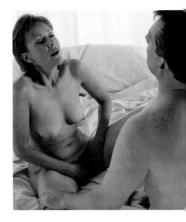

sharing sensuality

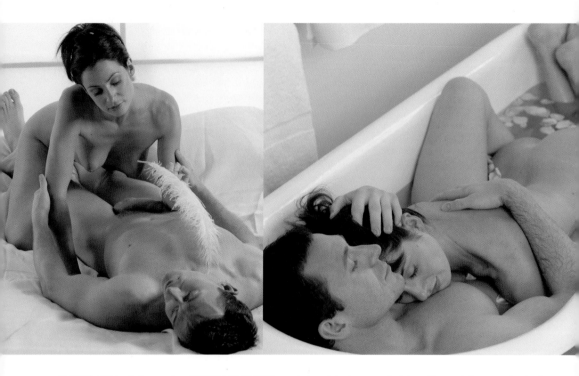

ABOVE | The light touch of a soft feather against bare skin is unbearably erotic.

ABOVE RIGHT | Get yourselves in the mood by sharing a warm, fragrant bath before an erotic session.

SHARING A WARM BATH is a perfect way to begin a massage and an evening of total indulgence and pampering. Many people associate water with relaxation and comfort and it is a wonderfully sensual stimulant. A warm, fragrant bath together is extremely erotic, as you luxuriate in the soft, silky textures of each other's bodies. The skin's responsiveness to touch is enhanced and the water's enveloping properties help you both to feel more united.

no touching

For added eroticism, give your partner a "hands free" massage. Tell your partner to close his or her eyes. The only rule is that you cannot touch one another with any part of your body. If you both have long hair, you can use it to caress one another. Make sure it is clean and smells nice.

Begin by putting your hair over your head and softly and slowly dragging it around your partner's body, starting from the head. You can add to the sensation by softly blowing on their skin at the same time. When you reach the most sensitive areas such as nipples, groin or armpits, allow your hair and breath to linger, gently circling and stroking to build anticipation.

Now try using a feather to caress your partner. Feathers are very sensuous, as the soft, light texture can be used in so many different ways. You can drag it slowly over the skin, following a path of your own choosing, or try a sharper, flicking motion, concentrating on specific areas. Whether you are male or female, being stroked by a feather is a delicious sensation. Make sure that your partner's eyes are tightly closed or that they are blindfolded before you start stroking them –

losing the use of one sense heightens all the others. Ask them to guess what it is you are using. If they guess correctly, reward them by spending extra long on their genital area. If they guess incorrectly, reprimand them by tickling their armpits or nose.

feathering

If you are stroking your man and he becomes aroused, ask him to lie on his back and place the feather between his hard penis and his stomach. Rub it up and down or forwards and backwards. Then get him to open his legs and, as you sit between them, run the feather up from his perineum, over his testicles and along the shaft before going back down again. Vary the sensation, so that on one stroke you keep the feather light, barely touching him, on another you use a firmer, circular motion, and on a third, you sweep it in quick sharp strokes, left and right, up and down.

Use your imagination to find other sensuous textures. Try the contrasting sensations of a bead necklace running over the skin, the softness of a leather glove, the barely there lightness of silk stockings or satin lingerie, the slight roughness of lace or the tactility of fake fur.

Another deliciously erotic sensation is the feel of ice against the skin. Run an ice cube over your lover's body and watch how their nipples harden as you gently circle the cube around them. Gently slide it around their genitals, holding it in your mouth at the same time, so they feel the heat from your breath and the chill from the ice. Be careful around the clitoris, as an ice cube may be too much for some women. Opt instead for running it over her inner labia for a more muffled chill.

Another way to excite the senses is to sprinkle the petals of your lover's favourite flower over their body so that they can luxuriate in the smell and the soft tickle of the velvety texture.

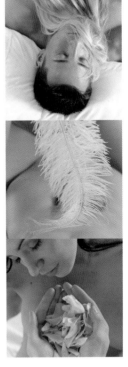

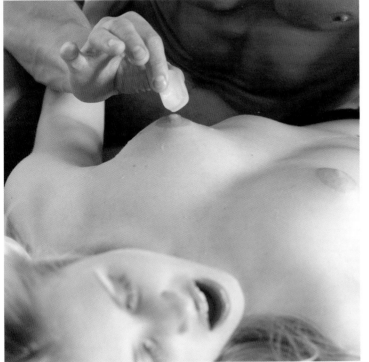

ABOVE TOP | If you have long, silky hair, brush it all over your lover's body for a unique "hands off" massage.

ABOVE CENTRE | Flick the feather over the aroused genitals for the full effect.

ABOVE BOTTOM | Showering your lover with fragrant petals is romantic and sensuous.

LEFT | An icy touch is a thrilling and tantalizing sensation.

mind games

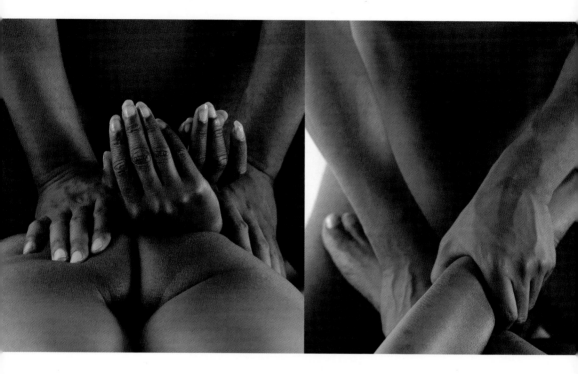

ABOVE | The woman can lie on her front while the man straddles her waist facing her bottom, restraining her hands together behind her back. He can then command her to wrap her restrained hands around his penis as he thrusts in and out of them.

ABOVE RIGHT | Hold your partner's legs bent and they won't be able to escape.

IN LONG-TERM RELATIONSHIPS, fantasies can play an important role in keeping the flames of passion burning. The difficulty often lies in sharing your fantasies with your partner, as many people are afraid of being judged. Most sexual fantasies range from the weird to the subversive and often people fantasize about things during the throes of passion that make them feel uncomfortable when they think of them out of the sexual context, but being unruly is a very human desire. An uninhibited and passionate session of being "naughty" with your partner is an expression of your innermost desires and an act of physical and emotional trust that can enhance a long-term relationship.

Your fantasies are personal and private and it is not necessary to divulge them, but there may be elements of them that you could bring up and explore with your partner. For example, a woman who fantasizes about having sex with two men at the same time could ask her partner to use a dildo or vibrator and double-penetrate her during sex.

restraint

Other common fantasies that couples can explore to spice up a long-term relationship involve restraint. These can range from holding hands or legs down while you stimulate each other, to being physically tied up. One advantage of restraining each other is that it helps you to communicate without actually having to speak. By holding your partner down you are telling them that you don't want them to worry about pleasing you, for now you are going to concentrate on them. All they need do is lie back and enjoy. It is fun to alternate playing the dominant role, in which you take charge of proceedings, with the submissive role, which takes the pressure off having to please and allows you to relinquish control to your partner's loving hands and kisses.

The great thing about restraint sex games is that they include a frisson of anxiety – which is immensely arousing – but do not have to include pain or fear. Forget the whip-cracking dominatrix and leather mask image of "heavy bondage" (unless that really is your thing) and concentrate on teasing and tantalizing. Loosely tie your partner's wrists and ankles to the bed with silk scarves, stockings or ties so that they are spread-eagled, or invest in a pair of furry handcuffs. Then slowly wreak havoc on their nervous system, by stimulating every inch of their body with your hands, tongue, genitals, a vibrator, a feather – whatever you like – repeatedly drawing back at the last possible moment. Remember, you are in control.

The idea of restraint can be intimidating, as however much you trust and love your partner the feeling and idea of helplessness is not always a pleasant one. To overcome this fear it is sensible to start with a few simple restraint positions such as holding down your partner's hands while covering their body with kisses, or tying your partner to the bed while you perform oral sex on them. Once you are aware of each other's boundaries and how far to take restraint, there are a number of different things that you can do.

Restraint can also be used within role-playing. Whatever your role-play fantasies are, whether it's doctors and nurses or parlour-maid and master, holding each other down or tying each other up can add to the element of excitement.

swinging

Previously known as wife-swapping in the 1950s, swinging has boomed into a lucrative alternative to straight sex. There are now swingers' clubs, swinging festivals and swingers' holidays available for like-minded couples who can go and fulfil their fantasies and desires in a relatively safe environment with other people who share their preferences. Swinging often culminates in group sex, as many swingers find the thrill lies in watching each other making love to different

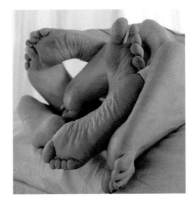

LEFT | Sex in a group is not to everyone's taste, but for some people it can be a great fantasy.

people. There are strict codes of practice and most partners have limits within their relationship as well. For example, usually if one partner does not want to have sex with a certain couple, then they choose not to as a couple, regardless of what the other partner may feel. It is almost always a joint decision. Swingers are usually very open people who are not interested in doing anything against anyone's will. Any couple interested in swinging should consider visiting one of the organized events to talk to other swingers and get more information before they decide whether or not they want to get involved.

see and be seen

Voyeurism and exhibitionism are other sexual activities that give some people a thrill. It is important to point out that watching someone else without his or her knowledge is both illegal and immoral. There is a current trend for car-park parties where people park their car, and allow others to watch them, and sometimes join in, having sex. This is aimed at voyeurs and exhibitionists as it is considered acceptable for other partygoers to wander around the car park, looking through windows and watching what is going on in each car. There are voyeur websites and some sex clubs have voyeuristic viewing rooms.

Obviously, there is an element of risk involved here, and by taking part you are laying yourself open to abuse. Not everyone who takes part in such activities will be as conscientious as you are.

BELOW TOP | Some positions require keeping a firm grip.

BELOW BOTTOM | Try different positions incorporating restraint. For example, he could lie on his back while she gets on top of him and forces him to surrender with her knees.

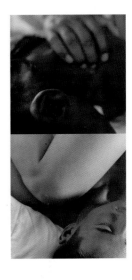

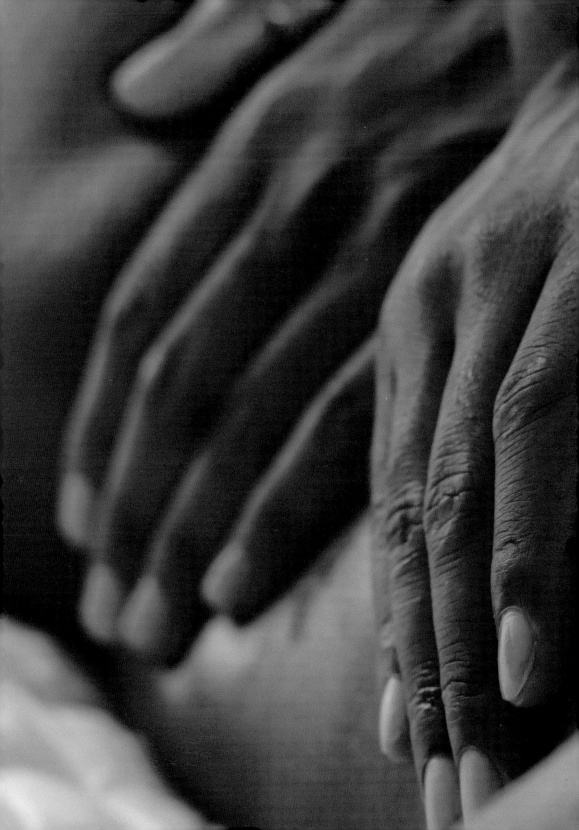

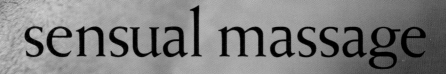

sensual massage

Touch is extremely important to our physical and emotional well-being, and regular massages will create a bond of trust. Arouse and satisfy the senses by caressing your partner's body with deliciously scented oils. Massage can be an erotic prelude to lovemaking or purely an end in itself, for sensual pampering, relaxing and revitalizing.

the loving touch

INTRODUCING SENSUAL MASSAGE as a regular event in a relationship is one of the most effective ways of enhancing physical and emotional communication. The loving and confident stroking of hands upon the skin, the way they mould into the body's curves, and the gentle palpation of muscles and tissues speak volumes in the silent language of touch about your innermost feelings for each other.

A sensual massage can help you and your partner unwind from the stresses of the day, creating a precious opportunity to relax and enjoy each other's company. A massage can be offered as a spontaneous gesture to ease a partner's pain or tension. You may want to give a soothing face massage, to relieve stress, anxiety or headache, or focus your strokes on the back, shoulders, and neck, to alleviate muscular aches and strains. You can pamper your partner by offering her a luxurious foot or hand massage.

The session may evolve into a truly sensuous affair, involving flowing caresses of the whole body from top to toe. A massage can include a variety of strokes, from soft, languid touches to firm, invigorating movements. The beauty of massage is that its motions are like notes of music or the steps of a dance, varied enough to enable you to always respond creatively to your partner's changing needs and moods.

It may become a prelude to a loving and sexual encounter so that the whole body is more ready and responsive to pleasure and erotic feelings.

RIGHT AND BELOW | Massage is a loving and therapeutic process which relieves tension in body and mind, and so allows more freedom to enjoy spontaneous interaction. By taking turns to massage each other, both partners can learn to enjoy sharing the roles of giving and receiving pleasure.

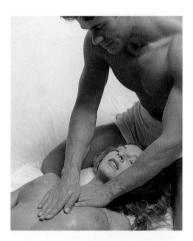

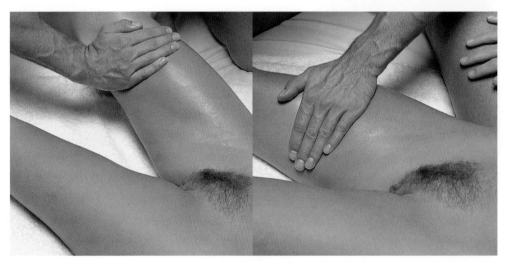

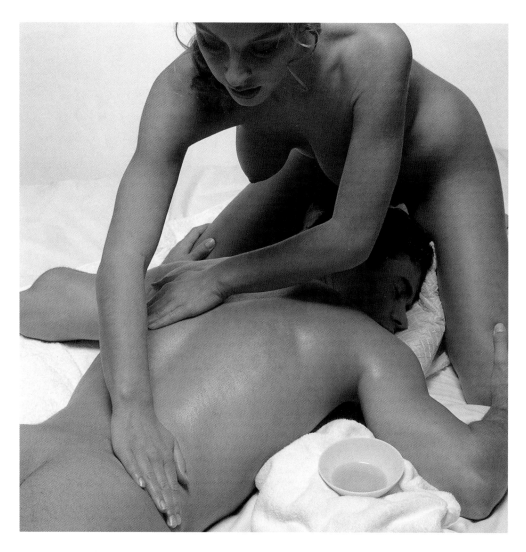

Sensual massage helps to build physical and emotional trust because one partner surrenders his or her body into the hands of the other, while the person giving the massage must learn to respect and tune in to its innate needs and responses.

emotional nourishment

Massage is the perfect medium for close physical contact at times when the libido of one or both partners is low, or there is a sexual dysfunction or physical condition that is inhibiting or preventing full sexual intercourse. By remaining in touch with one another's bodies, the essential emotional nourishment which ensues from physical intimacy can continue, thus avoiding a build-up of frustration, need and feelings of isolation. The strokes can release muscular tension from those areas of the body closely associated with sexual response, helping your partner to feel more alive and receptive to his or her sexual feelings.

ABOVE | Your movements as you spread the oil will warm the muscles, boost the circulation, and prepare the body's tissues for other strokes. There is no need to hurry this part of the massage as it will give you both time to relax, focus your attention, and tune in to one another.

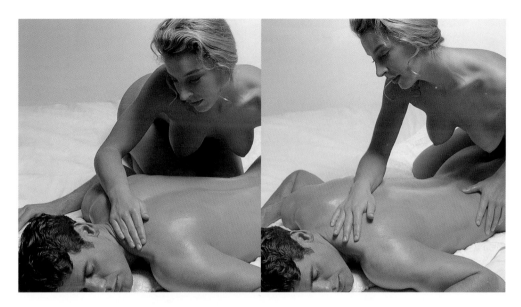

touch as a healing force

ABOVE | By opening your heart and pouring tenderness into your hands as you stroke each part of his or her body, you can impart a deeply nurturing sense of love and care which will increase his feelings of physical well-being and of self-worth. Massage expresses and heightens emotional bonding in a unique way.

ABOVE RIGHT | In an intimate and sensual massage, use your hands, forearms, and other parts of your body to stroke the skin, letting the touches flow like water over the body. At times it will seem as if the two bodies have melted and merged into one another, dissolving the physical boundaries between you.

The most important healing element in any massage is the power of loving touch. Touch is known as the mother of the senses, being the first to develop in the human embryo and in all other species, and the one on which all the other senses are based. The tactile sense resides in the skin, that miraculous organ covering the entire body. By means of its countless nerve endings, which respond to a whole variety of pressures from pain to pleasure, the skin relays messages through the central nervous system to the brain, transmitting information about the external world beyond its frontiers. A loving touch which brings reassurance and joy to the skin will ultimately infuse the whole body with a feeling of well-being.

Touch is an essential form of nourishment for the psychosomatic processes of body, mind and spirit throughout our lives. Adequate loving touch, in the form of affectionate caressing, hugging, stroking, cuddling and kissing, is vital in the early stages of infancy for the healthy development of a growing child. Through these pleasurable skin sensations, the infant can begin to define its sense of self-worth, and to develop an understanding and an appreciation of its own body.

Touch deprivation in early childhood can retard physical and emotional growth, potentially leading to behavioural and sexual problems in later years. Lack of adequate touch, even in adulthood, can rob someone of the feelings of vitality and ease within the body. This will often manifest itself as an inability to express or receive affection adequately.

Loving touch, through the medium of massage, will help to heal old emotional wounds whose memories remain locked within the body, forming a new and positive sense of body image, confidence and responsiveness to physical sensuality.

When couples experiment with touch techniques they discover that to give a massage is as satisfying as receiving one. This is because by touching and using your feeling senses, you open up the depths of your own emotions, and have a means to express them. Within a massage sequence, you can be playful, tender, strong, creative and loving. By coming to know and understand another's body, you begin to become more aware of your own physical needs.

It is important, however, to give massage only when willing to do so, for it is a caring act and the message imparted from your hands always conveys your innermost feelings.

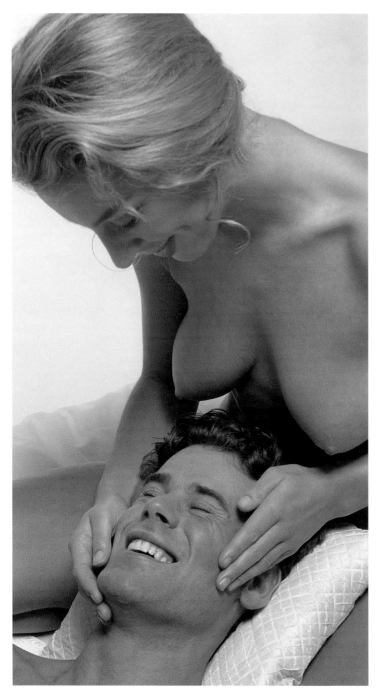

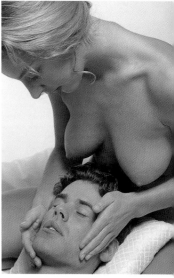

overture to lovemaking

Naturally, if there is mutual consent, a massage may transform from one experience into the other, but it is wrong to use the situation as a means of seduction if your partner has not given you clear signals of consent. If the massage is intended purely to soothe, comfort and relax, or your partner is unwilling to engage in sexual activity, then it is better to avoid direct contact with the genitalia or other erogenous areas which could provoke an unwanted sexual response in either of you.

Learning to receive massage is also a helpful process for those people who predominantly identify with the role of the main giver in a relationship, often unconsciously taking control of events and denying the other partner the chance to reciprocate love and concern. To receive massage is one of the few occasions in life where all you need to do is become totally receptive. Even in lovemaking, there is usually a constant interaction of activity.

BELOW | Allow all the tension to leave your hands so that they are able to glide, melt and sculpt the underlying contours and curves of your partner's body and bring to both him and yourself a much clearer definition of its shape and structure.

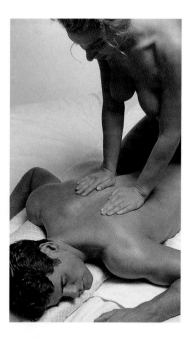

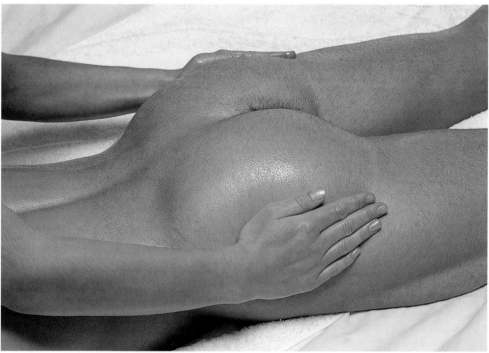

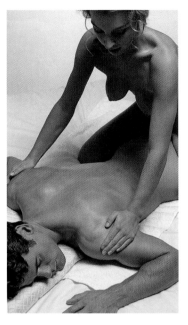

To allow yourself to become passive, and simply receive touch, means you must open yourself up to a certain degree of trust and vulnerability and this, in itself, is a gift which you can offer to your partner. It is important that you take it in turns to give and receive massage so that you can both learn from all aspects of the experience.

If both of you are clear that a sensual massage is a luxurious prelude to lovemaking, then once you have warmed and relaxed the whole body, you can stroke over the erogenous areas to increase excitement.

By straddling your partner, you can comfortably enfold the circumference of his or her back in one long flowing sweep, stroking your hands up along the spine, over the shoulders and back down the sides of the body. Your physical closeness will add to the sensuality of the massage, but you will also need to take care to support your own weight.

LEFT AND FAR LEFT | Sensual massage movements should be smooth and rounded and never finish abruptly mid-way on the body. Always glide your hands around the body's contours, such as the shoulders or hips, or sweep them out along the limbs.

BELOW | If you are proceeding to lovemaking, begin to stroke the erogenous areas.

selecting the oils

Choose a light, preferably unrefined vegetable oil for lubrication, such as grape seed, safflower or sunflower oil, to which you can add a much richer oil, such as almond, avocado or jojoba.

Learn about the soothing, romantic and erotic qualities of essential oils, so that you can create aromatic blends to enhance the sensuous mood of your massage. Place your oil in a ceramic bowl or a bottle that will allow you to pour the right amount into your hands. Warm the oil before applying it. Keep tissues or towels nearby for oil spillage or to wipe your hands.

If your partner does not like oil on his or her skin, then use a body lotion with nourishing skin properties. Talcum powder can also be used, though its dryness will prevent you from performing the flowing, soporific motions of a truly sensual massage.

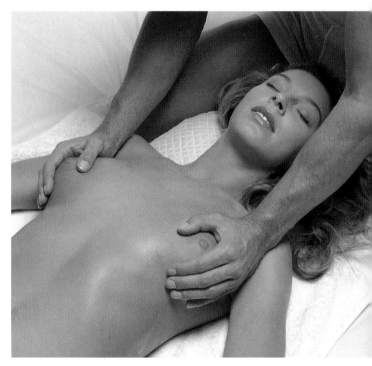

the strokes of massage

BELOW | Fanning motions
can be applied upwards or
downwards. Once your hands
have reached the base of
the back on a downwards
sequence, return to the top of
the spine by gliding them up
along the sides of the ribcage.

Confidence, quality of touch in your hands and
sensitivity to your partner's body are essential if
the massage is to be mutually pleasurable. But do
give each other scope to experiment with different
strokes, pressures and touches. Treat the whole
experience as a game, make it fun, and tell each
other what feels good. Give one another a chance
to explore the techniques without being too
directive, but make your feelings clear to your

partner if you do not feel comfortable with what is
happening to your body.

By learning how to apply different movements
and pressures you will be able to give the right
massage for the occasion. You can also read massage
manuals, or participate in a massage workshop.

The first step is to lubricate the area of the
body you are about to massage. Pour a little oil
into one palm and then rub both hands together
to warm it before spreading it with soft, free-
flowing motions, using the flat surface of your
palms. Apply sufficient oil to ensure your hands
slide sensuously over the skin. These strokes will
help your partner forget any stressful thoughts and
become more receptive to your touch.

You can create a truly relaxing and sensual
massage using only soft gliding strokes in a variety
of unbroken and flowing motions that embrace
the whole body. By letting your hands slide from
the back to the legs in simple easy stretches, or,
when stroking the front of the body, from the
thighs to the belly, you will bring a sense of unity
and integration to your partner's body.

circle and fan strokes

Circle and fan strokes stretch and ease the tension
out of the body's soft tissues, bringing a lovely
fluid and hypnotic movement.

Circle strokes are applied to any broad surface
area of the body, such as the back and sides of the
body, the thighs, belly and chest. The art of this
stroke is to keep it constantly spiralling over the
skin until you are ready to move with an unbroken
motion into the next sequence of strokes.

Fan strokes are applied to most areas of the
body with an upward, flowing and steady pressure
using the surface of both palms. One fan stroke
should merge into the next in a constant upward
movement, which boosts the circulation towards
the heart. When your hands reach to the top of a
body part, fan them out to the sides and slide
them back down to repeat the sequence.

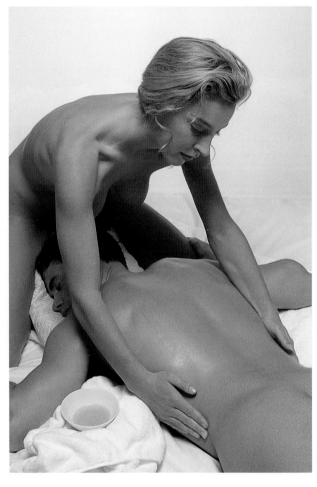

circle strokes

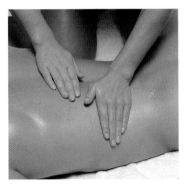 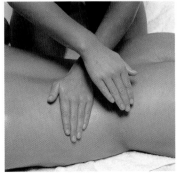 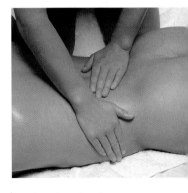

1 | To circle stroke, place both hands flat and parallel on the body. Your hands should be about 10cm/4in apart. With a steady pressure, begin to slide both hands in a circular clockwise motion with your right hand leading the movement.

2 | Lift and pass: Lift your right hand slightly away from the body, crossing it over the top of your left which continues to circle underneath.

3 | Completing the circle: As your left hand completes its circle, your right hand drops down to perform a half-circle, then gently lifts off again to let your left hand pass. Now repeat this sequence until you are ready to move on.

fan strokes

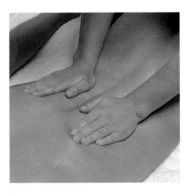 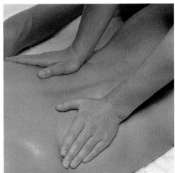 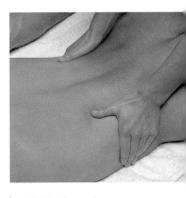

1 | Finger caresses: To fan upwards, place both hands flat and parellel, pointing to the head, on each side of the lower end of the spine. Apply gentle and even pressure with the fingers.

2 | Fanning out: Glide both your hands slowly upwards on the back for a distance of about 15cm/6in before fanning them out towards the sides of the body.

3 | Gliding downwards: Mould both hands firmly to the sides of the body and pull downwards. Then, with a turn of the wrists, glide your hands towards the centre of the back before stroking upwards once more.

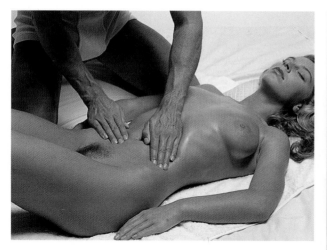

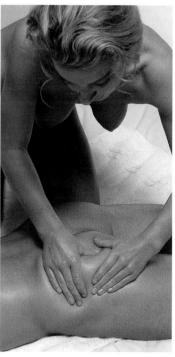

ABOVE | Always approach the abdomen sensitively as it is a vulnerable area.

ABOVE RIGHT | Fleshy zones: Kneading strokes are perfect for the fleshy erogenous zones of the buttocks and thighs, as the invigorating action helps to release tension from their large muscles and stimulate the sensory nerves that affect sexual response. When massaging the buttocks, begin with smooth, gliding motions that shape their ample contours, and then proceed with the kneading.

invigorating strokes

Different strokes add variety and spice to your sensual massage. They have a revitalizing effect on the system, boosting the blood circulation, loosening stiff muscles and ridding the tissues of trapped toxins.

Your partner will enjoy the stimulating effect and the sensation of different pressures of the hands and fingers. Introduce friction, kneading and percussion strokes to the massage, once the muscles are warm and relaxed.

maintain good posture

Whether you are kneeling, sitting or standing while massaging your partner, it is always important to take care of your own posture, pausing to relax and breathe deeply whenever you feel tense. By remaining at ease in your body and breathing, your own vitality is sustained throughout the massage. This boosts your enjoyment of giving the massage and brings a comforting warmth and vitality to your hands. As a consequence, good posture improves the quality of your massage strokes.

Always precede and follow invigorating movements with sensual strokes to soothe the skin and to integrate the part of the body under focus with the surrounding area. Friction grinds the tissue towards the bone and is excellent for relieving specific areas of tension. Pressure is applied slowly and sensitively from the heels of the hand, the thumbs, fingertips, or knuckles. The movement can be a steady slide, a short stretch, or small circular motions in which the pressure is greater on the outward half of the circle. Use friction whenever you are working close to the bone, such as alongside the spine, around the shoulder blades, under or over the scalp, or on the hands, feet and face.

Kneading is applied to the fleshy parts of the body such as the shoulders, sides of the body, buttocks and thighs. Kneading, as the name suggests, replicates the action of a baker kneading dough, and is performed by scooping up and squeezing a portion of flesh between the fingers,

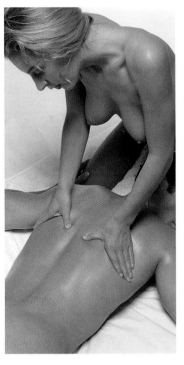

heel and thumb of one hand before pushing it towards the other hand. The waiting hand then repeats the action, and in this way the flesh is rolled back and forth between both hands. Work thoroughly over an area, ensuring that your wrists and shoulders remain relaxed.

Percussion strokes are rapid, vibratory movements used to revitalize the system and tone up the skin by enriching the blood supply to its nerve endings. There are a variety of percussion strokes, all made with one hand following the other in quick succession to strike the flesh briskly before flicking immediately back off the skin. They feel best when applied to fleshy areas and should never be used directly over the bones.

Pummelling is done by rhythmically striking the sides of loosely made fists against the body, while hacking is performed with a series of gentle chopping movements made from the sides of open, straight hands. Large circle strokes on the abdomen are very soothing, helping your partner breathe more deeply, so that she is more in touch with her sexual and emotional feelings.

LEFT | Apply friction on either side of the spine, using your thumbs.

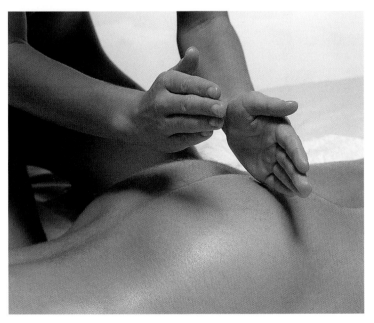

LEFT | Brisk strokes: The brisk staccato movements of hacking can be a fun addition to sensual massage, particularly over the buttocks and thighs, as they enliven the skin and may even stimulate your partner erotically.

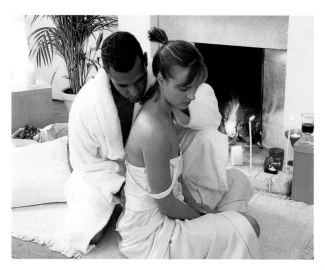

keep extra sheets and towels close by in case your partner gets cold. Have your favourite romantic style of music playing softly in the background but take care not to let the sounds invade the natural rhythm of your massage strokes.

Choose the setting for massage carefully, so both of you can relax fully. The room must be warm and draught-free if clothes are to be removed. Try to ensure privacy so the person receiving the massage has a chance to relax completely and put all concerns aside, and the

ABOVE | Creating the mood is an important part of a sensual massage.

RIGHT | A few candles will help to create soft relaxing lighting in the room. Scented candles will often help to lift the mood, too.

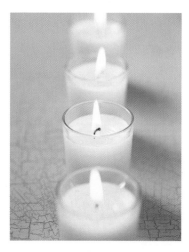

mood setting

When you set the scene for a luxurious and sensual massage, take time to create a romantic ambience so that your partner will know this is a special occasion. Place flowers around the room for their delicate aroma and colourful effects, and light candles to create a mellow mood, putting them at a safe distance from the place you are giving the massage.

You should cover the mattress or surface you are working on with fresh, clean sheets, and also

the gossamer touch

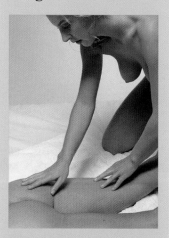

Feather touches are a sensual, skin-teasing way to carry out a series of strokes over any area. Using only the minimum of pressure from your fingertips, stroke very lightly over the skin, one hand following the other, and moving in one direction at a time. This will activate the skin's peripheral nerve endings, exquisitely heightening its sensitivity. Some people may find the feather touch just too light and ticklish, while others love its euphoric effects and would quite happily surrender to a whole body massage of these strokes alone.

essential oils

All that is necessary for sensual massage is a basic carrier oil, such as sunflower or almond oil. But by blending in a few drops of one or more essential oils you can make the massage a truly memorable experience. Essential oils have their own unique therapeutic qualities – some are highly beneficial in relieving stress, for example. You and your partner should both decide on the blend of essential oils, otherwise if one of you finds an aroma unpleasant the massage will not be so pleasurable. Some oils such as rose, jasmine, sandalwood, rosewood, and the exotic ylang ylang enjoy a widespread appeal.

Warning: Essential oils are highly concentrated and should never be spread directly on to the skin. Always blend them with a suitable carrier oil first. For a whole body massage, add 10–15 drops of one to three essential oils for five teaspoons of base carrier oil.

BELOW LEFT AND RIGHT |
A massage table gives greater freedom of movement and is more comfortable for the person being massaged.

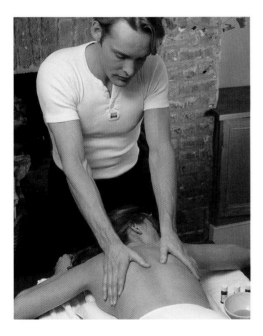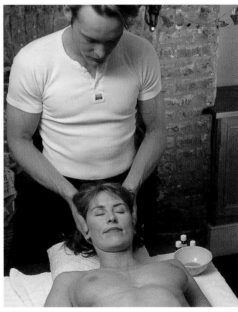

one giving it can devote his or her attention to the massage session.

In a full-body massage, both partners need a firm base such as a futon, a layer of foam, or a strong mattress to support their body weight under the pressure of strokes and movements. Folded blankets, a covered sleeping bag or firm cushions laid on the floor will also suffice. Towels and oils should be kept close at hand.

massage table

You can use a table for a massage base if it is sufficiently long and strong to take the size and weight of your partner, and narrow enough for you to reach her body. Pad it with blankets or cushions for comfort. A table of the right height and dimensions has the advantage of allowing you more freedom of movement, although it will inhibit close physical contact.

spontaneous massage

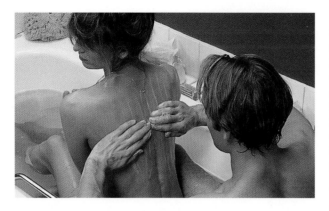

If you have a fireplace, take the opportunity to massage your partner in front of a lighted hearth at the end of the evening or after a bath. The heat of a fire adds a primal earthiness to your nakedness and physical contact, and you can give a full body sensual massage to your partner as he or she lies on folded blankets or a thin mattress in front of the flickering flames. Or simply take it in turns to give a head, neck and shoulder massage to relax your partner before going to sleep.

ABOVE | Apply friction strokes with your fingertips to relieve tension in the spine.

DIFFERENT LOCATIONS can turn a massage into a spontaneous treat. For instance, when bathing together you have the perfect opportunity for an impromptu massage, especially as your skin-to-skin contact will feel natural and uninhibited. In the bath, take turns to give each other a shoulder and neck massage. Your soothing strokes will assist the therapeutic qualities of warm water as it draws the tension out of the muscles.

bathing

In the bath, soapy lather on skin acts as a lubricant for you to glide your hands soothingly over the top of his or her back and shoulders. Then relax the spine with friction strokes. Hook your fingers over your partner's shoulders and work your thumbs in small circular motions up alongside the bones. Use a loofah or soap glove to massage the skin. The gentle friction leaves it soft and glowing. Rub over the chest and arms, and then the back and shoulders. Bathing together can be a treat.

giving a back, neck and head massage

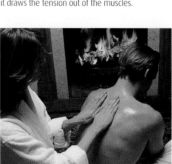

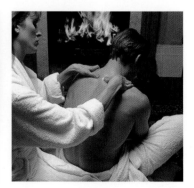

1 | You can add a few drops of essential oils into your basic oil to increase the relaxing effect of this fireside massage. Use soft, sensual strokes to sculpt the upper back and ease the tension from the shoulders and neck.

2 | Focus on tight areas between the shoulder blades, and at the base of the neck. Hook your fingers over his shoulders, and sink your thumb pads into the muscles, then use small circular motions over each tense spot in turn.

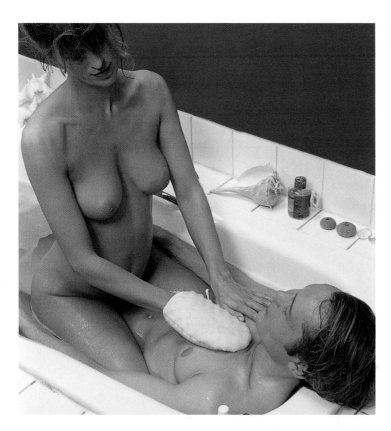

LEFT | Gently massage the skin with small circular strokes.

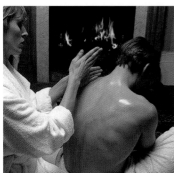

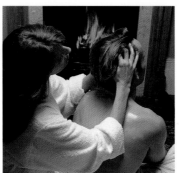

3 | Hack briskly over the top of the shoulders and down along the sides of the shoulder blades, but avoid striking the spine. The rapid vibrations will loosen stiff shoulders and leave the skin flushed and tingling.

4 | A head massage can calm the mind when your partner is feeling under stress. Firmly circle the fingertips of both hands over his entire scalp, then comb your fingers through his hair to complete your fireside massage.

a loving foot massage

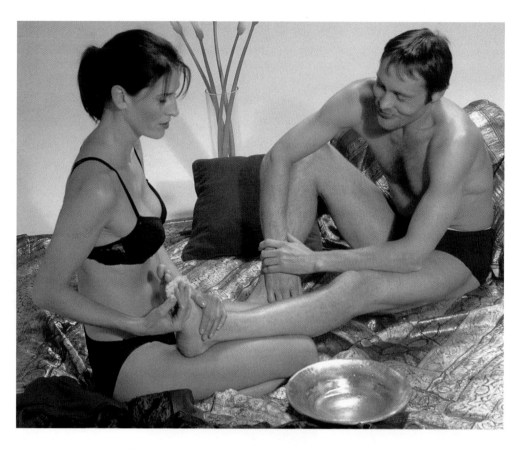

ABOVE | Take it in turns to offer each other a relaxing foot massage, ensuring that both of you benefit from receiving its stimulating and soothing effects.

BATHING AND MASSAGING your lover's feet can become one of your special rituals, serving not only to relax and refresh your partner, but also as a gift of love and devotion.

A foot massage will dissolve stress and soothe body and mind. The soft strokes over the feet have a calming effect, while the stronger pressures will boost low energy levels. Massage one foot at a time, and spread a little lotion over the top and sole with gliding, sensual strokes. When the foot is warm and supple, stroke your fingertips or thumb pads around the sides, front and back of the ankle to release any tension. Press or slide your thumbs

firmly all over the sole to stimulate its countless nerve endings.

Pay attention to the toes as touch here is surprisingly sensual. Palpate each toe gently between thumb and finger, then slide your little finger between each toe and rub the soft webs of skin with little corkscrew motions. Add the strokes shown here to your massage and then repeat them all on the other foot.

Take a bowl that is large enough to fit both feet and fill it two-thirds full with warm water. For a luxurious touch, add up to four drops of essential oil – relaxing lavender or cooling peppermint

giving a foot massage

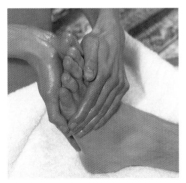

1 | Cradle each foot between your hands for up to 30 seconds to create a relaxing warmth and the feeling of caring tactile connection.

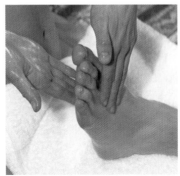

2 | Sweep your hands smoothly several times from the toes up to and around the ankle, gliding your fingers back down over the foot.

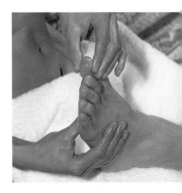

3 | Supporting the foot, stretch each toe by gripping it between your thumb and index finger and sliding firmly from the base to the tip.

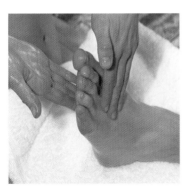

4 | Press gently all over the sole of the foot to stimulate the nerve endings.

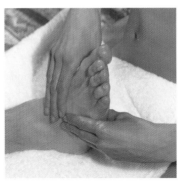

5 | Complete the foot massage with feather strokes, drawing your fingertips in soft motions down over the foot and towards the toes.

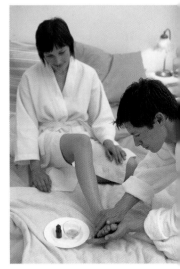

essences are perfect choices for a foot bath. For a more sensual blend, add two drop of patchouli mixed with two drops of lavender essence. Find a comfortable position for your partner to sit in and allow him or her to soak their feet for at least 10 minutes.

Taking one foot at a time, lather it with soap, gently squeezing and pressing the foot all over to release any tension. Then pat each foot dry with a soft, warm towel. Now massage one foot and then the other, ensuring your partner's legs are comfortably supported and relaxed.

ABOVE | Try using oils such as geranium or sandalwood, diluted in almond or another carrier oil, in your foot massage. Place a towel on the bedcover to protect it from the oil.

a loving face massage

A FACE MASSAGE IS ONE of the most intimate and loving ways to give pleasure through touch. Use soft caresses to calm and reassure, and steady, firm pressures to relieve tension spots in this most revealed and revealing part of the body. Every thought and emotion expresses itself in the face and, often, its muscles tighten to present an acceptable mask to the world. When your lover comes home, help him or her to become more vulnerable and allow their true feelings to rise to the surface by stroking away the stress.

To give a face massage, kneel or sit behind your partner's head so that it rests between your legs. Place a cushion under their head to take the strain off the back of the neck. Begin by cupping your hands very lightly over each side of the jaw and letting them rest there in a calm and still hold

for up to a count of ten. Then stroke with the palms of both hands continuously, one after the other, along the jawbone from the chin to the ear until you feel the whole area relaxing under these loving caresses.

Take the lobes of the ears between thumbs and fingertips and gently press them, then make tiny circle strokes all along the rims of the ears. Sweep your fingers in outward-flowing circles over both cheeks to move and loosen tense muscles. Follow this by tracing the fingertip of one hand lightly round and round the sensuous curves of the lips.

Using the tips of the first two fingers of each hand, stroke deftly around the eye socket up to ten times from the outer bridge of the nose to the edge of the temples, continuing lightly over the top of the cheekbones back towards the sides of the nose.

BELOW | Apply steady pressure as you move over tension areas such as under the cheekbones.

BELOW RIGHT | Draw your thumbs outwards over the brow to relieve stress and headaches.

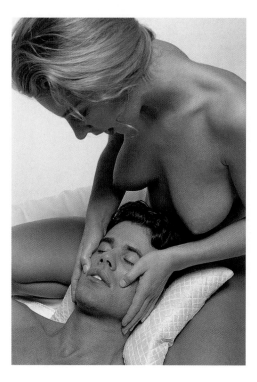

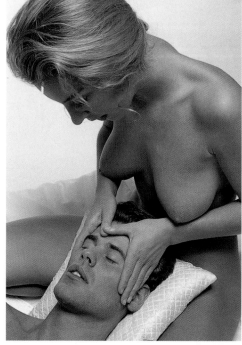

Glide your fingertips smoothly in clockwise motions around the temples, increasing the pressure slightly on the outward sweep. Now soothe the brow by softly drawing each hand consecutively across the forehead from the opposite-side temple, repeating these hypnotic movements for up to two minutes. Then work the fingertips of both hands simultaneously in small circles over the scalp as if shampooing the hair.

Complete the face massage with a still and tender hold by placing your thumbs over the centre of his crown, so that his head nestles between your hands and your fingers lay symmetrically over his temples. Close your eyes and focus your attention on your hands to pour your loving feelings into them. After a minute or two, slowly withdraw your hands from the head but sit quietly with your partner so you can both enjoy these precious and peaceful moments together.

steady pressure

When massaging the face, your strokes should be smooth, steady and consistent. Apply a gentle but firm pressure as you move over tension areas, such as directly under the cheekbones. In this movement, your hands softly clasp the sides of his face while your thumbs slide down the edges of the nose and continue stretching outwards under the bone. Lighten the pressure as you get closer to the ears. Draw your hands lightly over the head before repeating the stroke twice more.

help for headaches

To relieve a tension headache, place your thumbs over the centre of the forehead just above the eyebrows while resting your hands on the sides of the face. Steadily draw your thumbs outwards over the brow, completing the stroke with a sweep of the temples. Continue repeating this stroke to cover the whole forehead, moving up a little at a time until you reach the hairline.

BELOW LEFT | Your partner will love the feeling as your fingers comb through his hair, as if they are drawing the last of the day's stresses out of his mind and body. It is a very soothing motion to add to the last few strokes of a face and head massage.

BELOW | Use a feather or your own hair (if it is long enough) and long luxurious strokes to caress away all the cares and tensions of the day. Should your partner find this ticklish, substitute the feather with some lingering finger-stroking up and across the face.

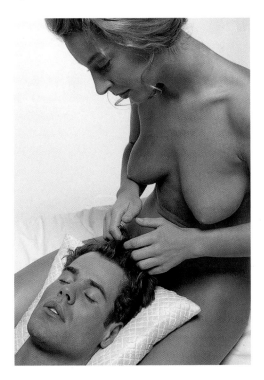

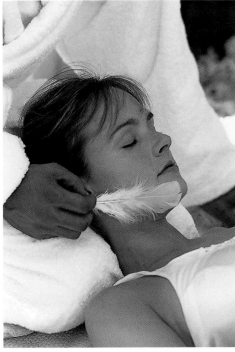

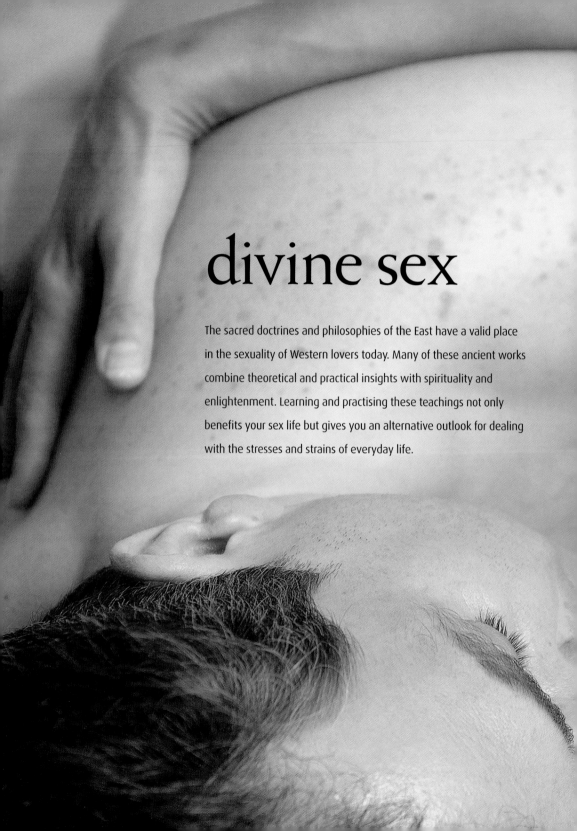

divine sex

The sacred doctrines and philosophies of the East have a valid place in the sexuality of Western lovers today. Many of these ancient works combine theoretical and practical insights with spirituality and enlightenment. Learning and practising these teachings not only benefits your sex life but gives you an alternative outlook for dealing with the stresses and strains of everyday life.

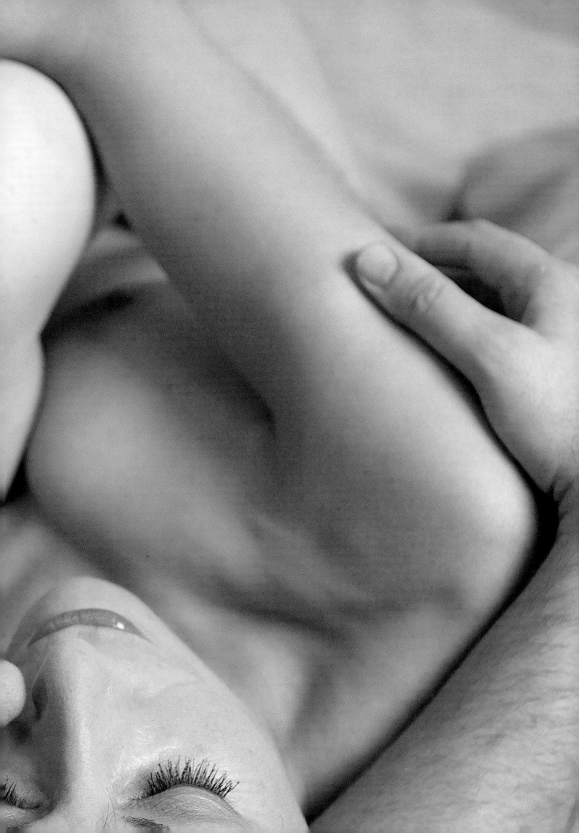

sex and philosophy

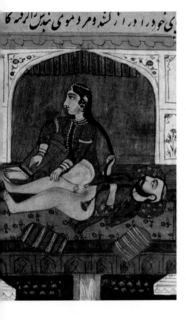

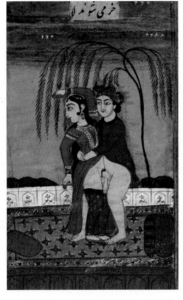

ABOVE | An 18th-century image from the Kama Sutra shows the woman on top while the man pulls her hair.

ABOVE RIGHT | Standing positions were most exalted.

SOME OF THE MOST FAMOUS ancient sex manuals originated in India many hundreds of years ago. The first, the Kama Sutra, is a collection of ancient Hindu writings on sex – known as Vedas – which were themselves based on an earlier oral tradition. It was followed by the Ananga Ranga and later by Tantric philosophy, both of which have used the Kama Sutra in their teachings as a sexual blueprint, adapting the positions and practices.

The Kama Sutra was put together by a student of religion and the divine, Mallanga Vatsayana, sometime between the 1st and 4th centuries AD. In its fearless and uninhibited approach to sexual passion it is more enlightening than the theories of many modern-day erotologists. Due to its explicit content and vivid descriptions of positions and potions intended to enhance lovemaking, it has often been misunderstood in the West as pornographic. In fact, it was intended as a guide to love, detailing courting practices, ways of treating marriage partners and consorts and more.

Over a thousand years after the Kama Sutra, Kalyana Malla's Ananga Ranga appeared. Although Malla used many of the Kama Sutra's sexual positions, embraces and other techniques, the Ananga Ranga had a different aim and content to the Kama Sutra. Whereas the Kama Sutra was associated with love and union, the Ananga Ranga was more orientated towards preventing the separation of husbands and wives and enhancing marriage longevity. Following up on this aim, Kalyana Malla describes the different types of men and women and catalogues their various seats of passion, characteristics and temperaments.

The origins of Tantra are harder to define. The oldest Tantric text seems to be the Buddhist Tantras that date back to around AD 600, but there are Tantric elements in the Vedas. More than a practice or step-by-step guide, Tantra is a philosophy, concerned with spirituality and divine energy, blending sacred sexuality, Eastern philosophy and the teachings of the Kama Sutra. It involves the use of meditation and yoga to master the ultimate goal of dissipating the ego and creating union with the divine energy that is within each of us.

Over the last three thousand years, Eastern cultures have worshipped and respected the power and life force of human sexual nature and recognized the importance of teaching this to the next generation. In the West, our social sexual development has been very different. Although contemporary Western society is more liberal and open than in the past, the arts of seduction, sensuality and wanton abandon have been underdeveloped by comparison with the East. By looking towards the East, we can borrow wisdom and teachings from a long history of enlightened sexual revolutionaries.

kama sutra

Although little is known of the compiler of the Kama Sutra, Mallanga Vatsayana, it is claimed that he was a student Brahmin, involved in the contemplation of the divine. He was probably based in the city of Pataliputra during a period of economic growth and social liberalism.

The Kama Sutra focuses around the three major concepts of Hinduism: *dharma* (the gaining of religious merit or righteousness and responsibility), *artha* (achieving goals, including personal wealth) and *kama* (love and the other sensual pleasures). The theory was that when one had attained these three goals, combining the moral, material and erotic, then one could aspire to acheiving *moksha*, or spiritual liberation.

The Kama Sutra is therefore not solely sexually focused and only a small portion of the text concentrates on the act of sex. In India it became a guide to human relations and interactions. It advises on other aspects of male-female relations such as courtship and marriage, the duties of wife and husband, enhancing beauty and attractiveness, and it provides a variety of recipes and incantations to help with sexual problems and difficulties.

Vatsayana's tone in the Kama Sutra is remarkably unprejudiced and liberal considering the time in which it was written. The emphasis is suggestive as opposed to dictatorial, frequently reminding couples that they should do whatever they feel is right for them at the time. It is a lover's guide, not a lover's law.

The West got wind of the Kama Sutra in the Victorian era, when women were not expected to enjoy sex and men did not therefore require any specific sexual skill or talent to please them. Its Victorian translators, F.F. Arbuthnot and Sir Richard Burton, published the book in English in 1883 for private circulation. It was not until 1963 that the first edition became available to the general public, a hiatus that greatly added to the mystique surrounding the Kama Sutra.

The Kama Sutra is in many ways a direct portal to the period and culture in which it was written. Although much of it is outdated, there are many underlying elements in the Kama Sutra that the Western world can still learn from. The most important of these is the sense of belonging to a civilized society that takes the pleasures of the mind and body extremely seriously.

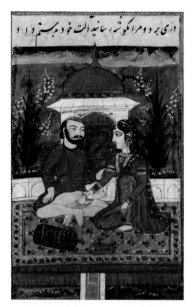

LEFT | In this 18th-century illustration, the woman is manipulating the lingham, or penis, of her partner.

BELOW | Illustrations of the Kama Sutra are often set in beautiful palaces, here complete with flowers, hand-woven rug and hookah.

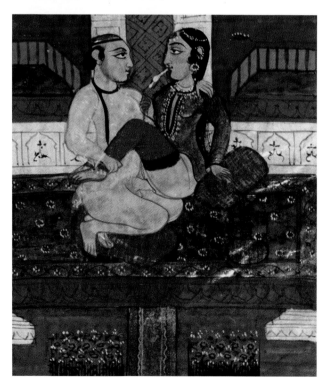

a modern kama sutra

THE KAMA SUTRA isn't just a list of exotic positions for sex. It describes in great detail the delicacy of foreplay and the importance of both parties being satisfied sexually, and also that they should share time together as a couple after congress.

the work of the man

In the Kama Sutra, the "work of the man" denotes any action that the man must do in order to give pleasure to the woman. Vatsayana suggests that when a man and a woman first come together, they begin by sitting on the bed talking about non-sexual topics and encourage each other to drink wine. While the woman is lying on the man's bed, engrossed by his captivating conversation, the man should loosen her undergarments and "overwhelm her" with kisses if she starts to protest.

When he becomes erect it is suggested that he should begin gently touching her with his hands. If she is shy or it is the first time they have had sex together, he should begin by placing his hands between her thighs. He should also caress her breasts, neck and armpits with his hands.

modern interpretation

The contemporary message of the concept of "the work of the man" is about the importance of foreplay. Take time to seduce each other in bed with words and actions and some good wine. The woman does not have to be passive; both should luxuriate in the sensuality of each other's body before actually having intercourse.

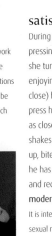

satisfying a woman

During sex, the man should concentrate on pressing the parts of the woman's body "on which she turns her eyes". Signs that a woman is enjoying herself are that she will turn (roll or close) her eyes, will become less shy and will press herself towards him to keep their sex organs as closely united as possible. When the woman shakes her hands, prevents the man from getting up, bites or kicks him, or continues writhing after he has orgasmed, it signifies that she is aroused and requires more satisfaction.

modern interpretation

It is interesting that Indian culture was so aware of the sexual needs of women at a time when the Western world seemed completely oblivious of them. Male reading of the body movements of women during intercourse allows you both to remain at the same tempo. If the man comes before his partner and ignores her need for sexual fulfilment he will invariably leave her frustrated.

sanskrit

The Kama Sutra was written in Sanskrit, the ancient and sacred language of India, in which Hindu literature from the Vedas downwards was composed.

Yoni is the Sanskrit word for the female genitalia, or vulva. The yoni is an object of veneration among Hindus as it is seen as a holy symbol of the goddess Shakti.

Lingham is the Sanskrit word for the phallus, which is worshipped among Hindus as a symbol of the god Shiva.

ABOVE RIGHT | The Kama Sutra was enlightened in its belief in foreplay and recommends that the man should begin by rubbing the woman's yoni with his fingers.

RIGHT | The woman can clutch the man, pulling him into her body, and demonstrating her physical pleasure.

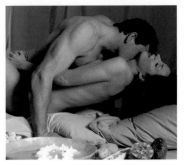

the end of congress

After sex, the two lovers must show modesty by
not looking at each other and by going separately
to the bathroom. They should eat betel leaves and
the man should anoint the woman's body with
sandalwood. He then must embrace her with his
left arm and hold a cup in his right, from which he
should encourage her to drink.

Together they should eat sweetmeats, soup,
mango juice or lemon juice mixed with sugar,
anything that is sweet and pure. The couple should
then sit outside on a balcony and enjoy the
moonlight, with her lying in his lap as they talk. As
they gaze at the night sky he should show her the
different constellations of stars and planets.

modern interpretation

Don't panic, most women today do not consider an
astronomy lesson an essential post-coital activity,
although if you do know a bit about stars and planets it
can be romantic to share it. Following the above advice
is actually a perfect way of spending time together after
you have had sex. Enjoy these moments – share a drink,
massage one another, feed each other with confectionery,
fruit or have a light meal, before cuddling up together for
a chat. Stargazing is optional.

the elephant woman

A Hastini, or elephant woman, is a woman with a
large vagina. According to Vatsayana, if a man is
unable to satisfy a Hastini, various forms of
congress are recommended where the woman
presses her thighs together, thus increasing the
sensations for both parties.

An alternative is to use an apadravyas, an
instrument put around or on the penis to make it
longer or thicker. Apadravyas should be made of
gold, silver, copper, iron, ivory, buffalo horn, various
kinds of wood, tin or lead and should be cool and
well fitted.

modern interpretation

Although it is not terribly polite to refer to women with
large vaginas as elephant women, it is a fact of nature
that with age and after childbirth, the vagina may lose
some of its tightness. Pelvic floor and Kegel exercises do
help to keep the vagina tight but for some women, it is
just the way they are. Luckily for contemporary lovers,
men no longer need to strap a buffalo horn to their
genitals in order to satisfy a woman who has lost her
grip. Today there is a wide range of gadgets that will
satisfy all shapes and sizes and incorporating them into
your sex lives can be great fun.

BELOW LEFT | At the end of
congress, sharing some
jasmine or mint tea with
some sweet food is a
marvellous way to bask in
the afterglow of sex.

BELOW | Turkish delight is a
modern equivalent to
Vatsayana's "sweetmeats".

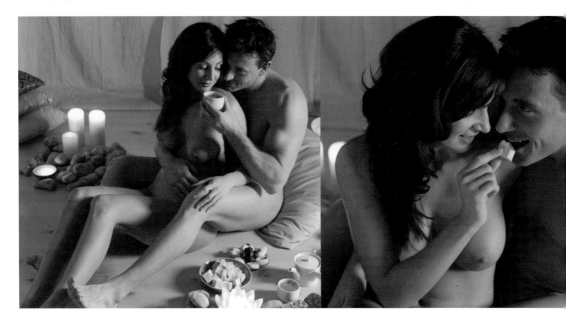

ananga ranga

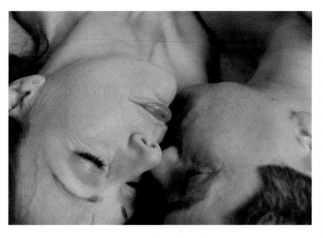

ABOVE AND BELOW | Closeness continues to be important in a long-term relationship. The Ananga Ranga sought to increase intimacy and rid marriages of any stagnation.

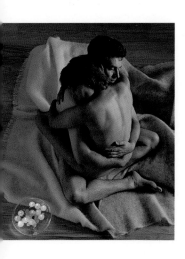

INDIAN LOVE SAGE KALYANA MALLA wrote the Ananga Ranga during the 16th century. It was aimed at keeping husbands and wives from separating when their relationship went wrong. Like the Kama Sutra, the book was translated into English in the late 1800s, but it was not made extensively available until the 1960s as it was considered too racy.

The Ananga Ranga aimed to define more clearly the distinction between monotony and monogamy, releasing one from the other, and relieving the tedium of marriage. Malla believed that the chief reason that husbands go off with other women, and wives with other men, is that sex becomes boring and mundane: "the monotony which follows possession". He wrote a long treatise of erotic work, which incorporated the much older Kama Sutra, describing a multitude of ways of kissing, embracing and sexual positions.

"Fully understanding the way in which such quarrels arise, I have in this book shown how the husband, by varying the enjoyment of his wife, may live with her as with thirty-two different women, ever varying the enjoyment of her, and rendering satiety impossible." The Ananga Ranga seeks to help couples to renew their desire for sex,

which in turn helps them to re-establish strong bonds, both of friendship and love. Although sex is clearly important to all loving relationships, Malla removes the emphasis from sex and argues instead that this should be the end result of all the teachings and techniques that can be introduced to the relationship via the Ananga Ranga. It defines the different types of men and women and their needs, what kind of sex they enjoy and how to hold each other physically, mentally and emotionally.

The contemporary significance of the Ananga Ranga lies in its insistence upon the importance of maintaining passion in long-term relationships and its practical suggestions for rejuvenating stagnant patterns. Despite its antiquity, the concepts and practices set out in the Ananga Ranga are relatively new to the West. By combining the elements of Eastern magic and mystery with what we already know, we can begin to understand how and why problems have arisen in our relationships and begin to take positive steps towards healing wounds and strengthening bonds.

thirty-two lovers

The Ananga Ranga differs from the Kama Sutra in its recognition that the ability to maintain erotic interest in an exclusive monogamous relationship is not simple.

The book defines the difference between intimacy and familiarity and encourages sexual partners to break down the patterns of laziness that are bred from familiarity and to reinvent and renew the possibilities of sustained eroticism that can be derived from true intimacy. It teaches couples to use their minds and imaginations to achieve a more sophisticated level of eroticism and aims to teach lovers to experience their partner as if they were thirty-two different lovers.

embracing techniques

The Ananga Ranga's chapter on the "treating of external enjoyments" concentrates on the importance of various preliminaries that should precede sex and internal enjoyment. These include the various types of kissing and embracing, biting, scratching and hair pulling. These acts, according to Malla, "affect the senses and divert the mind from coyness and coldness." Foreplay is an essential part of all sexual encounters, as it helps to relax and acquaint the partners with each other's bodies and erogenous zones, allowing both to reach the same levels of excitement before penetration.

Malla recommends these techniques for embracing in relationships where cuddling has ceased to be spontaneous. Touching is one of the mutually satisfying ways for men and women to show their affection for each other – not just when they are going to have sex, but at other times as well. The types of pressure to be used are described as pressing, touching, piercing and rubbing. Once tried, these techniques might arouse interest in further contact, or can just be enjoyed in their own right.

vrikshadhirudha

This is often referred to as the embrace that simulates climbing a tree. The woman places one foot on the man's foot and raises her other leg, resting her foot upon his thigh. She puts her arms around his back and holds him tightly.

modern interpretation

With the woman's legs parted in this fashion, and the man's hands relatively free, this embrace gives the man good access to the woman's breasts and genitals for light stroking and caressing, while she showers him with passionate kisses.

tila-tandula

The man and woman stand in front of each other and hold each other closely around the waist.

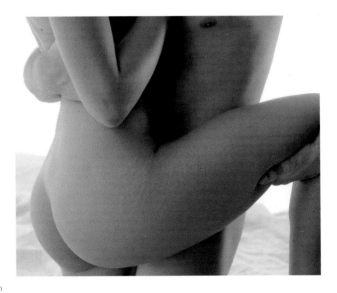

Then, being careful to remain still, he should allow his penis to come into contact with her vagina, with only the veil of her skirt between the two. They should remain like this for a time.

modern interpretation

This embrace is best achieved if the woman is wearing loose clothing made of soft fabric, as the sensation of the material against both the man's and the woman's private parts will add to the experience. It may be hard to remain like this for a long time, as the sensation of each other's genitals in such close proximity is arousing, and can be too much for some.

urupaguha

The man and woman stand in front of each other and he places her closed legs between his own, so that his inside thigh touches her outside thigh. As with all the embraces, the couple should also experiment with kissing at the same time.

modern interpretation

A good embrace if the man is taller than the woman. The squeezing of her thighs provides gentle stimulation of her clitoris and his genitals are pressed against her.

ABOVE | Climbing a tree – it is as if the woman is trying to reach up for a kiss.

BELOW | Embracing doesn't have to be done by the book – if you are lucky it will happen spontaneously.

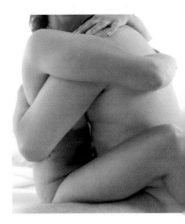

ananga ranga kissing techniques

THE ANANGA RANGA described osculations, or kissing, as particular styles to be studied and which were to be practised with the embracing techniques. "There are seven places highly proper for osculation, in fact, where all the world kisses." These are the lower lip, both the eyes, both cheeks, the head, the mouth, the breasts and lastly, the shoulders. Of course there is no reason why you should stop there.

nlita kissing

When the woman is angry, the man should forcibly cover her lips with his own and continue until her anger has subsided.

modern interpretation

This type of kissing can be a fantastic means of ending an argument in which there is simply nothing more that can be said. Couples who have been together for a long time often find themselves arguing over petty annoyances.

These arguments are usually cyclical in content and it can be hard to walk away or end the quarrel. A kiss such as this requires no words. It says, "Let's forget this, we are arguing over trivia and I love you."

sphrita kissing

The woman leans in to kiss her partner, who kisses her lower lip while she jerks her mouth away without returning the kiss.

modern interpretation

This is a playful, teasing kiss. When you move in to kiss your partner, allow him or her a taste of your lower lip before withdrawing and not allowing the kiss to continue. This is a great one to do in a quiet corner in the company of others. It tells your partner that you are feeling playful and frisky, but that he or she will have to wait until you decide when play will commence. It guarantees anticipation and excitement in your partner and is a seductive means of communicating without words.

BELOW | Nlita kissing – a great way of putting a stop to petty squabbles.

BELOW RIGHT | The teasing sphrita kiss can be initiated by either partner.

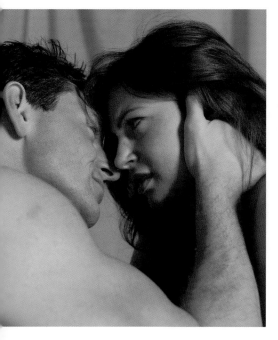

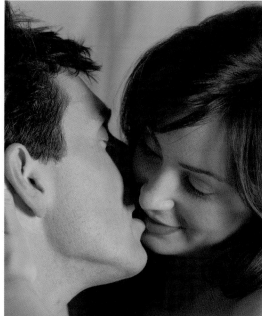

ghatika kissing

The man covers his partner's eyes with his hands and closes his own eyes before thrusting his tongue into his partner's mouth, moving it to and fro using a slow, pleasant motion that suggests another form of enjoyment.

modern interpretation

By removing one sense, in this case sight, the partners' bodies become more attuned to other sensations. In this case, sex is simulated with the mouth, building anticipation about how each will pleasure the other genitally. It is a provocative yet romantic method of kissing, ideal as a precursory invitation to a night of sensational sexual activity.

uttaroshtha

The man gently bites and nibbles his partner's lower lip while the woman reciprocates on his upper lip, then they swap over, both exciting themselves to the height of passion.

modern interpretation

This is like foreplay for kissing. With each other's mouths, the partners tease the nerve endings, so that by the time they begin a more passionate kiss, including tongues, all the sensory organs in the area will be in overdrive, and aroused beyond words.

pratibodha

When one partner is sleeping the other should fix their lips over their sleeping partner's lips, and gradually increase the pressure until sleep turns into desire.

modern interpretation

This kiss ignites passion first thing in the morning, and there is, after all, no better way to begin the day. Begin by gently kissing your partner, gradually increasing the pressure, sucking on his or her lips until they wake up.

tiryak kissing

The man places his hand beneath the woman's chin, and raises it, until he has made her face look up to the sky; then he takes her lower lip between his teeth, gently biting and chewing it.

modern interpretation

It would feel wonderful for a woman to surrender to this gently forceful kiss from a man.

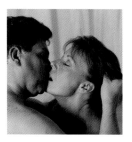

ABOVE | Here, playfully nibbling the lip is combined with pulling the hair.

BELOW LEFT | Ghatika kissing – this is a very suggestive way to arouse your partner's desire for more.

BELOW | Uttaroshtha kissing – he bites her lip, and she bites his; just be sure not to bite too hard…

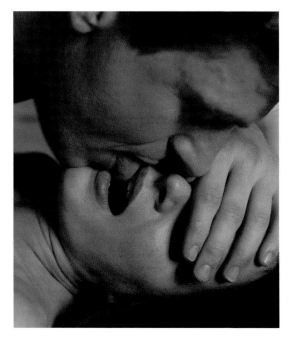

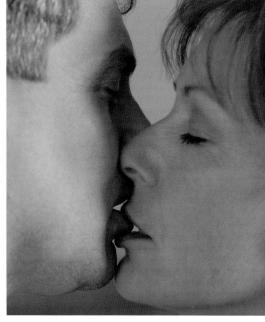

scratching, biting and hair-pulling

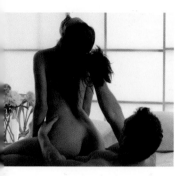

SCRATCHING AND BITING are, both the Ananga Ranga and the Kama Sutra suggest, to be tried only when love becomes intense. Description is given of the preferred, clean state of nails and teeth, and the willingness of both parties, before commencing.

scratching

The Ananga Ranga defines specific times when this type of sex play is advisable. Some examples include: when one partner is about to go away for a long period of time, or when both are "excited with desire of congress". It appears to have been done as a form of remembrance, so that when they are separated there will be a mark on the body to remind them of each other.

churit-nakhadana – gentle scratches

This involves the light scratching of the nails around the cheek, lower lip and breasts. The scratching should be light enough that it leaves no marks.

ABOVE | The ancient texts were witness to the effect that a woman's hair can have on a man.

BELOW | Light scratching can be extremely erotic if both partners are willing.

modern interpretation

The scratching described here is so light that it is more of a caress. The soft use of nails, however, indicates greater passion and energy than a more delicate touch.

the peacock's foot

For this specialist imprint the thumb is placed on the nipple and four fingers are spread adjacent to this on the breast. The nails are dug in to leave an indentation similar to that of a peacock footprint.

modern interpretation

Most women love to have their breasts caressed and squeezed during lovemaking. The preferred pressure and sensation is individual to each woman, with some having very sensitive breasts, especially around menstruation. Before digging your nails into your partner's breasts it is advisable to find out how much stimulation she prefers.

anvartha-nakhadana – to remember

Marks or scratches three deep are made by the first three fingers on the woman's back, breasts or genitals. It is most commonly done as a token of remembrance before the man leaves to go abroad.

modern interpretation

Many men and women really enjoy scratching if it is done correctly, as it is a form of sensual massage and can be very relaxing. Remember to be gentle and do not do anything that may cause pain. As with all these techniques, keep your nails smooth, clean and reasonably short.

biting

The Ananga Ranga suggests that biting should be done in similar places to scratching but lovers should avoid the eyes, upper lip and tongue. It also suggests that the pressure should be increased until the recipient protests, after which enough has been done. Neither party will be in particular favour if they bite the other too hard; soft nibbling is more advisable. Take cues from each other, rising to a passionate moment with appropriate strength, and a lighter touch when called for.

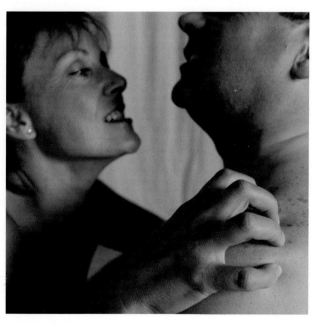

uchun-dashana – biting

This is the generic term to describe biting any part of the woman's lips or cheeks.

modern interpretation

Gently nibbling around each other's faces can be very sensual. Be careful around the bony areas like the cheeks, as they bruise easily. The lips should be handled with care too, as they are only protected by a thin layer of skin.

bindhu-dashana – teeth marks

This is the mark left by the man's two front teeth on the woman's lower lip.

modern interpretation

The lower lip is very supple and elastic and gentle sucking and nibbling on it is very pleasurable. In the days when the Ananga Ranga was written it was probably pretty acceptable for women to bear the marks of their husband's desire. Any imprint of passion today is reminiscent of the adolescent love bite, and not particularly desirable, so facial markings should be avoided.

kolacharcha – on departing

These are the deep, lasting marks left on the woman's body in the heat of passion and the grief of departure when her husband is going away.

modern interpretation

The fleshier parts of the body such as the thighs and buttocks can withstand more pain than the more sensitive areas around the face. They also have the added advantage of being hidden by clothing. Biting each other is a common outlet of sexual energy when in the throes of orgasm and many people, male and female, claim that they have been surprised at the depth of a bite afterwards. Many people enjoy sharp pain at the height of passion to enhance the powerful shudders of pleasure that they experience during orgasm.

hair-pulling

Softly pulling the hair of a woman, states the Ananga Ranga, is a good method of kindling a lasting desire.

samahastakakeshagrahana – stroking

The man strokes his partner's hair between the palms of his hands, at the same time kissing her with passion.

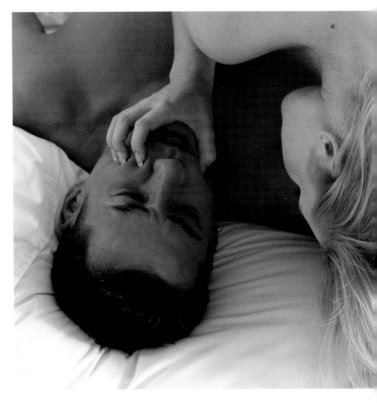

modern interpretation

Gentle pulling and playing with a woman's hair is very erotic and sensual. When pulling hair, make sure you get a good handful, as pulling at a small number of hairs can be very painful. Why not take this a stage further and gently pull tufts of each other's pubic hair – you are sure to bring each other to a state of excitement.

kamavatansakeshagrahana – pulling

This is done during sexual intercourse, when each partner grabs the other's hair above the ears as they kiss passionately.

modern interpretation

This type of hair pulling is ideal in the throes of passion when the body's touch sensors are dulled by the other erotic sensations that are flowing around. Stroking and massaging this area, including the temples, can be very seductive, especially if you whisper in each other's ears at the same time.

ABOVE | Churit-nakhadana – light scratching around the face – shouldn't leave a mark.

BELOW | He grabs her hair in kamavatansakeshagrahana.

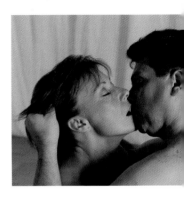

ananga ranga positions

MANY OF THE SEXUAL POSITIONS in the Ananga Ranga were adapted by Malla from the original work of Vatsayana's Kama Sutra. However, Malla's text was written in a very different social climate, where extramarital sex was frowned upon, so the emphasis is on variety with one partner.

the crab embrace

The man and woman lie on their sides facing each other. The man enters the woman and lies between her legs. One of her legs passes over his body (at about the level of his navel) while the other remains beneath his legs.

modern interpretation

The position provides deep penetration and increased friction. The man's movement is limited although the woman has more freedom. This position may be good when one partner is tired but both are still passionate.

kama's wheel

The man sits with his legs outstretched. The woman lowers herself on to his penis, facing him. She also extends her legs. He then stretches his arms out along either side of her body to support her. This forms the wheel-like figure for which this position is named.

modern interpretation

It is said that this position combines sex and meditation to create a higher level of awareness. It is meant to help the partners to obtain a balance of mind that is clear, calm and happy.

the ascending position

The man lies on his back while the woman sits cross-legged upon his thighs. The woman grasps his penis and inserts it into her, moving her waist backward and forward as they make love.

BELOW TOP | Kama's wheel – this is a great transitional position. Try it after ascending or before the placid embrace.

BELOW BOTTOM | The ascending position – this posture can give added satisfaction to the woman.

BELOW RIGHT | The crab embrace, lying side by side, enables plenty of physical contact along the body.

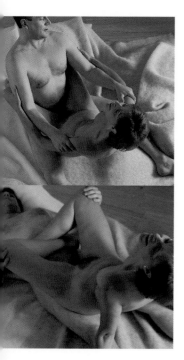

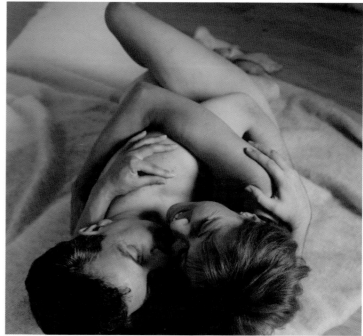

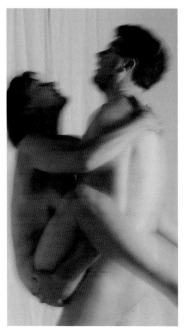

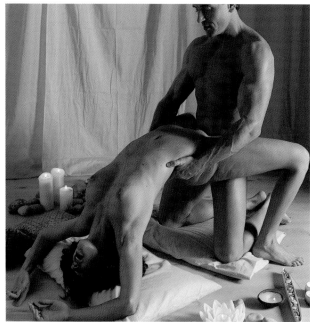

modern interpretation

The woman on top can control the movements and depth of penetration. By moving herself forward and back, her clitoris also receives stimulation from the gentle rubbing action against her partner's body. This is recommended for women who have not found satisfaction in other positions.

suspended congress

Both partners stand opposite one another. The man passes two arms under his partner's knees, supporting her by gripping her inner elbow or her bottom. He then raises her waist high and penetrates her while she clasps her hands around his neck.

modern interpretation

This one could be tricky, as its success depends on many factors such as the strength of the man, the weight of the woman, and the height of them both. It may be easier if the woman gets on a chair first, so that the man does not have to lift her from the ground and risk back injury. It may also help to be near a wall or rail to maintain balance. Good luck!

placid embrace

The man kneels and raises his partner to him by grasping her around the waist so that her head falls towards the floor. She in turn wraps her legs about his middle and lets her head fall freely.

modern interpretation

This position allows the woman to retain some control – by extending and flexing the grip of her legs she can draw her partner closer. Hanging with the head upside-down can also contribute a feeling of ecstasy and otherworldliness. Try this after kama's wheel.

ABOVE LEFT | Suspended congress – this one isn't for you if you have a bad back.

ABOVE | The placid embrace allows the woman to let herself go completely.

BELOW | You may have tried the crab embrace before without realizing it.

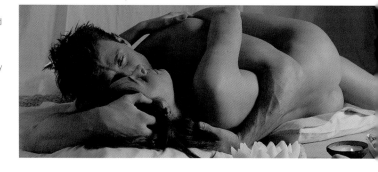

the art of tantric sex

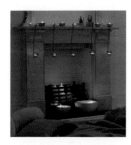

TANTRA FOCUSES on honouring and respecting your partner as the other half of yourself. Although Tantrists believe that sex is a divine gift that should be celebrated, Tantra is not a religion but a tradition, which can be practised by people of any faith or by non-religious people.

The word Tantra is derived from the Indian Sanskrit meaning, "liberation through expression". Based on early Hindu and Buddhist teachings, or tantras, Tantra unites elements of meditation, yoga and worship to provide practitioners with a more wholesome and intense sexual experience.

Tantra has many dimensions that can take years of study to fully appreciate. This does not mean, however, that people interested in Tantric sex must immerse themselves in study. Instead, it is perfectly valid to take some elements of Tantra and incorporate them into existing sex lives.

In Tantric sex the vagina becomes a sacred space (yoni) and the penis (or lingham) is a "wand of light". Kundalini denotes the life force and sexual energy that flows between sexual partners as they make love. Breathing and visualization exercises help to harmonize this energy. Tantric sex takes the emphasis away from the physicality

of the orgasm and concentrates more on spirituality, intimacy and connection. Men are often taught to suppress their orgasm, a Tantric skill known as maithuna, in order to devote their attention to the woman's sexual pleasure. If this all sounds rather pointless from the male perspective, it is worth remembering that once it is mastered, men reap the rewards, keeping sexually active for anything up to an hour with the promise of increased orgasm when it comes. It can also increase the chance of multiple orgasms for their partner and enable the man to "virtually experience" their lover's orgasm as well as their own.

tantra western style

Tantra cannot cure a failing relationship but it's a good prescription for a loving respectful relationship that has become a bit dull. Most people would prefer to tackle the problem of bedroom boredom rather than bailing out of a relationship. According to Tantra, boredom sets in when people make love with only their genitals, not their hearts and minds.

A couple should begin Tantric lovemaking with an idea of what they want and, more importantly, the genuine desire to give their partner what he or

ABOVE | Create a harmonious environment to share.

BELOW | Place your hand on your lover's heart so you can merge together.

BELOW RIGHT | Meditate with your partner, concentrating on each chakra in turn.

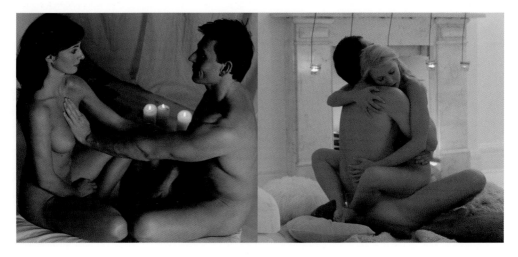

she wants. Tantric sex has no time limit: it can last minutes or hours, and it gives you and your partner the freedom and opportunity to explore each other's bodies and pleasure zones.

Much of Tantric lovemaking involves ritualistic foreplay that excites all the senses. Massage and the use of aromatherapy oils stimulate the senses of smell and touch. By caressing each other slowly and languidly the scene is set for a relaxed session of lovemaking, allowing time to explore each other's bodies and become more comfortable with each other's nudity.

meditation and breathing

Meditation in Tantra is an important principle, as it allows couples to move away from frantic passion, and emphasize tranquillity and harmony.

Dedicate an area for meditation and Tantric lovemaking and set aside a specific portion of uninterrupted time for you to either meditate alone, or with your partner. Make sure that the area is calm and warm, close the curtains, remove distractions, use aromatherapy fragrances such as cedarwood or frankincense, and light some scented candles to add to the atmosphere.

Begin by sitting on the floor with your legs crossed, back straight and hands resting in your lap. Ensure that you are comfortable before closing your eyes and focusing on your breathing. Breathe in through your nose and out through your mouth and become conscious of the soft rise and fall of your diaphragm with each breath. Try to concentrate on your breathing, and every time your mind wanders gently bring it back to your breath. With practice, meditation will create peace and tranquillity and leave you feeling refreshed and calm. Your meditation sessions will become longer, provided you remember to keep patient and relaxed.

tantra to share

Sit in front of each other and look each other in the eye as you place your hands on each other's hearts. As you breathe out, imagine that you are breathing the energy from your heart into your partner's heart. As you breathe in, imagine you are inhaling their energy into your heart. The physical

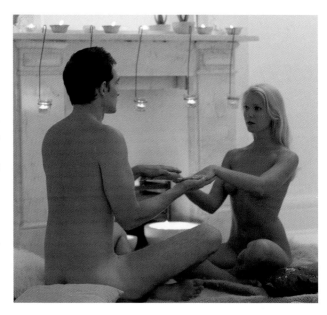

connection allows a circuit of energy to pass between you, so that energy flows from your heart, through your body to your partner's heart, and vice versa. Once you feel comfortable, begin alternating your breathing pattern with your partner's so that as they breathe in, you breathe out and so on. This should cause the energy to circulate evenly and harmoniously between you.

Sit before each other again, but this time merge your energy by placing your palms together, creating an electrical circuit. You can continue with the same breathing techniques or try chakra meditation, in which you concentrate on each chakra, breathing energy into each for two or three minutes. Begin at the base chakra and move up towards the crown, opening up each energy centre as you go. This may take some practice as each of you may require a different amount of time on each chakra, but be patient and before long both your sets of chakras will become harmonized with each other.

Don't be afraid to laugh! The point of this is not to reinvent you as Tantric gurus but to bring you closer together. Collapsing in giggles will not detach you from the spirit of what you are trying to achieve.

ABOVE | Create a circuit of energy between you – merge together for 15 minutes, allowing your breathing to synchronize naturally.

BELOW | A calming and private space in which to meditate will enable you to concentrate and not be distracted by external elements.

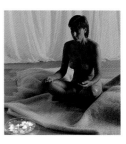

meditation in a relationship

It will be helpful for you and your partner to practise meditation both alone and together. Meditation helps focus your full attention into the present moment, away from the endless distractions of thoughts which course through your mind. The purpose of meditation is not to suppress these thoughts and feelings, but to harness all this potential energy and bring it to one focal point. Then, whatever you are doing in a meditative way has a different quality about it.

You are able to function more spontaneously and creatively, trusting yourself more and responding intuitively, letting one moment give birth to the next, without the constant interference of your mind. When this quality of totality enters into your lovemaking it can become more spontaneous and a true vehicle for mystical experience.

Awareness of breath is one of the basic tools of meditation. By focusing total awareness onto the breathing cycle, it becomes easier to detach from all mental images. Breathing is a natural, involuntary process, our most fundamental link to life and the doorway between the internal self and the external environment.

However, our breathing is largely affected by our thoughts, physical tensions and emotional states. When we are under stress, breathing may become too rapid or shallow. By focusing

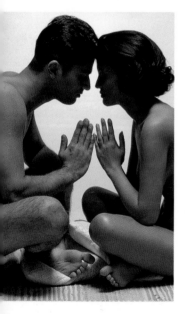

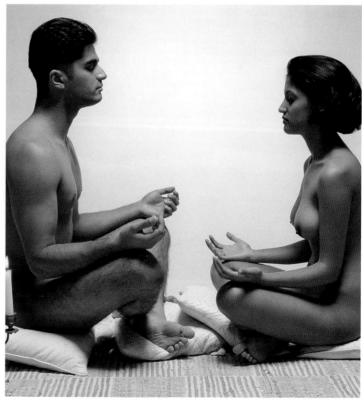

ABOVE | The traditional namaste greeting, used at the end of each meditation.

RIGHT | The basic meditation position, palms facing upwards.

awareness on the breath during meditation, we begin to breathe in a more relaxed and calming way, creating greater equilibrium between inhalation and exhalation. Meditative breathing brings harmony and balance to the body, mind and spirit.

Do not try to change or force your breathing in any way. First, close your eyes and focus attention on the sensation of breath as it is drawn into your nostrils, and then exhaled out of your nostrils or mouth. After about five minutes, start to focus on the subtle movement of your abdomen as it rises with each inhalation, and falls back with each exhalation. When thoughts and feelings distract you, bring your attention back to your breathing. It is actually quite difficult to remain focused on your breathing. Do not worry about this. Each time your attention begins to meander, lead it gently back. Gradually, your mind will become calmer and allow a transcendental quality of consciousness to arise within you.

Make a commitment to meditate together at least once to three times a week, setting aside a regular time when you can sit together, undisturbed and in total privacy. Try to meditate even if you feel preoccupied. Sitting with your partner will calm and refresh you both. However, do not try to force each other to sit and meditate. If your partner is unable to meditate with you, then be happy to meditate alone.

If you have never meditated before, start off with 15-minute sessions. The ideal position for meditation is to sit cross-legged on the floor, with your hands relaxed, palms facing upwards, on your thighs. Avoid slumping by placing a cushion beneath your buttocks, tilting your pelvis to support your upper body. Keep your spine straight but relaxed, and let your neck and head extend gracefully above your spine. If sitting on the floor is too uncomfortable, then sit on a straight-backed chair.

synchronize your breathing

Meditation can take your emotional and sexual relationship with your partner deeper and beyond its everyday parameters. Gradually extend your

meditation time to between 40 minutes and one hour as you learn to escape the hustle and bustle of your lives and enjoy a new tranquillity and serenity.

Initially, your focus will be on your own breathing, but after some time, as you continue to meditate together, your breathing patterns may begin to synchronize without effort.

signal your respect

In the East, people place the palms of their hands together in the position of prayer, and incline towards each other as a gesture of respect. This is the beautiful traditional greeting of namaste, also used to signify gratitude, and recognition of the divine self within each person. At the end of each meditation, acknowledge each other with this ritual.

BELOW | Visualize yourselves joining together to form a balanced circuit of energy through mutual breathing and contact.

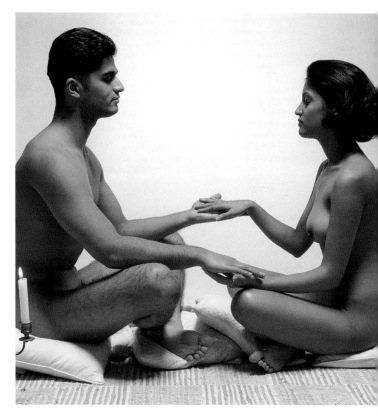

connecting and merging

The three meditation exercises which follow all involve a degree of physical interaction to deepen your mutual bond and intimacy. They will heighten your sensitivity and encourage you to open your hearts to one another so that your sense of merging energetically becomes stronger. This fusion of body and spirit is what Tantric, or sacred, sex is all about. Tantra teaches that when the male and female energies merge harmoniously, their union creates a powerful, moving, loving and transforming force.

meditation exercises

Use the following exercises on a regular basis to connect with one another on subtle levels, especially at times when the pressures of everyday life have caused an emotional or

physical distance to open up between you. In the first meditation for merging, both of you contemplate this union of opposite polarities, while connecting palm to palm, for up to 15 minutes, allowing your breathing to synchronize naturally. To complete this meditation, open your eyes, and slowly perform the namaste ritual which is designed to honour one another's intrinsic divinity.

The second exercise is an eye-gazing technique which gives truth to the saying, "The eyes are the windows of the soul". By looking softly into each other's eyes for periods of between 10 and 20 minutes, you can both see and be seen. It will create trust and deep intimacy as you look within each other, and let go of your normal defences to reveal your inner vulnerability.

During the eye-gazing meditation, breathe gently into whatever feelings arise, letting them come and go without trying to analyse them. Remain relaxed, and allow yourself to be seen by your loved one. At the same time, look deep within your partner's being as you continue to gaze steadily and softly into his eyes.

Make palm-to-palm contact so that you feel connected on the physical level. Focus attention on your breathing, your body and the tactile contact of your hands. If your face becomes tense, relax the muscles, particularly around the jaw and mouth. Do not out-stare or try to dominate your partner with your gaze; keep your eyes softly focused.

At first, you may feel exposed, as different emotions emerge, such as embarrassment, fear, happiness, sadness, love and joy. Do not suppress these feelings or try to change them, but stay with the eye contact and breath. When you are ready to complete the eye-gazing meditation, close your eyes and release your palm-to-palm contact slowly so your hands rest against your lap. Focus on your breathing and body sensations. After some minutes, open your eyes and thank your partner with the namaste bow.

The third exercise has four five-minute stages and connects you directly, heart to heart, with one

BELOW | Tune in to your heart. Place your right hand very lightly over your heart. Take some moments to bring full awareness to the physical sensations of your heart pumping beneath your hand. Now tune in more deeply to the feelings of the heart. Imagine your heart centre becoming more open and vulnerable as you breathe out any tensions.

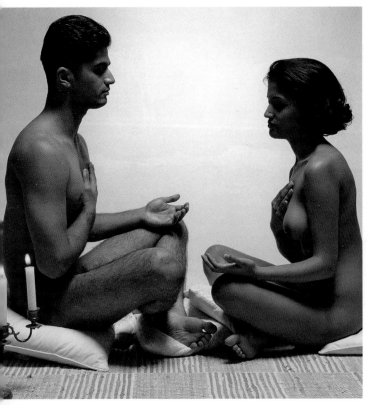

another. When we are "in our hearts" we long to share and merge with each other. The first step is to sit facing your partner in a meditative posture, close your eyes and begin to focus on your breathing. During the second stage of the exercise, you bring your attention to the feelings within your heart and allow yourself to become more open, vulnerable and receptive. In the third stage, you make contact with each other to allow a fusion of heart-to-heart loving energy.

The fourth step is to draw your hands very slowly away from one another's heart centre and to bring that sense of merging back within yourself by placing your hand back on to your own heart. Only when you are completely ready, open your eyes and give the namaste salutation to each other to conclude this meditation.

creating a meditative ambience

Set aside a room especially for meditation, or if this is not possible, create a specific area in your bedroom or living room which is dedicated to your Tantric rituals. Treat this space as a temple to your love. Place flowers, light candles and burn incense, or carry out any ritual which is appropriate and meaningful to you both, to make yourselves feel as if you are on consecrated ground.

Try to ensure you and your partner have complete privacy, and plan a time when you know you will be left undisturbed. Place a clock with a soft-sounding alarm some distance away from you, or have it muffled beneath a pillow, to alert you when your allotted time for meditation is over.

Be prepared to give yourselves at least 5 to 15 minutes for re-orientation back to a normal functioning state of consciousness. You may want to lie down on the floor next to each other, bringing your full attention to your body as it rests on the ground.

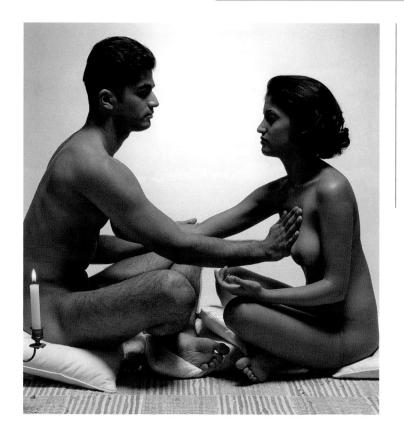

LEFT | Feel yourselves merge. Now stretch out to place your right hand gently over your lover's heart. Take some moments to feel the warmth of the skin, the beat of the heart and the rhythm of the breath. Connect to the feelings within your partner's heart and pour yourselves into this contact, so you both merge on a heart-to-heart level.

RIGHT | Balance the pathway.
To balance the Kundalini
Pathway, ask your partner
to curl up on her side into a
comforting foetal position
which exposes her back and
spine. Hold one hand above
the crown of her head,
while the other hovers
over the base of her spine.
Pour breath and love into
your hands.

opening the body's energy channels

Tantra teaches that within the human body resides
a vast and dynamic psychic energy known as the
Kundalini. Tantrikas, or exponents of Tantra,
believe that in normal circumstances, when
human beings are concerned only with the basic
matters of survival, the Kundalini power is a
dormant energy, symbolically portrayed as a coiled
serpent sleeping at the base of the spine.

The potential of its powerful and transforming
effects on the psycho-physiological processes may
never be realized. When the Kundalini energy is
awakened, through yoga, meditation and sexual

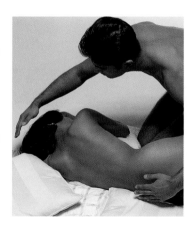

the seven energy centres of the body

Tantra originated the science of the seven chakras, or subtle energy centres,
within the human body, all of which are associated with different psycho-
physiological aspects of human nature. Each chakra is located in a different
area of the body, and is associated with one of the rainbow colours in the
spectrum of light. In everyday life, we experience the chakras on subtle
psychological and physical levels, and while we may be unaware of their
source or full potency, we are aware of their effects. We talk about our "gut"
level feelings when we experience strong, instinctive emotions, we feel the
bitter-sweet pain of love in the heart centre, and we trust the "sixth sense" of
our intuitive faculties.

The base chakra: Located at the base of the sex organs. Associated with
sex drive, survival, pain, pleasure, elimination. Colour: Red.

The belly chakra: Located just below the navel. Centre of gravity and
balance in the body and source of vital life energy. Associated with emotion,
reproduction, vitality. Colour: Orange.

The solar plexus chakra: Located at the centre point at the base of the
front of the ribcage. Associated with intellect, self-confidence, power and
action. Colour: Yellow.

The heart chakra: Located between the breasts or nipples. Associated
with love, empathy, vulnerability, joy and external merging. This chakra is
the point where the earthly instincts unite with the higher spiritual
conscious. Colour: Green.

The throat chakra: Located in the throat. Associated with
communication, self-understanding and self-expression. Colour: Blue.

The brow chakra: Located at the point between the eyebrows, and
sometimes called the "third eye". Associated with intuition, insight,
cognitive faculties, compassion for all things. Colour: Indigo.

The crown chakra: Located above the crown of the head. Associated
with the higher mind, self-realization, harmony of body, mind and spirit, and
merging with cosmic consciousness. Colour: Violet-white.

practices, it arises to travel upwards along a central
pathway in the body where it interacts with, and
transforms, the subtle energy centres, releasing
new levels of consciousness at each stage. At its
ultimate pinnacle, the Kundalini energy opens the
crown chakra, which is slightly above the head, to
bring the disciple into communion with cosmic
consciousness.

Tantra teaches that all seven energy centres
of the body must be fully open and engaged for
spiritual transformation. This is why it regards
sexuality as a potential path to higher
consciousness.

The following programme can guide you
towards becoming more aware and sensitive to
the subtle energy vibrations within the body. The
simple hands-on techniques will show you how
to bring balance and harmony between the
energy chakras.

First, return to the section on Sensual
Massage. When using massage as part of your
Tantric ritual, ensure that you touch each other
without sexual desire. Let massage become a
meditation in itself, functioning from a place of
asexual and infinite love. Trust your hands,
allowing them to move and stroke over your
lover's body in response to the messages you are
intuitively picking up. The more you trust yourself
as you touch the body, the more sensitive your
hands become, not only to the physical body but
also to its energetic essence.

When you massage meditatively, the physical boundaries between you seem to dissolve, and you experience a meeting and merging of energies. If you are receiving the session, try to relax deeply and focus your breath and attention towards the healing quality of the touch that you are getting from your lover. The more attuned you become to one another through massage, the more you experience the pulsation of energy within the body. You may feel this as a flowing stream, a current, or vibrations of energy. At other times, if your partner is tired, or under stress, the chakra centres may feel undercharged or overcharged with energy. Use the following hands-on techniques to restore equilibrium to body, mind and spirit, and balance within the chakras.

Lay your hands lightly and meditatively over the chakra centres, or slightly above them. Trust your intuition and let your hands rest softly over the areas to which they are drawn. You can also ask your partner to guide you. Or you can do a complete energy-balancing session, working slowly over all the chakras. If you sense your partner needs to come "down to earth", follow a sequence moving down the body.

Alternatively, if your partner's spirit needs to be more uplifted, then work up the body towards the head. Spend up to three minutes with each hold, letting your intuition direct you as to when and where to sensitively approach the body and when to withdraw from it. When you both feel that, through meditation, massage and energy balancing practice, you are more in harmony with each other physically, mentally and energetically, you are ready to begin to experiment with the following chakra alignment exercise.

BELOW | Use massage as a part of your programme of honouring each other's bodies. Let the massage become an act of meditation as if your hands are worshipping his or her body. As you receive the massage, surrender your body to your lover. Breathe towards his or her hands as they stroke your skin.

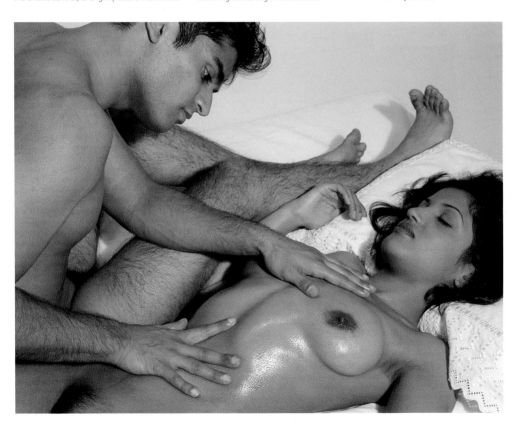

RIGHT | Your partner can lean her weight into the support of your body as you put one hand over her belly and the other on her chest. This contact with her belly will reassure and comfort her, especially in times of stress.

BELOW | Work at balancing the energy centres while in the sitting position. Place one hand over the heart and rest the other hand over the solar plexus. Gentle contact here dispels feelings of insecurity, fear and jealousy.

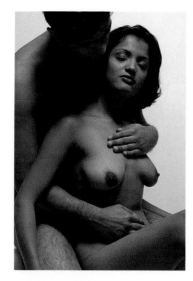

practice

In this practice, the female sits astride the man's lap. Use a chair if it is necessary. Relax and lengthen your spines so the Kundalini Pathway is without tension. If there is some sexual arousal, the man can enter his penis into the woman's vagina, and both partners can move slightly to sustain the erection, taking care not to become sexually over-stimulated. Otherwise, the penis can remain flaccid close to the entrance of the vagina. Gradually, naturally and easily let your breathing synchronize.

When you feel in harmony with your partner, direct your breathing towards the base chakra around the centre of your perineum, the area between your genitals and anus, for about 60 seconds. Visualize this chakra opening up and becoming charged with warmth and light with

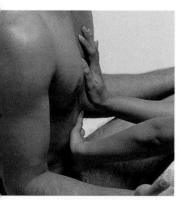

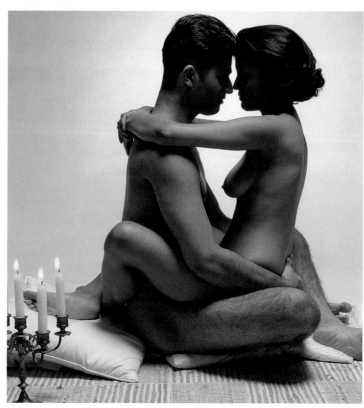

RIGHT | Aligning the energy centres. This chakra meditation helps bring you both into close proximity so that your energy centres become aligned.

your in-breath, and relaxing deeply with your out-breath. (Don't force your breathing, just imagine it flowing gently towards the chakra.) Breathe together through each chakra for about one minute, then visualize your breath and energy pouring into the crown centre above your head. As your bodies become increasingly charged with energy, let them vibrate and move together.

When you have completed the cycle of breathing, remain in the sitting position in a close embrace for up to five minutes, allowing yourselves to feel the pulsating sensations within. Then, slowly lie down next to each other for up to 15 minutes to rest and complete the meditation. You may need to set aside a quiet time after these exercises before you have to resume your normal activities.

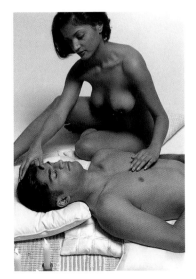

LEFT | Lay your hands tenderly over the heart and brow to integrate mind and body and to encourage more connection between the centre of love and the centre of intuition.

BELOW LEFT AND RIGHT | Release all tension so your bodies relax and mould together. Bring your attention to the sensations of skin-to-skin contact, the sound and rhythm of inhalation and exhalation, the beating of the hearts, the throb of the pulses. Remain bonded and secure in each other's arms.

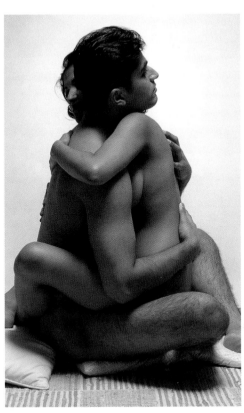

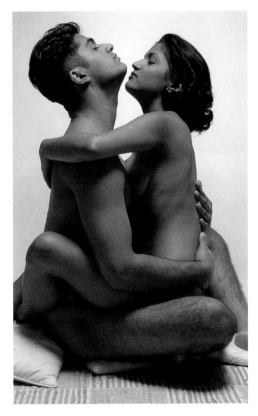

RIGHT | Respecting the male
principle. The male organ
is the symbol of cosmic
consciousness. The woman
can show her respect for the
male principle by kneeling
before her man to drop the
rose petals on to his lap.

BELOW | Symbol of creativity.
The woman's sexual organs
embody the divine principle
of cosmic creativity. Kneel
before her and scatter petals
on to her sexual area as a way
of honouring her intrinsic
feminine power.

honouring the sacred body

All mystical sex practices regard the sexual act
between men and women as something beyond
the purpose of pure physical gratification or
procreation. For instance, great honour is given to
the symbolism of the sexual organs, both male
and female. In more ancient cultures, images of
sexual organs were sculpted in wood and stone
and became shrines of worship.

These have been commonly regarded by
modern societies as ancient fertility symbols
erected to incite Nature to bestow her blessings in
the form of a good harvest or a healthy brood of
children. In fact, these symbols often represented
something more profound, and acknowledged
that sexual union of the opposites could lead
towards cosmic consciousness. Throughout India
there are many thousands of shrines, some simple
and some elaborate, which have stone images of

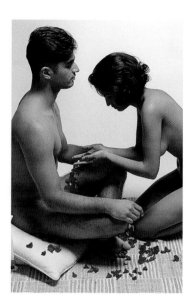

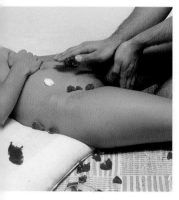

RIGHT | Honour her with rose
petals. In this ritual, you
honour her whole body as a
manifestation of her inner and
outer beauty. As she lies with
her legs wrapped around your
waist so your genital organs
are in close proximity, scatter
scented rose petals over her
entire body.

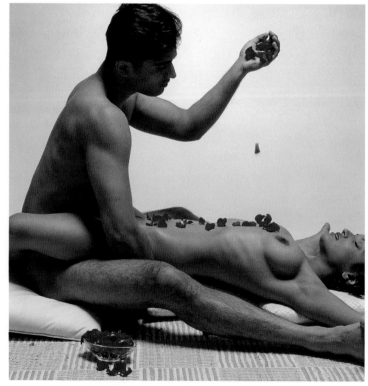

the linga and yoni, which symbolize a divine male phallus set within a divine female vagina. These symbols are objects of great devotion and worship.

To regard the most intimate sexual organs of the body with this degree of honour and respect drastically transforms an intimate relationship. You can create some beautiful rituals together in which you honour completely your own and your partner's body. Make up your own rituals, or use some of the ideas in the photographs shown here, to add this new element to the previous meditation exercises.

In the shrines in India devotees often spread petals and flowers around the sacred phallic sites. To make your ritual more special, use scented petals such as those of the delicate rose whose perfume is known to be spiritually, emotionally and sexually uplifting. Take it in turns to perform the ritual, scattering the petals over your partner's

body, and to acknowledge through touch and words that you honour each part of the other's body. Make the phrases simple, such as "I honour your beauty/skin/breasts", and so on. Or, "I have the deepest respect for your inner feminine/masculine power". Kneel before your partner's penis or vagina, and say something like "I worship your most intimate part as a manifestation of the god/goddess within".

When the ritual of honouring each other's body is over, lie together in an embrace. If it feels right, stimulate the penis so it is erect enough to enter and remain in the vagina.

Try to stay together in this meditative position for as long as you both want, focusing only on the present moment of your union, without becoming too excited. The idea is not to go full steam ahead into lovemaking or orgasm but simply to be united as one.

BELOW | Experiencing the cosmic union. The entry of the penis into the vagina symbolises the union of the male and female cosmic polarities through which joy and ecstasy can be attained. Immerse yourselves into this union, and to feel fully the depth of your physical, emotional and psychic connection.

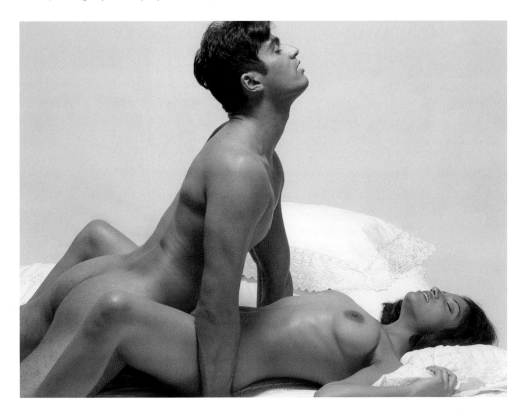

tantra lying down

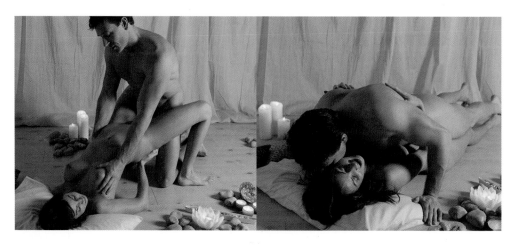

ABOVE | The flower in bloom, blossoming.

ABOVE RIGHT | The jewel case.

BELOW | Aphrodite's delight requires supple legs.

BELOW RIGHT | Dear to Cupid.

TANTRIC UNION IS A SEXUAL BOND that transcends the purely physical. Partners can forget their daily cares or status and concentrate though discipline on their being one with another person, thus achieving a higher state of ecstasy.

The positions of Tantra are based on those of the Kama Sutra. Here are a few examples translated into a more contemporary style, beginning with the supine, or lying down positions.

flower in bloom

The woman lies back, with bent knees, and spreads her legs wide, digging her heels in as close to her hips as she can. Then, placing her hands under her buttocks, she cups and lifts them with her palms, offering her yoni as a "flower in bloom". The man then enters her from between her thighs, and gently caresses her breasts. This may require some stamina and flexibility.

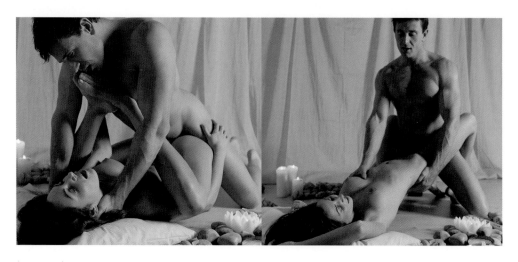

aphrodite's delight

This also requires quite a bit of flexibility from the woman. She lies back and the man clasps her feet, raising them to her breasts so that her legs form a rough circle. He then enters her, keeping her legs in place with the weight of his body, and clasps her around the neck as they make love.

dear to cupid

The woman lies back with her knees bent and the man kneels before her. He hooks her legs around his thighs and gently fondles and caresses her breasts as they make love.

the jewel case

This position is recommended for men with smaller penises. The man lies on top of the woman with his legs on top of hers, so that their legs caress each other from thighs to toes. This can either be done with the woman below the man, or side by side, in which case she should always lie to the left.

love's noose

The woman lies back as the man enters her. With her thighs pressed tightly together he encircles the woman's legs with his own. He should then squeeze and grip her thighs – very good for added clitoral stimulation.

the bud

The woman lies back and draws her legs up, clasping her knees to her breasts. This exposes her yoni (vagina) "like an opening bud" to her partner.

the mare's trick

The woman sits astride the man facing either way, and during penetration, rhythmically squeezes his penis, "milking it" with her PC muscle.

splitting the bamboo

The woman lies on her back and raises one leg over her partner's shoulder as he enters her. After a time she lowers that leg and raises the other.

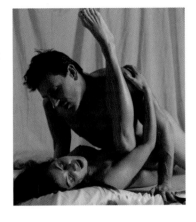

vadavaka

The art of vadavaka, or milking the man's penis, is a difficult one to be mistress of without significant practice. It can be tried in any sexual position, although some, like the mare's trick, will be easier than others where the woman is not in control.

Squeeze the PC (puboccygeus) muscle as if trying to halt the flow of urine. Pulsating in this way will heighten the pleasure of both parties. The grip may be improved by catching the glans of the lingham, or penis, behind the pubic bone, with the added advantage that it will be pushed up against the G spot here too.

ABOVE LEFT | Splitting the bamboo – this may not be comfortable for the woman for a long time, so vary the posture or move to another.

LEFT | Love's noose – this is an advanced version of the jewel case and you may find you can move between these postures quite easily.

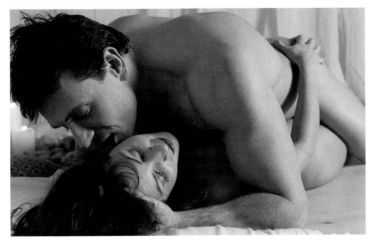

sitting tantra

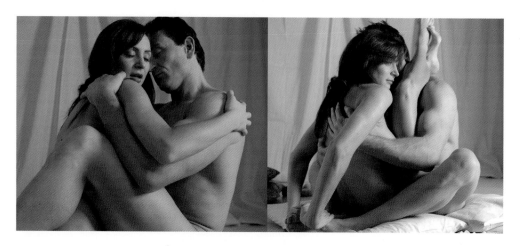

ABOVE | The feet yoke – this will be fun, once you have worked out how to do it.

ABOVE RIGHT | The lotus – it may be hard for the woman to keep her feet linked, but it isn't essential.

MANY OF THE SITTING POSITIONS are intended for long-drawn-out sex, where the couple become truly intertwined in mind as well as body.

the feet yoke

For this position you must both have reasonably flexible knees in order to achieve deeper penetration. The woman sits erect with one leg bent and the knee pulled in to her body, and the other leg straight out in front of her. The man does the same with opposing legs and penetrates her. If you cannot get close enough, then slip each straight leg beneath your partner's bent one, and gently pull one another closer together.

the circle

The woman sits with her left leg extended and encircles the man's waist with her right leg, laying the ankle across her left thigh. He mirrors this so that they are both entwined in a circle as they make love.

the peacock

This requires extreme female mobility! The woman sits and raises one foot to point vertically over her head, steadying it with her hand. In this position she offers up her yoni to her partner for lovemaking.

the lotus

The man and woman sit in front of each other, with his legs wrapped around the woman's waist. He then grips her ankles and locks them around the back of his neck like the link of a chain. She grips his toes or feet to steady herself as they make love.

awakening the chakras

The theory of chakras is that they are energy centres within the body that control our physical and psychological wellbeing. Kundalini energy is activated by the root chakra and allows spiritual energy to flow to the crown chakra, helping the body to achieve an ecstatic plane of consciousness.

There are seven chakras in the body. The first three, related to basic survival, are: root, associated with sexuality, pleasure and pain; belly, the central core of balance relating to sexual drive and reproduction, and solar plexus, concerned with power, intellect, will and ego. The four higher chakras relate to the mind, intellect and spirituality. The heart chakra is between the nipples, and being near the heart is associated with love, empathy and joy; the fifth, throat chakra, is associated with purity and expression; the sixth chakra, between the eyes, is often known as the third eye and is associated with intuition, compassion and intellect; the seventh chakra is the crown chakra, found at the top of the head. It is associated with cosmic consciousness, bliss and unity.

the swing

She sits in his lap, and the man and woman hold each other's arms and take it in turns to lean backwards, until a swinging or seesaw-like rhythm is achieved. This position restricts thrusting, so is good for when the man is tired, and also for allowing both the man and woman to have an equal role in lovemaking.

striking

The woman sits astride the man, and as they make love, he strikes her chest. Suggesting that the couple hit each other may seem odd to a modern audience. In the Kama Sutra, intercourse is likened to a quarrel "on account of the contrarieties of love and its tendency to dispute." Here the striking is almost a formalized kind of role-playing, where each partner strikes the other as if in anger, increasing the blows until orgasm.

Four different types of striking are described: striking with the back of the hand; striking with fingers contracted; striking with the fist; and striking with the palm of the hand. Different sounds should be made by the recipient of the blows, such as cooing or hissing, and they should then strike back in return. Even Vatsayana was scornful of the fashion for using implements to abuse each other, calling this "painful, barbarous and base, and quite unworthy of imitation." Striking was considered another form of "external enjoyment" to be used in the throes of passion, according to the strength and the proclivities of the parties involved. Obviously, this should not be undertaken without the informed consent of one's partner.

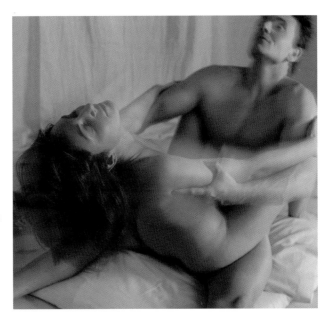

yab-yum

Yab-yum is the quintessential form of sexual union in Tantric lovemaking. It translates as "mother and father union", aligning all the energy centres (chakras) within the body, allowing kundalini energy to rise and a more spiritual level to be reached. The woman should sit on her partner's lap, facing him. Her legs should be wrapped around his waist and arms wrapped around each other. The idea is that the couple stay still and visualize, in the mind's eye, the energy rising from the root chakra to the crown, despite the temptation, of course, to move and thrust.

ABOVE | The swing can be fun once you get into the rhythm.

BELOW LEFT | Striking should be a passionate, rather than a painful, experience.

BELOW CENTRE | Yab-yum is one of the most loving poses allowing maximum contact.

BELOW | The temptation to be active can be strong.

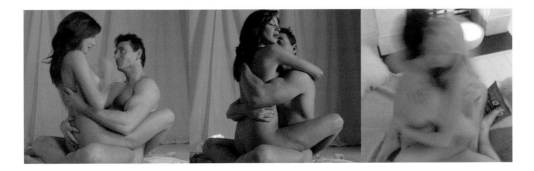

standing and rear tantra

STANDING POSITIONS were considered by Brahmins like Vatsayana to be a high form of congress, and they are depicted in numerous works of art. Rear entry postions were also enjoyed, taking their inspiration from the animal kingdom.

BELOW LEFT | The tripod – this is a position that could be done anywhere, but try next to the bed the first time, in case you lose your balance.

BELOW RIGHT | The ass – if the woman is not flexible enough to reach the floor, she could rest her hands on a chair.

please her yoni

It is the man's duty to please his partner and here are some suggested techniques.

manthana – churning
Grind your penis in circles once inside her, avoiding thrusting.

piditaka – pressing
Press your penis hard towards her womb and hold before withdrawing and repeating.

varahaghata – the boar's blow
Provide continuous pressure on one side of her vagina during penetration.

vrishaghata – the bull's blow
Thrust wildly in every direction while you penetrate her.

chatakavilasa – sparrow sport
Quiver your penis while it is inside her.

suspended

This posture requires quite a bit of strength from the man. He begins by standing with his back to a wall, but not leaning against it. The woman sits in his cradled arms with her thighs gripping his waist, feet flat against the wall and arms wrapped around his neck. As they make love she pushes back and forth against the wall.

the tripod

This requires a good sense of balance. He holds one of her knees firmly in his hand and stands, without support. As they make love she can caress and explore his body with her hands.

the dog

This is similar to the doggy position, in which the woman goes on all fours and the man enters her

from behind. In Tantra, however, the woman should turn her head and gaze into her partner's eyes as they make love.

the ass

The woman stands with her legs slightly apart and bends forward, gripping her thighs with her hands, or with hands on the floor. The man then enters her from behind. Height differences can be combated by the width that she spreads her legs. For shorter men, she should spread her legs wider.

the stride

This is another one for the more adventurous and agile couple. The woman stands on her palms and feet so her body forms a triangle. From behind he lifts one of her feet to his shoulder, driving his lingham into her yoni with vigorous strokes.

the elephant

This is similar to spoons, in which the woman lies on her side facing away from the man. She offers her buttocks to him and he penetrates from behind, using his hands to gently caress the other parts of her body.

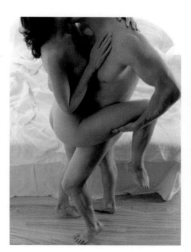

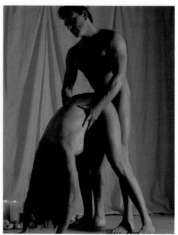

oral tantra

KNOWN AS "MOUTH CONGRESS" in the Kama Sutra, oral sex was considered a base activity practised by wanton women and eunuchs. These days it is a healthy part of most loving relationships, although some lovers are not sure how to go about it.

fellatio

There are different techniques described by Vatsayana for performing fellatio on a man. You don't have to put the whole thing in your mouth – the head is the most sensitive part.

nimitta – touching

Holding his penis with one hand, the woman shapes her mouth into an "O" and places it on the tip of her partner's penis. She moves her head in tiny circles, maintaining a light touch.

parshvatoddashta – biting to the sides

Holding the head of the penis in her hand, the woman clamps her lips lightly above the shaft, first on one side and then the other, being careful to keep her teeth hidden so as not to cause any pain.

antaha-samdansha – the inner pincers

The woman takes the whole of the head of the penis into her mouth. She then presses the shaft firmly between her lips and holds it for a few seconds before pulling away.

parimrshtaka – striking at the tip

The woman begins by flicking her tongue all over his penis, using a hard pointed tongue. Then she concentrates on the sensitive tip of the glans, striking it continually to evoke a heightened sexual sensation.

sangara – swallowed whole

This is done when the man is close to orgasm. The woman takes the whole of the penis into her mouth and sucks, working her tongue and lips until the man comes.

cunnilingus

Oral sex performed on a woman doesn't get much of a write-up in the ancient texts – it was considered just another form of kissing.

jihva-bhramanaka – the circling tongue

The man uses his nose to spread the woman's vaginal lips and then gently probes her yoni with his tongue. Then, with his nose, lips and chin, he moves in gentle circles all around her vaginal area.

chushita – sucked

The man fastens his lips to the woman's vaginal lips and nibbles at her before sucking on her clitoris. He uses varying degrees of pressure as he sucks on her clitoris until he finds one that she is comfortable with and, more importantly, one that gives her pleasure.

uchchushita – sucked up

The man cups and lifts his partner's buttocks, and uses his tongue to gently massage her navel, working down to her genitals. Once between her legs he should use his tongue to gently lap up her love juices.

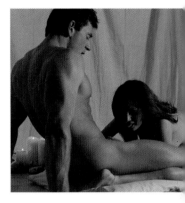

ABOVE | Striking at the tip – you don't have to put the whole penis in your mouth. The head is the most sensitive part, so concentrate here.

BELOW | Sucked up – hopefully, the tantalizing sensations will be almost unbearable by the time he reaches his destination.

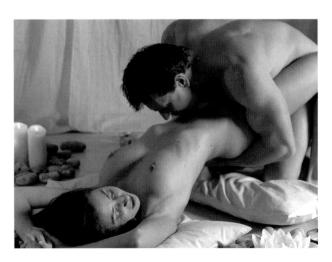

suppressing orgasm

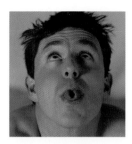

ABOVE | Controlling your breathing may help you orgasm without ejaculation.

RIGHT | Suppressing your orgasms may enable you to find an ecstatic plateau.

BELOW | Saluting one another acknowledges the other's body as the bridge to the spiritual world.

ACHIEVING ORGASM is often seen as the *sine qua non* of modern sex. Without that emphasis, lovemaking can become more relaxed and less goal-orientated. So sex without orgasm can be an activity in itself. Each partner tries not to reach orgasm for as long as possible.

The Tantric skill of maithuna is a technique for controlling response, designed to help intensify orgasm and also to help men to delay their orgasm to keep in harmony with their partner's sexual tempo. The technique is designed to help the flow of sexual energy and to ensure men feel energized after sex as opposed to exhausted.

● When you feel like you are about to come, breathe deeply. Many people hold their breath, as if forcing the orgasm to come out. By keeping the breathing regular the orgasm will become more intense as you flow with and not against it.

● Keep the tip of your tongue on the roof of your mouth or roll it into a "straw" to breathe through. This can help to circulate the energy and help men to withhold their orgasm.

● When you begin to orgasm, imagine the energy is flowing away from your genitals and up your spine. Do not contort yourself to try and help this physically. This is purely a visualization to

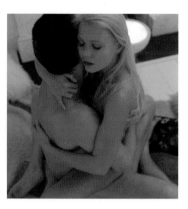

prolong orgasm. The more control a man has over his own sexual responses, the more he will be able to offer his partner.

saluting one another

At the culmination of your time together, you should sit before each other and salute each other, saying words such as,"You are a god/goddess." This acknowledges the other's body and gives praise for awakening each other's senses, and thanks for helping each other in the unity of spiritual Tantric lovemaking.

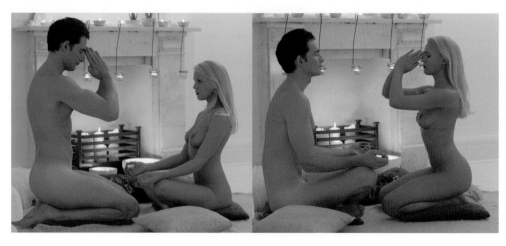

sex without orgasm

This last Tantric ritual can be practised regularly in your relationship and can keep you intimately connected, even when you do not have the time or will for a full lovemaking session. For instance, when you awake in the morning and you must soon go separate ways, you can lie together for 5 to 15 minutes just holding each other in this intimate conjugal embrace.

All mystical sex practices have upheld the importance of containing ejaculation and orgasm during lovemaking. The concept of non-orgasm while making love is considerably different from most edicts of modern sexology with their emphasis on achieving great orgasms. In fact, orgasm is usually seen as the ultimate goal of sex. This can make the man afraid of ejaculating prematurely before his partner has reached her climax, and leave the woman concerned about not having an orgasm before the lovemaking session is over. Some women fake orgasms in order to protect their lover's ego.

The pressure in modern sexual relationships is for bigger, better orgasms, simultaneous orgasms,

and even multiple orgasms. There is no doubt that an orgasmic capacity enormously increases the pleasure and satisfaction of lovemaking. Yet the whole physical and psychological pressure on achieving orgasm can rob sexual intercourse of its natural spontaneity, its deep sensuality and tenderness, and the exploration of its intrinsic spiritual dimension.

When orgasm becomes the main goal of sex it is almost impossible to remain with the pure sensual feeling of the present moment. Orgasm-orientated sex has a finite purpose and is in danger of becoming a performance-related programme aimed mostly at achieving a satisfactory conclusion.

The essence of meditation in sex is when two people pour body, heart and soul into that which is actually happening spontaneously and intuitively between them, without purpose or goal. When this happens, all the bodily senses become heightened and movement, breath and mutual interaction start to flow effortlessly, without interference from thoughts, fantasies and pre-conceived expectations.

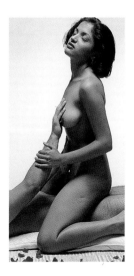

ABOVE | Slowing the pace
The woman-on-top position helps the man slow his pace of lovemaking. In this position, he is also more able to touch, and remain sensitive to, her whole body.

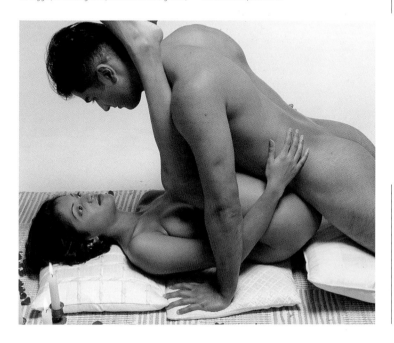

LEFT | Achieving true harmony
Tantric lovemaking does not preclude any sexual position or behaviour but it does add a more intuitive and spontaneous quality of effortless movement because the lovers are in harmony with each other's bodily responses.

tantric energy orgasms

THE TANTRIC IDEA OF CONTAINING ORGASM during sex applies to both men and women as it is seen as a way to prolong lovemaking and to create a force of transforming energy within the body, without dissipating it through ejaculation and climax.

The following are some of the benefits:

● A couple can make love for as long as they want as they do not become exhausted by effort or orgasm.

● Lovemaking becomes a continuous, unbroken theme to the relationship, so that the couple can interrupt sex when necessary and begin again when convenient, without feeling frustrated, because they remain deeply sexually connected.

● Mental thoughts, judgements, goals and expectations which interfere with the intimacy of sexual bonding can be dropped so that the truly natural and spontaneous body and feeling responses take over.

● The uncomfortable sense of using each other's bodies for sexual gratification disappears. Mutual honour and deep respect develops for the body and its inherent sexuality as they are both perceived as divine sources of transformation.

When practising Tantric lovemaking, the following suggestions are important to remember:

● Ensure that this sexual exploration is a mutual decision, otherwise it may become a subtle means of controlling one another. If you or your partner want passionate sex and orgasm then go ahead and enjoy yourselves. Respect each other's needs, as this is just as important as any ideal.

● Do not turn the containment of orgasm into another mental programme of sexual achievement. Remember, that "being together" rather than "doing together" is what it is all about.

● Tantric sex means making love meditatively. It is "cool" sex rather than "hot" sex. You should slow down long before you reach the orgasmic point of no return. Stop moving, if necessary, or change positions if you are getting too excited. Lie

together in a still embrace, breathe together, or look into each other's eyes.

Energy orgasms cleanse the body of repression, emotional pain and sexual blocks and barricades. It is a Tantric masturbation technique that requires deep concentration, visualization and lots of practice. Energy orgasms can vary in strength – extra time put into building energy generally leads to a more powerful orgasm. It is for men and women, and is said to be very different from an ordinary orgasm and may or may not feel sexual.

move like a butterfly

Begin by lying on a flat hard surface and bend your knees up. Start to take a few deeper breaths, empty your mind and release the tension in your mind and body. As you inhale, arch your lower

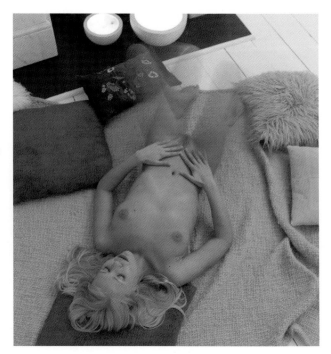

BELOW | It may be helpful to do some further research on the chakras so that you will know what you are trying to visualize. Each chakra is distinguished by a colour and a frequency of vibration which will become familiar to you as you practise.

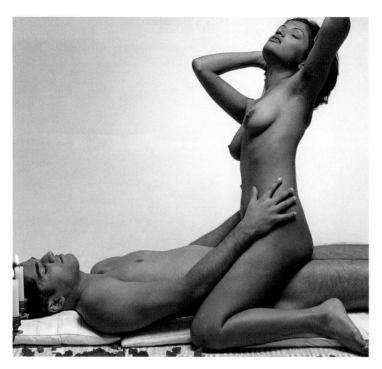

LEFT | The orgasmic energy which arises during Tantric lovemaking continues to pulsate throughout your body for as long as you want. You may feel that your individual egos are disappearing and that you and your lover are merging into one being.

BELOW | The sense of closeness during the union of lovemaking can continue as you rest peacefully together.

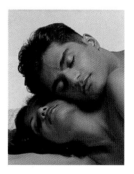

back to rock your pelvis, and as you exhale, squeeze your PC (pelvic floor) muscle. By squeezing these muscles you are stimulating the G spot and clitoris or penis and testicles, and at the same time you are helping to pump energy throughout your body. Let your breathing and contractions be erotic and as you repeat the circular breathing technique, fan your legs open as you inhale and close as you exhale, like butterfly wings, to help to keep the energy flowing and maintain your rhythm.

Your energy will follow your thought processes, so visualize drawing energy in from the atmosphere and into the perineum area, between your genitals and anus. Build strong fires of energy in the sex centres of the first and second chakras and circulate this energy back and forth. Once the energy feels powerful and strong, move it up and continue circulating it from the genital area to the belly area, the first and second chakras. Again, once you feel that the energy is strong, let it flow from the belly to the heart, the fourth chakra, via

the solar plexus, the third. Then move the circulating energy on from the heart to the fifth, throat, chakra. You may find it helpful to consciously make sounds, opening the throat and allowing energy to then circulate upwards from the throat to the third eye, circulating between the fifth and sixth chakras.

Finally, visualize the energy flowing between the third eye and the top of the head, the seventh, crown, chakra. Now you should start to feel the energy shoot from the top of your head and a full body orgasm will hopefully begin stirring. Follow the flow of the orgasm. Your breathing patterns may change and with practice you will learn to ride the waves of your orgasm and allow them to keep it going for longer and longer periods of time.

Don't worry if you don't reach orgasm first time round. This is a technique that requires a lot of practice. The breathing exercises alone will reap their own benefits by cleansing your mind of mental blocks and hurtful memories, clearing the path for more positive orgasmic experiences.

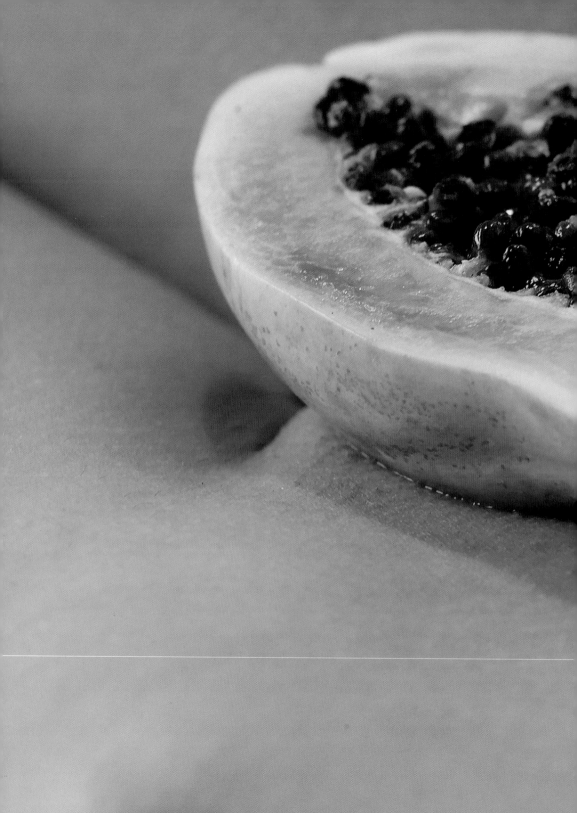

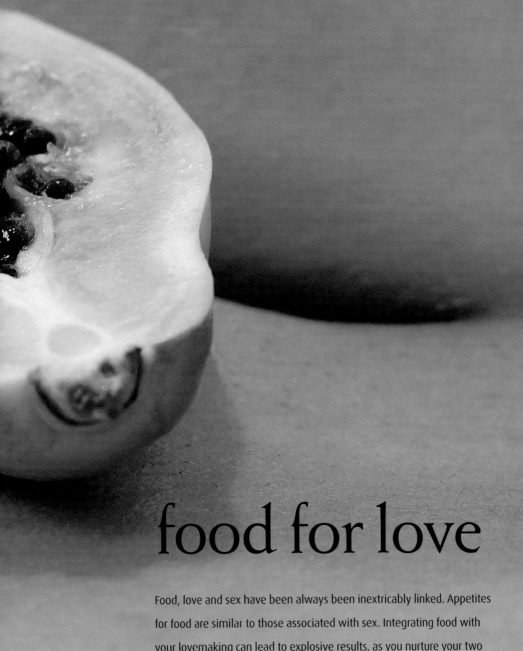

food for love

Food, love and sex have been always been inextricably linked. Appetites for food are similar to those associated with sex. Integrating food with your lovemaking can lead to explosive results, as you nurture your two most basic needs simultaneously.

food and sex

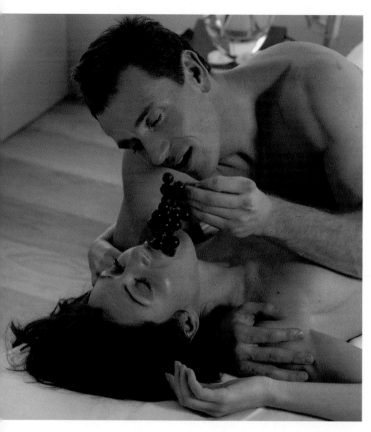

Part of the excitement of courtship is finding out about each other. You can tell so much about the person you are with from the food they buy, the method in which they cook and present it, what they choose from the menu in a restaurant and how they eat it. People with hearty appetites who really enjoy their food often have a healthy appetite for sex as well.

We use our mouths for many different things – talking, kissing, sucking, smiling, laughing, as well as eating – so watching your partner slide the flesh of an oyster into their mouth and imagining the salty, silken texture slipping down their throat can be very arousing. Eating draws attention to the mouth. The tongue, the lips and genitals all have the same neural receptors, called Kraus's end bulbs, which make them supersensitive to stimulation. This is why kissing is such an important part of the prelude to lovemaking.

a lovers' menu

Of course, we eat with our eyes as well as our mouths. The shape of certain foods can be very erotic and can conjure up all manner of suggestive images; a downy peach looks like a voluptuous bottom, oysters and figs are reminiscent of a woman's vulva, and bananas, celery and asparagus are phallic. Some foods just look irresistible – think of sashimi or chocolate cake.

In fact all the senses come into play. The pervasive aroma of truffles is astonishingly sensuous, while the sweet scent of strawberries or mangoes makes the mouth water. Texture is as important as flavour and intrinsically sexy foods include: caviar that just bursts on the tongue; anything that you eat with your fingers from a chicken drumstick to edamame (soya beans); most shellfish from scallops to crayfish, although not anything you have to remove with a pin. The sound of food sizzling stirs the appetites. There is something strangely erotic about the crunch when your lover bites into an apple.

ABOVE | Food and sex are inextricably linked and sharing food with your partner is one of the most intimate things you can do.

WHERE WOULD ROMANCE BE without the element of food? We even use foodie words to describe people we are attracted to: she's a peach, or he's really tasty, scrumptious or delicious. Honey, sugar and my sweet are terms of endearment. The reason that food has always played a part in the rituals of courtship is that both eating and sex are two of our strongest instincts and a combination of both can prove irresistible. Food, like sex, is another way of stimulating the senses. The flavour and taste, the texture and touch, the visual appearance, the aromas and even sound of food cooking, all play a part in its sensual appeal.

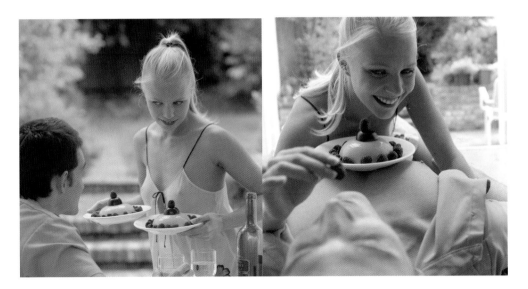

Don't forget that what you drink matters, too. Champagne is a turn-on for most people, cocktails are glamorous and even a mug of creamy hot chocolate after a brisk walk on a windy day can stir the senses. The light sparkling on beautiful crystal glasses adds to the sensuous pleasure of good wine, while many men find the sight of their partners drinking "designer" beer straight from the bottle very arousing. Drinking tequila the traditional way is sexy and fun: place a little salt on the back of your hand between your index finger and thumb and hold a wedge of lime in the same hand, then lick the salt, down a shot of tequila in one and then suck the lime.

saucy snacks

Sex shops sell a range of naughty nibbles, including chocolate body paint and penis-, bottom- and breast-shaped chocolates, combining everybody's favourite aphrodisiac with an element of fun. You can even buy edible underwear.

With a little imagination, you can create your own suggestive dishes. How about setting pink blancmange in shallow, 15cm/6in dishes and, when they're turned out, topping with them with glacé (candied) cherry nipples? Then just try serving them without a sly smile.

sexy cocktails

Why not dress up for cocktail hour? One of you can be the bartender, and the other the Hollywood starlet. Each of these recipes will make one cocktail.

- **slippery nipple** – Stir 1 measure Bailey's Irish Cream with ice. Strain into a cocktail glass and float 1 tsp Sambuca on top.
- **sex on the beach** – Pour 2 measures vodka, 1 measure peach brandy, 2 measures cranberry juice and 1 measure mixed orange and pineapple juice into a cocktail shaker over ice. Shake vigorously, then strain into a tall glass and decorate with a slice of orange.
- **slow comfortable screw up against the wall** – Fill a highball glass with ice cubes, then pour in 2 measures sloe gin and top up with fresh orange juice. Float 1 tsp Galliano on top.
- **bosom caresser** – Dash a little Cointreau over ice in a jug, pour in 1 measure brandy and 1 measure Madeira. Stir and strain into a glass.

ABOVE | Provocative, if not subtle: create your own range of suggestive snacks and find imaginative ways of serving and eating them.

BELOW | Why not try a slow comfortable screw up against the wall – then you'll really need a drink.

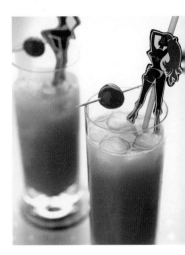

aphrodisiacs

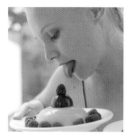

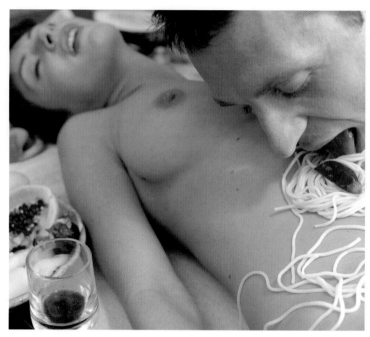

ABOVE | Food can be about more than nutrition.

RIGHT | Any Italian will tell you that spaghetti is one of the sexiest foods around, even if one of the messiest.

SINCE TIME IMMEMORIAL, men and women have been obsessive in their search for the ultimate aphrodisiac to help flagging libidos, improve their sexual performance and generally enhance the act of lovemaking.

Ayurvedic medicine, which originated in ancient India, so valued the importance of sex that a whole branch of medicine was dedicated to it called "Vajikarana", and there is a wide spectrum of preparations in use around the world that use animals and insects to enhance sexual performance. The Romans ate the penises, wombs and testes of animals such as monkeys, pigs, cockerels and goats, and lizards used to be pulverized and the powder taken with sweet white wine by the Arabs and southern Europeans. The Chinese today often use the genitals of animals and insects to increase the strength of reproductive organs, believing that ingesting substances with sexual properties will impart those properties to the person consuming them. Snake blood is still consumed in east Asian countries and the gallstones of animals are used in Asian countries alongside ginseng and royal jelly.

chocoholic

Of course, it's debatable whether any aphrodisiacs actually work – there's certainly very little scientific evidence – but most people would draw the line at powdered reptiles and foul-tasting herbs. Fortunately, there is an extensive range of far more palatable options.

On the Richter scale of aphrodisiacs, chocolate is up there among the top three, alongside champagne and oysters. People are passionate about it. The Aztecs brewed cocoa like coffee, and Aztec leader Montezuma is alleged to have drunk up to 50 cups a day so that he could keep going with his harem of 600 women. It may have gained its reputation because the Aztecs believed the cacao pod was a symbol of the human heart. The notorious Marquis de Sade is said to have demanded chocolate cake while imprisoned. Chocolate lovers will gladly eat it before, during and after sex and some even choose it instead of sex. But what is it about chocolate that is so special? It's questionable that it can really affect sexual performance, but it does possess certain stimulating properties. As you swallow it, a chemical called phenylethylamine and the feel-good neurotransmitter serotonin are released in your brain, spreading a feeling of tranquillity. Then, the theobromine in chocolate kicks in to create the high feeling that you have when you are in love. Chocolate also contains other stimulants, such as caffeine, which excite the central nervous system, but all these properties exist in such tiny amounts that you would have to consume vast quantities for it to have any real sexual effect. What is certain is that chocolate contains sugar, which provides energy, and that, combined with its pleasurable texture and flavour, may explain why so many people find it so addictive. For many women, the fact that it is a "forbidden food" is also exciting.

foods for sex

Champagne, of course, like any alcoholic drink, reduces inhibitions, but too much will cause a downturn in your sex life. Oysters, on the other hand, have a long-standing reputation for stimulating the libido. This is undoubtedly much to do with their appearance and texture, but, interestingly, they are extremely rich in zinc, "the sex mineral" essential for the production of healthy sperm and fertility. Scallops also contain high levels of zinc and have a reputation for increasing the sex drive in women. In fact, aphrodisiac qualities have been ascribed to seafood of various sorts, including lobsters and caviar, while Chinese medicine recommends mussels and shrimps for increasing the libido.

Many foods, such as asparagus, morel mushrooms, figs and avocados, have been thought to possess such properties simply as a result of their appearance. Others, such as salmon and pigeon, seem to have been designated as aphrodisiacs because of the living creature's courtship rituals. The reasons for the reputation of still further foods are even more mysterious. The Romans swore by bread, which may have been because eating a lot of it tends to make you want to lie down. However, eating a lot of it also promotes flatulence, which is distinctly unsexy. When tomatoes were first imported into Europe, the French called them love apples for their heart-like shape. Nevertheless, tomatoes are high in lycopene, which is essential for prostate health. The Chinese recommend ginger and this too has a grain of validity in that it promotes healthy circulation, especially to the genitals.

So do aphrodisiacs really work? It seems unlikely, but their placebo effect can work wonders and, as we all know, the most powerful aphrodisiac that exists is the imagination.

BELOW | In different cultures and throughout history, a range of foods have been thought to raise the libido. Certainly some foods have an erotic sensuousness and sharing them with your lover can be very arousing.

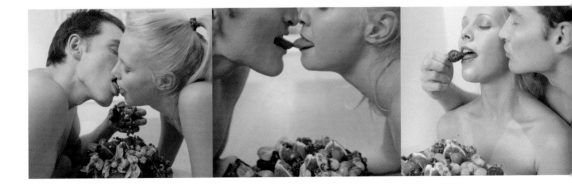

foodplay

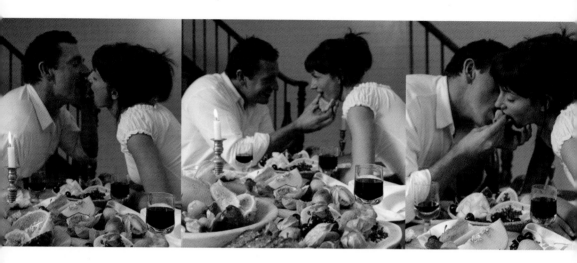

WHEN PLANNING A PASSIONATE evening with your partner, think of your meal as part of the foreplay to your lovemaking. Never underestimate the importance of food and wine in the enjoyment of a romantic evening. Teasing each other across a candlelit table can be so tantalizing. The cardinal rules for eating before sex are never to eat too much and never to select food that is too heavy. No one wants to make love on a full stomach – their own or someone else's.

Sharing your food and feeding each other is a potent form of foreplay. Having a romantic meal in the privacy of your own home is a wonderful opportunity for you to be outrageous flirts and to act out your seductive desires. You both know what's coming, but so much of the enjoyment is in the getting there.

Set the scene beforehand. Make the table look enticing with a lovely cloth, some flowers and candles, but don't use your best china as it may get swept to the floor in the heat of the moment.

Because no one else is there, you can act out your romantic fantasies and pull out all the seductive stops. Remember all those scenes in movies which you have always wanted to try out?

Well, now here's your chance. Think Jennifer Beals in *Flashdance* or Mickey Rourke and Kim Basinger in *9½ Weeks*, rather than Meg Ryan in *When Harry Met Sally*. It's also a perfect opportunity to tell each other things that you don't necessarily say over the breakfast cereal. In this romantic setting you remind one another just how much you still desire each other. Don't forget the music. It should be romantic, sexy and not too loud, something that is meaningful to both of you.

gourmet sex

The whole process of eating can be incorporated into the art of seduction. Start your sensuous feast with pre-dinner drinks and little canapés as light as butterfly kisses. Next, the appetizer should be a tantalizing treat, promising much more and seducing you with its textures and flavours. The main course is the climax of the meal, satisfying but not satiating your appetite, while dessert is a pause for refreshment.

Playing with the stem of your glass, running your fingertips around the rim and stroking the stem has its own connotations. Locking eyes with your lover over your glass of wine, caressing his or her hand across the table, making soft moans and sighs of pleasure as you enjoy an asparagus tip dripping with butter, even the way you butter your roll, can all create a tremendous sexual tension between the two of you. As the meal progresses and the wine diminishes, you can become bolder, eating off each other's plates or kissing the traces of food from each other's lips. End this wonderful meal by feeding each other delicious morsels of fresh fruit, passing them from mouth to mouth and allowing the juices to flow. Lots of action can take place under the table as well as on top. Kick off your shoes and caress each other's feet and legs.

finger foods

There is always something especially sexy about eating with your fingers, perhaps because we were always told not to do it when we were children. The only places where it is acceptable are fast food outlets, which must be among the least seductive locations on the planet.

If you're not in the mood for a three-course meal, then prepare a mini-banquet of succulent snacks that you can eat with your fingers – or better still, feed each other with your fingers. In fact, why not keep a ready supply of enticing nibbles in the refrigerator for just such occasions?

Include your partner's favourite rude food as well as your own. For the purposes of erotic eating, you can interpret the words "finger food" very loosely. Fruit is a perfect choice. Try wedges of watermelon or slices of mango and then lick the juices that have run over your partner's hands or chin. Bite into a strawberry or lychee and then offer your mouth to your partner.

weekend break

At the other end of the day, treating yourselves to a leisurely breakfast in bed at the weekend is a deliciously indulgent experience. It needs a little advanced planning, otherwise by the time it is ready, the mood will have been lost. The night before, prepare a tray with cups, saucers and plates, knives, spoons, marmalade or jam and, perhaps, a single flower in a small vase. Set the coffee maker ready to switch on and make sure that you have some croissants or rolls to pop into the oven in the morning. Avoid bowls of cereal, both messy and unromantic, and toast, which produces uncomfortable crumbs.

Don't take the newspapers back to bed with you and forget morning television, although some quiet background music could be atmospheric. That way, when you have finished eating, you'll have to think of something else to do.

fruity

Of all the food groups, it is fruit that is most closely associated with sensual pleasure. Grapes, the fleshy fruit, are associated with the ancient gods Dionysus, Priapus and Bacchus, the true connoisseurs of sex and pleasure. Across North Africa and the Middle East, dates are believed to increase erotic potency in men and desire in women. Coconuts are believed in India to increase the quality and quantity of semen. Strawberries and raspberries invite you to feed your lover, piece by piece. But it is fleshy fruits such as papaya, mango, peaches and apricots which spill over into true, and outrageously sticky, sensuality.

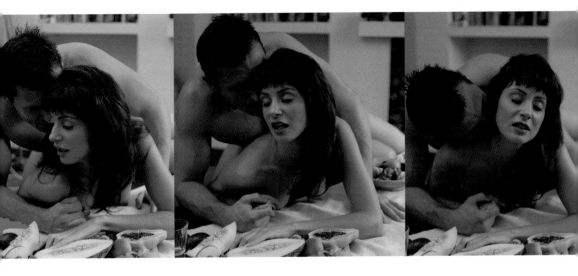

cooking with your lover

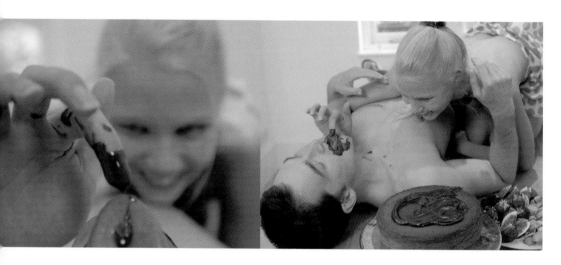

ABOVE | Nothing quite comes close to the taste and texture of molten chocolate.

ABOVE RIGHT | Making a cake to share with your partner can be just as much fun as eating it afterwards.

BELOW | Once the main course is cooking in the oven and the dessert is prepared, it's time to turn up the heat.

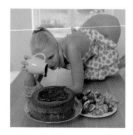

COOKING TOGETHER can bring an extra romantic dimension and sense of intimacy to the whole process of eating. Lots of people don't really enjoy the nitty gritty of food preparation, but when it's done together, you can make it much more fun. Put on some music, open a bottle of wine and get your ingredients together.

Choosing the ingredients that suit your mood at the time adds to the joy of sharing the cooking experience. It's fun to shop together, especially at an outdoor market, where you can handle the produce and ponder over which particular item you think is best. You can linger over plump, bright red tomatoes and let yourselves be seduced by the smell of ripe cantaloupe melons or fresh juicy mangoes.

If you are adventurous, it's a great turn-on to try to cook something totally different. Leave plenty of time for the preparation and have an adventure in the kitchen while you are chopping, slicing and stirring.

This is a wonderful opportunity for some serious love play as well, as you add a pinch of seduction to the list of ingredients. While the chocolate cake is rising in the oven you could be stripping down to your sexy underwear or negligee. For the truly adventurous, why not strip off totally and cook wearing nothing more than an apron? Take Isabel Allende's advice in her book *Aphrodite*: "Everything cooked for a lover is sensual, but it is even more so if both take part in the preparation and seize the opportunity to naughtily shed a garment or two as the onions are peeled or leaves stripped from the artichokes."

man about the house

Recent research has revealed that women are turned on by men who cook and you have only to think of the devoted female following of the many male celebrity chefs on television to see a clear manifestation of this. Women undoubtedly have a more emotional attitude towards food than men, so when a man is wielding a whisk or chopping a chilli, he is not just entering traditional female physical territory, but also her psychological home ground, which can be very alluring.

Another study by the Smell and Taste Treatment and Research Center in Chicago may provide an additional incentive to any men reluctant to enter the kitchen until the meal is on the table. The aroma of different foods as they cook has, apparently, a profound effect on the libido and, in particular, the smell of meat cooking significantly increases the flow of blood to the penis. This fact could make basting the Sunday roast a whole lot more fun.

feasting the senses

Cooking shouldn't be a chore, but it can often seem to be, particularly when it's a routine responsibility. Cooking with your partner can change this, especially if you tackle the task with a new attitude, actively relishing the textures, colours, smells and flavours of your ingredients. Preparing food can be as sensuous as eating it, especially when you are sharing the experience. Try out some new recipes, adding your own special touches, inhaling the aromas and tasting as you go. Does the chocolate mousse need more

orange juice? Dip in your finger and hold it out for your partner to decide. By the time they've finished licking it clean, they will probably have forgotten the question. Waft a spoonful of your newly created sauce beneath their nose, but tantalizingly deny them a taste until they have guessed at least three of the spices that flavour it.

Enjoy sharing the sensations of cooking and encourage each other to be daring in the kitchen. If you've never attempted to toss a pancake, try it and see who can catch it. Ice a cake together – literally, if you like, squeezing your partner's hands and the icing bag at the same time. Messy, but fun. Get out the food colouring and see who can create the most outrageous masterpiece with the mashed potatoes. Food is one of our most basic needs, and we all know how important it is to have a balanced diet, but you can still have a lot of fun together while you are preparing it.

BELOW | Experimenting together and tasting the fruits of each other's labours makes cooking together fun.

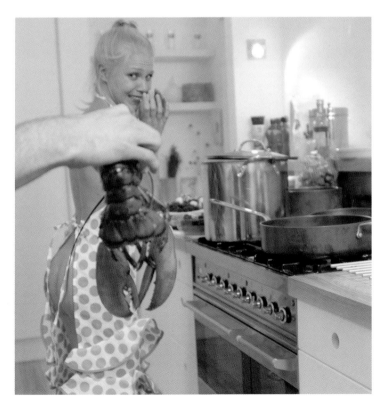

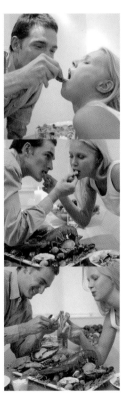

food without plates

THE MOST EROTIC WAY to share food with a lover is when you are both totally naked, so that you can eat from each other's bodies. It's a mutual experience. Where one enjoys the sensation of having food eaten from their body, the other enjoys the application and the subsequent pleasure of eating off their lover's body without using their hands.

What food you use is a question of personal taste. Many people enjoy the cool, silky sensation of cream or yogurt being drizzled over their body before being slowly licked off. Honey is another favourite, especially when massaged into the breasts before being nuzzled off. Smooth peanut butter can be warmed and smoothed over the penis (avoiding the urethral opening). Take your time slowly to suck it and lick it off. If you have a sweet tooth, you may prefer to use vanilla ice cream or strawberry jam. (These might prompt a much more dramatic response, as neurological research has shown that the smells of these two substances increase penile blood flow by anything up to 40 per cent.) Be creative when laying the food across the skin. Use a mixture of flavours, textures, aromas, tastes and temperatures. Cover your lover's naked body with slices of your favourite fruit or vegetables or make patterns with melted chocolate and eat them off.

If you really want to go for it and have a full body banquet, one of you can be the main course and the other the dessert. Don't eat very much the day before, make sure you have everything within easy reach and leave yourselves plenty of time. In between courses, you can have a long leisurely bath together, to be relaxed and receptive for the next course. Be especially mindful when you come to the more sensitive, delicate regions of the body such as the eyes, the vagina and the penis. Avoid any acidic, astringent irritants, such as vinegar, pickles or lemon juice, and particularly never use any form of chilli where it may sting.

BELOW | Asparagus is an age-old sexual remedy for men and there is nutritional evidence that it can assist in regulating hormonal balance. Mushrooms are a good source of the vitamin B complex, while truffles smell fantastic.

BELOW RIGHT AND OPPOSITE | Turn your partner into a banqueting table and feast off their bare body before offering your own for dessert.

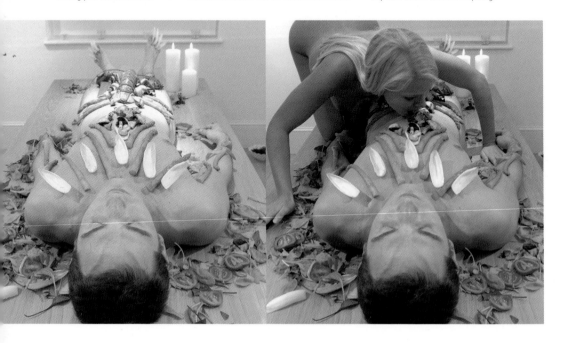

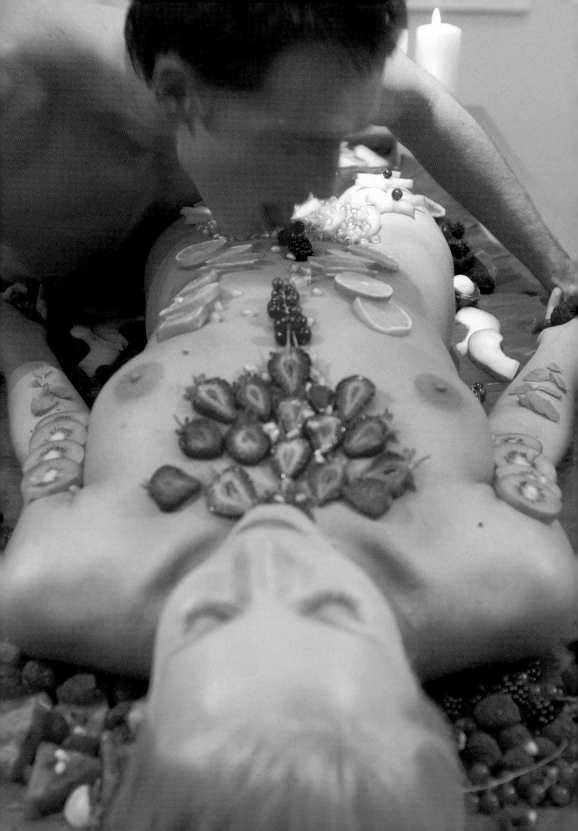

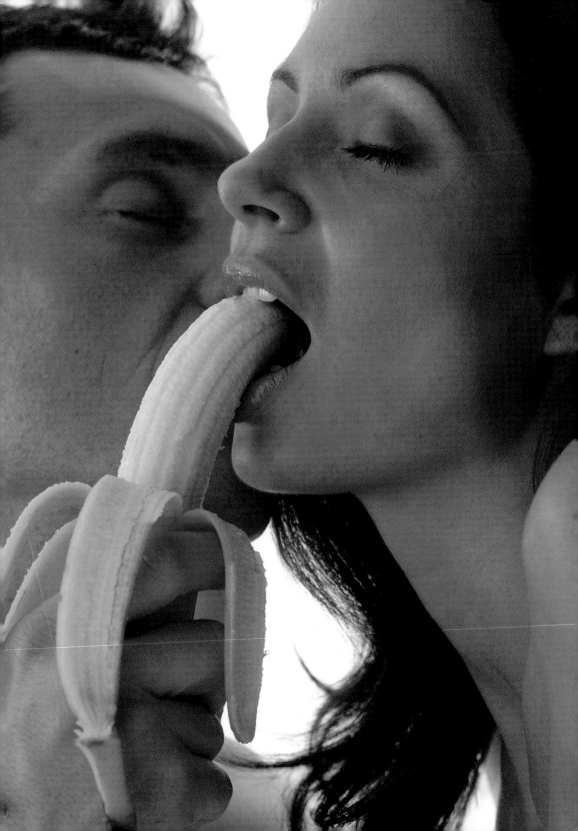

good food, good sex

FOOD ISN'T JUST FOR FUN AND SEX – it helps your body to stay on top of things. Eating well is essential to good sexual health and function. There are many, many reasons for loss of libido and impaired sexual function, but often one of the primary reasons is the balance of our sex hormones. However, this balance is also linked to our metabolic hormones, and these rely on a constant supply of certain nutrients that we provide through our diet.

minerals

Important dietary minerals include iron, zinc, magnesium, calcium, iodine, selenium, chromium, arginine, co-enzyme Q10 and essential fatty acids (EFAs). There are many food sources that are rich in these minerals. For example, chicken and red meat are rich in iron, which is needed for haemoglobin production in blood, essential for arousal, erection and lubrication. Nuts, brown rice, eggs and cheese all contain zinc, from which the sperm's tail is formed, so helping with fertility and sexual performance. Shellfish, dried fruit and dairy produce all contain calcium, crucial for bone growth and cardiovascular health and an essential ingredient for arousal, as it plays a part in sending messages to the nerves, enabling the sensation of touch. It is also needed for the contractions of muscle during male and female orgasm.

vitamins

In helping to maintain physical and sexual health, vitamins such as vitamin A, vitamin B complex (including B_1, B_2, B_3, B_5, B_6, B_{12} and choline), vitamin C and vitamin E all have their own roles.

Spinach, watercress, dairy produce and oily fish all contain vitamin A, which is vital for healthy eyes and strong bones and teeth. It is also an antioxidant required for cardiovascular health. Pulses, nuts, avocados and meat contain vitamin B complex such as B_3, which helps the circulation, allowing more blood to specific areas, such as the penis during erection; B_6, which plays an important role in regulating sex hormone function such as testosterone in men; and choline, which helps with transmission of nerve impulses necessary for boosting libido and energy during sex. Vitamin C helps to boost sex drive and strengthen male and female sex organs and can be found in food such as potatoes, ginger, beetroot (beet), citrus fruit and sprouted beans. Vitamin E is essential for healthy skin and its protective nature makes it vital for sexual health and vitality. It can be found in avocados, spinach, wheatgerm and all leafy green vegetables.

A good basic principle is to always have a balanced diet and to eat small portions regularly. Sex on a very full stomach is never a good idea.

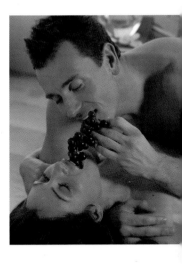

ABOVE AND OPPOSITE | it's the way that you eat it that counts.

BELOW | There are certain elements which are crucial to keep body and soul together, and without which a healthy sex life would be impossible. Nutritionally speaking, fruit and seafood are some of the richest foods.

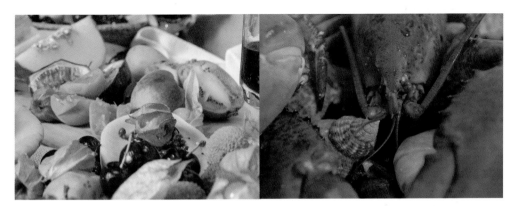

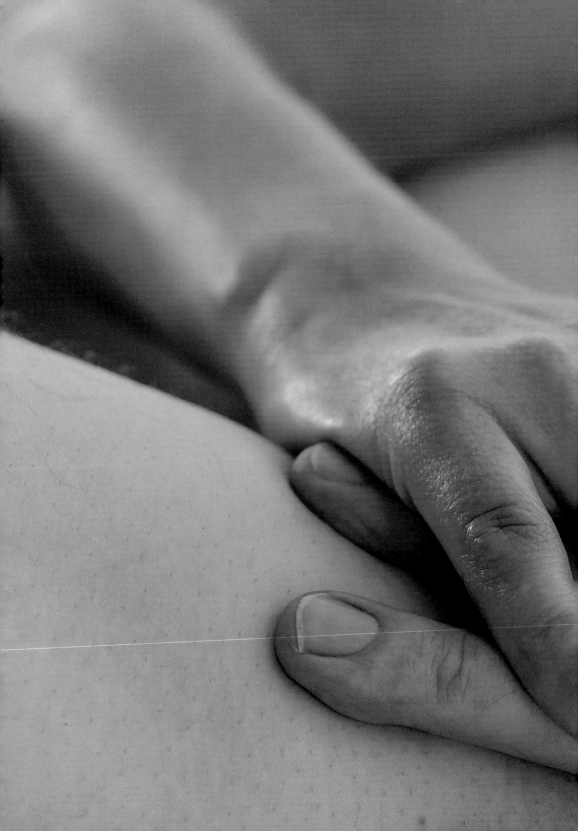

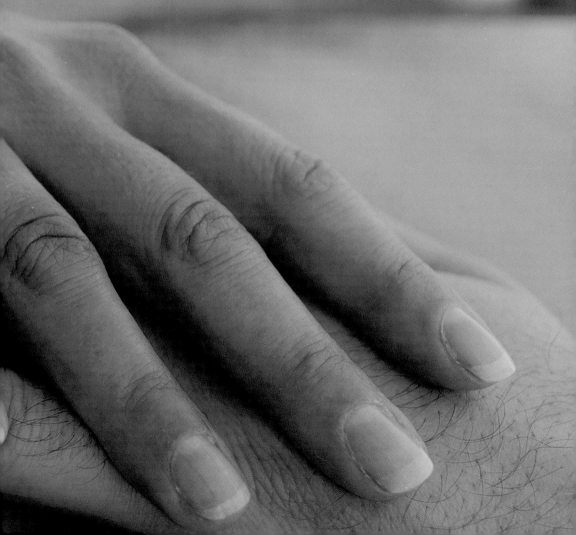

seasons

A long-term relationship is constantly subject to change, with ebbs and flows, ups and downs. As you journey through your lives together your relationship changes and matures, as do the seasons of the year, from the exciting, carefree years of early spring to the more laid-back and contented golden winter years. Your sexual needs and desires follow these ebbs and flows, but are the essence of what keeps your relationship youthful and timeless.

long-term lovers

A RELATIONSHIP CAN BE LIKENED TO THE SEASONS of the year, with spring, summer, autumn and winter each bringing with them their own qualities and climatic changes. Even the strongest relationships tend to be cyclical, with ups and downs, good times and bad. This is worth remembering as you go through your journey together, so that when there are stormy bad times you can weather them by looking forward to better, sunnier times to come.

spring

The season of spring is the beginning of your relationship with your partner, the first few years when you meet, fall in love, before you decide whether to marry or cohabit. This is often the most carefree time, in which you spend a lot of time getting to know one another and allowing your roots to entwine, building the foundations on which you will grow as a team. With little to tie you, this is often a romantic season in which you feel truly secure in the knowledge that you will cope with anything life throws at you, because you have each other.

Springtime sex lives are exciting and adventurous. You can rarely take your hands off one another and use every spare moment together in making love and being romantic. If things become tougher in the future, it will be this era that you will refer back to. You will be able to

RIGHT AND BELOW |
In the springtime of your relationship, you are endlessly fascinated with your lover and want to be with them all the time.

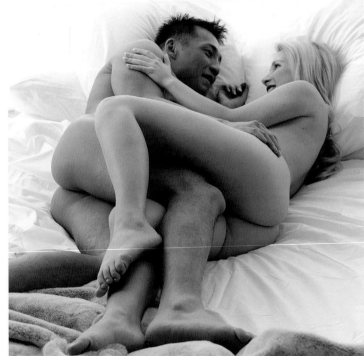

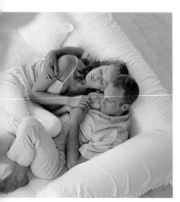

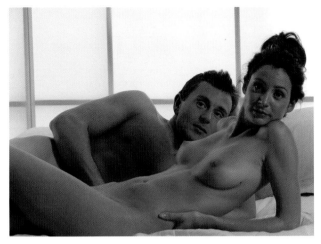
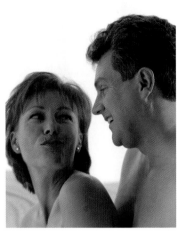

remind each other of how much love you have shared – you are building a scrapbook of memories that you can call on in the future.

summer

The summer of a relationship signifies a settling down period in which you begin to build a nest, find a home together, plan your futures and realize your dreams. Deciding on children will cause you both to re-evaluate your priorities over careers, social lives and sex lives. Sex changes during this season, as the emphasis is upon making love and creating another human being together, rather than having sex just for fun. Having a baby together is one of the most powerful and bonding things any two people can do. With a bit of time both of you will adjust to the changes and enjoy your new roles as mum and dad, providing you don't ignore the fact that you are also still lovers with sexual needs and desires.

autumn

Autumn is represented as the time when the kids fly the nest and lovers return to being just two again. This can be a difficult time for parents who have devoted the last couple of decades to their children. It is difficult to remember what life was like before the children came on the scene, and so it is important that a couple discuss the issues well

in advance. This is a time to plan your future together once again, to start talking about retirement and to make plans to finally fulfil your long-term dreams. Sexually this is a time of rediscovery, confirming each other's sexuality and using the stability and confidence in yourself and each other that you have built over the years to create better sex.

winter

The onset of winter signifies the beginning of another distinct, golden season as you share your retirement and, for many, grandchildren. You can enjoy each other's company with all the stresses and strains of work and dependent children finally put behind you. Most people do not associate senior citizens with sexuality, but in many cases this is an important and precious aspect of a long-standing relationship. You may no longer be swinging from the chandeliers but sex and touch are still important. Although there may be more health challenges to face as you age and libidos may not be what they once were, romance and seduction never age. By continuing to regard each other and your relationship as challenging and fun, you can maintain excitement and indulge each other with the frivolity that the freedom of old age can bring, working together to make your relationship both timeless and ageless.

ABOVE | In the summer and autumn of your relationship you can face anything if you keep communicating.

changing sexual needs

YOUR SEXUAL RELATIONSHIP may improve with time as you and your partner become increasingly compatible on an emotional and physical level. As intimacy grows between you, and the relationship becomes stable, you may be better able to relax together in every way. In these circumstances, your sexual relationship can mature with age like a vintage wine.

Many women are only able to open up sexually once they feel emotionally secure, finally reaching their true orgasmic potential when they trust that they are truly loved. For some men, the early stages of a relationship can be fraught with tension, particularly the pressure to perform well in bed. They may be so nervous and excited in the early stages of a relationship that they engage in intercourse with undue haste and ejaculate prematurely. Only when they have relaxed into a sexual relationship can they allow the more sensual side of their nature to shine through in their lovemaking.

Time and familiarity will allow you and your partner to know each other's arousal responses, to tune in to your mutual sexual needs, and to feel increasingly comfortable with your own and each other's bodies. As sex is an expression of caring as well as desire, your lasting and loving relationship can, by its very nature, enrich your sexual exchange.

Knowing and trusting each other well gives you the opportunity to explore new avenues within your sexual preferences. The safety of the relationship may allow you to reveal and act out you sexual fantasies and this can add an extra erotic input into your conjugal activities. This is also a good way to pep up your sex life when things have become dull and routine.

changing patterns

If you are in a long-term relationship, your sexuality may pass through a variety of phases, and it would be highly unusual if it never changed in content or style from your early days of romance.

For the reasons mentioned above, it can steadily improve, and it may enhance in quality if not in quantity. However, there may come a time when the frequency of your sexual activity declines after you have lived together for more than a few years.

Seeing each other every day, and concerning yourselves with the other important demands in your lives, you may no longer have the time, energy, wish or need to make love with the same intensity as when you first met. Quite naturally, like any two people who begin to build a home together, juggle finances and improve on their

BELOW | Intimacy, deepening companionship, and knowledge of each other's bodies and physical responses can enhance your sex life in a long-term relationship. As both of you relax deeply into your sexuality, it can become more expansive, creative and loving.

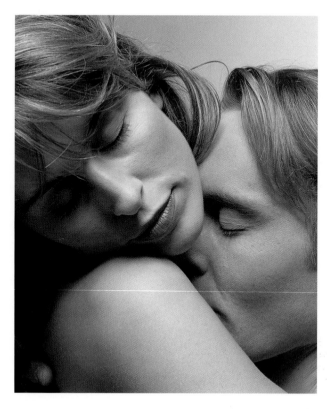

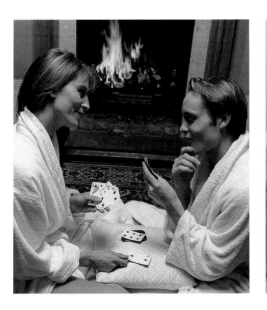

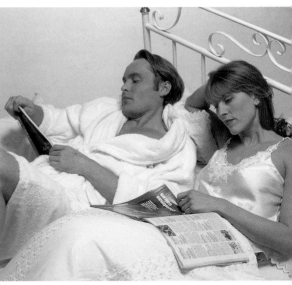

careers, or decide to start a family, you may focus your attention on other matters of mutual and personal concern.

The passion which drew you together and ignited the flame of your love is unlikely to sustain itself with the same degree of desire throughout the duration of your long-term relationship. The familiarity which makes your partnership so comfortable and supportive can be the very thing which erases the excitement of the earlier days, when just the sight of each other would be sufficient to arouse you. Seeing your lover every day, and sharing the hard times as well as the good, may create a supportive and nurturing relationship, but does not necessarily arouse the libido to the same extent as before.

Often, these changing patterns of sexual behaviour will settle into an easy and compatible rhythm which happily satisfies you both. There will be times when your sexual interest rises, and periods when it subsides, and this will largely be affected by outside pressures, such as stress, the needs of your children, the demands of your work and career, moving home or changing jobs and the general accord between you both in other areas of your lives.

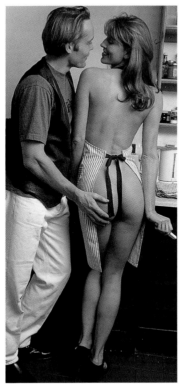

ABOVE | It is perfectly normal for the frequency of sexual activity to subside after some years in an established relationship as passion gives way to closeness and intimacy of a different nature. This can be a mutually satisfying situation if there is no great disparity in your sexual needs. Just being together, relaxed and aware of each other, while quietly involved in your own activities, can be a very nourishing experience in itself.

LEFT | Confidence in the relationship, and trust with each other, may inspire you to reveal and experiment with some of your more playful sexual fantasies. A little kitchen erotica may convince him that there is more on the menu than just supper!

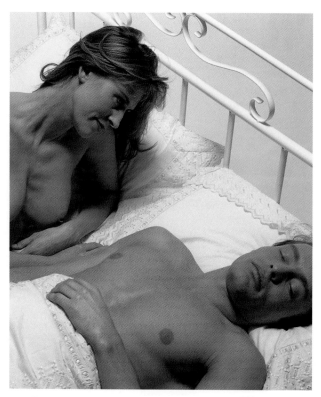

together for a number of years, or following illness, child-birth, the loss of a parent, or promotion to a more stressful job. The emerging differences in sexual needs can create a severe problem if you do not look at the issues, adapt to the changes, and reach a mutually satisfying arrangement that suits your varying levels of libido.

The one who is more deprived can feel aggrieved, and personally rejected. If you are in this position, you may begin to put pressure on your partner, berating the person you love, and you may feel demeaned by your unsatisfied sexual needs.

If you are the one who has lost interest in sex, you may resent your partner's desires, and even begin to feel that he or she is making unreasonable demands on your time and intimacy. A situation like this, if it is allowed to develop unchecked, can eventually become a vicious circle. One of you will become increasingly obsessed with the need for sex, while the other may withdraw and become even less romantically inclined.

A couple may allow a long period of time to pass before realizing the extent of the problem or feeling sufficiently resolved to face up to its issues. This dilemma may be compounded by the difficulty of talking about sexual matters – a subject in which egos can so easily be bruised. Tact, diplomacy and negotiation, however, are needed to approach and address the subject. If you are facing this situation, you will need to develop your communication skills so that you can explore and discuss your varying sexual needs and feelings. You may then discover the root cause of your differences and find new ways to resolve the imbalance.

To rekindle the flames of passion, you could start off by experimenting with making love in parts of the house other than the bedroom so that the change of setting inspires new and delightful ways of lovemaking. If you have one, light the fire in your living-room hearth and abandon yourselves before its flames. By breaking old patterns of sexual behaviour, you can keep your relationship very much alive.

ABOVE | At various times, and for different reasons, a low libido can affect either one of you. If this affects the happiness of your relationship, you will need to find some way to improve the situation.

OPPOSITE | After a time, you may seek to change the quality of your lovemaking into something that is more sensual and spiritually and emotionally uplifting. If you are able to make love in a more meditative way, your intimacy and bonding will continue to flower.

differing sexual needs

Problems may occur in an established partnership, however, if you and your mate develop very different patterns of sexual need. One of you may lose interest in sex altogether, or be content with occasional sexual episodes. What one of you might regard as a normal or adequate level of lovemaking might be vastly different from the other's expectations.

There is no rule that dictates how often a couple should make love. You may feel deprived if you are not having sex every day, whereas your partner may think that three times a week is a normal and happy routine. The disparity could be even greater, with one of you believing that once a week is sufficient for your needs while the other is rarely interested in making love more than once a month. One of you might even lose interest in sex altogether, especially when you have been

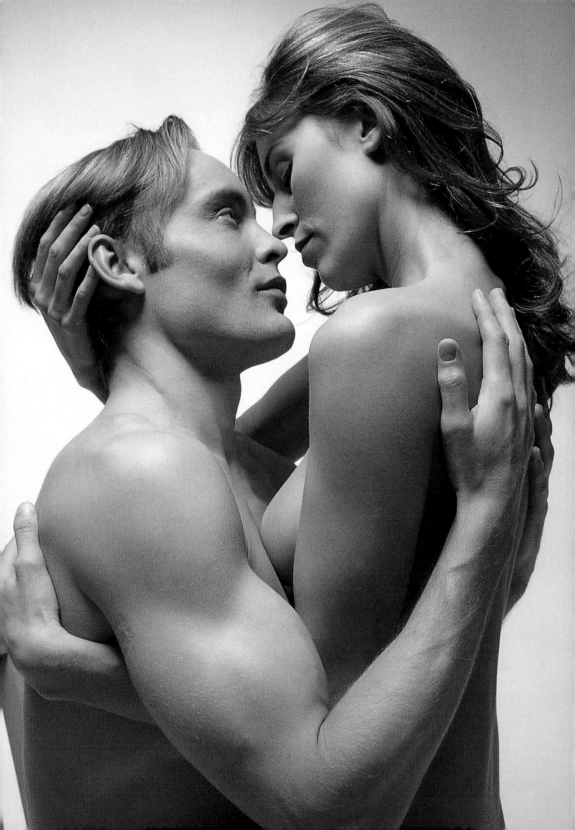

starting a family

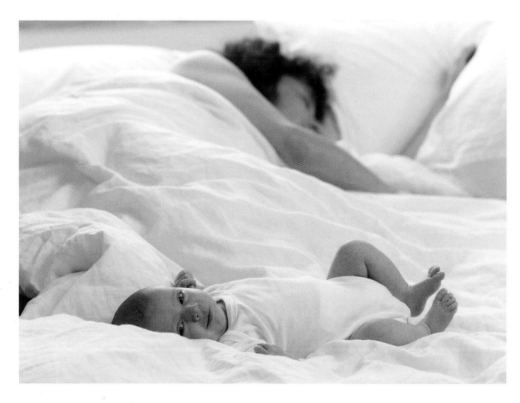

ABOVE | For many couples a long-term relationship is a welcome reprieve from the singles circuit. However, once you decide to start a family, your bed will never be your own again.

FOR MOST COUPLES, the first few years of marriage or cohabitation are an exciting time. You have finally escaped the dating scene and are confident and content that you have discovered the person who makes you happy. This can be a unique time for many relationships where you can concentrate on each other's sexual needs without any other forms of distraction, such as children or responsibility for elderly parents. The next stage for many couples is starting a family. This said, the introduction of a third set of feet in your home brings with it a total rearrangement of your priorities, your social life and, yes, your sex life.

Sex is often the last thing on the minds of new parents until their baby settles into a routine of sleeping through the night. There are numerous emotional problems that are common to almost every couple during this time. New mothers can become both physically and emotionally exhausted. Many feel their role as a sexual woman has been totally replaced by that of a child-bearer who is constantly cleaning, feeding, bathing and nurturing her new baby, with no time for nurturing herself. Men may feel neglected or even left out of this new regime. These are all very common issues that new parents face as their lives go through one of the biggest transitions. It's important to remember that these changes are occurring to you as a couple and not as individuals and you need to talk about it together.

During your child's early years he or she will require a lot of your time and attention and it is all

sex during pregnancy and after the birth

With a normal, healthy pregnancy, there is absolutely no reason why you should not continue to have a normal, healthy sex life, unless advised otherwise by your doctor. You cannot hurt the baby, who is comfortably cushioned in the amniotic fluid. As the pregnancy progresses, man-on-top positions are likely to become uncomfortable, even impossible. Experiment with positions that suit the two of you. "Spoons" is often a favourite and some women favour rear entry positions. It is a myth that lovemaking will bring on a premature labour, although there is some evidence that substances present in semen may encourage labour at full-term.

For reasons of health, women are usually advised not to have penetrative sex for six weeks after giving birth. If an episiotomy scar hurts or the birth itself was very painful, a woman may be afraid that lovemaking will also hurt.

Gentleness and patience will probably overcome this. If the woman is breastfeeding, sore or cracked nipples may mean this is definitely not an erogenous zone. This is a difficult time for men as well, who may be tired after waking with the baby in the night if you are taking turns in getting out of bed. This is a major life adjustment for both of you – sharing the burden will unite you.

too easy to put your sex life to one side, or neglect the need for time out to be a couple. Try to set aside some time once a week to make a date with each other. Get a babysitter or ask grandparents to take the kids once a week. Use this time to get out of the house and spend some romantic time together discussing issues that have been on your mind, but try to avoid constantly discussing your children. This is a perfect opportunity to talk freely about sex and how you can both work to improve things. If the kids can stay away overnight from time to time it's even better, as you can enjoy each other in a more uninhibited manner.

families today

There are many different relationships and family structures nowadays that work equally as well as the stereotypical married couple. Many couples prefer to remain unmarried, even though they have a family together, and some couples even choose to live apart as they can be a happier unit when they are together by keeping their own space. More same-sex couples are setting up home together and choosing to adopt children or find surrogate mothers or fathers or sperm donors, to help them have their own.

Relationships can be complicated whichever sexual path you follow. Not all couples who get together stay together for the rest of their lives. Often people separate or divorce and begin life

with a new person. Starting again with someone new, when either you or your partner already have kids from a past relationship, can be tricky as you have to integrate yourself or your partner into a ready-made family. Children are understandably fiercely loyal to both their parents and often a new partner on the scene can cause problems.

Children of blended families (couples who both have children) and stepchildren will invariably need plenty of reassurance and understanding when a new relationship begins. Any stresses and strains in a relationship will affect its sex life. Ultimately, given time, much joy and happiness can be found in these kinds of relationships.

One of the most important roles of a parent is to make sure that your children become confident and unafraid of sex and their developing sexuality. This can be harder than it seems and much of their attitude towards it will stem from how you react to their questions.

It is very common for children to walk in while you are making love, and you need to prepare for it before it happens or else you may react in a way that you will regret.Try just covering up slowly, without making it appear like you were doing something that you shouldn't. Often children think that sex looks like "daddy was hurting mummy" and so it is important to emphasize that what you were doing was positive, and something that two people do when they love each other.

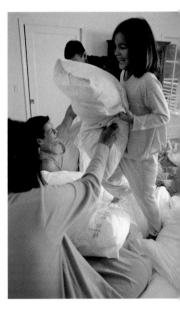

ABOVE | Family life can often be a battle – but making time for a healthy sex life will help maintain the balance in the equation.

pregnancy and your sex life

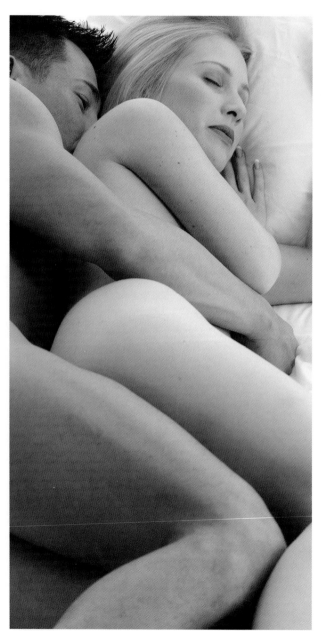

THE MOST COMMONLY ASKED QUESTION about making love in pregnancy is whether or not it is safe. Experts say that it is – and there is no evidence to suggest that it might not be. A pregnancy is actually much more robust than some of us believe. Some consultants even say that it is safe to go riding – something that women are usually advised to avoid. They maintain that if the pregnancy were to be lost in this way then it was going to be lost in any case; in other words, that the pregnancy was frail. So, you need not fear causing miscarriage through the act of lovemaking.

The next big question is whether or not both you and your partner feel like making love. Some women go off sex during their pregnancy while others enjoy sex more than ever before. Similarly, some men find that their partner seems even more attractive when she is pregnant. Others are nervous of making love once their partner is visibly pregnant and prefer to wait until after the baby has arrived. However, for many couples the frequency of lovemaking does not change substantially whether or not the woman is pregnant.

If you lost interest in sex early on in your pregnancy, as many women who suffer with morning sickness do, your sex drive will probably return later on. Some women find arousal easier and orgasm more intense during pregnancy. It may be that the pregnancy hormones are responsible for this, but general feelings of well-being and happiness may also be a factor.

LEFT | Pregnancy can often have an impact on your sex life, but it is not necessarily a negative one. This is the time to experiment with different positions to find the most comfortable. The spoons position is a good option.

good positions in pregnancy

Now that you are getting larger, you will probably need to experiment with different positions in which to make love. Lying on your back will probably not feel comfortable. Experiment with different positions until you find some that work well for you and your partner.

One good position to try is the spoons position, in which both partners lie on their sides. You lie with your back to your partner, who lies curled around you and facing your back. He can then enter you from behind without putting any pressure on your abdomen. You may also find it easier to use the doggy position, with you on your hands and knees and your partner behind you. Another good position in pregnancy is with the woman on top, when again there is no pressure on her abdomen.

if you go off sex

If your sex drive has diminished, try to show your partner love and affection in other ways. Of course, your partner will respect your wishes but he may feel rejected or alienated all the same. Showing that you love him is all the more important at this time. Reassure him of your feelings in thoughtful ways. Give him a glorious pampering massage, cook deliciously for him, send him a card, e-mail him during the day if he is at work.

if he goes off sex

Lovemaking necessarily involves respecting one another's wishes. You may naturally find it disturbing if your partner rejects you sexually while you are pregnant, particularly if your sex life was very active beforehand. Try talking to him when he is neither tired nor busy and explain how you feel. Ask him to talk about he feels, too.

Show your partner that you cherish him in ways that are unrelated to sex. For a start, make sure that you are paying him as much attention as you are paying your pregnancy and your unborn baby. It may be that your partner has started to feel a little left out while you are, inevitably, receiving a lot of attention.

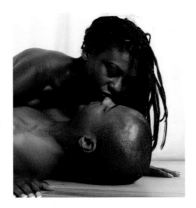

LEFT | The woman-on-top position is popular during pregnancy.

BELOW | Massage can be a wonderful way of achieving physical closeness, and relaxing together.

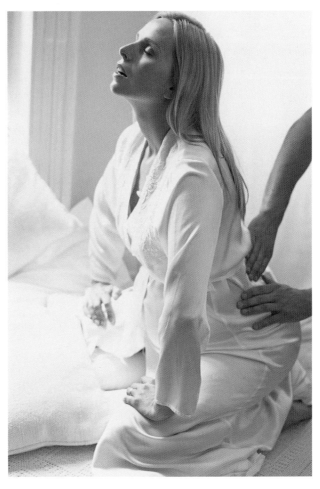

middle years

IF YOU HAVE CHILDREN, then sometime you will experience the "Empty Nest Syndrome". One or all of your babies will have flown away – to university, jobs or into marriage – and you are left alone in your house with your partner. This period in your life often creeps up on you and you don't realize the impact until it happens. What was a longed-for dream of more time together may turn out to be a period of incredible emotional emptiness until you get used to the absence of the children and to spending so much time together.

Once you get used to the idea, it can be a very exciting time. If your sex life has been on the back burner for some years, now is the time to get to know each other again and become sexually reacquainted. You have more time and tend to be more relaxed and positive about having sex.

Another aspect of having more leisure time is that there will be more time to exercise. Whilst physically you will be slowing down, this is a great opportunity to take control and become fitter – start going to those yoga classes! This is crucial because as we age, we need to remain active, not only for our health but also for a good sex life.

time of life

It is the period when women may be going through the menopause, the end of their reproductive life. This causes emotional and physical challenges, so talk to your partner about how it makes you feel so he understands the process. Many women find that taking HRT (hormone replacement therapy) can help them through this period of change – lessening the hot

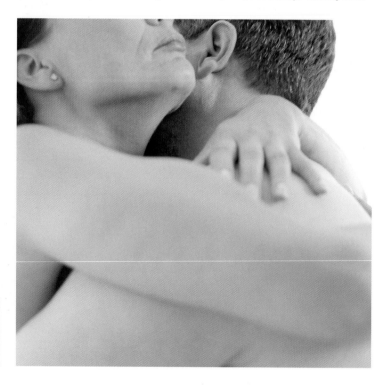

RIGHT AND OPPOSITE | Once the children have flown the nest, you will have more time to spend alone with each other.

flushes, mood swings and forgetfulness. Sexual desire or libido varies greatly in every woman whether pre- or post-menopausal. Hormone levels determine sex drive and diminished hormone levels undoubtedly interfere with sexual desire. Although oestrogen plays a part, the hormone that has been shown to be most closely associated with sex drive is testosterone. The ovary, although capable of producing oestrogen after a "natural" menopause, may continue to produce significant amounts of testosterone for several years. This is the reason why many women maintain a good sex drive for a considerable length of time. These testosterone levels provide additional benefits to the naturally menopausal woman. Tissues of the body are able to convert some of this circulating testosterone to oestrogen.

When women undergo a hysterectomy where the ovaries are also removed, this benefit may be lost. Some women even find that their sexual desire increases after menopause (if their ovaries are left) as they are free from pain and excessive bleeding.

mid-life crisis

Men also may well be experiencing a slow-down in their sexual response time, taking longer to become aroused as they approach middle age. In fact, both men and women may need more stimulation to become aroused and to orgasm. But, since you will hopefully be able to spend more time together, take advantage of this. Talk to each other about what pleases you. If you have difficulty communicating, or are not able to take that step forward together, then you may well need to speak to a therapist.

It is at this stage that men may have a "mid-life crisis". This can manifest itself in seeking reinforcement in a younger girlfriend or a new motorbike when he normally drives a family car. This is just a glance back at his youth and women often have similar feelings. Patience is required during this time, on the part of both of you. It can be frightening to let go of the younger part of you that you are accustomed to – however, you are exchanging it for the confidence and experience that can only come with age.

looking lively

It is important for both men and women to make an effort to look attractive for their partner and for their own self-respect. Perhaps you can get into the routine of spending an hour or so having a long bath and pampering yourself. Invest in some glamorous nightwear that makes you feel sensuous. Give yourselves the time to feel sexy as adults and not just parents or workers.

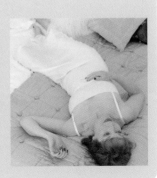

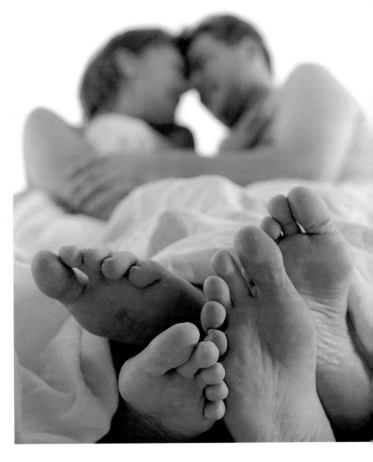

golden years

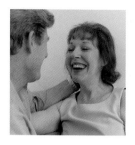

IT IS A MYTH THAT YOU STOP HAVING SEX when you are in your "golden years". Just because you are older, it does not mean that you don't need the same physical and emotional intimacy that you demanded when you were young. Intimacy is an important part of your life at any age.

An active sex life will keep you mentally fit and healthy, and having a good companion whom you can share your life with is said to be the key to living longer. The emphasis on the necessity of regular exercise promoted over the last couple of decades means that older people will be fitter

than ever. Having a positive attitude is crucial for a good sex life. Your body may be ageing, but for many your desires certainly aren't. If the man is experiencing problems having erections on a long-term basis, you can ask your doctor for their advice. Older men may need more stimulation in order to achieve erection – a little manual assistance is sometimes necessary. In these cases oral sex and mutual masturbation can be an enjoyable path to explore together. The time that you make love can be an important factor in later years as well. It is frequently recommended that

ABOVE | Companionship has many mutual benefits.

RIGHT AND BELOW | Taking up a hobby such as dancing or learning a musical instrument with your partner can be one way to rekindle romance.

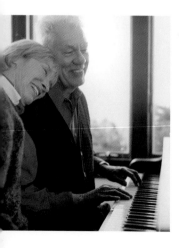

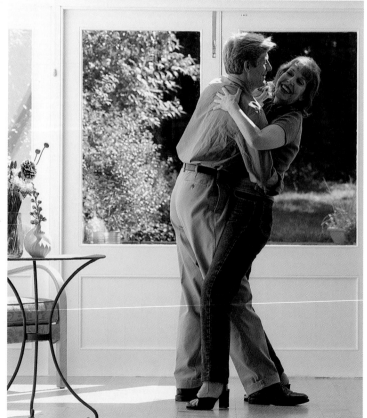

older adults should try making love in the morning, as older men are more likely to have a firm erection in the morning after a good night's sleep. There are also unexpected advantages for men as you get older; you can delay ejaculation for longer, and your partner will love you for this.

freedom years

By their golden years, women have finished with the menopause and can experience a new sense of sexual liberation. There are some physiological changes of course such as vaginal lubrication, which instead of taking only 15 to 30 seconds when younger can now take up to five minutes. There are plenty of lubricants, and even hormonal treatments that can help. Women who continue to have sex after the menopause finishes will remain fitter and their vaginas will remain more elastic than those women who do not.

A woman's sex drive over the age of 65 is more stable than a man's. In fact a woman reaches her peak in her late twenties or thirties and remains on that plateau until her sixties. A woman of 80 has the same physical potential for orgasm as a woman of 20.

Even if sexual desire has abated, intimacy is still an important part of any loving relationship, regardless of age. Touching and cuddling up together and learning how to massage each other can be extremely sensual. Setting aside time to visit galleries together or to go for long walks – perhaps joining a dance class – can give you that extra contact outside the home that you need. To stay young you have to feel young, regardless of what your body is doing. Being active together, and remaining tactile with each other, will help to keep your relationship as fresh and exciting as in the early days when you had only just met each other.

going it alone

As women tend to live longer than men, the major problem is often having a partner to share their sexuality with. Many older people have to come to terms with the loss of their loved one and one of the important issues is how you deal with the loss of intimacy and sex that was part of a

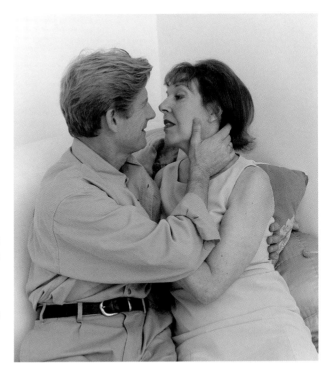

loving relationship. Sexual desire and drive do not die with your partner. Masturbation can be especially helpful in these circumstances and will help you to keep your sexual identity and sexuality alive.

You are never too old to fall in love, and on a happier note, many older people can find new love and companionship in their golden years. This can bring comfort to them, their new partners and their extended families alike.

Society's image of "old people" is that they are too sagging, wrinkly and unattractive to even think about having a sex life. It is up to all of us to resist subscribing to that kind of ageism, not just mature people themselves, but also younger generations. As the baby-boomer generation comes of age, attitudes will surely have to change – there are going to be a lot of healthy pensioners out there.

We owe it to our children and those who come after us to claim our sexuality in old age. If we don't do it, how will they?

sex in maturity

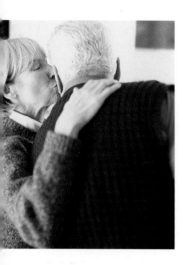

ABOVE | The twilight years of a relationship may allow a couple to discover a new level of intimacy.

SEXUALITY IS NOT SOLELY THE PREROGATIVE of the young and there is no reason why people in their more mature years should not continue to enjoy a happy and rewarding sex life. Indeed, there are aspects of aging that may actually enhance a sexual relationship, and research shows that even very elderly people can retain a healthy libido. While certain changes do occur in the sexual responses and reproductive organs of men and women as they grow older, if people can accept and adapt to them both physically and psychologically, then age itself does not preclude the capacity to be sexually fulfilled.

If a woman is past the menopause and no longer concerned about issues of pregnancy or contraception, she may feel more free to enjoy sex. Studies show that many women actually become more orgasmic in the later years of their lives, compared to when they were younger. However, as a man gets older he will often need more time and extra stimulation before he is able to get an erection.

If his partner is able to respond positively to this natural process of change, she may enjoy taking a more active and creative role than ever before in initiating the love play between them.

As people age, particularly if couples have been in a relationship for many years, their sexuality often becomes less focused on the act of penetration alone and more open to other forms of sensual and tactile contact, such as hugging, kissing and loving caresses.

Even if a couple no longer desire penetrative intercourse, or if it is no longer possible because of impotence or other health reasons, they can still continue to pleasure each other with alternative forms of erotic love, such as oral sex, sensual massage and masturbation.

In ways such as these, the physical intimacy between partners can actually develop as they grow older together and embrace a whole new sensuality that may have been missing in their earlier days.

overcoming taboos

One of the main problems facing the older generation is society's attitude towards sex and aging. It is as if sex is seen as the domain of the young and beautiful alone, and that there is something indecent or embarrassing in acknowledging that older people may also have sexual needs.

Many older people feel embarrassed about revealing their sexual needs, finding it easier to repress them, and resign themselves to the commonly held opinion that at their age they should be "beyond it". Unfortunately, this view may prevent a mature couple seeking the specialist help they may need to resolve their physical and psychological sexual concerns. Even in long-term relationships, partners may give up all forms of physical intimacy because they feel unable to surmount these problems.

Many members of the older generation may believe that certain practices, such as oral sex and masturbation, are harmful, disgusting or even perverted. It is unlikely that, at this point in their lives, their views are going to change. However, oral sex is an excellent addition to a couple's love life, when sexual functioning is otherwise impaired by the aging process or arousal responses have begun to slow down. An older man may find that he is more easily aroused and can maintain his erection better if his partner is willing to perform fellatio on him or to apply manual stimulation, strokes and caresses to his penis and testicles.

In a woman's case, after the menopause, her vagina may undergo various physical changes, losing much of its lubrication and elasticity. This can cause her discomfort in penetrative intercourse and reduce her enjoyment of sex. These changes are not related to her libido, which can still function healthily, and aging should not affect the responsiveness of her clitoris, which is her most erotically sensitive organ. Cunnilingus is an excellent option in lovemaking, and one way that her partner can continue to give her sexual satisfaction.

changing sexual health

Health issues are the most significant factor in causing diminished sexual response as we grow older. It is natural for some people, as they age, to become less interested in sex. However, a sudden loss of libido, in men or women, could be due to illness or other physiological factors, and this should always be checked out with a doctor. Certain medications can inhibit sexual response, as can medical conditions such as diabetes, cardio-vascular diseases and prostate disorders. Some women experience a loss of sexual feeling after the menopause, but this is by no means inevitable, and many women actually feel more sexual at this time than they did before.

However, there are natural changes in sexual response and functioning which occur as part of the aging process. In themselves these do not necessarily prevent men or women from continuing to enjoy a happy sex life, especially if they are able to adapt to these changes and have an understanding partner who is also willing to explore new ways of enhancing the sexual relationship.

A man's reproductive capacity can remain throughout his life, although a decline in testosterone levels in later years may decrease his sperm production. However, as some famous men, such as Clint Eastwood or Anthony Quinn, have demonstrated in recent years, age is no bar to becoming a father. As he gets older, a man may find that he is slower to become aroused, and that his erection is less firm. He may take longer to ejaculate when making love, and may ejaculate with less frequency than when he was younger. Also, the refractory, or recovery, phase between each ejaculation will increase, and it may take several hours or even days before he can be aroused again.

There may also be psychological reasons for a man's changing sexual responses as he gets older. Many men equate their sense of virility and potency with their earning capacity and careers. When a man retires from work, he may feel that he is no longer useful and this can adversely affect his sexual performance. It is important for a man

to maintain and develop absorbing or worthwhile interests, and take up pursuits which will help him re-establish his self-esteem. Talking over these issues with an understanding partner, who can reassure him that he is still a real man in her regard, or discussing his problems with a counsellor, can help him to come to terms with his new role in life.

BELOW | Massage, no matter at what age, is a good way to rediscover the areas of your partner's body which enjoy the attention the most, and to retain an intimate bond.

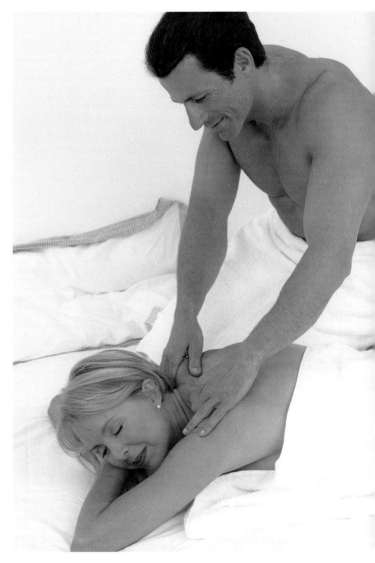

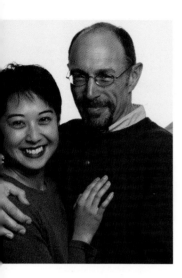

changes in a woman's body

A woman will experience far more dramatic hormonal changes than a man as she ages. This change can herald a whole new phase in her life, and can instil in her a range of emotions. She may feel that she is finally her own woman; many women consider the post-menopausal years to be the best time of their lives. This may also be tinged with a sense of loss that a certain aspect of her feminine role has gone for ever.

On average, the onset of the menopause occurs at around the age of 50 (although it can begin much earlier or later) and takes around two to five years to complete. During this time, there will be hormonal fluctuations in the woman's body, and her oestrogen levels will steadily decline. Menstruation often becomes irregular, and there may be times when her periods are close together with a heavier than usual menstrual flow, and then more widely spaced, with only a very light showing of blood. Excessive bleeding or other menstrual problems should be investigated by a doctor to rule out possible disorders.

The menopause can affect women very differently, partly due to psychological factors such as whether they are mentally well prepared for the change, their attitude towards growing older and no longer being fertile, and the symptoms experienced during this process. Some women travel through this time without a backward glance, and suffer few of the more uncomfortable side-effects.

Many women, however, experience one or more unpleasant physical and psychological symptoms. These can include hot flushes and night sweats, palpitations and anxiety attacks, loss of concentration, mood swings, lethargy, vaginal dryness and thinning of the vaginal tissues. In some women, the reduced oestrogen levels lead to osteoporosis, a thinning of the bones caused by calcium loss, leading to increased risk of fractures.

However, it is important that women realize the menopause in itself is not an illness but a natural part of the female life process. At the same time, no woman should hesitate in seeking medical advice if she is suffering from any of the debilitating symptoms described above.

HRT

Many doctors recommend that women take hormone replacement therapy (HRT) to safeguard their health during the menopause, while other medical experts disagree. The pros and cons of HRT are still being debated in the medical world. HRT will usually alleviate the physical side-effects of menopause, and is effective in reducing the risk of developing osteoporosis and heart disease.

Whether or not a woman chooses to take HRT, she should ensure that her lifestyle is balanced and healthy. A good nutritious diet, plenty of exercise, avoiding smoking and keeping alcohol intake to sensible levels will all enhance her state of well-being at this special time in her life.

As a woman ages, she may notice some change in her sexual organs and sexual responses. As oestrogen levels drop, it is possible that her vaginal secretions will decrease, and the vaginal lining will become thinner and so more vulnerable to tears and infection. To reduce friction and soreness during intercourse, she can use a lubricating jelly or obtain a locally applied oestrogen cream. She may also notice that, as she ages, her arousal responses are less intense, not because of a lack of desire, but because of physiological changes. There is no reason for her to become less orgasmic, although her climaxes may not seem as powerful as when she was younger.

hysterectomy

For various medical reasons, a doctor may recommend that a woman undergoes a hysterectomy, but it is advisable to seek a second medical opinion regarding the suitability of this operation in her circumstances. While a hysterectomy is more common once women have reached their forties and beyond, it may sometimes be necessary to carry out this procedure in a younger woman.

Once a woman has had a hysterectomy she is no longer able to have children, and if both ovaries are removed, she will become menopausal. In these circumstances, hormone replacement therapy is usually offered to the woman by her doctor. While a hysterectomy is a major surgical procedure, a healthy woman should recover well within six weeks of the operation if she is able to receive the adequate aftercare and rest she needs.

A hysterectomy does not have to mean the end of a woman's sex life or capacity to enjoy sexual or orgasmic pleasure, although in some cases, women do report that the intensity of their orgasmic contractions reduces slightly. If a woman has a hysterectomy, it is important that she realizes the operation does not make her less feminine.

life without sex

For some people, sexual passion declines quite naturally after a certain age, and not only are they happy to accept this, they may even find it a relief. The freedom from being driven by sexual desires which had to be fulfilled can open up a whole new vista on life, allowing that person time to relax into other pleasures and pursuits. If this happens mutually within a partnership, the couple may find that their relationship changes to allow greater compatibility in other areas of their lives.

If one partner loses the sex drive completely, while the other retains an active libido, they need to talk about their incompatible desires and try to find a compromise. A couple who face this dilemma may also benefit from counselling to help them confront the changing nature of their intimate relationship and enable them to acknowledge their own and each other's needs.

There are circumstances, of course, when the loss of a sex life in the later years of life is not a matter of choice. Death, divorce, or separation may leave one partner alone, and often as we grow older, it becomes less possible or desirable to form new partnerships. Many people, from middle age to elderly years, face the prospect of spending the rest of their lives without a sexual companion. In a situation like this it is important to assess one's real needs and hopes, rather than abandon the idea of finding a new partner.

Some people take active measures, joining dating agencies or broadening their recreational activities to make new acquaintances. Others learn to accept their single status. Even so, it is possible to keep the flame of sexual energy burning bright.

Dancing, having fun, sharing good times with friends, receiving a massage, cuddles and hugs from people who care, all help to keep sensual vitality alive. Masturbation is a way to achieve release from sexual tension, but it can also be much more than that. Getting older, with or without a partner, does not mean that you can no longer enjoy the sensual and sexual pleasures of your body if you so desire. It is good and healthy for you to acknowledge and enjoy your sexuality, whatever your age.

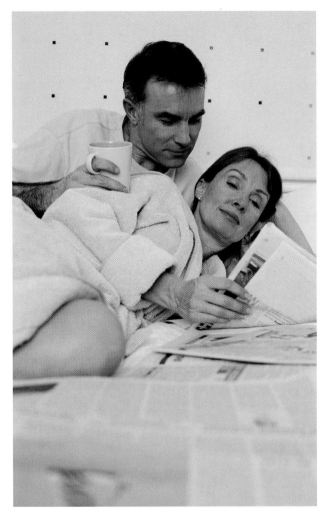

BELOW | Many couples, in their later years, have the opportunity to spend more leisure time together, free from work pressures or the demands of childrearing. This gives them more chance to enjoy each other's company so that their bond of affection and intimacy can deepen.

rediscovery

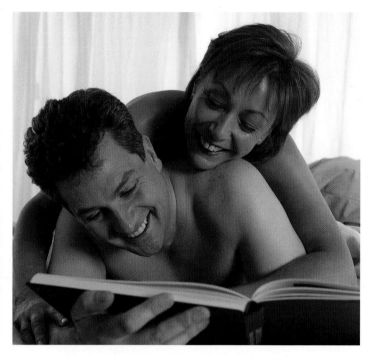

ABOVE | Life is tough and sometimes your sex life can suffer, becoming dull or non-existent. It is time to take action, read a book about sex together and share your laughter.

THERE INEVITABLY COMES A TIME in most couples' lives when the emphasis of their relationship is no longer on sex, and in fact has not been for quite some time. It is easy for this to happen to couples who have been together for a while and have devoted their partnership to their kids, careers, home-building and the multitude of other tasks, whatever their age. Standard patterns and routines somehow appear over the years, often without you realizing it. Sex may be dull, and many feel that they have worn out the possibility of ever having exciting, exhilarating sensual sex again.

It is never too late to reawaken each other's sensuality. Good sex is the magic ingredient to a great relationship. There is joy in store for some, perhaps discovering orgasm for the first time after a lifetime of frustration and disappointment. To get all your sexual fantasies fulfilled in the later stages

of a relationship can be heartening. The lesson is that it is never too late to start.

Rediscovering your own and your partner's sexuality is a journey through known territory that will invariably lead you to a new destination. Remember a particular place where you both felt passionate – revisit it. If there is a particular song that invokes special memories for you both, play it while you cuddle or massage each other. Perhaps there is one dish or type of wine that reminds you of a particularly memorable evening. Each of these may reawaken the spontaneity that you may have lost over the years, but the main focus should be on setting aside some time for you both to talk and appreciate each other's needs and wants.

The biggest erogenous zone is the brain, so this is a good place to start stimulating each other's sensuality. Talk to each other, avoiding selfless topics such as the children. Visit museums or cinemas together, share interesting extracts from a book, or create meals together in a new style.

practical steps

The following are some hints and tips that couples can incorporate into their relationship to help them to rediscover each other's sexuality, and their own. An understanding of trust and respect is paramount in all loving relationships, and as you age and mature together you need to develop an element of flexibility to allow for personal growth and development. This may involve taking practical steps to nurture, listen to and act on one another's needs:

● Talk to your partner about making time for lovemaking and if you lead very busy lives, clear a space in the diary. Don't rush sexual activity and make time for the post-coital cuddles, too.
● You may well both be feeling horny at different times, so that will have to be negotiated. There's no prescribed perfect frequency of lovemaking – how often you do it, or how infrequently – it just has to work for both of you.

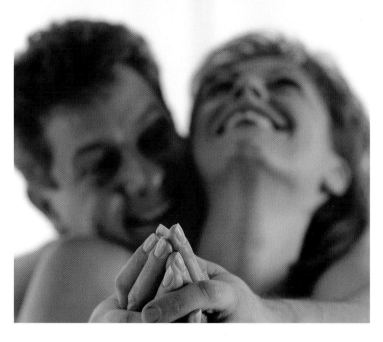

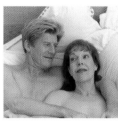

ABOVE | No matter how long you have been together, it is never too late to change things for the better.

LEFT | Trying something new together might end up just being a laugh, but then wasn't that part of the idea?

● Talk about sexual fantasies together and see whether it is possible to carry some of them out. If you find you are falling into a routine, take stock and try something different for a change. "How about trying this today?"

● Many people see sex as a way of making up after an argument, which can be very exciting, as well as an easy way of keeping emotionally close to their partner. But the potential for misunderstanding the real problem that caused the argument in the first place is enormous. Try to understand how you both function emotionally, talk about it and see how you can progress.

● Many people feel that they are not fully satisfying their lover, and worry about it. Make yourself feel better by addressing some of the things that concern you and discuss your sexual performance with your partner, asking them how you can make sex better for them.

● Familiarity can breed contempt in a long-term relationship, so try to retain some of the mystery and your own personal privacy. For example, the bathroom can be a great place to shower and bathe together but it should also be a private space sometimes. You need to be able to tell each other when you need some privacy and your own separate space and time.

● And lastly, be romantic and thoughtful towards each other. Kiss each other before you say goodbye and when you see each other again. Remember the thank yous and the small pleasantries. Buy each other small gifts or tokens – after all, it's the little things that matter.

keeping the bedroom hot

Here's how to maintain the spice:
● Use soft sexy music, dim lighting and candles or try covering the bed and floor with rose petals to create a more sensual space.
● Reorganize the bedroom every now and again to make a change in the surroundings – perhaps move the bed to a different position or bring in furniture from other rooms.
● Brighten up the room with flowers, or change some of the pictures in the photo frames. You could even buy a new print or painting to hang on the wall.
● Use sexy bed linen, perhaps silk sheets or a new bed-throw of fake fur.

● Experiment using different coloured light bulbs or change your net curtains for lightly-dyed sheer fabric: a change of light intensity or colour can completely alter the ambience of a room.
● If you have a television in the room, try taking it out for a while. A recent study showed that couples were having more sex in the 1950s than they are today, and one of the reasons was because of today's reliance on television for entertainment. By taking it out of the bedroom you will have to be creative and work on entertaining each other in different ways.

long-term tactics

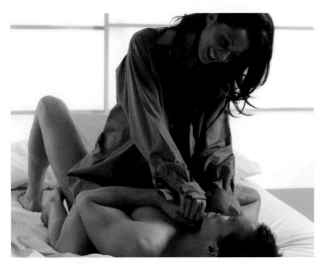

sex appeal

Rediscovering your sex appeal is about building your confidence. If you feel ashamed or embarrassed about your body then you will not be able to go full throttle during sex. If your body image is inhibiting your sex life then you have to take positive steps to do something about it.

Start doing more exercise; take time to dress up, wear sexy underwear. Go out together somewhere smart that requires you both to dress up a bit.

SOME OF THE MOST SUCCESSFUL long-term relationships cite humour and being best friends as the essential ingredients that make it work. Great friendship involves respectful behaviour towards each other, friendly gestures, lots of touching and cuddling and of course good sex. If you can have a great laugh together as well, all the better. A loving relationship should be a mutual appreciation society, to coin a phrase. Respect your differences and remember, you can't change the other person. Only they can change themselves.

Studies show that laughter is seriously good for your health. It lowers blood pressure, reduces stress and boosts your immune system. It also triggers the release of endorphins, chemicals that provide a natural painkiller for the body, and produce that "feel-good factor".

If we all looked at the physical mechanics of the way people make love, the mess they get themselves into, the funny faces they pull when having an orgasm, the fumbling, farting and funny noises that emanate from the bed, no one would ever be able to keep a straight face while having sex. Although sex is seriously fun, it has its

ridiculous side. There's a good reason why we say that laughter is the best medicine and this applies equally to your sexual relationship.

buying gifts

Buying each other sexy gifts is another fantastic way of reawakening each other's sexuality. Everyone loves both receiving and giving gifts, especially if they are spontaneous. Men can buy their partner some sexy lingerie or underwear from specialist boutiques. It is important that he buys something that will suit her taste – if in doubt then ask the shop assistant, they are usually only too keen to help! It is important also to buy it in the right context. If he buys it because he secretly wants her to look more sexy, or feels that their sex life is boring and wants to spice it up, she will invariably pick up on this and may feel offended or hurt. A better approach is for him to gently discuss with her beforehand the possibility of spicing things up, saying things like: "I would really love to spend more time with you sexually, perhaps we can try some new things together." Then she will be more prepared for her new gift, and the likelihood is that it will be better received.

More adventurous gifts such as dildos, vibrators and other sex toys must also be handled with sensitivity. If a couple has got into a pattern of rather repetitive and mundane sex and then one springs a vibrator on the other, it may be a bit of a shock, regardless of the intentions. Again, it is important to establish through discussion that you both want to try something new – there's no room here for unilateral action.

sex talk

For some reason couples often find talking about sex together really difficult regardless of how long they have been together. One reason for this may be that although sex is something that you do together, often the experience is pretty personal. During orgasm, for example, individuals often disappear temporarily into their own intense world of pleasure, and even building up to orgasm requires an element of personal concentration.

Another reason couples may find it tricky to talk about sex is fear that they may upset or offend their partner by telling them what they like, and, more importantly, what they do not like. This is especially true for couples in long-term relationships who may have spent years doing it in a specific way that is not necessarily giving one or both of them enough satisfaction.

The important thing to remember is that when you love one another, the need to satisfy and please each other sexually is crucial. All you need to do is approach the subject sensitively, avoiding direct criticism. A good technique is to use the question and answer method. When you are in

bed together, spend time trying to rediscover areas of sensuality on your partner's body by asking questions such as "May I touch you here?" or "Can I stroke you there?" The recipient should avoid responding with negative responses such as "No that feels awful." Try "That feels great, but if you do it this way it feels even better."

A tricky situation is when your partner is doing something to you that you really don't like, but are unsure how to deal with it without hurting them. Try focusing on the positive by saying things such as "I like it when you do that but I much prefer it when you do this", or "I love giving you a blow-job and I love the way you taste, but I find it uncomfortable when you thrust too deeply into my mouth, perhaps we could try a different position."

BELOW LEFT | Don't force anything on your partner you feel they won't like.

BELOW | Make a pact to buy each other something you would like to try: "I have heard that using a vibrator during sex can be really fun, I'm quite keen to try this, what do you think about it?" Even if they are not keen, the door has been opened for a discussion on your sex life.

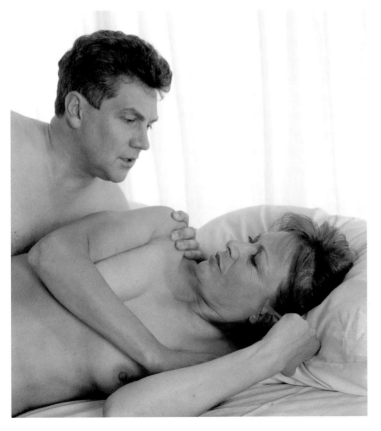

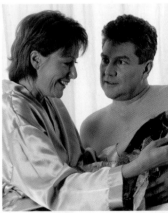

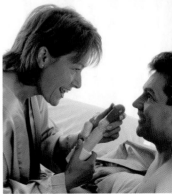

talking and listening

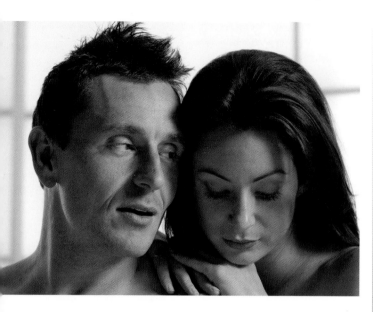

ABOVE | Making a connection with your partner is more than just a physical thing – talking and listening are crucial to keep a relationship strong and healthy. If you stop communicating, things can only get worse.

ONE OF THE MAIN PROBLEMS that couples experiencing difficulty have in common is an inability to talk effectively. Communication is the key to getting what you want out of a relationship. If done with sufficient sensitivity, it can help you to air grievances with one another and to stop one partner doing something that the other feels is annoying, hurtful or aggravating. Communication is a learned skill and blocks often occur from situations that have happened in an individual's past. It is important that each couple works together to find out what their communication strengths and weaknesses are in order to understand what makes them react to each other in the way that they do.

learning to listen

Listening is paramount in successful communication. Often people who do not listen to their partners find themselves cutting in on them, or remaining silent. Inwardly they may be thinking about what they are going to say next, without actually paying attention to what their partner is saying. Listening is one of the most valuable skills that a therapist can teach. Often couples learn this by noting how their therapist listens to each of them when they speak, and the positive effect this has on them. Therapists can encourage individuals to listen more openly and not to feel defensive when their partner is speaking, thus reducing the need to attack. By listening, couples learn to give each other time for self-expression, taking away the bad feeling or resentment that is engendered when we believe we are not being heard.

Some of the listening techniques that counsellors may advise are as follows:
● Give your full attention to your partner when they are talking by focusing on their face and voice.
● If other thoughts intrude into your mind allow them to gradually fade as you gently swing your attention back round to what is being said to you.

• Once they have finished, don't jump in immediately, give yourself a couple of seconds to evaluate what has been said and ultimately make them feel you are taking stock of what they have been saying to you.

• Listening is not all about being quiet and maintaining eye contact, it is also about encouraging your partner to speak and open up to you. The person listening should try to keep their body language as open as possible by turning towards their partner and not blocking them with gestures. They should keep their face turned towards them and look interested in what they are saying.

• Acknowledgement signals are very helpful, a nod or encouraging "yes" or "okay" all tell the partner that their words have been heard, and although you may not necessarily agree, you are accepting what they are saying. If they pause, use words that will encourage them to elaborate. Phrases such as "That incident must have made you very angry," or "You must have felt very upset when that happened to you," will help your partner to say more about their feelings and emotions.

talking to each other

Talking is also an important skill that therapists will help couples to learn. When a relationship is in its early stages, couples tend to talk a lot together to learn more about one another. As they continue, this talk becomes less and less since they already know each other and so don't feel the need to ask as much. Conversations can become short-lived and stagnant, discussing mundane issues such as "What do you want for breakfast?" as opposed to "How do you feel this morning?"

The worst thing a couple can do when they talk together is attack one another. Often when people feel passionate about something their choice of words is instantly on the offensive and confrontational, making them feel like they are getting their point across but leaving their partner feeling defensive.

The following are some common phrases and constructions that often trigger arguments, and some alternative ways of addressing the issue that may be less explosive.

blame "You ruined my evening when you told everyone that story." Instead of blaming your partner try to describe how you feel: "I felt uncomfortable and didn't enjoy myself this evening."

accusation "You made me feel furious when you forgot to pay the gas bill." Admit to your feelings by saying: "I felt..." instead of "you made me feel..."

nagging "I have asked you hundreds of times to do the dishes." Try a more constructive approach such as "Shall we do the dishes together?"

shouting Try not to raise your voice and point your finger to get your message across. Shouting will evoke an immediate defensive response. Instead, try using a softer tone and less harsh hand gestures.

BELOW | Sometimes we need to go back to school, and unlearn some bad habits.

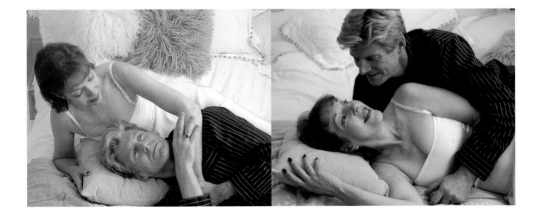

seeking help

COMMUNICATING WITH ONE ANOTHER is one of the most useful tools for ensuring success in a relationship. Sadly, successful communication is not as easy as many people may think. As a relationship progresses and other factors and influences take over such as work pressures and children, many couples find themselves communicating less and less often, unwittingly building barriers that eventually seem impossible to break down.

Therapy and counselling can be a huge benefit here. Many therapists say that a lot of couples come to them thinking that their relationship has already ended and that they have lost faith in their love and are trying therapy as a "last resort". The encouraging news is that all too often this is not the case. The use of sexual and relationship therapy has become increasingly popular as couples are less inclined to settle for an unsatisfactory love life and quite rightly seek to better their alliance on both an emotional and physical level.

The therapist will take time with the couple to re-evaluate the communication skills, find the root of the problem and help them to change their approach to each other so that their conversations become more positive and encouraging. Often communication problems stem from learned patterns picked up as children. A child whose parent was non-communicative or even abusive can carry the emotional effects of this over into their relationship in adult life, often without realizing it. This is a very common problem and once it has been identified, it can be worked through and with the help of the therapist the couple can begin working on developing more effective methods of communication.

visiting a therapist

The majority of couples who visit a therapist do so because they believe that their relationship is in trouble. Often they are unsure of how bad things

BELOW AND RIGHT | Whatever you do or don't do in bed with your partner, it is crucial to keep the channels of communication open. Masters and Johnson, through their research, popularized the concept of sexual therapy and openly talking about sex.

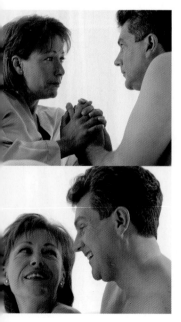

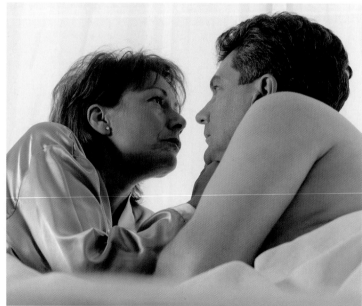

hot off the press

In 1948 Alfred Kinsey published his mass study on the human sexual male, followed in 1953 by that of the female. He shocked America by producing statistics such as 50 per cent of males had cheated on their wives, and 25 per cent of women had done the same to their husbands. *Playboy* hit the news-stands in 1953, and in the 1960s William Masters and Virginia Johnson published the first serious study on the physiology of orgasms and arousal.

In 1976, Shere Hite published *The Hite Report: A Nation-wide Study of Female Sexuality*. Hite's book contained statistical analysis, which was questioned and supported by statisticians and other scientific reviewers alike, causing much academic debate and controversy. It also contained anecdotes from women on their opinions and complaints relating to their sex lives. It became an instant bestseller.

Dr Alex Comfort broke down many barriers in the West with his 1972 publication *The Joy of Sex: a Gourmet Guide to Love Making*. This book and his other later sex manuals allowed couples to explore their sexuality with more freedom and to push out the boundaries without feeling guilty. Studies of sex have come a long way and there is today a constant stream of new information and books, like this one.

ABOVE | When you wake up with the same person every day, it is hard to maintain any mystery.

BELOW | Try to talk clearly using unthreatening gestures and positive language so you won't start an argument, and remember to listen as well.

are and need an external voice to help them to get back on track. People who no longer feel good about each other or rarely talk except to row have often built up barriers over time that they alone cannot break down.

Relationship support organizations have trained counsellors who will help couples to feel more positive about each other. Choosing and deciding to see a counsellor is often the first and hardest step for any couple experiencing difficulty, and it relies on a real desire from both parties to work together to sort out their problems. Often people are nervous, as they are unsure of what to expect from their first visit. The main purpose of the counsellor will be to provide a safe and supportive environment in which to help you rebuild your relationship. They aim to help you find the external point of reference that you need to see in order to re-evaluate your relationship.

The appointment with the therapist usually takes place in a private room where the couple can relax with the therapist and be guided to talk about their problems. A wide range of approaches and individual techniques are used, so that there is no fixed formula. They look at each individual's past to help provide meanings and answers for problems that may be occurring. They use their interactions and conversations with couples to help highlight or reflect on the roots of some of the problems and they also suggest some practical exercises that couples can try together to take a more active approach towards improving their relationship.

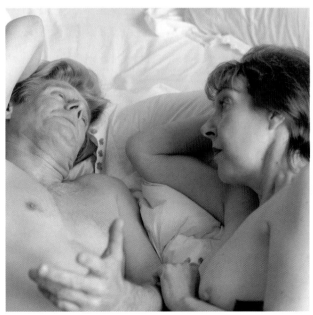

differently abled

BODY IMAGE is one the hardest things that most disabled people have to contend with, whether they have physical or learning difficulties. Other people's attitudes towards them and their own attitudes towards themselves can be a barrier in their social interactions. Other people constantly reinforce a negative attitude and most able-bodied people do not associate sexuality with the physically challenged. This perception has a knock-on effect and can inhibit a disabled person's ability to be sexual. Not only do people with disabilities have to fight the prejudices in society that do not recognize them as sexual beings, they have to learn to accept themselves and become confident. They have exactly the same needs as able-bodied people.

effects of disability

Many disabled people have limited contact with the outside world, so it can be difficult to meet other members of their peer group. Shyness and a lack of confidence can add to the problem.

One of the most frequently asked questions about disability is whether men in wheelchairs get hard-ons. The answer to this is more often than not yes. Usually a man who has no feeling in the genital area will not be able to get erect from visual stimulation alone, although they can still feel aroused. Direct physical stimulation of the genitals is normally needed in order to get an erection, and here vacuum pumps, injections and implants can be of help.

Those with high-level spinal cord injuries often get reflex erections when their genitals are touched although these are usually not associated with arousal. These reflex reactions usually go down once the touching stops but couples can learn to use these reflex erections by keeping the stimulation going in order to have intercourse. Learning to read their body signals in order to know when they are feeling aroused is a valuable skill as an erection is not always a reliable sign. Other arousal signals are hardened nipples, goose

bumps, heavier breathing and an increased heart rate – much the same as able-bodied people.

Many men who are paralysed, especially those with more serious spinal cord injuries, experience problems ejaculating. Physicians can relatively successfully "milk the prostate" by placing electrodes into the rectum and shocking the nerves in the prostate, but this is somewhat invasive if not a bit dramatic. Some men with serious spinal cord injuries claim that they are able to ejaculate with the help of a vibrator on the penis.

Another common question people have is whether women in wheelchairs can experience orgasm. In 1976 Bregman and Hadley interviewed a number of women with spinal cord injuries. Their findings concluded that their descriptions of orgasm were much the same as non-disabled women's experiences, heartening news considering many non-disabled women have such difficulty achieving orgasm, too. Women with spinal cord injuries may find that the sexual lubrication in their vagina is either lessened or absent, and may find the assistance of extra lubrication can benefit them and help them to achieve orgasm. Also some people with spinal cord injuries report having what are known as para-orgasms, which are different from the genital variety, as they occur from stimulation of other areas of the body. Para-orgasms can be so strong that some women need to be aware of, and monitor, rapid changes in their blood pressure.

Most women with disabilities are able to become pregnant even if they are paralysed from the shoulders down. It is important, therefore, that they continue to use birth control unless they are trying to have a baby.

disability and illness

There are illnesses that can lead to disability of varying degrees, all of which can have a knock-on effect on your sex life. Diabetes, for example, can cause men to lose the ability to have an erection;

BELOW | Attitudes towards disability are slowly changing, and the prejudices of the past are giving way to a greater understanding and fuller appreciation that the emotional and sexual needs of disabled and able-bodied people largely coincide.

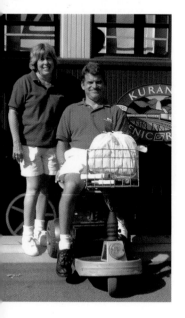

with arthritis, joints become so painful that it is not possible to masturbate or touch yourself. Multiple sclerosis can make you so fatigued that you no longer have the energy to do anything and some sufferers lose the ability to orgasm due to excess nerve damage. With some treatments for other illnesses your libido may be either dulled, or lost altogether. People experiencing these difficulties should consult their doctor who may be able to prescribe alternative treatments to help them. For example, Viagra and apomorphine have helped many male diabetes sufferers and there is some research to suggest that these treatments have positive sexual effects on women too.

practical solutions

Men and women with physical difficulties commonly use vibrators. They can supply the necessary stimulation when a hand is unable to. If your hands cannot grip a regular vibrator then a ball-shaped one is available which may be easier to handle. Also it is possible to get vibrators with longer shafts if it is difficult to reach between your legs. A rechargeable or battery-operated vibrator is usually better if you are incontinent as plug-in models could pose an electric shock risk, although these are pretty outmoded today.

Able-bodied people all too often forfeit better sex because of their inability to communicate their wants and needs to their partner, often relying on their genitals too much for sexual arousal, totally or partially ignoring other sexually sensitive areas. For a disabled person, this is not an option. A disabled person needs to tell their lover how to touch them, where and how to lie with them, what to do with their hands, legs and mouths, how not to hurt them and how to make sure they do not hurt their partner.

Although this may seem clinical and complicated, it doesn't have to be like that. Communication is the key to all great sex, so sexually confident disabled people often make the most wonderful lovers – in many cases they achieve equal, balanced and open relationships, the dynamics of which many able-bodied people could learn from.

learning difficulties

It is not just the physically disabled, but also adults with learning difficulties who have the right to a sex life. Some people may regard those who are mentally challenged as not having the emotional maturity to be able to control their own sexuality. This is a mistaken attitude and one that creates many barriers for a disabled couple. There is usually no good reason why they should not have a healthy sex life, and live fulfilled and independent lives.

looking after the carers

Most carers are devoted to the people they look after, but caring comes with some hidden agendas, especially when caring for your own relatives at home. The commitment to being a carer can leave very little time for your own needs, emotional, physical and sexual. So it is important for you to try to balance your life and get time off and space to be a sexual being for yourself. Whether you are caring for an elderly parent, disabled child or partner, often you may feel like you are in a constant state of red alert. It can be very exhausting both physically and mentally, so it is imperative that you take time out to care for yourself as well. There are many support groups available to carers, so make sure you get the necessary assistance and advice that is available to you.

getting support

Social clubs and dating organizations offer those with physical and social disabilities the chance to gain confidence, make new friends and potentially, find a partner. It is all too easy to become isolated and feel like an outsider if you do not have any support. There are charities which can offer practical suggestions for meeting, seducing, and having sex with people. They can help you find new ways to experiment, try new positions and combat a lack of confidence.

At times, it must feel as if the obstacles to a normal life are insurmountable, but once you have overcome your own inhibitions and your partner can do the same, then you will be more able to relax, laugh and have some good sex.

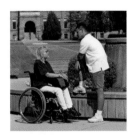

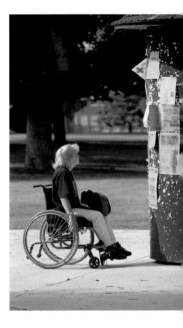

ABOVE | Being confined to a wheelchair is just the most obvious obstacle a disabled person will face.

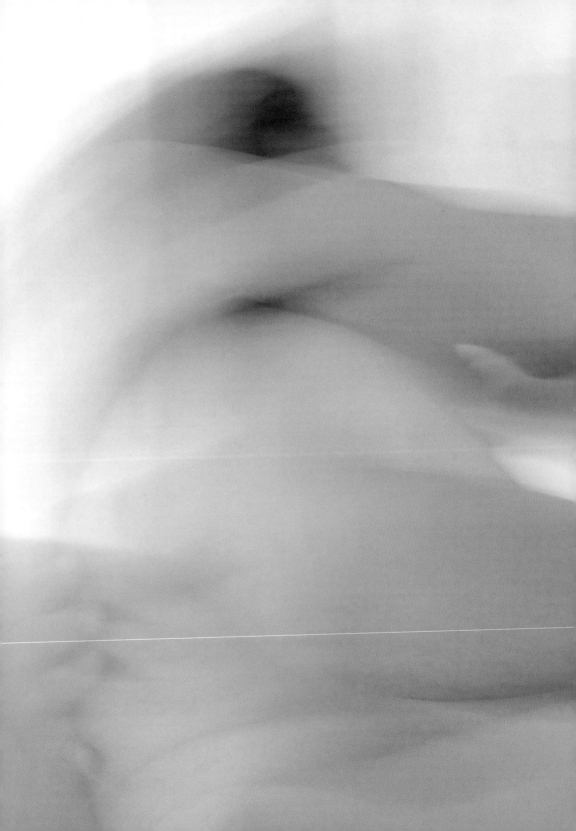

sexercises

Good sex is usually invigorating and energetic and therefore needs to be backed up by a fit body. Eating the right food and taking plenty of exercise can help people cope with life's challenges, maintaining energy and vitality in their sex lives. Taking responsibility for contraception and practising safer sex are also important to staying healthy.

bedroom workout

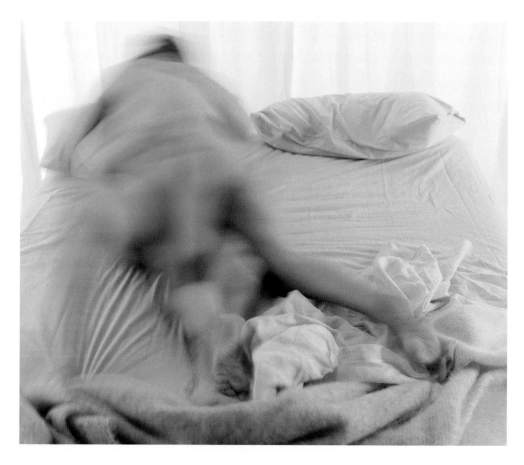

ABOVE | Lovemaking is a workout in itself, but it will be all the more pleasurable – and frequent – if you exercise to keep yourself fit and supple.

GOOD HEALTH MEANS GOOD SEX. Regular exercise promotes energy and stamina. If you are feeling good about yourself and your body, then you can feel good about your sex life, whatever age you happen to be.

There appears to be a direct relationship between being a couch potato and a lack of sexual potency. Research in the USA on a group of middle-aged men who led sedentary lives found that just one hour of exercise three times a week greatly improved their sexual function in terms of frequency, orgasm and satisfaction. Similarly, a

study of women in their forties who exercised regularly revealed that they had more frequent and enjoyable sex than women of the same age who did not exercise.

Sex is, of course, a form of exercise in itself, needing cardiovascular and muscle fitness, so exercise is important for that reason alone. And one of the many benefits of sex is that it is actually a fantastic workout that helps to keep you fit. The average person's heartbeat is around 70 beats per minute, and during lovemaking this can increase to up to 150 beats per minute, about the same as an athlete's heart rate during maximum effort. Really vigorous sex is the equivalent of 15–20 minutes on the running machine, and burns around 200 calories, which is why many people feel hungry after sex. The contractions of your pelvic and other muscles during sex also help to strengthen and tone these muscles.

fitness regime

In order to maintain an active sex life as we age and slow down, it is necessary to supplement our carnal workout with other fitness regimes. Vigorous exercise, such as running or swimming, for half an hour or more, three times a week, helps to keep everyone mentally and physically fitter. Your level of mobility and state of health will dictate the sort of activities that you should do. Whether it is a brisk walk or cycle, or a trip to the gym to use equipment such as the treadmill or rowing machine, all will help to increase your own personal fitness level.

A regular fitness regime not only helps to keep your muscular and cardiac systems healthy but also has many other benefits – helping to lower stress and blood cholesterol levels and reducing the risk of heart disease, high blood pressure, strokes and diabetes. It also increases your muscle and bone strength, and your flexibility. These benefits not only help you keep sexually active for longer, but also help you to practise positions that may previously have been too difficult for you to try.

It is never too late to start exercising, although it is better to start a regime before you actually experience problems. People can begin exercising at different levels at any time in their lives. If you are unsure about how much and what sort of exercise you should do, it's a good idea to pay a visit to your doctor for advice, especially if you have any medical conditions or you haven't taken much exercise since you left school.

Exercise programmes are available for everyone – pregnant women, seniors and disabled people alike. Age-related symptoms are often alleviated by increased mobility and activity, and many recreation facilities have specialized classes for people who may have mobility problems or

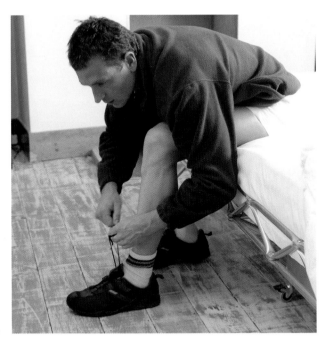

special needs. It is well worth visiting your local gym or recreation facility and talking to a trained professional about the options available and their suitability to your particular needs. Fitness professionals are extremely welcoming and motivating to everyone who is interested in increasing their fitness levels, and the chances are that they will give you the utmost support to help you achieve your goals.

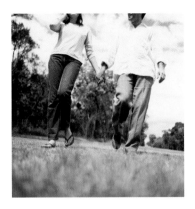

ABOVE | Running is a great way to get fit and increase your stamina and, apart from the cost of a pair of good, supportive running shoes, it's completely free.

LEFT | There are many kinds of exercise you can try, whatever your age. Just taking a walk in the open air together whenever you can will keep you in shape.

warming up

Physical exercises that concentrate on the key sexual areas of the pelvis, lower back, buttocks, abdomen and thighs can release the tension in body and mind that prevents you achieving your full orgasmic potential. These exercises allow you to achieve the strength, suppleness and mobility you need to explore and express fully the physical aspects of lovemaking, and when combined with correctly focused breathing techniques, they open up energy channels in your body which will enhance your enjoyment of sex, and enable you and your partner to achieve a feeling of greater spiritual harmony and union.

Sex is fundamentally a physical activity, so if it is to be enjoyed to the full it is important to ensure that the muscle groups, tendons and joints that come into play during healthy vigorous lovemaking are supple and well conditioned.

The positions and movements involved in the various forms of sexual intercourse put muscles and joints under pressure in a way that is totally different from that encountered during routine daily activities.

Unless you keep your body supple and pliant you are liable to suffer muscle cramps and strains during sexual intercourse as you and your partner try to achieve the different angles and changes of position you are seeking in order to obtain mutual sexual satisfaction. By conditioning the areas of the body that are most actively involved in lovemaking – most notably the muscles of the buttocks, abdomen, thighs, lower back and pelvic floor – you will extend your range of motion and enhance your ability to move smoothly and with control, enabling a wider variety of pelvic movements and allowing more comfortable lovemaking.

PELVIC SWING

RIGHT | Stand with your feet a shoulder-width apart, knees slightly flexed. Place your arms by your side with your palms open forwards. Breathe in and draw your pelvis back.

FAR RIGHT | Breathe out and swing your pelvis forwards, allowing arms, hands and genitals to swing up. Repeat this for up to five minutes as a continuous pelvic motion.

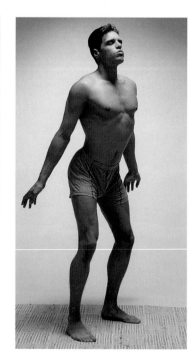
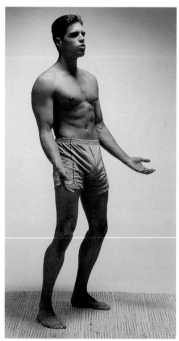

When you are sexually fit you have the suppleness, mobility and enthusiasm to throw your mind and body into the passion of the moment. You will also be able to explore new positions and hitherto undiscovered heights of ecstasy.

By relieving tension you are also helping to fight the stress that often prevents you getting into the relaxed and giving mood needed to achieve a satisfying sexual encounter. Tension in the pelvis, legs, lower back and abdomen restricts the flow of sexual energy and vitality and reduces your inclination for and total enjoyment of lovemaking. Repressed feelings here can upset the wholeness and unity of the body and act as a barrier between the mind, the emotions and the physical responses. Exercises combined with breathing techniques, that you can carry out alone or with your partner, will release the tension in these key areas, and help to release the flow of sexual energy so that you can achieve your full orgasmic potential.

gentle warm-up

As with all physical exercises, ensure you are fully warmed up before you try these routines to reduce the risk of minor strains and sprains. Exercise is best carried out after a warm bath or shower so that relaxing warmth is transmitted deep into the muscle fibres. Put on some loose, comfortable clothing, choose a room that is draught-free and fairly warm (but not too warm), and ensure you have a soft floor surface to lie on.

Start off the session with some loosening movements and gentle stretches to free the muscles and tendons. Try a simple warm-up routine such as marching on the spot while circling your arms above your head. Remember to fill your lungs with air when you start an exercise to ensure your body gets all the oxygen it needs, and then expel your breath on the exertion to rid the body of the waste products it has accumulated.

The following simple routines can help release tension in the abdomen, lower back and pelvis.

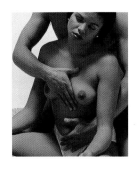

ABOVE | Deep breathing brings oxygen to nourish the body, and eases emotional tension by relaxing the muscles. Your partner can kneel behind and encourage the tension to melt by placing his or her hands softly over the key areas.

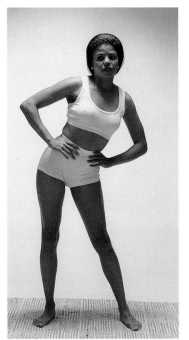

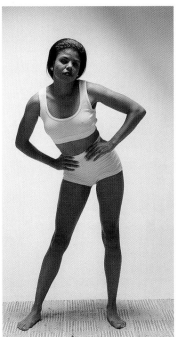

PELVIC CIRCLES
FAR LEFT | Stand with your feet a shoulder-width apart and knees slightly flexed. Place your hands on your hips. Mentally focus inside to the inner shape of your pelvic bowl.

LEFT | Rotate your pelvis slowly in wide circles – ten times to the right and then ten times to the left. Breathe in to the movement and consciously allow any tension to relax.

RIGHT | Breathe into your chest and abdomen. Imagine your breath to be reaching your genitals. Breathe in and out.

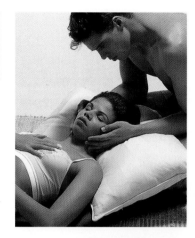

breathing

Correct breathing is a vital part of these exercises. Your breathing is directly affected by your emotional state as a result of external worries and pressures. When you are tense and under stress your breathing becomes rapid and shallow and your body cannot get all the air it needs for normal healthy functioning.

By focusing on your breathing you can draw the air deep down into your abdomen to fill the lungs to capacity. This saturates the blood with life-giving oxygen, which is then pumped round the body to restore the tissues and replenish the energy reserves depleted during physical activity. When you breathe out, aim to empty your lungs completely to rid your body of the waste products that have built up. This slowly releases the emotional tension, leaving you feeling relaxed, more alive and vital.

Pent-up feelings of anger, anxiety, or fear can also lead to tension in the key energy centres of the body – the chest and abdomen. Inhalation and exhalation can be combined with the healing power of touch to help you direct your breathing into each part in turn, to unblock the energy channels and release the sexual tension.

RIGHT | Place your arms by your side. Breathe in – draw your thighs together. Imagine your in-breath to be pulling your legs in.

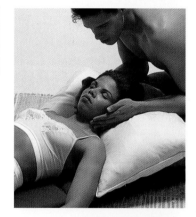

Place your hands softly over the chest and abdomen and imagine that the warmth and contact of your hands is melting these areas. Encourage the tension to drain away as you focus your awareness into every inhalation and exhalation.

genital release exercise with partner

This simple exercise helps to release sexual tension in the pelvic and genital area and increases vitality.

RIGHT | Breathe out – let your legs flop open – to open up the genitals and relax the thigh muscles and groin. Then breathe in again.

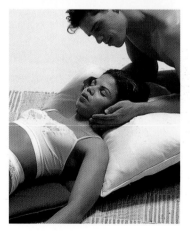

Lie down comfortably on your back, with your feet on the ground and knees raised. Your partner gently supports your head. Place your hands over your chest and abdomen to encourage breathing and aid relaxation. Repeat this exercise for up to five minutes, then rest for five minutes – feel the vibrations in your legs and body and acknowledge any rising feelings.

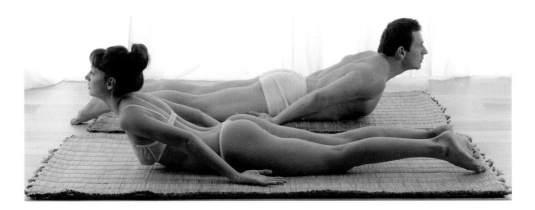

ABOVE | The dart is a gentle exercise that tones all the muscles of the back and neck.

BELOW | Scissors is a Pilates exercise that will improve the condition of your legs and stomach muscles.

BELOW RIGHT | The bridge is quite a demanding pose. Continue with regular practice of these basic exercises, and it will become easier very quickly.

scissors

Lie on a mat, bend your knees to your chest and hold your right leg behind the thigh. Breathe in to prepare. Breathe out and zip up and hollow. Breathe in and straighten both legs in the air, pointing the toes. Breathe out, lengthen and lower the left leg, stopping just above the floor. Breathe in and raise the leg as straight as possible. Breathe out and change legs, crossing over like scissors. This movement strengthens the abdominals and improves the flexibility of the hamstrings.

the bridge

Lay on your back with your knees bent and your feet flat on the floor close to your body and parallel to each other. Rest your arms alongside your body with your palms facing down. As you exhale, rotate your pelvis back and push the small of your back into the floor. As you inhale, lift your back off the floor, vertebra by vertebra, starting at the tailbone.

Hold the pose for 15 to 30 seconds, or until you feel discomfort. Bring your spine back down to the floor in the same way, beginning with your upper back and stretching your spine towards your heels.

the dart

This position strengthens the back extensor muscles and shoulder blades and works the deep neck flexes. Lie on your front with your arms by your sides and palms facing upwards. Keep your legs together, point your toes and lengthen your neck. Prepare by breathing in, tucking in your chin and lengthening your spine. As you breathe out, zip up your pelvic floor muscles and hollow your shoulder blades, pulling them down into your back. At the same time lengthen your fingers towards your feet and keep looking straight down at the floor. Avoid tipping your head back but squeeze your inner thigh muscles together., keeping your feet on the floor.

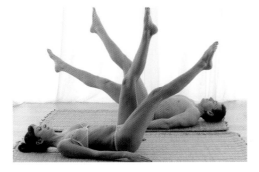

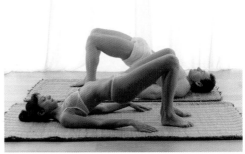

strengthening the pelvic floor

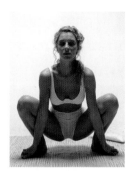

ABOVE | Squat on your haunches. Breathe in five short breaths (don't exhale), tightening the pelvic floor muscles, as if pulling your vagina up step by step. Then give five short out-breaths (don't inhale), releasing your pelvic floor muscle.

RIGHT | Pelvic curls are good for strengthening the pelvis and thighs. Do this exercise five times. Lie with your back on the ground with the whole of the spine touching the floor. Place the soles of your feet flat on the floor, shoulder-width apart. Put your arms by your side. Breathe out and roll your spine upwards, using your buttocks and lower abdominal muscles to curl your tailbone up off the floor. Tighten your buttocks and inside thigh muscles. Breathe in and roll your spine down to the floor, uncurling your tail-bone and relaxing your thigh and buttock muscles.

YOU CAN GREATLY ENHANCE YOUR SEX LIFE by learning exercises to strengthen the pelvic floor. This is the collection of muscles and ligaments at the base of the abdomen that supports the bladder, vagina, uterus and rectum. Childbirth and aging can weaken this part of the body, reducing control over the vaginal and pelvic muscles and blunting the nerve responses. A weakened pelvic floor can also lead to serious medical problems such as a prolapsed uterus and urinary incontinence and is often the underlying cause for women who are having difficulty achieving an orgasm. Regular pelvic floor exercises will ensure that these muscles and ligaments remain taut and well toned, so that you have adequate structural support for the uterus and vagina, and will be able to continue to enjoy sex.

Many women also find that by toning up the muscles of the pelvic floor they are able to climax more freely and to experience stronger or more intense orgasms. Improving the strength and flexibility of these muscles will extend your range of movement and make those positions that involve squatting over your partner, or wrapping your legs round him, easier and more comfortable to adopt. Your vagina will also be able to grip your partner's penis more firmly during lovemaking, which will enhance the enjoyment for both of you.

You can discover your pelvic floor by imagining you need to urinate but are trying to hold it back. The part of the body that tightens as you do this is your pelvic floor. In addition to the exercises in this section, there is a simple pelvic floor exercise that you can practise at any time, as no one can see you do it. Slowly contract the pelvic floor muscles, ten times, pulling the muscles up inside in slow stages each time. Breathe normally as you do this exercise. Practise two to three times daily for at least a month. Another exercise you could try on your own is to place two fingers inside the vagina and try to squeeze them by contracting the pelvic floor muscles.

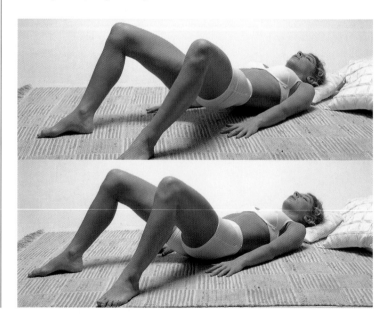

pelvic floor exercises

The following exercises will tone and strengthen the pelvic floor. They are particularly important after childbirth, but all women will derive some benefit from them. You will particularly notice the effect during lovemaking when you find that your vagina is better able to clasp your partner's penis.

pelvic tilt

This is a marvellous exercise to flatten your stomach muscles and keep you feeling good about your body. Lie on your back, placing your hands on your pelvis with the fingertips on the pubic bone and the pads of your hands resting on the pelvic bones. Breathe in and lengthen through the top of your head. Breathe out and draw up the pelvic floor muscles and pull the lower abdominals back towards the spine, hollowing out your lower stomach (this is referred to as zip up and hollow, which is a requirement for almost all the exercises). Keep your tailbone on the floor lengthening away and do not push into the spine or tuck under the pelvis. You are in neutral position. Breathe in and then relax.

Try this again, with your legs flat on the floor. Lie on your back, lengthening your spine through your head. Your legs should be shoulder-width apart and totally relaxed. Your arms should be by your side with palms facing up. Breathe in to prepare, breathe out and zip up and hollow from the pelvic floor. Your tailbone should be on the floor lengthening away. Breathe in and relax.

It is a good idea to start any new exercise regime by attending a class such as Pilates or yoga

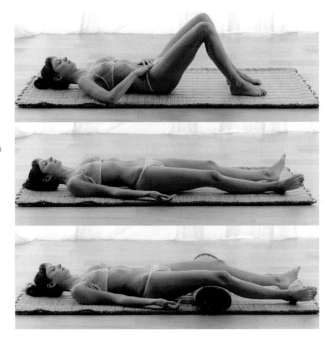

before you try to do it by yourself. Find one that suits you and try to go at least once a week. Once you have learned some of the positions, you can practise at home with the aid of a book or a video. With good teaching, you are unlikely to suffer injuries. Working on some of the postures, like hip openers, will help you to achieve more complex sexual positions than you thought you would ever do again. It really is possible at the age of 55 to bend forward, hook your big toes with your fingers and rest your head on your straight knees.

ABOVE | The pelvic tilt helps to build up strength and stamina around the pelvic girdle, vital for an active sex life. If you have lower-back problems you can use a cushion or rolled-up mat placed under your knees, which will release any pressure around the lower back area.

feel-good factor

The body responds to physical exercise by releasing more of the hormone adrenaline. After exercise the come-down after the adrenaline rush makes you feel relaxed and often also increases feelings of arousal, making some kind of fitness regime an excellent idea for people who may have flagging libidos.

The body also releases "feel-good" hormones from the brain called endorphins, the body's natural equivalent to morphine. Endorphins block out pain and make you feel exhilarated, energized, invigorated and generally happy and calm. In other words, they create a perfect physical

and emotional state for lovemaking. As exercise also encourages the flow of blood through all the organs of the body, this can help with arousal, heightened sensation and lubrication. An increased blood flow also helps to make orgasm more intense. In short, the fitter you are, the better the sex.

increasing flexibility

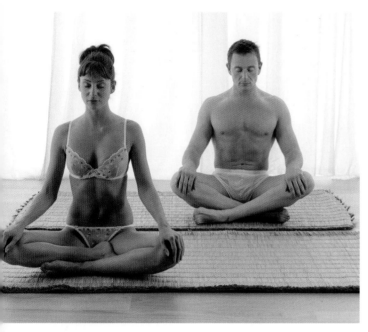

ABOVE | Practising yoga increases suppleness and flexibility, which makes for great sex. PC exercises contract the anal muscles, pelvic floor muscle and navel into the body, increasing energy, while strengthening other muscles in the area.

A GREAT SEX LIFE is dependent on good health, and one aspect of keeping well is keeping fit. You will benefit by keeping your heart and lungs strong and your muscles toned.

for her

There are certain exercises that women in particular need to do to keep themselves sexually fit. As they get older, muscles become flabbier if they are not worked and when women hit the menopause, the muscles begin to weaken even more. This also applies to the PC (puboccygeus) muscle. This is the pelvic floor muscle that runs between the legs from the anus to the genitals in both men and women and is the muscle that contracts at a rate of just under once a second during orgasm.

Women who have given birth will probably remember the midwife telling them not to forget their pelvic floor exercise. She was referring to the

PC muscle, which will have been stretched when the baby was born. There are good reasons for doing the exercises: to avoid problems with bladder control (sneezing and coughing causing leaks, for example) and uterine prolapse in later life. The exercises also help keep a tight vagina for sexual activity. Pelvic exercises are also essential for young women and those who have never given birth, just to keep the muscle toned.

Sexercises were practised in the ancient civilizations of China and India, but it was an American, Dr Kegel, who developed the famous Kegel exercises in the 1950s which are now widely used for pelvic exercising. The quickest way to find your PC muscle is to stop and start when you are urinating, although it is important not to do Kegel exercises during urination. Once you have found it, exercise the PC muscle daily by tightening and relaxing the muscle in turn, starting with 20 times at one session, twice a day. Build up to 60 or so a day and when you have accomplished this, try prolonging the squeeze to five seconds at a time up to 200 times a day.

These exercises can be done while waiting at the bus stop. Even better, while having sex, a woman can squeeze her vagina around her partner's penis and he'll love it. This used to be called Cleopatra's kiss and certain royal courtesans were famous for it. Alternatively, exercise your PC muscle while you are masturbating. One of the results will be to help you and your partner to intensify and prolong orgasms.

for him

If a man has a strong PC muscle, it will help him control the timing of his orgasm, but it won't make his erection any harder. An additional exercise for men is to place a small wet towel on their erect penis and then practise moving it up and down. Once they have achieved this, they can use a bigger towel. This exercise is also excellent for strengthening the muscles of the lower abdomen.

yoga and pilates

Yoga and Pilates are extremely beneficial and holistic forms of exercise for both men and women, young and old. Because sex can require stamina, flexibility and muscular endurance (holding your partner up around your waist for half an hour, for example), both yoga and Pilates will positively help. Making a regular space with your partner to do these exercises every few days will help you to stay relaxed, supple and optimally fit. Doing it together will give you the incentive you need to keep at it.

wall slide

The aim of this exercise is to lengthen the base of the spine without over-tilting the pelvis or tucking it under too far. At the same time it will strengthen the thigh muscles and stretch the Achilles tendon. Stand with your back against the wall and your feet hip-width apart and parallel, 15cm/6in from the wall. Place hands on hips or by your side. Lean back against the wall and breathe in, lengthening through the spine. Breathe out, pull up the pelvic floor and draw your lower abdominals back to the spine (this is also termed zip up and hollow). Slide about 30cm/12in down the wall. Breathe in as you slide up. Repeat eight times.

the full hundred

Lie on the floor, or a comfortable mat or rug, with your knees bent and feet flat on the floor. Your arms should be by your side, palms down. Breathe in and prepare. Breathe out, zip up and hollow. Tuck the chin in slightly and curl the upper body off the floor, at the same time straightening one leg into the air. Reach through the fingertips, lengthening the shoulder blades down the back. Turn out your legs from the hips and flex the feet, lengthening through the heels, so you feel the stretch on the inside of your legs. Squeeze your inner thighs together and engage the pelvic floor. Breathe in for a count of five beats of the arms, then breathe out for five beats, moving the arms as if you were patting the floor. Continue for 100 beats then repeat with the other leg. For beginners, release the head and rest it on the floor.

the half hundred

This is a slightly more advanced version. Breathe in and prepare, breathe out, zip up and hollow. Tuck in the chin slightly and curl the upper body off the floor, or rest your head on the floor. This time bend both knees at the same time while you repeat the movements above. Keep this up regularly, and you will feel an improvement very quickly.

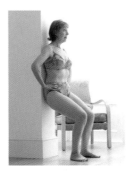

ABOVE | The wall slide will strengthen your legs and stomach muscles.

BELOW LEFT | The full hundred, with straight legs.

BELOW RIGHT | The half hundred, with knees bent.

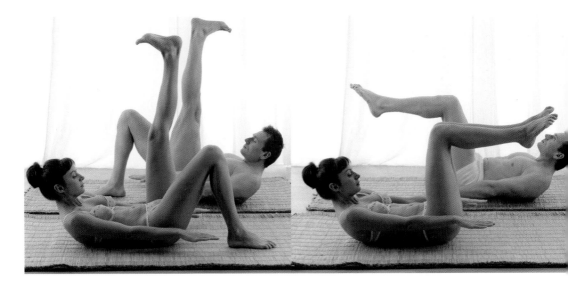

games and exercises

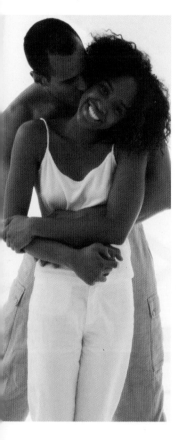

GAMES AND EXERCISES OFFER a great opportunity for you and your partner to relax and have fun together, while renewing your physical vitality as you breathe more deeply, tone up your muscles and stretch your joints. It is a chance to enjoy your own and your lover's body outside of sexual contact.

The warming-up exercises shown here provide a non-threatening and playful opportunity in which to discover whether there are any subtle physical and psychological tensions within yourself and your relationship that may be inhibiting harmonious and spontaneous interaction. Tension often reflects an internal state of mind, such as a fear of letting go or of losing control, which shows itself outwardly as hesitation, resistance or even aggression. The games will help you find a point of balance in yourself where you are at ease and

exercise one

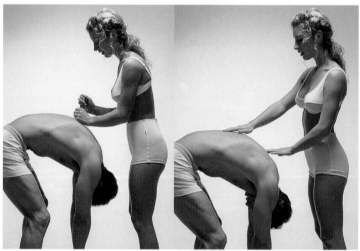

ABOVE | Games and exercises can make you feel more relaxed with each other and confident in your relationship.

1 | PUMMEL THE SPINE

Get the passive partner to stand in a balanced posture, feet shoulder-width apart and knees flexed, taking a few moments to relax all joints. He then drops his head forwards and leans his upper body towards the ground. The head and neck hang relaxed between the shoulders, and his arms dangle loosely down. As the active partner, pummel briskly, one hand following the other, up along each side of his spine, and between the shoulder blades. Take care not to strike the spine itself.

2 | SOOTHE THE SPINE

After the invigorating pummelling, soothe your partner's spine and back with overlapping strokes from the fingers of each hand. Start the motion from the lower back, drawing one hand after the other up along the spine and over the neck. Repeat this action several times.

relaxed within your body and mind. From this position you then co-operate with your partner to find a mutual point of harmony and balance between you.

Before attempting the games, warm up with one or both of the two ten-minute tactile contact programmes shown here. The first exercise uses some of the percussion strokes explained in Sensual Massage to enliven the body and help ease strain from the back, shoulders and chest.

The second exercise, illustrated on the following pages, encourages greater relaxation and more fullness of breath, while helping you to make a deeper connection with the abdominal and pelvic area, the centre of gravity and balance in your body.

Physical relaxation and emotional trust come from a sense of being at ease with your body and feelings, so you can trust your basic instincts. Those feelings are deeply rooted in the body, in particular within the abdominal region.

After each game, take some time to assimilate its effects, and discuss honestly with each other what thoughts, feelings or sensations occurred. Then you can reverse the roles to receive maximum benefit.

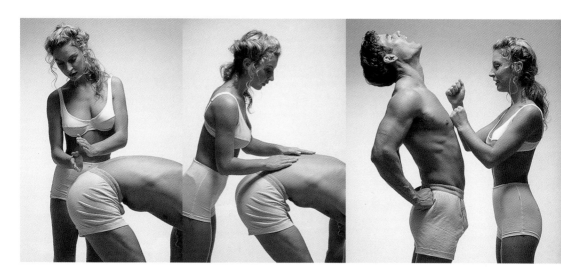

3 | STIMULATING STROKES

Move to your partner's side and hack briskly over the large muscles of the buttocks to invigorate and stimulate this area and to loosen its tension. Aim for the fleshy areas, taking care not to strike the lower spine or pelvic bones. You can continue this hacking motion down to the thighs.

4 | FRICTION RUB

Position yourself behind his posterior, and apply a friction rub over the kidney area to warm and revitalize the whole body. Using the flat surface of each hand alternately, briskly rub them back and forth for about 30 seconds to generate a tingling heat. Then, soothe the back with some sensual strokes. Now ask your passive partner to extend his upper body, uncoiling the spine slowly from its base, vertebra by vertebra. The last area to lift is the neck and head.

5 | CLEAR THE CHEST

Now ask your partner to expand his chest, by pushing his fists into his lower back while letting his shoulders and head drop backwards. Encourage him to clear tension from his throat by emitting sounds while you pummel thoroughly over the chest. The pummelling dispels carbon dioxide from the lungs, helping him to breathe more deeply and releasing sensations of tightness in the ribcage. When you have completed these stokes, your partner should stand straight and shake his arms and hands.

exercise two

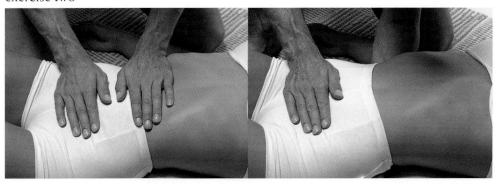

1 | EXPERIENCE CONTACT

The partner who is lying down first relaxes her whole body, and then focuses her breath and attention softly towards her abdomen. Lay your hands gently but with total presence on her belly to develop warmth and contact. Encourage her to become aware of her belly's expansion towards your hands with each inhalation, and its contraction with each exhalation.

2 | TAKE THE WEIGHT

Cradle your partner's pelvis and lower abdomen between the reassuring contact of your hands, by slipping one hand beneath the lower back, and the other just above the pubic bone. Wait patiently for her to drop the weight of her back and pelvis into the support of your lower hand, while she directs her breathing and mental concentration to her pelvic girdle and genitals, allowing those areas to relax more with each cycle of breath.

developing trust and synchronicity

The following games centre on developing trust and attaining synchronicity. Both factors represent a huge dynamic in any relationship. Our basis of trust develops within us as children through the experiences of our primary relationships, and is generally replayed unconsciously in other relationships throughout our adult lives. Learning to trust more does not mean that we must throw caution to the wind; our inner self-protection mechanisms have developed for good reason and need to be respected.

Through physical game-playing we can become aware of our fears about developing real trust – and the body is the most manifest place for this observation – and can sometimes gain insights into our earlier childhood experiences. We can then begin to undo some of our fears and inhibitions, while regaining more natural spontaneity. Awareness occurs the moment we draw something from the unconscious into our conscious minds, and is always the first point of any change.

By playing these games, you also learn how to become aware of whatever is happening, both within yourself and your partner. You cannot expect your lover to relax and trust in the situation if you are self-absorbed, or your attention is wandering, or if you are not receptive to the mental and bodily signals he or she is giving out.

Try not to overpower your partner, or demand results, and be patient whenever you meet a moment of resistance. Explore those experiences together and learn from them. These games are intended to be fun and should not become a serious encounter, even if they evoke some profound feelings. They are an experiment, allowing you both to interchange constantly between passive and active roles, and to become confident and attuned to your bodies, so that you can develop a more harmonious relationship.

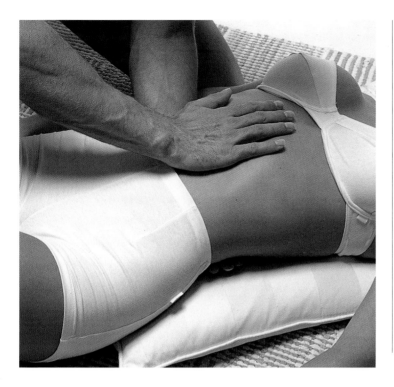

Stress causes the diaphragm, the sheath of muscle separating the chest and the abdominal cavity, to tighten, constricting breathing, increasing feelings of anxiety and cutting you off from basic emotions. Scoop the hand which is closest to your partner's head under her body to rest beneath the middle of her back. Encourage her to consciously release the tension in her back towards this hand. Place the other hand softly over the diaphragm area, above the solar plexus, and just below the ribcage. Ask your partner to breathe gently into the area between your hands and allow her tension to melt with each exhalation.

A successful relationship between two people also results when synchronicity is attained on energetic, physical and mental levels. Many couples are drawn to each other in the first place because of a certain rapport. There is a kind of ebb and flow in a happy relationship, where a balance exists between knowing when to take the lead and when to yield.

Synchronicity is the moment when these two facets of the one phenomenon come together and form a unity of thought and action. This can be witnessed when two people dance together and their bodies flow as one motion, because they are able to respond equally to one another's subliminal signals indicating when to take the initiative and when to surrender to the movement.

This fine tuning manifests itself in bed too, when lovemaking can become a congruent interplay of mind, heart and body or, adversely, a battleground of subtle domination, control, resistance or submission.

Synchronicity, which tends to exist naturally in the first stages of a relationship, should not be taken for granted. It can be lost as the individual personalities and egos emerge, or when either one or both partners becomes enmeshed in the normal stresses and strains of daily life.

The four games in this section will help you become more attuned to each other, as they require both trust and synchronicity while finding a balance between taking passive and active roles.

The first game involves squatting, the importance of which as a pelvic floor exercise has already been explained. The next two games use a push-and-let-go technique, which requires the active person to take charge of moving the other's body, while the passive partner yields to the movement. The motions must be confident but gentle so your partner can relax. You must become sensitive to his or her body movements. If you are jerky, or too aggressive, your partner will resist and tighten up. The last game is a trust game.

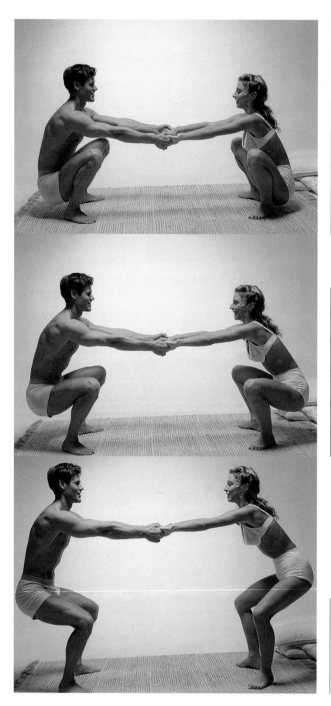

developing synchronicity

1 | SYNCHRONIZING

Both of you should squat, facing each other and maintaining eye contact, but with enough distance to let your arms stretch out to make contact. Keep your backs straight, and your neck and head relaxed. Focus your breath and attention on your pelvic region to allow this point of gravity to give you balance. Let the genital area and the anus, relax, and drop the weight of your buttocks towards the floor. Weight should be distributed evenly through the feet. Once you feel comfortable reach out and clasp each other's hands or wrists.

2 | PUSH AND PULL

When you are ready, begin to lever yourselves upwards from the squatting position. The thrust of the upwards movement should come from your leg muscles and hips, so always keep your spine lengthened and your shoulders relaxed. The art of this exercise is to find a mutual point of balance between you as you gently push and pull on each other to rise upwards. Too much or too little assertion from either partner will tip this delicate balance, causing one or both of you to topple over.

3 | LIFT AND DESCEND

Raise up your bodies until you are both standing, then begin the process again as you lower yourselves back down to a squatting position. Repeat the exercise several times until you have found a fluid balance of movement between you.

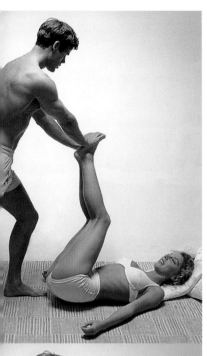

developing mobility

◄ 1 | LETTING GO

In this exercise, your partner lies on the floor with her back relaxed and her legs raised in the air. Gently, but firmly, push both legs to one side of her body and then remove your hands.

► 2 | BACK SWING ►

When you have released contact, she then swings her legs back to a central position. At this point, decide on the direction of the next push so that one movement flows into another.

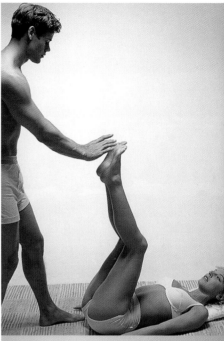

◄ 3 | CHANGE DIRECTIONS

Try to use a whole range of directions, this time pushing the legs to the other side of the body. The side-to-side and back-and-forth movements of the legs will exercise and strengthen the abdominal muscles. Gently make her aware of whether she is resisting or aiding you as she should be yielding to these passive movements.

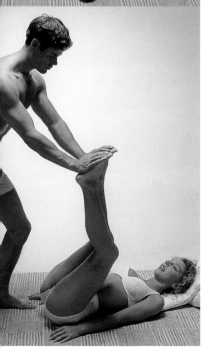

► 4 | REVERSE ROLES

When you have completed a whole range of movements, swap roles. By pushing the legs towards the body you are giving a stretch to the lower back and hip joints.

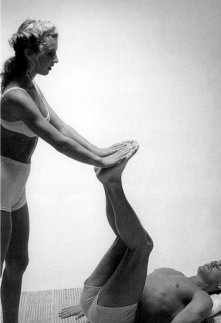

learning to relax

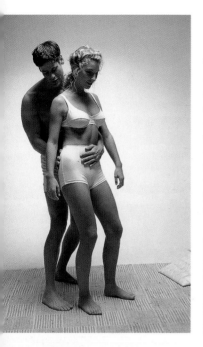

◄ 1 | TAKING CHARGE

This exercise is performed in a standing position. Ask your partner to stand in a relaxed posture so that she feels secure and balanced. She should close her eyes and focus on her breath and the sensations of movement. Position yourself behind her body and, very lightly, begin to direct her, pushing her to the side with one hand, and catching her with the other. Stay relaxed as you take charge of her movements.

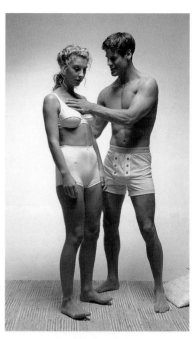

► 2 | GENTLE ROLLING

Gracefully and quietly move around her body so that she is unable to guess the angle of the next movement. Roll her gently from side to side and back and forth, so that her body falls easily from one hand into the other.

◄ 3 | LOOSENING CIRCLES

Help her to loosen the hips and pelvis by circling this area between your hands. As she relaxes, and yields and allows her whole body to surrender to your hand directions, the movements can be gradually enlarged.

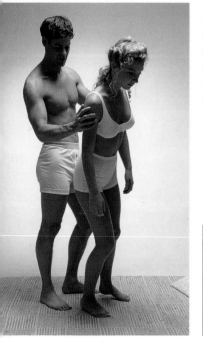

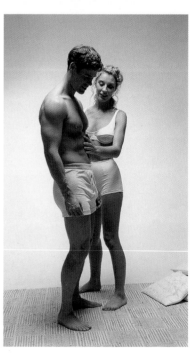

► 4 | LEARNING TO SURRENDER

Initially, your man may find it difficult to surrender his body to these movements, fearing he is too big or heavy to let you take charge. If he is able to relax and release his body rigidity, you will be able to move him with ease.

developing trust

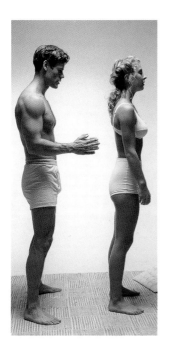

◀ 1 | TRUST

This game is definitely about trust, and also requires the total attention of the active partner; only play it if you are confident about catching and supporting the weight of your partner's body. Ask her to stand in front of you, fully relaxed and with eyes closed. Position yourself behind, allowing enough space for her to fall back into your arms.

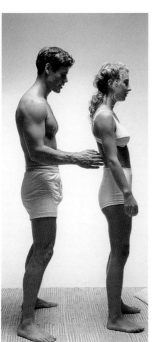

◀ 2 | FALLING FOR YOU

When she is ready, she allows herself to fall slowly backwards, trusting that you are there for her. The more physically relaxed she is able to remain, the easier it is for her to fall.

▶ 3 | SAFE CATCH

As she tilts back, catch her securely in your arms, so that her upper back is supported and her head and neck rest against your chest or shoulder. Hold her against you so she becomes aware of what she is feeling, then gently ease her back to a standing position. Repeat the exercise twice more.

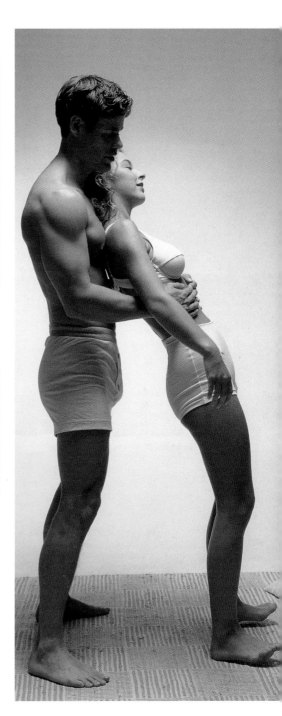

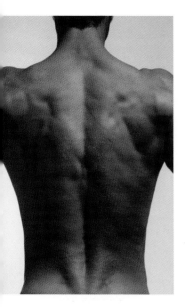

back to back

Most of the time we relate to others face to face. We spend inordinate amounts of time taking care of the front, ensuring we present a good image to our partners or to the world at large. Normally, we have very little sense of ourselves as viewed from the backs of our bodies. It is to correct such a gap in our self-knowledge that this book has emphasized the great importance of touching, stroking and making sensual contact with the back of the body during foreplay and lovemaking, as well as dealing with the more obvious intimate and directly sexual areas located at the front.

The back acts as a protective shell, often harbouring tensions which shield a deeper level of vulnerability. If you have practised your sensual massage strokes on each other, you may have noticed how, once the muscles of the back are relaxed, the whole body seems to become more alive and sensitive. Often, touch, massage and contact to the back can help someone let go of their inner emotional tensions.

Here are some exercises you can enjoy with your partner to develop more familiarity with your own and each other's back. Through them, you develop a clearer feeling of its shape and structure and, therefore, a stronger sense of your body image.

In addition, these back-to-back exercises can help you dissolve the tensions which tend to keep you rigid, and allow you both to merge more with each other, both physically and emotionally.

Again, you need to be sensitive to each other and find a mutual point of balance, where your weight and movement are evenly and gently distributed. (It is not advisable to do these exercises if you are suffering from back problems of an acute or chronic nature.) Begin by sitting with your backs to each other on a firm and

ABOVE | A healthy back is important for posture and will help your sexual performance.

RIGHT | Fitting together: Bend your knees to lower your body so that she can fit her buttocks comfortably into the small of your back. Before moving, ensure that she is ready and relaxed for the lift.

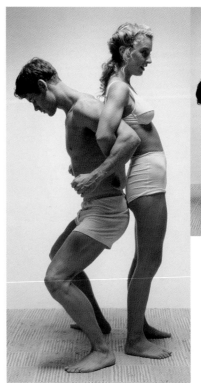

1 | SPINAL STRETCH
As you tilt from your hips to lower your upper body, the passive partner sinks her back down on to yours, allowing her head and neck to relax backwards. Check that she is feeling safe before you lift her upwards.

supportive base, so that the surface of your backs and your spines are in comfortable contact. How much contact depends, of course, on the differences in your size and structure. It is important not to slump, but to keep your spines relaxed yet extended upwards.

Link your arms loosely together, and spend about three minutes directing your awareness and breath to areas of the back which feel tight and withholding, gradually allowing the tensions to melt.

Lean gently into each other, taking care not to burden your partner with your weight, especially if he or she is smaller or lighter than you. Close your eyes and begin to focus on the skin-to-skin contact of your backs, the shape and structure, how and where they fit together perfectly, and where there is tension. Imagine those tensions are beginning to dissolve so that both backs are merging together.

Start to sway gently together, finding a natural rhythm to your motion, and becoming more aware of the moments when the movements jar. Change the rhythm every so often, but always aim to remain harmoniously in tune with your partner's body.

Try to stay aware of any feelings which arise in you or which you may be picking up from your partner as you let go of muscular tensions.

Now sit silently together, eyes closed, but staying as deeply in tune with each other as possible for at least a minute. Once you are ready to separate, it is a good idea to discuss with each other what you experienced during this exercise, in relation to both your own body and your partner's body.

This back-to-back attunement will prepare you for the spinal stretch exercise shown here, in which one partner lifts the other on to his or her back and balances the weight.

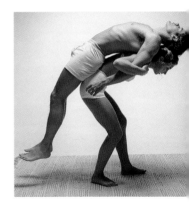

ABOVE | It is possible for two people of different sizes to do this provided you maintain stability and relaxation. However, common sense will guide you as to whether the weight or height differences are too great to attempt it. The first priority is to ensure that there is no danger of you straining your back or spine.

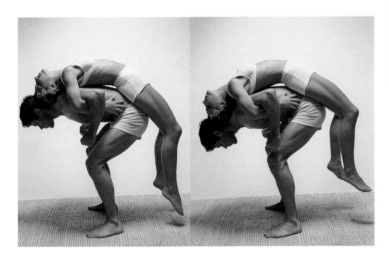

2 | LOWER YOUR TORSO

Begin to lower your torso to lift your partner's feet away from the ground so the full weight of her back is released towards your body. It is important for her shoulders and neck to remain relaxed. Move very slowly and in tune with her. Stay balanced on your feet and legs, and breathe easily.

3 | LIFTING OFF

As you lift her higher off the ground, her spine receives a good slow stretch. She should breathe fully into her chest and abdomen. Remain in this position for some moments, and then slowly put her back down, by extending gently upwards from your hips. Her feet need firm contact with the floor before you straighten up.

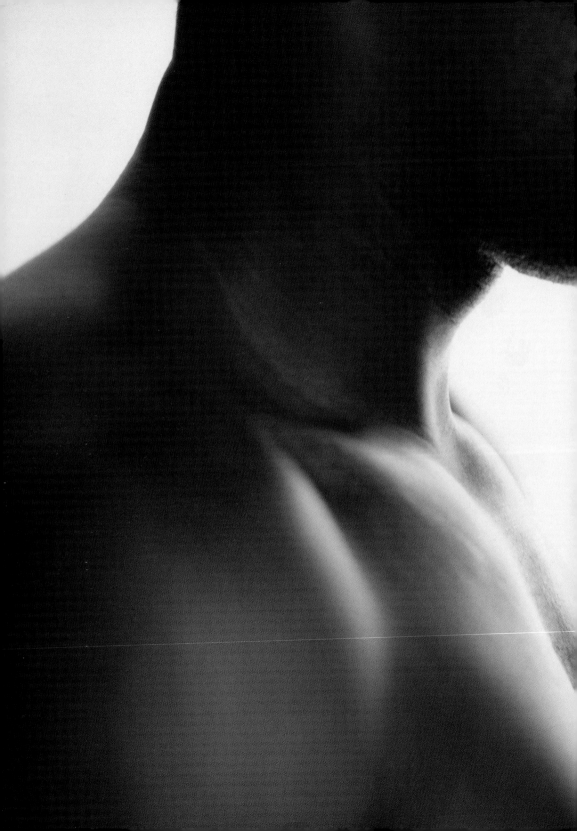

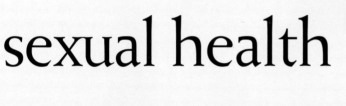

sexual health

Good sex involves caring for your body and respecting your partner's.
It includes taking responsibility for contraception, and practising safer
sex is a vital part of staying healthy.

sexual health awareness

SEXUAL HEALTH AWARENESS is about developing a deeper understanding of the sexual self and discovering how the mind and body interact to achieve true fulfilment. It involves a commitment to a regular health regime, to include sexual hygiene, medical check-ups and a programme of physical and mental exercises, as well as an awareness of the sexual body and of the way it changes and develops at different stages throughout life. By following a sexual health awareness programme you can learn how to become attuned to your basic physical, emotional and psychological needs, thus helping you to achieve more satisfying and fulfilling relationships and a feeling of personal well-being.

The first step towards sexual health awareness is the confidence that comes with the knowledge that your body is clean and wholesome and free from illness and disease. This will help you to feel more relaxed in mind and body and boost your self-esteem because you will be able to feel assured that you are physically appealing to the opposite sex. Your sexual health routine should include an understanding of the way your sexual

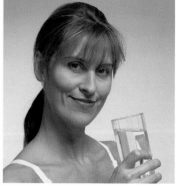

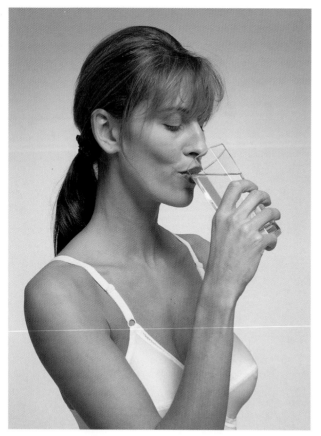

body looks and feels on a day-to-day level so that medical disorders, if they arise, are identified at an early stage, when they can be more easily treated. This approach is particularly important for a woman because the hormonal fluctuations that routinely occur throughout the menstrual cycle cause physical changes which may mask possible medical disorders unless she is totally in tune with the many different facets of her body.

sexual hygiene for women

The sense of smell is powerfully evocative and so it is to be expected that many women feel self-conscious about their natural aroma. In fact, this is an exaggerated worry as a woman's basic scent is a potent turn-on for men and does not need to be masked by pungent fragrances and perfumes. Plain water and a mild unscented soap are perfectly adequate for daily washing.

Many women are over-zealous about their sexual hygiene, often scrubbing too vigorously and using highly scented, antiseptic soaps, bath salts and bubble baths. These preparations can cause skin irritation and may even lead to an allergic reaction in serious cases. It is only necessary for women to wash the external part of the genitalia, as the vagina itself is self-cleansing. In particular, douches or vaginal deodorants are to be avoided, except on medical advice, as these can irritate the vagina's sensitive lining, and upset its delicate bacterial and chemical balance. This can lead to conditions such as thrush (candidiasis).

The most important sexual hygiene rule is to always wash the bottom from front to back, to avoid spreading infection. If you use flannels, keep one solely for the genital/anal area, be sure to wash it out after use and leave it open on a radiator to dry thoroughly. A damp flannel provides a perfect breeding ground for germs.

It is important to learn the look and pattern of your normal vaginal secretions so that you can recognize if an abnormal pattern develops. These secretions usually increase during sexual arousal and at the mid-point in the menstrual cycle, around the time of ovulation.

If you develop a discharge that seems out of the ordinary, particularly if it is accompanied by soreness or itching of the genital area, it may indicate an infection, and you should see a doctor as soon as possible.

Signs of infection include a copious watery secretion that is greenish or greyish in colour, possibly with a fishy smell, or a discharge that has the creamy consistency of cottage cheese. Other signs include sores, inflammation, rash, pain in the lower abdomen, pain or discomfort when urinating, and blood in the urine. You should avoid having sex until the condition has been identified and successfully treated.

Some sexually transmitted diseases cause symptoms in men but not in women, although

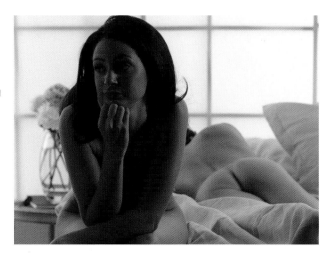

they may still lead to infertility or other serious conditions. If a sexual partner complains of symptoms such as difficulty urinating or abnormal discharge from the penis, encourage him to see his doctor and also seek medical advice yourself.

Because the urethra, the tube that carries urine out of the body, is so much shorter in women they are at much greater risk of infections spreading to the bladder, causing the painful condition cystitis. Sufferers develop a pain in the lower abdomen and find urination painful. In severe cases the urine may be cloudy and the woman may feel feverish. Cystitis can also be caused by soaps, gels and deodorants and even by bruising as a result of over-enthusiastic lovemaking.

Always see your doctor if the symptoms are severe or persist for longer than a few days as the condition may lead to kidney infection, if left untreated. In the meantime, drink plenty of fluid, and ask your doctor or pharmicist to recommend a suitable painkiller. A hot-water bottle held against the abdomen may help to ease the pain. If you do not suffer from high blood pressure, drinking a solution of baking powder (sodium bicarbonate) can reduce the acidity in the urine and ease the stinging sensation as well as helping to flush out any bacteria, or there are several over-the-counter medicines that may help.

ABOVE | If intercourse is painful, you may need to see a doctor.

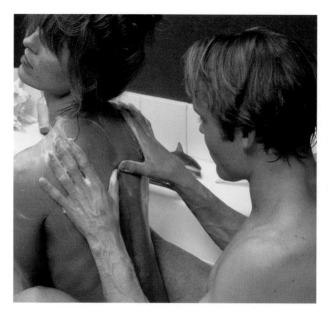

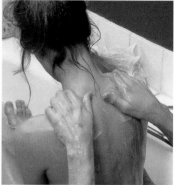

LEFT AND ABOVE | Bath-time is a good time for both sensual exploration and making regular health checks.

sexual hygiene for men

While the natural musky male smell is attractive to many women, the basic masculine aroma should not be confused with the odour of an unwashed body, which is a positive turn-off. Fresh sweat has no smell, but after six hours bacteria on the skin act on sweat causing the release of unpleasant odours. A regular shower or bath is necessary, and it is particularly important to wash the anal and genital area daily, or more often if necessary.

Uncircumcised men should take particular care to wash the glans (head of the penis) regularly, pulling back the foreskin to ensure it is really clean. This is necessary to prevent the build-up of an oily secretion called smegma which develops under the foreskin.

Smegma is a white substance produced by the sebaceous – or oil-producing – glands under the foreskin that helps it to retract smoothly. Without regular washing, smegma can build up and become a source of infection, which can lead to inflammation of the glans, a condition known as *balanitis*. It has also been linked with cancer of the penis and may be a possible cause of cervical cancer in female partners.

Men should also be alert to any signs which could indicate a sexually transmitted disease, or other serious condition. Signs of infection include pain or discomfort when urinating, abnormal discharge from the penis, or inflammation, sores or a rash around the genitals. It is important to seek medical advice immediately if you notice any of these signs because delay can lead to a worsening of the condition and risks infertility. Abstain from sex until the condition has been identified and successfully treated.

testicular awareness

Just as women should learn to recognize the normal shape and feel of their breasts so that abnormalities can be detected straight away, men, too, should get into the habit of examining their testicles regularly so that they can spot a cancerous growth or other problem as early as possible to increase the likelihood of effective treatment.

Testicular cancer is one of the most common cancers in men in the 20–34 age range. It does not usually cause any pain in the early stages and so self-examination is vital if it is to be detected.

However, most lumps turn out to be benign conditions, such as a harmless cyst. You should not notice any pain during the examination, provided you are not squeezing too hard, but if there is discomfort, especially if you notice any swelling, you should seek medical advice. There are several conditions that could cause pain and swelling in the testicles, such as infection or injury, that are unconnected with cancer but which may still require treatment. A simple testicular examination takes only a few minutes and is best carried out during a warm bath or shower while the scrotal skin is most relaxed.

testicular self-examination

Make a point of examining your testicles once a month while you are having a bath or shower. Ensure the scrotum is well-covered with soapy lather and then roll each testicle gently between the fingers of both hands. Learn to recognize its normal shape and consistency. Carefully probe for any pea-sized lumps, or nodules, or any swelling or other changes. After your bath or shower, stand in front of a full-length mirror, hold your penis up out of the way and carry out a visual inspection of your scrotum looking for any change in size and shape. Be aware of any pain or sensations of heaviness in the groin or lower abdomen. Report any problems to your doctor.

LEFT | Regular self-examination is as important for men as it is for women.

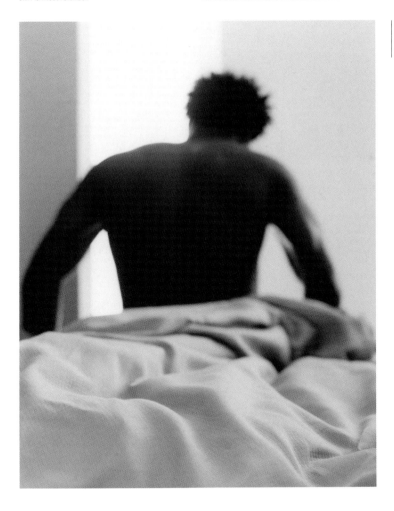

breast care

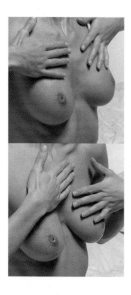

ABOVE | Breasts are a major sexual characteristic and are central to a woman's femininity. Learn to examine your breasts regularly for lumps or any signs of change, and use a rich moisturizer to help keep the skin supple. To avoid sagging, use an upward motion, as you would on your face.

Caring for your breasts should be an important part of your sexual health regime. Managing your stress levels, and keeping to a diet that is low in saturated fats and refined sugar is thought to promote healthy breasts. Exercise can help strengthen the underlying muscle and so help prevent sagging, although the best way to keep breasts firm is to wear a well-fitting support bra, particularly when playing sport, or during pregnancy and when breastfeeding.

Change your bra size as often as seems necessary and be sure to try a bra on before you buy it. A surprising number of women wear a bra that does not fit properly. After washing your breasts, pat them dry with an upward motion to prevent sagging and use a moisturizer to help keep the skin smooth and supple – again using upward movements.

The breasts usually become slightly enlarged in the second half of the menstrual cycle, mainly as a result of hormonal changes, giving a sensation of heaviness and fullness. They may also feel lumpy. One-third of women suffer breast tenderness as a result of these hormonal changes, which can make many activities, including sport, lovemaking and even walking up stairs, very uncomfortable. A cause of this is benign breast disease (see below), but the pain may also be due to a bruised or strained chest muscle.

Self-help measures include cutting down on stimulant drinks, such as tea or coffee, and taking evening primrose capsules and vitamin B6 (pyridoxine) in the second half of the menstrual cycle. Wearing a support bra day and night might also help. If the pain persists, or affects one side only, you should see your doctor.

breast awareness

Breast cancer is the most common form of cancer in women and is most likely to be successfully treated if it is diagnosed at an early stage. Many breast cancers are first detected by the woman

herself, so it is important to get to know the normal shape and feel of your breasts throughout the menstrual cycle.

Benign, or harmless, breast lumps are far more common than malignant, or cancerous, ones. The most common type of lump is a cyst in a blocked gland or duct. Such lumps are most likely to occur in the second half of the menstrual cycle and they usually subside completely after a while. Monthly lumpiness which does not go away, especially if it is tender, is called benign breast disease. This condition, although harmless, may be very painful.

breast self-examination

Get into the habit of carrying out a monthly breast examination. If you menstruate, a good time to do this is a week after the first day of your period. Undress to the waist and, with your arms at your sides, inspect your breasts in the mirror, from the side as well as the front. Look for any changes of appearance, such as changes in the outline, puckering or dimpling of the skin (like orange peel). Squeeze the nipple to check for bleeding or discharge.

Next, raise your hands over your head and look to see if any puckering or dimpling appears. Put your hands on your hips and push, again looking for puckering or dimpling.

Now, examine your breasts while lying down on the bed. Place a folded towel under one shoulder and raise your arm on that side above your head to stretch the breast. With the flat of the hand only, gently feel the breast using a circular movement and working from the outer edge to the nipple. Also feel for lumps under the armpit. Repeat with the other breast.

Another form of benign breast lump is a fibroadenoma, or fibrous tumour, sometimes known as a "breast mouse" because it can be moved around in the breast tissue. A malignant lump is usually not tender and is not mobile.

Because the breasts alter in size and lumpiness throughout the menstrual cycle, it is important to examine your breasts regularly so that you become familiar with these changes. All breasts have normally lumpy areas – so try to discover what is normal for you. During a shower or bath is a good time, particularly when the breasts are soapy.

In addition, at least once a month, you should examine your breasts more systematically. Aim to do this at the same time in your menstrual cycle.

If you notice any abnormalities, contact your doctor as soon as possible. If a lump does turn out to be malignant there is a far better chance of a cure if it is detected early.

medical screening for women

Many conditions affecting women can be diagnosed early through regular medical screening checks. One of the most important of these is a cervical smear test which can detect cells that will become cancerous before other signs would become apparent. Treatment at this pre-cancerous stage is fairly simple and has a high success rate. During a smear test, a thin layer of cells is scraped from the cervix and smeared on to a glass slide so they can be examined under a microscope. If abnormal cells are found there will be follow-up tests and, if necessary, treatment.

Doctors recommend that women have a cervical smear test at least every three years. But those in high-risk groups should have annual tests. Women most at risk include those suffering from genital warts (or whose partners have the condition), smokers, and those with multiple sexual partners or who began an active sex life at an early age.

Smear tests are often carried out during routine gynaecological check-ups. During the examination, the doctor will look at the external genital area and into the vagina to check for

signs of infection or other abnormalities. The doctor will also feel the lower abdomen to detect possible swelling or tenderness which might indicate a disorder.

Women should also have a breast examination by their doctor at least every three years, if under 40, or annually, if older. Women over the age of 50 are usually screened for breast cancer every three years using a form of X-ray called mammography. However, this method of screening is less effective in younger women because their breast tissue is more dense and any growths do not show up as clearly on the X-ray.

ABOVE | Many breast lumps are benign, or harmless. Get any lumps checked out by a doctor immediately to avoid any unnecessary worry.

safer sex

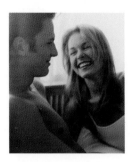

ABOVE | Many men and women have longed for a return to old-fashioned courtship. As awareness grows around safer sex issues, romance is coming back into fashion. The wish to form monogamous relationships is popular again. Many couples now prefer to become better acquainted with each other before embarking on full sexual intimacy. Casual encounters or multiple sex partners are definitely not a good idea in terms of safer sex, and this provides an excellent excuse to modify sexual behaviour if you have previously allowed yourself to be pressured into casual sexual encounters.

RIGHT | Kissing, cuddling and hugging are safer sex practices through which new partners can discover if they are physically and sexually attuned.

NOWADAYS, THE PHRASE "SAFER SEX" is generally used wherever sexuality is written or spoken about. Safer sex practices help lovers to care for their own and each other's health while enjoying an exciting and joyful sex life. The term "safer sex" generally refers to all sexual activity which avoids the exchange of body fluids, such as semen, vaginal juices and blood, between partners. It is a way of modifying sexual practices to help prevent the risk of infection from the HIV virus and other sexually transmitted infections. Safer sex practices apply to all members of the community, both homosexual and heterosexual.

Safer sex is essential to the art of love at the present time when the HIV/AIDS virus continues to spread through the world's heterosexual and homosexual population. HIV can remain in an otherwise healthy person for many years without causing symptoms, and any sexual acts that involve contact with the person's blood, semen or vaginal fluids put lovers at risk of catching the disease.

Safer sex means taking adequate precautions against the exchange of these body fluids, and abstaining from high-risk sexual activities which allow this to happen. For instance, the sensual and erotic massage programmes described in this book are examples of safer sex practices.

If you are making love with your partner in any way that involves penetrative sex, then you should consider using condoms. If used correctly, condoms reduce the risk of the spread of the HIV virus and other sexually transmitted diseases. Initially, you may feel that condoms inhibit the spontaneity of lovemaking, but by simply knowing they are the best method available of protecting yourself and your partner, you can begin to consider them as an integral part of lovemaking. Safer sex, like massage, is a way of showing how much you care for the well-being of the body, mind and spirit of both yourself and your lover.

how to discuss safer sex

Anyone who is contemplating a sexual relationship, or who is already involved in one, should consider safer sex. However, since sexual issues are invariably difficult to discuss, you may find it embarrassing to raise the subject of safer sex practices or to reach an agreement about it with a new partner.

The best way forward is to develop a clear, responsible attitude towards your own health and sexual practices, rather than relying on anyone else's responses. This clarity will enable you to stand firm on your decisions, and may also help your partner to resolve his or her own conflicts.

If you meet a negative response, be patient but firm. Your partner may believe, mistakenly, that safer sex practices are relevant only to people who belong to high-risk groups. He or she may insist that they have had only a few sexual partners and, therefore, present no risk. The truth is that it is often impossible to know the sexual history of all the other people who have been linked in a sexual chain of partners.

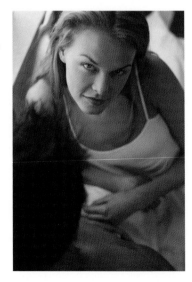

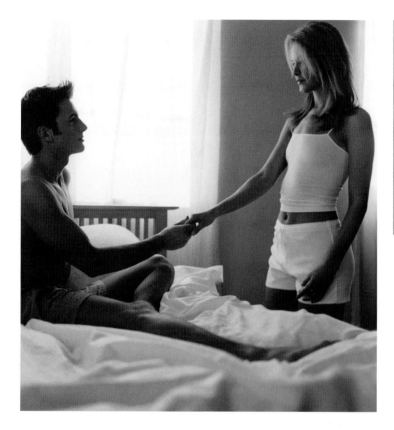

For instance, a previous lover may have had a relationship with someone who, at another time, had sex, unknowingly, with a person from an HIV high-risk group. Making love only once with someone who carries the HIV virus presents sufficient risk of becoming infected yourself. People can be HIV-infected without knowing it and remain in good health for a very long period of time, showing no outward sign of the infection. Also, there are many other sexually transmitted diseases which need to be considered and many people do not show symptoms, especially in cases of chlamydia, which can cause infertility in women if left untreated.

Some women, in particular, find it difficult to assert themselves in sexual issues. Old attitudes persist, despite the dramatic changes in sexual mores and gender roles over the last few decades.

Women are still generally more conditioned than men to please others, and often feel shy to take the initiative on safer sex issues, particularly if there is resistance. As a woman, you may be worried that you will be deemed too sexually forward if you produce a packet of condoms at the opportune moment.

Remind yourself that you have as much right to self-determination over your sexual health as you would, nowadays, expect to have over your choices of contraception.

The bottom line is: if you want to use safer sex methods and your potential lover refuses, for whatever reason, you will need to delay any sexual activity involving the exchange of body fluids until you have reached a mutual agreement; or even be prepared to forgo a full sexual relationship with that person.

long-term relationships

If you are already in an established relationship, you may believe that you do not need to consider safer sex issues. This is so only if the relationship is truly monogamous and you are both absolutely sure of the safety of each other's sexual and drug-related past. For the various reasons mentioned before, it is virtually impossible to know the whole truth because you can rarely vouch for the sexual history of all previous partners who have been linked by sexual activity. As a couple, you should examine and discuss all the implications involved before making a decision on whether or not to start or abandon safer sex practices.

the HIV test

The HIV antibody can take up to three months to develop and be detected in a blood test after the virus has been transmitted. HIV testing is one possibility for couples who are willing to commit and be monogamous with each other, and who want a sexual relationship without using safer sex practices. There are, however, quite contrasting professional views as to whether this is an advisable or necessary step to take.

It is not a decision to be taken lightly, and all people testing for HIV should first receive proper counselling as to its advisability in their particular situation. This help can usually be obtained from health specialists attached to sexually transmitted infection clinics or specialized hospital departments. The decision to test for HIV must be an individual one, and no one should allow themselves to be coerced into taking it.

risky behaviour

While considering safer sex issues, it is important not to become over-anxious or alarmist. The HIV virus has a low infectivity rate, cannot survive long outside the human body, and is spread only when it enters the bloodstream through the exchange of body fluids. You cannot catch it from sharing utensils such as cups, knives and forks with an infected person, or from normal physical contact such as hugging or holding hands.

Transmission of the virus from sexual activity is only possible if either you or your partner are already infected.

However, it is essential for all sexually active people to become well acquainted with the facts of the disease and to put into practice safer sex methods whenever there is even the slight risk of infection.

The following activities are considered to present the highest risk:
- Anal intercourse without condoms: The blood vessels in the rectum can easily rupture with the friction of sexual activity, creating a high risk of infection if one or other partner carries the virus.

BELOW | Close physical contact which does not involve the exchange of body fluids is perfectly safe. You can caress and explore each other's bodies with peace of mind.

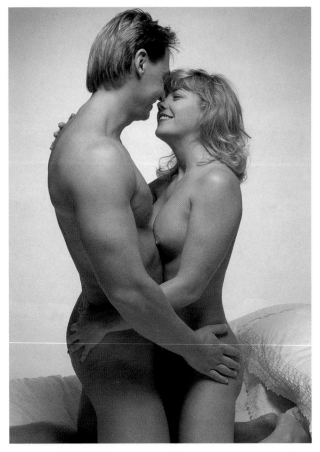

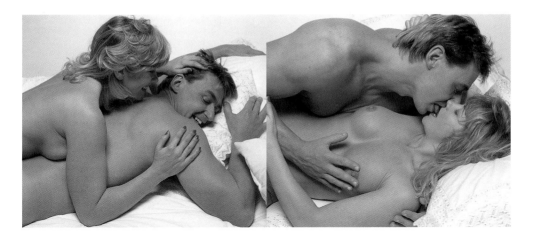

• Vaginal intercourse without condoms: Vaginal fluids and semen can both contain the HIV virus, as can the menstrual blood flow. Broken blood vessels, and small abrasions either in the vagina or on the penis can allow the virus to enter the bloodstream.

• Multiple partners and casual sex: The more sexual partners someone has, the greater exposure to the risk of infection. In the case of casual sex affairs, it is unlikely that you will know the full sexual history of that person.

• Sharing needles: Anyone who has been an intravenous drug user and has ever shared a contaminated syringe or needle with another person has a high risk of HIV infection. That person's sexual partners are also at risk if safer sex precautions are not used.

The following sexual activities carry less but still some risk of infection:

• Oral sex: The HIV virus in semen and vaginal fluids will normally be destroyed by stomach acids if ingested. However, the risk of infection increases if the partner giving fellatio or cunnilingus has any small cuts, sores or ulcers in the mouth, or bleeding gums. To minimize risk, condoms should be used during fellatio and latex barriers can be used during cunnilingus.

• Intercourse with condoms: The use of condoms and other barrier methods reduces the risk of

disease transmission by 98 per cent, so long as all the safer sex precautions are used. The risk lies in not following the proper procedures for barrier method protection, or in the accidental tearing of the rubber causing a spillage of semen or vaginal fluids.

• Sharing sex toys: You should not share a sex toy with your partner because of the risk of cross-infection.

safer sex activities

The following suggestions should present no risk so long as there are no open sores or cuts to the skin which could allow cross-infection. To be extra safe, cover any open wounds on the skin, however small, with adhesive plaster.

• Cuddling, hugging and caressing: These are all perfectly safe and wonderful ways to make physical contact.

• Kissing: Mouth to mouth or dry kissing is fine. Deep or "French" kissing and saliva exchange is only minimally risky if there are open cuts, bleeding gums or ulcers in the mouth.

• Licking, nibbling and sucking: Go ahead and enjoy yourselves, but ensure that you do not bite so hard that you break the skin.

• Masturbation: Self-masturbation is fine. So is mutual masturbation, so long as you take care that body fluids do not penetrate the skin. Keep all skin abrasions covered.

ABOVE LEFT | Safer sex need not mean boring sex. Couples can explore and enjoy a whole range of exciting sensual and sexual practices. By stroking, massaging and caressing each other you will become more familiar with your partner's body and its unique erogenous responses.

ABOVE | Kissing, licking, nuzzling and touching are all safer sex practices which can only add greater pleasure to your sexual relationship as well as extending your range of foreplay techniques. As your relationship develops, you will learn how your lover likes to be caressed.

sexually transmitted infections

THE MAIN CONTRIBUTORS to unsafe sex are drugs and alcohol, which prevent normally sane adults from making responsible decisions. Many sexual encounters happen when the protagonists are either inebriated or high, which enhances their libido but definitely impairs their judgement and performance.

There have been plenty of awareness campaigns in recent years about the dangers of being infected with the HIV virus and the need to practise safer sex. But HIV is only one of a number of infections that can be caught through engaging in unprotected sex – gay or straight. A passionate situation can develop at any time and it is worth remembering that people with a sexually transmitted infection look just like anybody else and may not say a word about it.

What many people still fail to realize is that many STIs can be contracted without penetrative sex. While condoms will protect you from STIs contracted through exchange of bodily fluids, they will not protect you against herpes, warts, pubic lice and scabies.

With sex between two women, the same principles apply. The use of a dental dam or condoms (if they are using dildos) is recommended as protection against the exchange of bodily fluids. Remember STIs can also be transmitted by sex toys.

When HIV and AIDS first came to public notice there was increased awareness of the need for safer sex, but there is now a developing tendency towards complacency. It is still vital to protect against STIs with condoms and dental dams.

Many people haven't a clue that they have contracted an STI. Sometimes there are no outward symptoms, such as with chlamydia, which may have disastrous effects. However, there are many other infections that do leave their calling card.

signs to look for

If you have any of these symptoms, check them out with your doctor:
- Blisters or bumps around the genital area or anywhere from your navel to your knees. Sometimes they are very painful.
- Persistent flu-like symptoms and painful urination.
- Burning or discoloured discharge from the vagina or penis, abnormal bleeding or pelvic pain, pain in the groin, stomach or testicles.
- Yellowing of the skin or whites of eyes, nausea, fever, discoloration of faeces or urine, itchy sores wherever there is hair on the body, itchy genitals, foul-smelling discharge.

If you display any of these symptoms, a trip to the doctor or GU (genito-urinary) clinic, however embarrassing, may be a life-saver or prevent you from becoming sterile. We all know our bodies pretty well, so anything that you think may not be normal should be checked.

human papilloma virus

There are over 50 strains of HPV. Some cause genital warts and the more dangerous ones can cause cervical cancer. HPV is spread by having vaginal or anal intercourse with an infected person. The warts are small painless cauliflower-like lumps that appear on the vulva, vagina, penis or anus. The doctor can successfully remove them, but you do need to take care of yourself and have regular check-ups as condoms are not complete protection.

BELOW | If you can't face having to tell other partners in person that you have an infection, some sexual health clinics provide a contact slip, which you can send anonymously and which, in turn, can be presented at any other clinic. The code will let the staff know precisely what they are looking for.

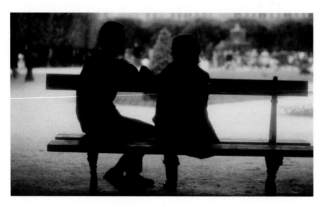

chlamydia

This is the commonest type of STI in the UK and USA. It causes widespread infection in the genital tracts of both men and women, but especially women. It can cause inflammation of the uterine neck, blockage of the fallopian tubes and inflammation of the glands that produce sexual fluids. In men it can cause inflammation of the urethra or tubular part of the testicles and joint or eye disorders in extreme cases. In women it often displays no symptoms but can lead to infertility, highlighting the necessity for regular gynaecological check-ups. If caught in the early stages it is easily rectified with antibiotics. If left, it can cause trachoma, which is a serious eye infection that can lead to blindness and from which 500 million people suffer today.

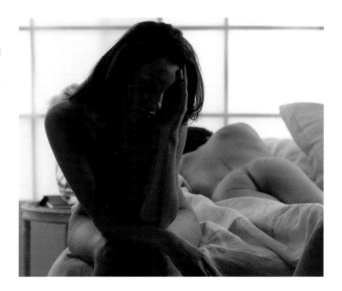

gonorrhoea

This is caused by the passing of bacteria from an infected individual which leads to infection that can spread via the bloodstream. It may not show any symptoms for a while, with an incubation period of two to ten days, and even after this no clear symptoms may present themselves.

Men may find discomfort when they urinate, or a whitish-yellowish discharge from the penis. Women may experience a green or yellow vaginal discharge, abdominal pain or disrupted menstruation patterns. If it is left untreated, gonorrhoea can lead to pelvic inflammatory disease (PID), or may close the fallopian tubes, causing infertility.

syphilis

This disease has become more common in men than in women over recent years and the majority of new cases occur in homosexual males. One-third of untreated sufferers die from brain, nerve or heart damage. It has an incubation period of about three weeks and can be treated successfully in its early phases with antibiotics. If it is untreated, a recurring bout can occur up to ten years later. The symptoms usually appear on the skin in rash-like lesions called chancres, which are painless.

genital herpes

This can be a completely symptom-free infection that is passed through genital contact with a partner who has an area of infection. Men may discover blisters on the penis, scrotum or surrounding area (blisters can be found on the navel and upper and lower thighs), which are often painful. Women may discover red bumps, which will turn into painful blisters. These are usually discovered in the labial folds, but can also be present in the cervix, anus or navel. Herpes can also induce flu-like symptoms in both men and women. Herpes has been associated with cervical cancer so if you find you are infected, it is important to follow treatment up with a smear.

hepatitis A, B and C

Hepatitis is an infection affecting the liver, and can be associated with excessive alcohol, drug or chemical consumption or infection by viruses. Hepatitis A is not usually transmitted through penetrative sex, but can be through anal sex. Hepatitis B is passed on via semen, mucus or blood. Hepatitis C is similar to B but is blood-borne so transmission is more common through sharing needles. Hepatitis B and C have incubation periods lasting from six weeks to six months, and may

ABOVE | A trip to your local sexual health clinic is the best way to deal with any fears that you may have about having contracted an STI. No matter how embarrassing it may be for you, you are merely one of thousands of people they help each week.

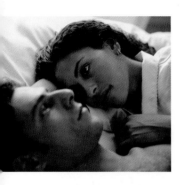

show either no symptoms or very severe ones. Symptoms for both include the yellowing of the skin, increased fatigue, darker urine and paler faeces. Unfortunately, like HIV and AIDS, it is caused by a virus and so there is no cure for hepatitis at the moment, although there are drug treatments available to help control the symptoms.

yeast infections

These are fairly common among women. Symptoms usually include itchy genitalia and a dense, clotted whitish discharge from the vagina. Yeast infections are not necessarily sexually transmitted but can be caused by antibiotics and wearing tight-fitting synthetic clothing that does not allow the skin to breathe. Men can suffer from yeast infections too, but it is less common.

Bacterial vaginosis (BV) has similar symptoms but the discharge usually has a fishy smell and is creamier. BV may also cause pain when urinating. Trichomoniasis affects men in their urethra and women usually in the vagina. It can have no symptoms, but a smelly discharge or pain when urinating can be a sign.

pubic lice (crabs) and scabies

These are particularly nasty little mites that are horrendously contagious. Scabies burrow under the skin of an infected individual, causing itchy sores, and crab lice congregate mainly in hairy areas of the body, usually the pubic area. Your pharmacist (druggist) or doctor can advise you on treatment but it is also important to wash all your clothes at a very high temperature. Anything that cannot be washed should be vacuum-packed in plastic for at least two weeks.

HIV and AIDS

Human Immunodeficiency Virus (HIV) is the primary virus that leads to Acquired Immunodeficiency Syndrome (AIDS). Since the 1980s epidemic, many have died. The reported number of people with HIV in industrialized countries increases each year because of the greater accuracy of diagnosis and decreasing deaths due to antiretroviral therapies. However, many cases are not diagnosed.

The majority of infections first reported are thought to have occurred through sex between men. After an initial reduction in new cases, increasing numbers of diagnoses are now occurring again each year. It is estimated that a quarter of HIV-infected men who have sex with other men have not been diagnosed.

Since 1999, there has been more diagnosis of heterosexual-acquired infection in First World countries, although 80 per cent of cases were infected elsewhere, particularly in Africa. Globally, women are becoming increasingly affected by HIV. Approximately 50 per cent, or 19.2 million, of the 38.6 million adults currently living with HIV or AIDS worldwide are women.

It is important that people are aware of HIV and AIDS, which is spread through exchange of bodily fluids such as semen, vaginal secretions and blood and very, very rarely through saliva. The effect AIDS has on the body is that it gradually breaks down the body's natural defence mechanisms until eventually it is no longer able to fight infection. This results in infected people dying from relatively simple and usually easily treatable infections, such as the flu or, particularly commonly, pneumonia.

The symptoms are often difficult to identify. In the first few weeks, only about half of infected people suffer from flu-like symptoms, such as fevers, tiredness or swollen glands. This is usually when the person is carrying HIV and doctors use combination drug therapies to keep people in this relatively "healthy" phase for as long as possible. If HIV progresses to AIDS, then the individual is liable to get much more ill, with consistently swollen glands, chronic diarrhoea, weight loss, fever and the development of skin lesions.

It is important – vital in fact – that people are constantly reminded of the risk, regardless of their sexuality, as it is still a very real, worrying and distressing problem. The main weapon against AIDS is education and myth-busting. It is not an act of some retributive deity punishing the human race for its sexual actions; it is a disease that can be prevented from spreading. The message is: use condoms.

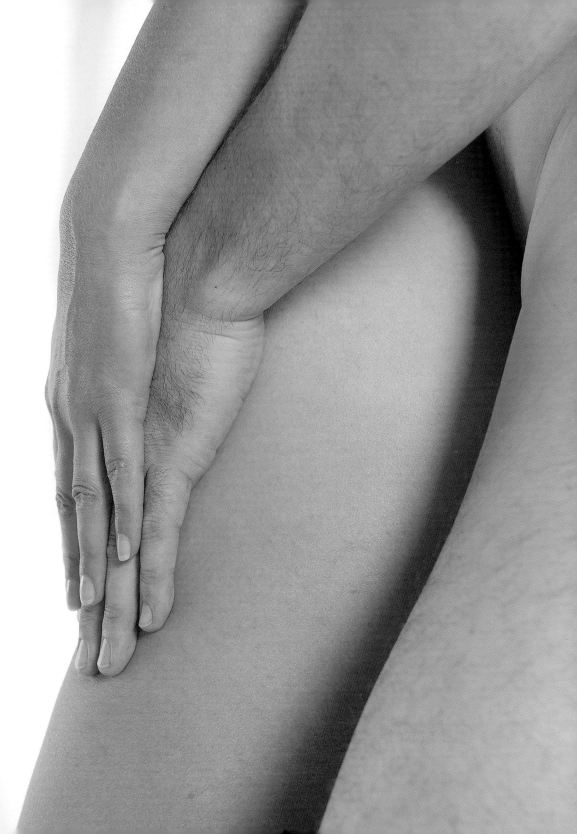

contraception and safer sex

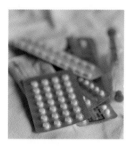

ABOVE | As well as the female pill, new male contraceptives are under development in the form of a transdermal gel and patch that rely on MENT™ (7a-methyl-19-nortestosterone), a synthetic steroid that resembles testosterone but lacks the unwanted side effect of an enlarged prostate.

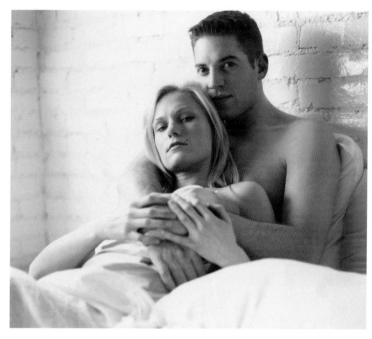

sex education

A survey carried out for the sexual health charity Marie Stopes International revealed that one in five parents believed their children would find out about sex for themselves.

Research has shown that one-third of under-16s are sexually active and every year 15,000 girls under 18 have an abortion. It is known that parents who discuss sex openly with their children will have more sexually responsible children who are less inclined to lose their virginity because of peer pressure.

CONTRACEPTION AND SAFER SEX precautions should be paramount to everyone who has sex, not just people who do not want to have babies. Everyone should have been told about the importance of safer sex and should be well aware of the measures that can be taken, but for some reason too many people are still willing to take the risk. As with so many things that are good in life, there is a downside. Just as cake can make you fat and alcohol gives you a hangover, sex can make you sick. And it starts from the first kiss. Even a seemingly innocent little kiss can lead to herpes viruses that never go away.

It is fairly hard to avoid this, but when beginning a new relationship it is important to evaluate what type of person it is that you intend to get intimate with. Never assume that other people are as responsible with their bodies as you are. You have no way of knowing their previous history and, in many cases, infection and disease is passed on unknowingly as many diseases can be carried without showing noticeable symptoms.

When deciding on suitable contraception methods there are several factors that should be considered: age, lifestyle, health, whether you have children, and whether you may want to have children in the future. The important thing to remember is that contraception is for *everyone*, whether male, female, married or single. When you are in a relationship, contraception should be seen as a mutual project and not the responsibility of the man or woman alone. Bearing this in mind will lead to a more fulfilling love life and a trusting partnership.

No contraceptive is 100 per cent effective but many are close. For extra peace of mind you can always use more than one product – such as the contraceptive pill combined with condoms.

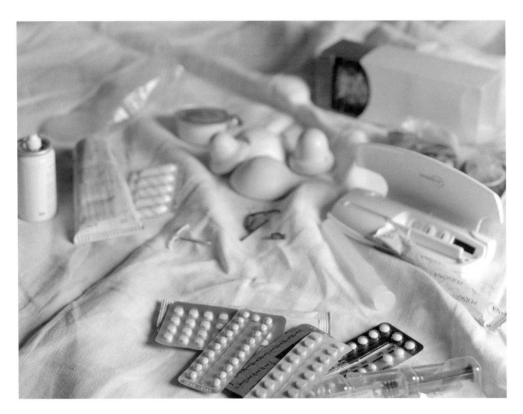

hormonal methods

The contraceptive pill is hormone-controlled contraception, which is either in the form of the combined pill or the progesterone-only pill.

The combined pill combines the two hormones oestrogen and progesterone to prevent the monthly release of an egg from the woman's ovary. If taken correctly, the combined pill is 99 per cent effective.

There is increasing evidence to support the theory that the pill may offer some protection against uterine or ovarian cancer. However, it is not always suitable for women who have conditions such as high blood pressure, circulatory disease or diabetes. Women over 35 who smoke or are overweight are usually advised to use another form of contraception.

The progesterone-only pill is also known as the minipill. The progesterone causes cervical mucus to form a thick barrier which prevents sperm from entering the uterus; it also makes the uterine lining thinner to prevent fertilized eggs from attaching to the wall. The minipill is advised for breastfeeding mothers, older women and women who smoke. This method is 98 per cent effective if taken correctly.

For longer-acting contraception, an injection is now available which is 99 per cent effective. It slowly releases progesterone into the body, preventing ovulation. Each injection lasts for 8–12 weeks. Side effects can include continual menstruation or no menstruation at all.

Implanon is a progesterone implant, which releases progesterone into the body. It is 99 per cent effective and lasts for three years, but can lead to irregular periods or cause them to stop altogether. Hormonal methods do not provide protection against sexually transmitted infections, so should be used with a barrier method.

ABOVE AND OPPOSITE |
The variety of contraceptives available on the market today means you do not have to remain with any contraception that does not suit you. Discuss any side effects, likes or dislikes with your partner and your doctor.

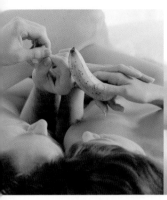
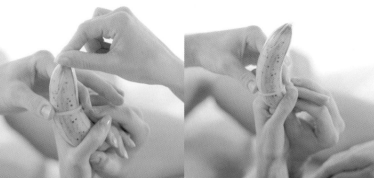

ABOVE | If you or your partner
have never used a condom
before, why not try putting
one on a banana or cucumber
before trying the real thing?
It is important to exclude the
air from the bubble on top,
otherwise it may burst later on.

barrier methods

Condoms are the most common forms of barrier method. If used properly they are 94–98 per cent effective, but always make sure they carry an official approval symbol. Condoms are usually made of latex or rubber and work by being placed over the erect penis. They should be placed on as soon as the penis is erect because it can drip semen before ejaculation. Although robust, they must be used with care as they can split or come off. Men must withdraw as soon as they ejaculate and make sure that they do not spill any semen.

Semen has immuno-suppressant qualities. These are important for vaginal penetration as they allow the sperm to enter the vaginal canal without being attacked by the woman's immune system. When sperm is swallowed, stomach acids break down these properties. Little is known about the effects they have in the anal passage so it is important to use condoms when performing anal sex, as well as to protect against sexually transmitted infections (STIs) such as HIV and AIDs. Anal sex without a condom can also result in faecal matter and bacteria becoming trapped in the man's urethral opening, which may not be removed by washing. This can lead to infections in the man, and in the woman if vaginal penetration follows anal sex.

Using lubrication or contraceptive jelly with condoms can also help prevent female urinary tract infections. Make sure you do not use oil-based products such as petroleum jelly, however, as they reduce the effectiveness of condoms by 90 per cent; water-based lubricants are best.

RIGHT | Condoms have a
high rate of effectiveness
as contraceptives and also
protect against sexually
transmitted infections.
However, they can tear,
burst or simply slip off.

FAR RIGHT | It is always
important to take extra care
when removing a condom
from its packaging to ensure
that your nails do not damage
it in any way.

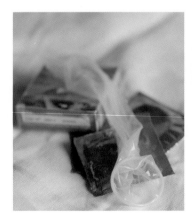
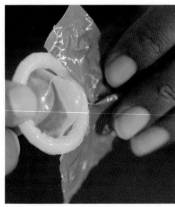

Female condoms are made of quite thin polyurethane plastic. They fit inside the vagina and around the surrounding area to prevent sperm from entering the vaginal environment. If used correctly, they are 95 per cent effective, but it is important that the penis enters the condom and does not get between the condom and the vagina, or it will fail to protect.

The diaphragm or cap is another method of barrier contraceptive, and is 92–96 per cent effective. It is a rubber dome that fits over the woman's cervix to prevent sperm from entering the uterus. It must be used in conjunction with spermicidal jelly or pessaries and should stay in place for six hours after sex. Your doctor will be able to measure you for the correct size and teach you how to insert it. This barrier method does not protect you from STIs, such as HIV and AIDS.

The dental dam is a very thin sheet of latex that is laid flat, covering the entire vulva and anal area. It is used in oral sex (anal or vaginal) by both gay and straight couples as a safer sex precaution to prevent transmission of STIs, although the risk can never be completely eliminated.

intrauterine methods

These methods of contraception fall into three categories: the intrauterine device (IUD), the intrauterine system (IUS) and the relatively new Gynefix. They all work in a similar way and are fitted, by a doctor, inside the uterus.

The IUD is a T-shaped plastic device that works by stopping the sperm from reaching the egg and preventing the egg from implanting in the uterus. IUDs can make periods heavier and more painful and are unsuitable for women who have more than one sexual partner as they can increase the risk of infection. Some women's bodies have rejected – and ejected – IUDs, but they have often not realized it until they became pregnant.

The IUS works in a similar way to the IUD, but contains the hormones progesterone and oestrogen, which are gradually released into the body. This system can reduce heavy periods and period pains and is over 99 per cent effective.

Gynefix works in a similar fashion to the IUD and IUS, except it has a more flexible frame. It is composed of a row of copper beads, which bend to fit snugly inside the uterus, and has a fine nylon thread attaching it to the uterine wall, so it is more secure and less likely to be expelled. It can also assist in relieving heavy and painful periods and has been shown to be more than 99 per cent effective as a contraceptive.

All three devices can remain inside a woman for up to five years and doctors teach women how to check for the threads of their IUDs or IUSs to make sure that they are still in place. This is critical and all women fitted with such devices should check regularly. None of them, however, protects against STIs, such as HIV and AIDS. So again, barrier methods are recommended.

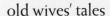

old wives' tales

Don't fall for myths that were exploded decades ago; people still do.

• Standing-up positions do not prevent a woman from conceiving.

• Breastfeeding reduces the likelihood of conceiving, but is by no means guaranteed to prevent it.

• Douches have no contraceptive effect and can increase the risk of infection in the woman.

• Jumping up and down after sex is just silly.

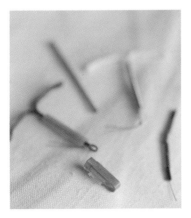

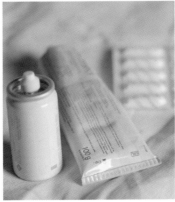

FAR LEFT | IUDs can last for five to ten years and are a good long-term contraceptive.

LEFT | A variety of spermicides are available in cream or pessary form.

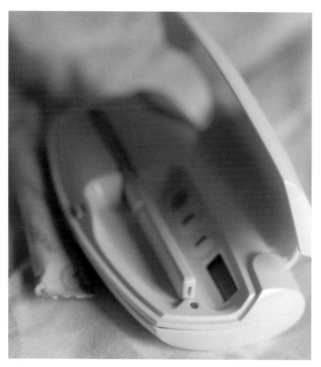

The sympto-thermal method involves taking the woman's temperature at waking every day and plotting the results on a chart. From these temperature changes, the time of ovulation can be calculated, and hence the times when the woman is more, or less, fertile. A special measuring device can be purchased to alleviate the need for complicated documentation.

Hormone testing monitors the levels in the woman's body to tell her which are her fertile days and which are not. A kit will contain disposable urine sample sticks and a hand-held monitor that displays a different colour when she is fertile and when she is not.

Checking dates and the longevity of the menstrual cycle may work better for women who have a regular cycle than those who don't. This method is best used in conjunction with another technique such as monitoring cervical secretions and other hormone-related changes such as breast changes or mood. Cervical secretions change in nature throughout a normal monthly cycle, with dryness directly after the bleeding phase and increased secretions during ovulation.

Many women prefer the natural method, as there are no side effects or chemicals involved. Its success relies not only on the organization and discipline of the couple but also may be affected by age, stress, illness, hormonal treatments, irregular periods and the menopause. Natural methods claim to be 94–98 per cent effective, as long as the instructions are carefully implemented. Once again, this form of contraception does not protect against STIs, such as HIV and AIDS.

natural methods

Using natural methods of contraception involves identifying the fertile days of the woman's menstrual cycle (the time from the first day of a period until the day before the next period starts) and abstaining from sex during these days or using another form of contraception. The fertile time is the time when she is ovulating (releasing an egg). Although the egg will only live for about 24 hours, sperm in a woman's body can survive for much longer, up to seven days in some instances, so sex a week before ovulation can still result in pregnancy.

Noting the different signs of ovulation can be done by using either a hormone-testing kit or the temperature method, or noting dates and cervical secretions. These methods are used as often by those attempting pregnancy as those seeking to avoid it and are more effective if the different methods are combined. If in any doubt about the efficacy of one of these natural methods, a barrier form of contraception should be used as well.

permanent methods

Male and female sterilization are permanent methods of contraception that some couples opt for if they believe they are sure they do not want children, or they already have all they want. They are not for people who may have doubts, however small, as they are usually not reversible.

Female sterilization is done by a doctor who makes a small incision below the navel to access the fallopian tubes, which are then either clipped, ringed or heat-treated to seal them. This prevents the sperm from meeting the egg. It is a relatively safe procedure that begins to work immediately and is 99 per cent effective.

Male sterilization seals the vas deferens, the tubes that carry the sperm to the penis from the testicles. When a man who has undergone vasectomy ejaculates, his ejaculate contains only semen and no sperm. Sperm continue to be produced but are merely reabsorbed. Unlike female sterilization, vasectomy takes a while to work, as there can often still be sperm in the semen for a few months after the procedure. It is necessary to use other contraceptives until the doctor gives the all-clear, and it is then considered to be 99 per cent effective. Neither male nor female sterilization provides protection against STIs, such as HIV or AIDS.

abortion

Many women become pregnant unintentionally and a surprisingly large proportion of these were using contraception of some sort. If you decide on termination, it is important to have a supportive circle of close friends or family to help. The availability of abortion varies from one country or state to another. The important thing to do is seek advice straight away from a reputable doctor or organization. If you do decide to have a termination, then it is best done early, when it's still a relatively simple procedure.

emergency contraception

It is possible to obtain the emergency contraceptive pill over the counter at a chemist's (drugstore) or from your doctor. It is expensive and is not the best method of contraception, but everyone can make mistakes: condoms split or slip off and sometimes people suffer from temporary insanity and don't use anything at all.

This emergency measure must be taken within 72 hours of unprotected sex, in the form of two pills, one 12 hours after the other. The pill may stop an egg from being released, prevent sperm from reaching the egg, or prevent the egg from implanting in the uterus. If a woman vomits up to two hours after taking the pill, then it is important that she takes the second one straight away and then purchases another. New versions of this medication mean that it won't automatically make you feel nauseous.

An IUD can also be fitted up to five days after unprotected sex to prevent pregnancy and can be left in as a longer-term method of contraception, or it can be removed after the next period.

BELOW | Sharing the responsibility for safer sex can increase the sexual trust and enjoyment in a relationship.

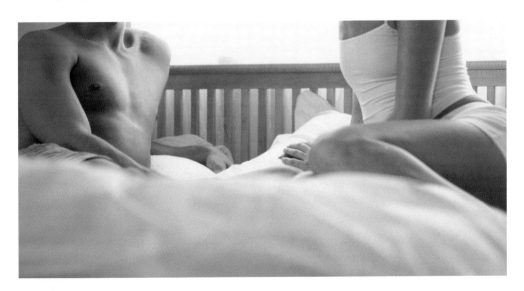

quick guide to contraception

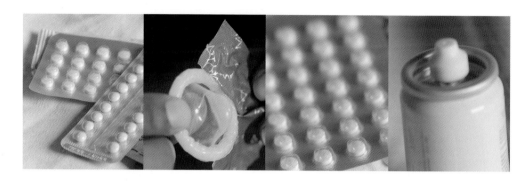

METHOD: THE COMBINED PILL

RISKS:
- ✗ Side-effects: mood swings, nausea, weight gain, loss of libido, headaches
- ✗ Increased risk of blood clots, especially in the overweight and smokers aged over 35
- ✗ Possible increased risk of cardiovascular disease, and liver, breast and cervical cancer

BENEFITS:
- ✔ Highly effective as a contraceptive
- ✔ Protection against cancer of the ovaries and endometrium
- ✔ Lighter periods
- ✔ Reduced risk of ovarian cysts
- ✔ Does not interrupt spontaneity of sexual intercourse

METHOD: THE MINI-PILL

RISKS:
- ✗ Small increased risk of ovarian cysts
- ✗ Less effective than the combined pill
- ✗ Possible increased risk of breast cancer

BENEFITS:
- ✔ Possible protection against ovarian cancer
- ✔ Side-effects are less severe than the combined pill
- ✔ Does not interrupt spontaneity of sexual intercourse

METHOD: HORMONAL IMPLANTS

RISKS:
- ✗ Complications have been reported in some women during insertion or removal of implants
- ✗ Heavy, irregular or absent periods
- ✗ Weight gain

BENEFITS:
- ✔ Does not interrupt spontaneity of sexual intercourse
- ✔ Provides effective contraception for up to five years or until removed

METHOD: HORMONAL INJECTION

RISKS:
- ✗ Heavy, irregular or absent periods
- ✗ Weight gain
- ✗ Delay in return of fertility

BENEFITS:
- ✔ Reduced risk of ovarian and endometrial cancer
- ✔ Reduced risk of ovarian cysts
- ✔ Does not interrupt spontaneity of sexual intercourse

METHOD: IUD

RISKS:
- ✗ Increased risk of pelvic infections
- ✗ Increased risk of ectopic pregnancy
- ✗ Heavier periods

BENEFITS:
- ✔ Very effective form of birth control
- ✔ Can be removed without delay in return of fertility

METHOD: CONDOM

RISKS:
- ✗ It may break or tear during intercourse
- ✗ Can interrupt spontaneity of sexual intercourse

BENEFITS:
- ✔ Protects against HIV and other sexually transmitted infections

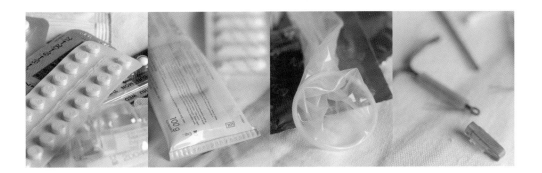

METHOD: DIAPHRAGM/CAP

RISKS:
✗ Slight risk of toxic shock syndrome
✗ Can interrupt spontaneity of sexual intercourse
✗ Not as effective without the use of a spermicide

BENEFITS:
✔ Does not interfere with a woman's hormonal balance
✔ Some protection against genital warts
✔ Some protection against cervical cancer
✔ Some protection against HIV and other sexually transmitted infections, particularly when used with spermicide

METHOD: THE SPONGE

RISKS:
✗ Relatively high failure rate

BENEFITS:
✔ Once in place it can be left for 24 hours

METHOD: VASECTOMY

RISKS:
✗ Psychological regret about loss of fertility
✗ Must generally be considered irreversible

BENEFITS:
✔ Freedom from fear of impregnating partner

METHOD: FEMALE STERILIZATION

RISKS:
✗ Psychological regret about loss of fertility
✗ Must generally be considered irreversible
✗ Some women experience heavier periods

BENEFITS:
✔ Freedom from fear of pregnancy

METHOD: NATURAL FAMILY PLANNING

RISKS:
✗ Without adequate tuition, motivation and commitment, this is an unreliable form of birth control

BENEFITS:
✔ Morally acceptable for couples who don't want to use artificial means of contraception
✔ Gives better insight into how a woman's body functions

METHOD: COITUS INTERRUPTUS

RISKS:
✗ Too unreliable

changing needs

THERE ARE VARIOUS FORMS OF CONTRACEPTION for different needs and different times of life. While your body changes throughout your life, one thing is certain: if you are fertile and sexually active, and don't want babies, you need to use some form of contraception. Your doctor, gynaecologist or family planning advisor will be able to give you the best advice for your age and health. Many of the more popular contraceptives are just not suitable for some people. The pill, for example, is not good for smokers. The coil (IUD) is not an ideal contraceptive for women who have not yet given birth; and the condom is not 100 per cent reliable. In fact, no form of contraception is 100 per cent reliable, so it is best to have another strategy just in case. For example, if you are on the pill, you should consider using condoms as well.

Couples should decide together about contraception. It is generally women who take responsibility – they are the ones who risk getting pregnant, and they also have a bigger choice of

BELOW | Couples need to offer mutual support and discuss changing contraceptive needs together.

contraception. Men are mostly limited to the condom or to having a vasectomy. (The male pill hasn't yet proved to be a great success.)

Male vasectomy is less risky than female sterilization. It is a big step, so it is wise to think about it very carefully and to consider all the implications. If you do go ahead, and subsequently start another relationship, don't forget that a vasectomy will not protect you from sexually transmitted infections.

When you reach the menopause, don't be fooled into thinking that you cannot conceive. Even if your periods are irregular, you must continue to use contraception until a year after your last period and until you are finally given the all-clear, through a hormone test.

infertility

As people age, fertility levels change, most notably in women. Women reach the menopause in mid-life, resulting in an inability to have any

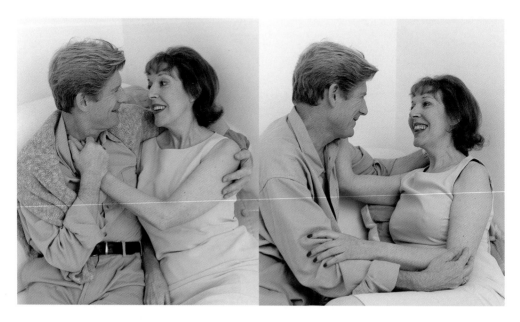

more children. Although men are normally able to father children throughout their lives, their fertility can be affected by problems such as low sperm count or age-related impotence and erectile difficulties. A young, fertile, healthy couple has an approximately one in four chance of conceiving a baby with each cycle. Once the woman reaches the age of 35, the odds of conceiving become greatly reduced, to 10 per cent each cycle. At this stage, some couples seek medical help in the form of hormone treatment or in-vitro fertilization (IVF). Couples trying for a baby need to be in tune with the woman's menstrual cycle, so that they are aware of when she is at her most fertile. The ovaries release an egg each month in the middle of the menstrual cycle, around the 14th day. A woman can be fertile for a few days before and 24 hours after she ovulates. Sperm has a better chance of reaching the egg, however, if it is ejaculated into the vagina 24 hours before the egg is released, as sperm can stay alive in the woman's body for two to three days.

During ovulation, the woman may notice that her mucus discharge is thinner and stringier than at other times. Another way of knowing when the egg is released is by using an ovulation tester kit that detects hormonal changes. An alternative method is to chart changes in the woman's body temperature using a basal body temperature thermometer. When the woman ovulates, her temperature rises by about 0.2 to 0.6 degrees and remains higher until her next period. When she becomes pregnant, her body maintains this increased temperature.

IVF

In-vitro fertilization is a procedure that stimulates egg production through drug and hormone therapy. The growth of ovarian follicles is checked by ultrasound and when the follicles reach the correct size, hormones are administered to cause the eggs to be released. The eggs are harvested using a fine needle guided by an ultrasound image. The eggs are then incubated at body temperature for four to six hours before sperm is added. The fertilized eggs are kept in a culture medium for around

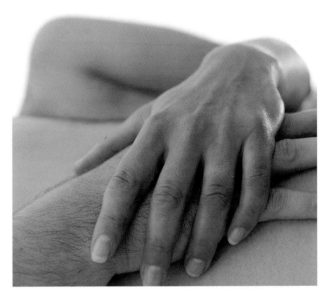

two days, before one or more is implanted in the woman's uterus using a fine needle. At present, this procedure is still fraught with difficulties and only around 10 per cent of attempts are successful, making it the least successful method of conceiving artificially. It is often seen as a last resort, not just because of its failure rate, but also because it is fairly unpleasant to undergo.

Another artificial method is used for couples where the man has a low sperm count. This involves injecting a single sperm directly into the ovary via a fine needle. This method has been highly criticized, as there is some evidence that it may increase the likelihood of birth defects. It is also suggested that it interferes with the natural selection process by which only the fittest sperm reach the egg, and that sperm taken from men with a very low sperm count may contain a genetic mutation that could pass on male infertility to future generations.

IVF is expensive, both financially and in terms of the couple's emotions. Couples considering IVF are required to consult a professional expert beforehand to go through their options and get all the information, support and counselling that they will need.

ABOVE | A course of IVF treatment can be an ordeal emotionally, physically and financially, so make sure you go into it together.

fertile ground

Many factors affect the fertility of both men and women. Over-eating, smoking, stress and drugs all have a negative effect on sperm production. The correction of mineral deficiencies and eating organic produce are thought by some to improve libido and fertility by up to about 86 per cent.

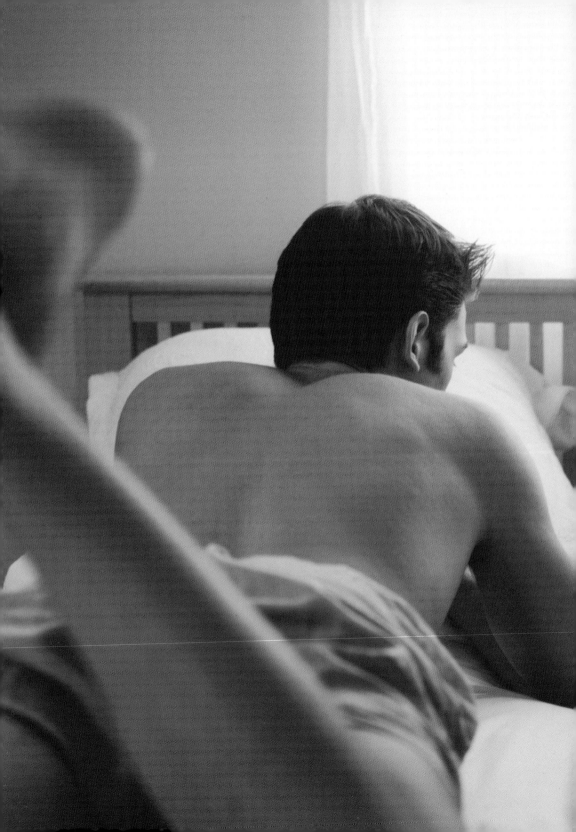

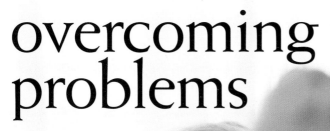

overcoming problems

A successful long-term relationship involves keeping the door open to discussion and negotiation as your needs change and develop. Any sexual problems should be talked about and dealt with together.

communication skills

COMMUNICATION AND LISTENING SKILLS are essential keys to unlock the tensions and problems which inevitably occur in any ongoing relationship. They enable you to verbalize those issues that are important to you, and help you to express your most vulnerable and emotive feelings, without descending into a tirade of blame and criticism that will only serve to alienate your partner.

Learning to listen carefully to your partner's thoughts, values, opinions and feelings without the need to become defensive or argumentative ensures that open and honest communication continues between you. If both of you determine to practise the communication and listening skills described in this section whenever problems arise, you may be able to respond more positively to difficult situations. In this way you can support,

understand and accommodate each other's needs and differing opinions.

No relationship is without its stresses and strains. In the beginning, when you first fall in love, the pull of your mutual attraction can mask aspects of your individuality and ego and also blind you to the truth about your partner's personality. Only when your relationship settles down do your personal views, values, needs and temperaments begin to emerge in detail. If you marry, or form a long-term relationship, create a home together, raise children and pursue demanding careers, inevitably these additional challenges will test your relationship in different ways. While you strive to make your relationship a secure and nurturing base from which you can both draw emotional and physical support, you

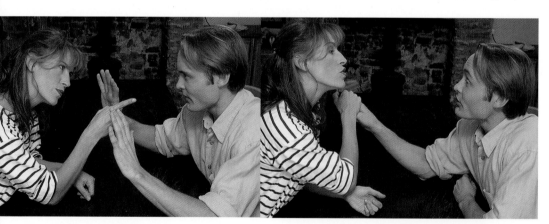

ABOVE | Avoid accusatory statements, harsh words and criticism. Be aware of body language – hardening your eyes and mouth or pointing your finger will make your partner defensive.

ABOVE | Bombarding each other with personal insults, shouting or talking louder than the other person, or aggressive words and actions will alienate you from each other, ensuring neither of you has a chance to communicate or even be heard above the din. Words spoken in the heat of the moment are often greatly regretted once your tempers have had a chance to cool down.

must also constantly adapt and respond to life's ever-changing realities.

Everyone evolves in mind, body and spirit as they mature. No one can expect a partner to remain exactly the same as when they first met. Nor can you stop the process of change within your own life, and you may come to realize that the things which made you happy or content in earlier years may no longer bring you such fulfilment. As in any partnership, there will be a constant need for negotiation if you wish to navigate your relationship safely and successfully through the turbulent waters of life.

areas of conflict

There are countless situations in which the needs and boundaries of a relationship have to be carefully re-examined and re-defined. Small issues can build up into a major area of conflict if you fail to communicate your needs, or listen to one another. For example, you might feel neglected by your husband because he watches football at the weekends, leaving you feeling aggrieved and abandoned. Perhaps your partner has forgotten your birthday, or a wedding anniversary, and you take that as a sign that he no longer cares about you. Maybe you feel your girlfriend criticizes and harasses you, she resents your friends, and that makes you feel she is trying to change you.

Issues can be intensely personal, such as the way you make love, whether you are honest with one another, the degree of intimacy you share, and whether you care enough about each other. Domestic problems can arise over the housework, parental responsibilities, and especially over the finances.

In almost every area of a relationship, some rules and boundaries need to be made to help it function well. Two mature adults should be able to make agreements which incorporate their mutual needs. Even so, those rules will be subject to change and renegotiation.

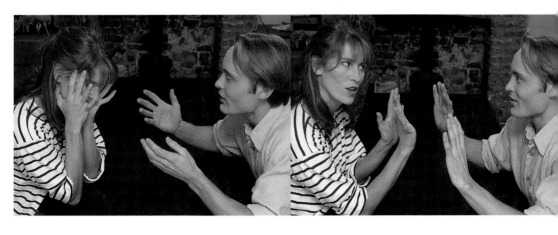

ABOVE | Don't undermine your partner's self-esteem in order to accentuate your point of view. It will only make them angry or hurt. Overwhelmed by these feelings, they will be totally incapable of hearing your side of the story. Here her body language demonstrates that she is virtually cutting off all her points of access, by covering her face, ears, eyes and mouth.

ABOVE | The body language here clearly indicates that both partners are saying "back-off". If you have failed to communicate and listen carefully, then you are probably going to reach a stalemate situation where nothing more is going to be resolved. Things may carry on relatively normally for a while, but both of you have become even more entrenched in your own points of view. Sooner or later the attack will begin again.

RIGHT | Take it in turns to discuss your feelings and needs, and state clearly what is bothering you about a certain situation. Take responsibility for how you feel, using "I" rather than the accusatory "You". Keep eye-contact and let your bodies be open and undefended towards each other, and remember to breathe deeply so you stay relaxed. Listen carefully to what your partner has to say to you, avoiding judgement or criticism.

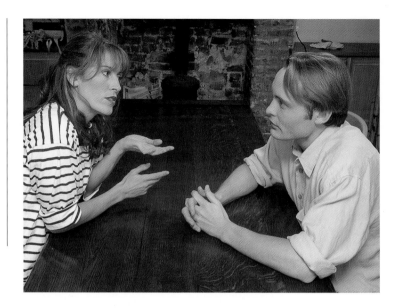

taking responsibility

Words of war will never heal a relationship or help you and your partner to find a solution to troublesome issues. In good communication, you need to take responsibility for your own feelings instead of blaming your partner for your emotional state. Accusation will force him or her into the mode of protection and the need to block your words, either by retaliating with a damaging counter-attack or by withdrawing.

Comparing your partner negatively or with derision to someone else is demeaning to that person, and can only result in more anger or bad feelings. Insulting your partner's family, friends or beliefs can deeply hurt his or her feelings and cause lasting damage to a relationship.

Manipulation may work in your favour temporarily, but your partner will know he has been duped. If you threaten your partner, you may gain a tentative victory, but revenge is likely to be in store. Making your mate feel guilty about who he is will guarantee defensive behaviour, and criticism can only serve to lower your lover's self-esteem.

Stubbornness demonstrates an unwillingness to work on a solution and an entrenched point of view. If you placate your partner, you are dismissing her needs and avoiding the real nature of the issue, and withdrawal is the ultimate weapon of power because your absence leaves the other person feeling helpless.

What you say is one thing, and how you say it is another. Shouting and raising your voice "deafens" your partner, and continually repeating yourself, nagging, complaining or whining is guaranteed to make your partner react in a negative way.

listening well

How you listen to your partner complements your communication skills. You can hear the words, but still not listen to their content. You can make your own judgements about what your partner is saying, while failing to comprehend what she is really trying to get across.

Listening to someone with an armoured or defended attitude which says "Here we go again" indicates that you are unwilling to be receptive. Imagining that you know what is best for your partner and your relationship means that you are unable to consider the other person's point of view. Thinking up a retaliatory statement while your

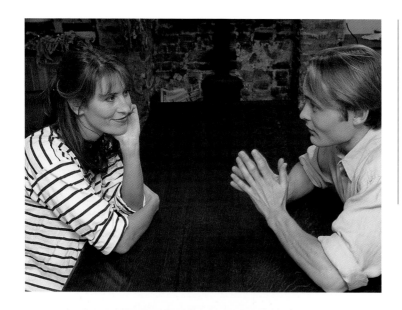

LEFT | Repeat back to your partner what you think you have heard him or her say so they can correct any misunderstandings that may have occurred. The fact that you have absorbed their words and are able to feed them back so succinctly will restore their confidence in the relationship because they will feel you have listened carefully to them.

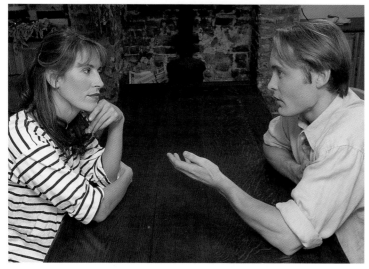

LEFT | Once you have expressed your needs and feelings and felt that your partner has fully understood them, allow him or her the chance to respond in a similar way. Now it is your turn to listen carefully to their point of view. If they don't think they are going to be criticized or judged, they may be able to reveal aspects of themselves they have previously felt unable to show. Focus carefully on what they have to say, nodding or smiling to show you have grasped its content. Even if you do not share their opinion, let them express it.

partner is speaking to you renders you incapable of listening at all. Tuning out is the aural version of physical withdrawal – you are not going to hear what your partner is saying if you have one eye on the television and the other on your newspaper.

All of the above are typical examples of relating patterns which any of us may employ when real communication breaks down. Instead, we may revert to our "parental voices", blaming and punishing. If we are on the receiving end of this critical tirade, the "child" within us is provoked and it is inevitable that the reaction that ensues will be petulant, hysterical, sullen, angry or argumentative.

communication exercise

COMMUNICATION BETWEEN TWO PEOPLE who love each other should never become a power struggle, or a battle to win at all costs. It should be a mutual search to try to understand and support each other, respectful of the needs of both the individual and the relationship. It takes courage to talk about your feelings honestly and to take responsibility for them, and diligent awareness to locate the true source of your emotions and unhappiness. It needs respect and empathy to listen carefully to what your partner is saying without immediately feeling threatened, or needing to defend your corner.

If you are experiencing communication problems within your relationship, you can try the following exercise which allows you to explain your needs and opinions clearly, and to listen empathically to your partner's truth. At first the exercise may seem awkward and too formal but this is because it is a new way of sharing with each other.

When an important issue is at stake, or whenever you are feeling hurt about something within the relationship, take the time to make an appointment with each other specifically to sit and talk it over. Resolve to do this calmly and without recrimination, and try to enter this communication exercise with an open heart and mind. Try to relax your body and breathe deeply so that you release some of the pent-up tensions before you begin.

Sit opposite your partner so you can maintain eye-to-eye contact. You may find it more comfortable to have a table between you which

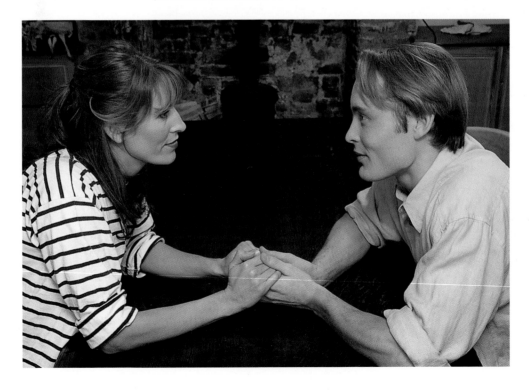

you can consider as a neutral arena. Uncross your arms and legs so your body language is not defensive, avoid using your eyes to intensify your words, or gritting your teeth, or tightening your jaw, and do not point your finger accusingly at your partner.

One partner takes five minutes to speak while the other's task is simply to listen. If you are the speaking partner, state clearly what your feelings are and what is bothering you. However, take responsibility for those feelings. Avoid phrases like: "You don't love or care about me any more. You are so selfish around the house and you never do your share of the chores. You make me feel like I'm the servant here."

Instead, try to phrase this in a different way, such as: "I realize that over the last weeks I have been getting very angry and snappy towards you. I am finding my work very stressful at the moment, so when I come home, I do not feel able to cope with the cooking and housework alone. Recently, I have been doing most of the tasks in the evenings. What I would like is for us to draw up a new agreement on how we can share the jobs."

In this way, you have spelt out your needs clearly. You have identified your emotions and put them in a context. In addition, you have explained, without accusation, why you need extra support at this time, and you have offered a framework for a solution.

As the listening partner, you do not interrupt or defend yourself, and this is made easier by the fact that you are not being blamed for the situation. You can show your partner that you are listening to her empathically by leaning towards her as she speaks, or nodding your head to show you are assimilating her words.

At the end of the five minutes, sum up for her what you believe you have heard her say. In this way you reflect back to her the content of her communication, and by repeating it, you absorb the information better. Your feedback enables her to correct any misunderstandings you may have gained as to what she actually said, and it assures her that you have been actively listening.

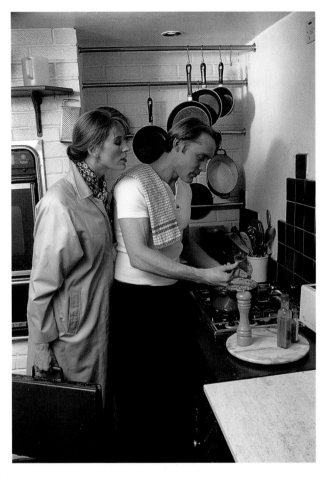

OPPOSITE | The communication exercise will enable both of you to move positively towards solving a tricky dilemma because you will have gained an understanding of each other's feelings and needs. This will provide you with the useful tools with which to tackle the issues involved, and hopefully find a suitable solution.

ABOVE | When both partners are working outside the home, household tasks need to be shared. How you negotiate that division of labour should take into consideration your needs and preferences, the time that either of you expects to put into the housework, and when any particular task should be done. There should be flexibility in the arrangement, so, for example, if your partner is working late, you may offer to cook the dinner – even if it isn't your turn.

swapping roles

Now it is the listening partner's turn to speak. If you do not feel ridiculed or criticized, you have a better chance of communicating your own version of the situation. In the past you may have retorted with something like: "You never stop nagging. Sometimes your complaining makes me so sick that I want to walk out. Anyway, the house looks perfectly fine to me – the problem is that you are neurotic." This reply is a defensive attack which manages to combine an accusation, a threat, a denial and an insult all in one delivery!

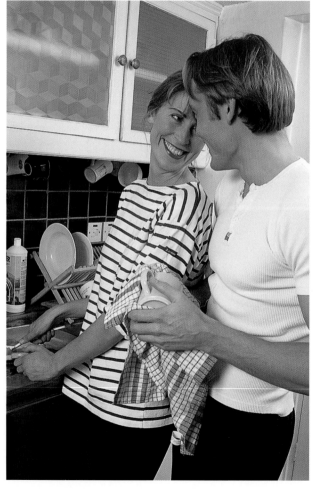

BELOW | Household jobs do not have to be turned into chores – they can be a great opportunity for you to spend some time together, joking and chatting over the day's events.

During this exercise, you have more chance to respond rather than to react in the manner above. You might say instead: "I've also had a lot of pressure at work recently, and when I come home, my immediate need is to take time to unwind. The difficulty between us seems to be that you like to get things done straight away while I prefer to do them later, or at the weekends. What usually happens is that you go straight ahead with the chores, and I usually skulk off feeling guilty. I am very willing to do my half of the work, but my main priority is that we make more time to relax and enjoy each other's company in the evenings."

If you are now the listening partner, you should summarize and reflect back what your partner has just told you and allow them to correct you if you have misheard any of their communication. If you need more time to continue your reciprocal communication exercise, then you can use its structure again. If you were to use the above example of the exercise, it would have enabled you to refrain from blame and criticism, while stating clearly your paramount needs.

You have established a framework in that you both agree that the housework needs to be done and the chores shared, but you now need to discuss how the jobs can be better divided and when is the best time to do them. You will need to negotiate a solution which encompasses the needs and wishes of both of you, but that will be far easier to do if neither of you feels angry or in the wrong.

Unless relationship issues are dealt with as they arise, their undercurrents are likely to affect other aspects of your lives. Sexual disharmony or reduced intimacy can often be a reflection of other unresolved issues, rather than being directly related to sexual problems. Good communication and listening skills are as important to the health, harmony and growth of your relationship as is the happiness of your sex life.

catharsis

Pent-up feelings of anger and frustration can become locked in your body's musculature, making you feel tense and irritable, and more

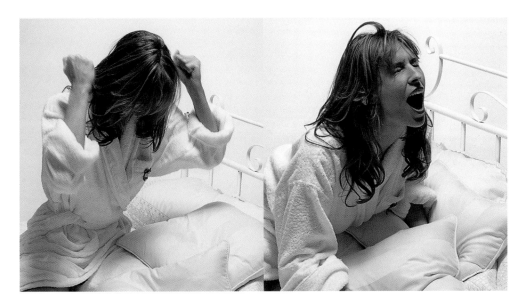

inclined to provoke arguments in the home. Sometimes the cause of these feelings is not directly related to anything that has happened between you and your partner, but your charged emotions spill out and you react negatively to the slightest comment. Perhaps you are under stress at work, or you have been angered or disappointed by a certain event, or maybe there are issues in your relationship that you are too wound up about to discuss rationally.

One way of helping to discharge this emotion in a safe way, without hurting or blaming any one else, is by catharsis. By acting out and giving vent to your feelings when you are alone, you can release your intense emotions.

Beating the cushions as shown here is a method that is sometimes used in therapy sessions, enabling clients to express their anger in a non-harmful way. You can do this in the privacy of your home, too, though it would be better to wait until you are alone. You can shout and yell at the same time, if you can do so without disturbing the neighbours.

Let rip for up to ten minutes, giving yourself permission to discharge your rage into the cushions by beating your fists against them. By

allowing yourself to feel and express your anger without judgement, it may transform itself into a wave of non-emotive energy which will leave you feeling full of vitality as your tension blocks are released.

Sometimes, sadness lies behind anger and you may get in touch with your more vulnerable feelings. If the anger turns into tears, then hug a cushion to your body, and allow yourself to cry until you feel a release from your pain. When you have experienced your catharsis, rest for at least five minutes, and breathe deeply so your whole body relaxes.

If this technique is suitable to you, then use it at times when you feel your body is completely racked with emotion but are you are unable to express your feelings adequately in words. This way no one else gets hurt, and you may find it a great relief.

If you cannot imagine yourself undergoing catharsis, another good way to release pent-up frustration is through strenuous physical activity, such as running, brisk walking or dancing. Try to breathe deeply and move your body freely in order to discharge all your tensions and regain a sense of equilibrium.

ABOVE LEFT | Build a pile of cushions in front of you on a supportive base such as your bed. Make fists and begin to pound the cushions. Get in touch with your emotions and allow them to gather momentum and express themselves through your body.

ABOVE | If you feel able to shout and yell without disturbing other people, this will help clear the emotional tension that has been "choking" you. You can even say all the nasty things you have been carrying in your mind. This will help you to dispel your more negative thoughts so that later you can approach your problems more calmly.

OPPOSITE | Hugging each
other is a very reassuring
non-sexual form of physical
contact.

being vulnerable

No matter how mature and responsible we have
become as adults, a part of us remains child-like,
retaining the vulnerable and playful elements of
our nature. If you accept that part of yourself, and
learn to love your "inner child", it will help make
you a more balanced person and better able to
respond to those aspects in your partner. The inner
child is the part of your personality that is magical
and inquisitive, but that also feels insecure and is
easily hurt. It is the part of you that sometimes
needs nourishment, comfort and reassurance.

In an adult relationship, there will be times
when the "child" within one partner will meet the
"parent" within the other. A balanced relationship
is one in which these roles can be shared, so
that you are able to respond to each other
appropriately in times of need.

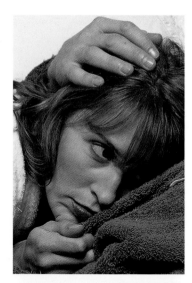

RIGHT AND ABOVE RIGHT |
Even as an adult there are
times when you will need to
be comforted and supported
by your mate. A partner who
is able to respond to your
"inner child", and is not afraid
of it, is secure in himself or
herself and in touch with their
own sensitive side.

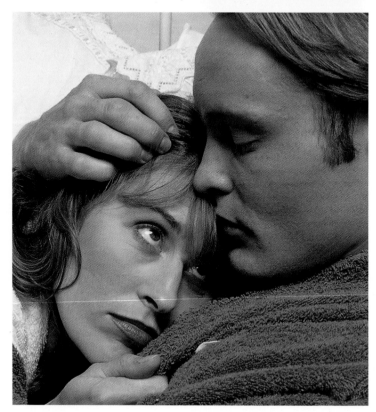

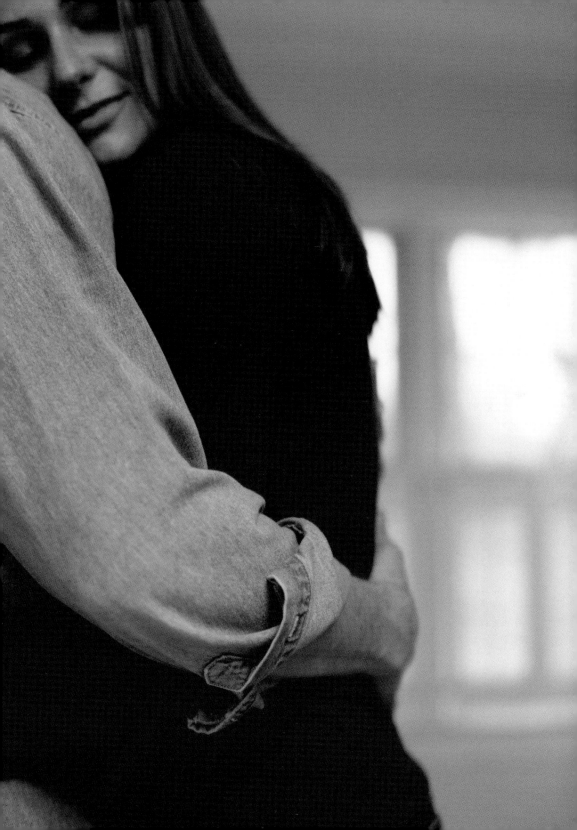

sexual health

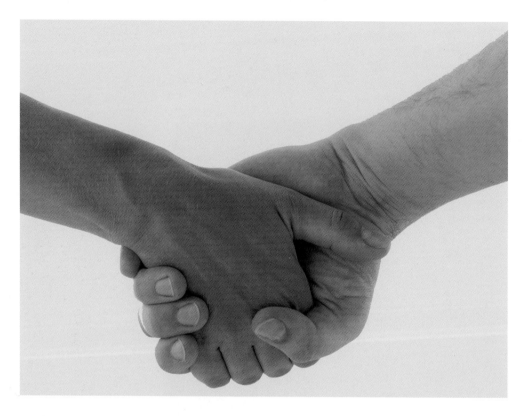

AT SOME POINT DURING YOUR LIFE, your sexual activity is likely to be interrupted and temporarily halted. This could either be as a result of physical illness, such as heart problems or major surgery, or the outcome of psychological challenges involving bereavement, breakdown of a relationship or depression, or a combination. This is equally applicable to both men and women, and it is crucial to get to the bottom of the problem by discussing it with your partner, a doctor or a sex therapist.

men's problems

Men can suffer from performance problems at any time during their life, either in the form of premature ejaculation, erectile dysfunction (failing to get an erection), or an inability to ejaculate. Although erectile dysfunction is more likely to occur later in life, men's penises can let them down even in their teens or early twenties. This can be owing to any number of reasons: anxiety about performance, fear of sex, or even excessive drink and drug use. A vicious circle can occur if, following an isolated incident of impotence, a man is so worried the next time he makes love that it occurs again. In this situation, an understanding partner is essential and a period of sexual abstinence until his normal sex drive reasserts itself will usually solve the problem.

Most men at some point in their lives will have experienced the odd difficulty in "getting it up". Erectile problems are generally considered to be mostly psychological in origin. However, if it occurs regularly, it is wise to consult a specialist. This condition is associated not only with aging, but also with diabetes, surgery for prostate cancer, damage to the nervous system, taking some medication, heavy drinking and smoking.

premature ejaculation

This is when a man is not able to control or delay his orgasm. This can be the result of anxiety over his performance, or related to a poor first sexual experience. This condition can contribute to a lack of self-confidence and, if it is a long-term problem, can lead to further difficulties in an existing sexual relationship. If it continues, a doctor or therapist should be consulted. Most commonly it is the result of persistent learned behaviour, which can in turn be unlearned, and new research shows that it is inherited in some cases.

Many men find it difficult to talk about their health problems, either with their partners or with a doctor. But it is important to do so. There is the possibility of Sildenafil (Viagra), the "wonder pill" that increases the penis's ability to achieve and maintain an erection once a man is sexually aroused. Every man who is thinking of taking such drugs should have a medical check-up first, as a number of serious side effects have been reported.

Practitioners of complementary medicine have been conducting research on a herbal "Viagra". Ginkgo biloba, the maidenhair tree, has long been used to stimulate the circulation to help treat a number of conditions. There is some anecdotal reportage that daily doses of the herb have led to significant improvements. Herbal practitioners will almost certainly also recommend changes to the diet, probably excluding saturated fats, coffee and alcohol. Smokers will be advised to give up. Acupressure, a Japanese system of applying finger pressure to specific points on the body, has also achieved success for some. Before taking any herbal remedies, you should consult a qualified practitioner. There is no evidence to suggest that alternative methods will work, but any improvement in overall health will help.

women's problems

There are several problems which are common amongst women. Pain while having sex, dyspareunia, may have physical or psychological causes. It can simply be the result of inadequate lubrication, especially with older women. In that case, the remedy is simple, so why not avail yourself of some of the exotic flavoured gels available from sex shops? If the pain is deep, then it could result from infection or cysts and you should consult your doctor. Psychological problems may vary in severity. Many can be resolved with the help of an understanding partner and a loving touch that stops short of penetration until the woman feels ready. More severe or long-term problems will require professional help.

As with men, women's sex lives will be affected by illnesses such as diabetes, heart disease or high blood pressure. Your doctor will be able to advise you and will almost certainly help you to resume a normal sex life.

BELOW | If one partner is suffering from sexual problems, it is extremely important that the other is both sympathetic and understanding. Keeping the lines of communication open and expressing your love will go a long way towards resolving the difficulty.

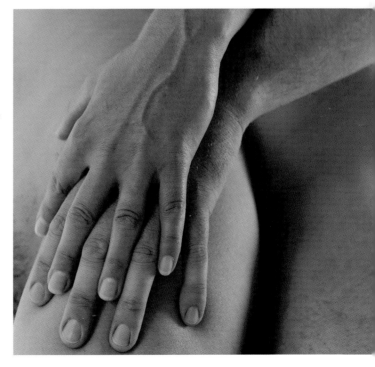

loss of libido and other problems

THE LOSS OF LIBIDO can affect both men and women and presents as a total lack of sexual interest. Sufferers of impotence usually feel frustrated as they still have the desire to have sex, but for one reason or another are unable to perform satisfactorily. To lose the desire to have sex is loss of libido and is just as frustrating but in a rather different way.

People who have a reduced libido tend to take steps to avoid lovemaking by either staying up later to watch television, starting an argument before bedtime or avoiding any form of affection with their partner, often leaving the partner feeling very confused and rejected.

The causes of low sex drive are often very common things, such as stress, depression, physical illness, overwork or relationship problems. In men, it is a fast-growing problem, owing in part to the strain of today's competitive workplace.

A recent American study showed that 33.4 per cent of women between the ages of 18 and 59

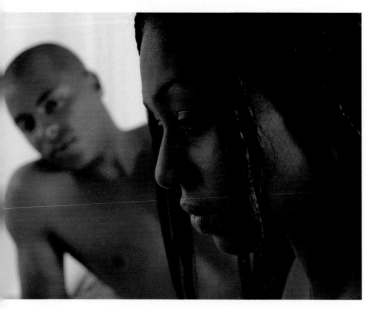

BELOW AND RIGHT |
A temporary loss of libido is very common in long-term relationships. It can be devastating for both partners when it happens, whether it is caused by emotional or physical problems. However, with the right help, it is usually overcome.

suffered from hypoactive sexual desire disorder (HSDD) or libido loss. The definition is vague because further research showed how varied are the levels of sexual interest among women in general. The causes of HSDD among women are dominated by the menstrual cycle and the stages of their reproductive life and hormone balance.

Many antidepressants such as Selective Serotonin Reuptake Inhibitors (SSRIs), like Prozac, are known to have a negative effect on sexual desire. It is important to continue any medication that you may feel is inhibiting your libido until you have consulted your doctor, who will be able to advise you and offer a possible alternative. Sometimes lack of libido is just a symptom of another problem that can be investigated.

painful intercourse

Sexual intercourse should not be painful, but therapists say that a large number of women suffer for some time before seeking help. Painful intercourse, or dyspareunia, can have a variety of causes from vaginismus (involuntary spasms of the vaginal walls) to lack of lubrication or arousal. The main thing is to take action, not to suffer in silence, as the solution may be simpler than you think.

premature ejaculation

One of the most common sexual problems for men is premature ejaculation. It is an inability to control the timing of their orgasms. Some men come as soon as they enter their partner's vagina, others within a few minutes, or within a period that they consider to be far too soon.

Many men experience premature ejaculation at some point, but it is most common in young or inexperienced men. Although no one knows exactly why it happens, most experts agree that the condition is probably psychological, as a result of anxiety about sex and whether they will do it right. Over the years, men generally learn to control their orgasms through experience – by having more sex. And the longer the gap between orgasms, the quicker a man will come the next time round.

If you feel you have a problem, you can train yourself to control your orgasm. Begin by masturbating and bring yourself close to ejaculation. Stop, relax and start again. Repeat until you can't control the orgasm any further. The point here is to learn when you are about to climax, so the more you practise, the more you are likely to be able to delay your orgasm to the exact point at which you want to come. Once you have accomplished this, experiment with your partner. While she is masturbating you, ask her to stop when you are about to ejaculate. Again, stop, relax and start again.

The squeeze technique is another way of achieving the same result. Either you or your partner can squeeze the tip of your penis just before climax. The squeeze forces the blood out of the penis and reduces the erection. Something else which might help is wearing a condom (or even two if necessary) because prophylactics reduce sexual sensation during sex. Alternatively, choose a sexual position in which you find it easier to relax. This is most likely to be one where your partner is on top, taking control.

delayed ejaculation

This occurs in some men who find it difficult to reach orgasm even though they may want to and are receiving the necessary stimulation. The reason it happens is either physiological – due to diseases such as diabetes or prostatic disease, or certain types of drug therapy – or psychological where some men may have become repressed or inhibited, with a real fear of women or of causing pregnancy. Psychosexual therapy can teach men how to overcome the inhibitory behaviour or fears that have become conditioned in them.

retrograde ejaculation

This occurs when men feel the sensation of ejaculation and orgasm but no fluid comes out. Semen is expelled from the testicles but instead of following the contractions and going through the urethra, it travels back into the bladder via the bladder neck. This is relatively common in men who have undergone prostatectomy. Other reasons for its occurrence are disruption of the nervous system caused by spinal cord injury, diabetes, multiple sclerosis and some prescription medications.

erectile dysfunction

During adolescence, young men are frequently embarrassed by how readily – and publicly – an erection occurs. The converse of this is that, with increasing age, it doesn't happen so often, it isn't so firm and it doesn't last so long. By the time this happens, most men should be mature enough to explore other options, from oral sex to a simple change of position.

Alcohol can be the culprit when the spirit is willing but the flesh is weak. Surprisingly, erectile problems as a result of drinking too much – sometimes known as brewer's droop – affect young men more frequently than older men.

Impotence may also be caused by a neurological disorder, where nerve signals are interrupted; problems with the blood flow; hormonal deficiency; diabetes or infection. Not surprisingly, perhaps, men are reluctant to seek help, although many treatments are available. One of the most widely known is Viagra (Sildenafil), although this is only effective for one-third of users. Other treatments include vacuum pumps used with a constricting ring, penile implants and urethral injections.

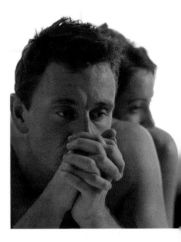

ABOVE | Ejaculation problems can be terribly frustrating but it is important to maintain a perspective on the situation. Sensitivity combined with humour can help, while removing the emphasis from penetration and concentrating on foreplay can divert attention away from the problem and restore confidence.

overcoming difficulties

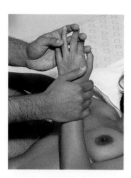

ABOVE | The palms and fingertips are the main tool in the following exercises.

LACK OF SEXUAL INTEREST shown by one or both partners is the most common form of sexual problem occurring within a relationship. There may be a number of factors that block the sexual response. Sometimes stress at work or in the home can cause fatigue or anxiety and consequently a diminished libido. If there is anger or other negative feelings between the partners, and a lack of clear communication skills, then the sexual relationship is ultimately bound to suffer.

Sadly, in many relationships, once the first flush of passion and excitement has subsided, lovemaking can become perfunctory, focused mainly on penetration and thrusting, and regarded more as a relief from sexual tension than a sensual, nurturing and fulfilling encounter. In these circumstances, either partner may withdraw from the sexual arena, and this can lead to a build-up of frustration within the relationship.

exercises

Sensate focus exercises are the backbone of psychosexual therapy, enabling couples to overcome their sexual difficulties and regain, or even discover, a more sensual and intimate side of their physical relationship. They work by helping the couple to change their focus away from penetrative sex, performance and sexual obligation. While a couple are working through these exercises, they make a commitment to ban all intercourse until the very last stage.

The point of sensate focus is to help people break old habits and patterns of sexual behaviour which have proved unsatisfying. The pressure is taken away from the need to initiate or respond to sexual overtures, giving the couple an opportunity to relax with each other's bodies and to recreate their sexual relationship in an entirely new way.

Sensate focus exercises, originally devised by sex researchers William Masters and Virginia Johnson, are based on encouraging couples to discover the joy and pleasure of sensual touching for its own sake, and not for an end result. This is a very important factor which may be missing from a sexual partnership.

In their haste to reach a climax, many individuals may not actually experience their own sensual pleasure and may completely miss their partner's sensual responses. If the sexual relationship falls into this mode over a long period of time, it is hardly surprising if one or other partner becomes disillusioned or resentful and eventually withdraws from physical contact.

The human body has an enormous capacity for sensual joy and pleasure, especially that experienced through the medium of touch, but this fundamental sense is often suppressed within us from an early stage of life. Young children are frequently told "not to touch" either their own bodies or the objects around them, thus inhibiting the development of their sensory perceptions. Touch, in western cultures, is generally associated with sexuality once we have reached adolescence. We forget how to communicate and feel through touch, how to enjoy its nurturing qualities and, by doing so, cut ourselves off from a vast dimension of tactile sensory awareness.

seeking help

If you and your partner are experiencing serious or long-term problems within your relationship, or your communication has begun to break down so that conflict ensues whenever sexual or emotional issues are discussed, you would probably benefit from seeking professional help from a qualified psychosexual therapist. The therapist will be trained to deal with a whole range of sexual disorders or dysfunctions, including premature ejaculation, loss of desire, erectile dysfunction, inability to achieve orgasm, fear of penetration, or intercourse avoidance.

He or she will also help you to improve your communication skills, so that you are able to relate to each other and negotiate solutions on difficult issues. It is very difficult for any couple who are experiencing relationship or sexual difficulties to gain a clear perspective of the situation for themselves, simply because they are too emotionally involved in the issues. A psychotherapist or sex counsellor will act as a mediator, providing practical advice and helping you reach your own understanding of the problems.

When a couple work through the sensate focus exercises with a therapist, the professional will be able to help them resolve physical and emotional conflicts which may arise between them at any stage of the process. What follows here is a programme of sensate focus exercises, adapted from the therapeutic model, but designed for couples to work with by themselves.

The success of these exercises depends upon a genuine commitment that you and your partner will make to follow the rules of each stage. Choose a specific time during the week when you can both give your full attention to the exercises, and decide which partner should initiate the session. Try to choose a time when you both feel generally relaxed and agreeable towards each other. Allocate 40 to 60 minutes per session, and ensure that you have complete privacy, picking a time when there will be no interruptions from the children, or visitors, and remembering to take the phone off the hook.

You need a warm room as you will both be naked, and a comfortable mattress or base to lie on. If possible, choose a room in the house other than a bedroom – somewhere where you are not reminded of the charged issues of your sexual relationship. You are trying to create something new between you, moving away from past patterns, expectations and memories.

BELOW | Carefully explore the angles and contours of your partner's face, feeling the difference between the firmness of the bones and the softness of the skin and muscles. The whole point of this touching experiment is for you to increase your sensory awareness and your sensitivity of touch.

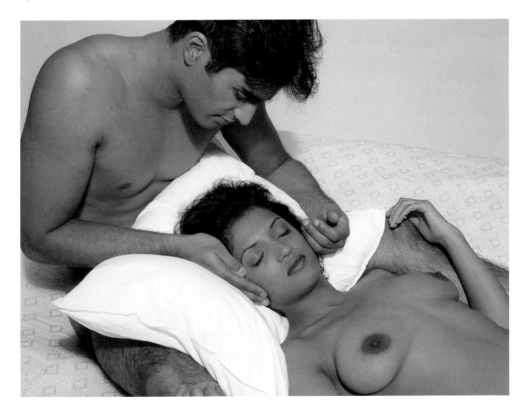

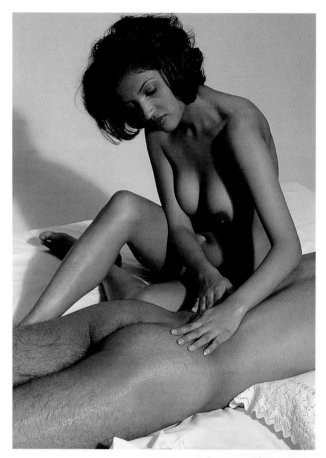

stage one: non-sexual touch

During the first weeks of your sensate focus exercises, you must refrain from sexual intercourse completely. This is the period when you will, instead, explore your sensual receptivity to one another's bodies, and develop your tactile communication. You will take turns to touch each other, as if you are discovering and exploring the human body for the first time. The person who is touching must remember that he or she is not aiming to arouse the partner, but is simply dedicated to developing his or her own sensory awareness.

You can touch anywhere on your partner's body except the genitals or other erogenous areas, such as the woman's breasts. You should allow yourself to feel through your hands and fingers all the different sensations of touch, texture and temperature of the skin. Vary how you apply your tactile contact, using your palms or fingertips, or even the backs of your hands.

You should experiment with using one hand at a time, or stroking with both hands, and keep taking note of the different sensations that you notice as they occur. The passive partner has only to lie there quietly and focus on the sensation of being touched.

Do not try to reciprocate touch, or go into any sexual fantasy. Both of you should try hard to avoid analysing the situation or making judgements, such as "this sensation feels good" or "am I doing it right?". All you have to do is focus your whole attention on the physical sensations you are experiencing, whether it is through touching or being touched.

Agree beforehand that if the passive partner is uncomfortable about the type of touch he or she is receiving, they can say so and the session can stop, to be resumed at another time. Each partner should spend up to 15 or 20 minutes giving and receiving touch before swapping roles. Do not go on for so long that you become bored or tired. When the exercise is over, you can share with each other the feelings and sensations that each of you has experienced.

ABOVE AND RIGHT | Stroke your partner's body with one hand, then with both hands, while he or she simply enjoys being touched.

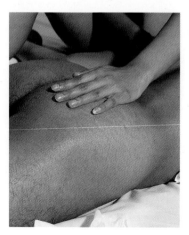

experiment with touch

Take the time to touch and feel your partner's body in a way you have never done before. You are not trying to please him or turn him on; this experiment is purely for your own sensation and discovery. Run your fingers around his nipple, and along the soft skin at the side of the ribcage, feeling the difference between bone and skin.

Explore his body with your touch, feeling each and every part including his limbs, neck, chest and back, except for the genital area. Move the joints, wiggling the fingers and toes. Notice the skin's temperature changes and its rougher and smoother parts.

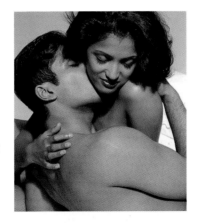

LEFT AND BELOW | Explore your partner's body, but do not try to arouse him or her.

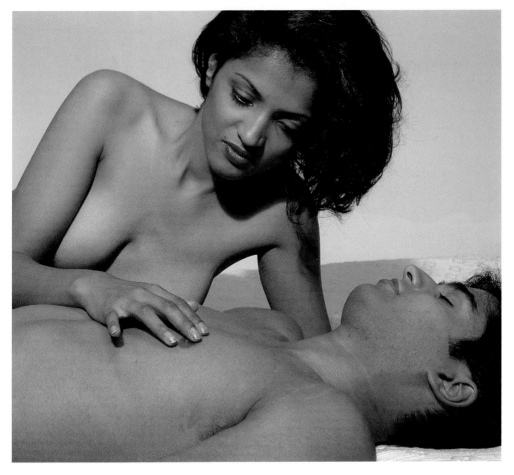

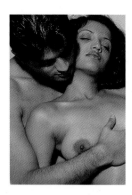

ABOVE | Reverse roles so that the other partner can explore the sense of touch.

stage two: adding lotion

You can continue to touch each other in the same way as before, but now, if you want, you can add oil or lotion. This is still a touching exercise, not a massage, as the point is to experience yet another dimension of touching, which may become more smooth and sensual, more flowing and soft with the addition of lubricant.

Remember, the purpose of these exercises, at this juncture, is not about pleasing the other person but about discovering new tactile responses for yourself. Stroke, knead and press the flesh, each time becoming aware of the different sensations of movement and touch, especially now that you have added the oi or lotion.

Feel the fluid quality of your hands as they slide over the skin and around the curves of the body. Use your fingers, thumbs, and the heels of your hands to make varying levels of pressure in your strokes. Stop moving occasionally, letting one hand rest on the heart and the other over the belly. See if you can feel his or her heartbeat under your hands, and sense the movement of breath.

Even though you can now make tactile contact with more sexual areas, such as the genitals and breasts, you should be stroking and caressing the erogenous zones in the same manner as you have been touching the other parts of the body – with a sense of wonder and innocence.

Your partner can now lay his or her hand over yours and give you a gentle direction of where to go, how firm or soft your pressure should be, when to move your hand to another place and when to return. See if you can pick up their signals through the receptivity of your skin. In this way, you are becoming more deeply attuned to their physical messages. You can also reverse the position of your hands, so that your hand lies on top and they can guide you.

Try to continue your non-sexual thoughts when it is your partner's turn to spread oil or lotion over you.

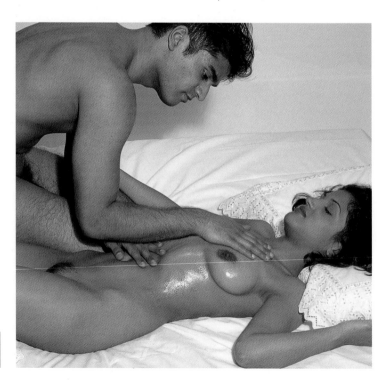

RIGHT | Stop occasionally, with one hand over the heart and one on the belly.

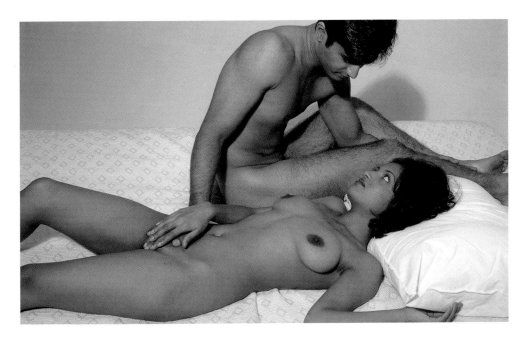

stage three:
touching the genitals

Once you both feel ready, you can progress to the stage of these exercises where you are allowed to include the genitals and breasts into your programme of exploratory touch. However, your tactile contact should not be intended to create sexual arousal, although this may happen inadvertently. Do not zone into the erogenous areas immediately but start with all-over-body touch as before, with or without lotion.

There is still no goal in mind except to fully experience the present moment of tactile awareness. If you find yourself becoming too excited, then move on to another area of the body, as you did in the first stage of this exercise. If you are the male active partner, you can use a sitting position during this phase, so your partner's back is leaning against you. Prop yourself against some pillows and reach comfortably around to touch the front of her body. Also, become aware of the feel of her back as it nestles against your skin. As the woman during the active phase, you can kneel between

your partner's legs to gain easier access to his genital area.

Once you are touching the genitals, the passive partner can also guide you by laying his or her hand over yours, and giving you silent cues as to how he or she likes to be touched there. Move your hands with synchronicity, and try to remain receptive to the passive partner's subtle directions. You can even swap the position of your hands, so that at some point, your hand overlays the hand of the receptive partner. Follow their movements, gauging how your partner likes to stroke himself or herself and what variations of pressure they may like to apply.

Your intention is not to arouse each other to orgasm, as your focus is still on gaining a greater sense of tactile awareness. Do not concentrate only on the genitals, but continue to touch other parts of the body as before. You should not kiss at this stage, or pursue any activity which may lead to intercourse. If, however, either partner does become orgasmic while being genitally stroked, you can continue your touching, with just your own hands, or with your combined hands, to allow orgasm to happen.

ABOVE | Progress to touching your partner's genitals, allowing him or her to guide your movements.

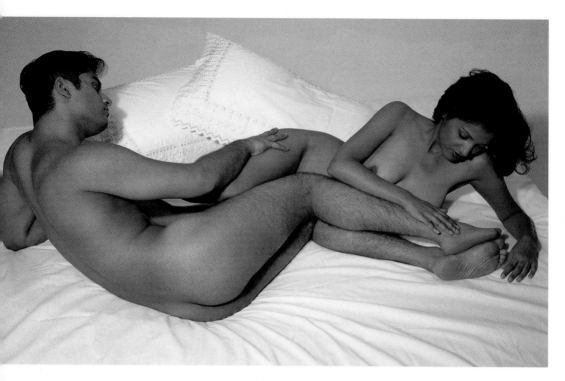

Lie comfortably close to each other so that you can simultaneously touch and explore each other's bodies with the sensual awareness that you have steadily been developing through this programme. Focus all your attention on the sensations that you are experiencing of touching each other and of being touched.

Slowly and gently begin to make love, with the woman kneeling on top of her partner.

stage four: touching each other

Mutual touching is now the new phase in your senate focus programme. Here you begin again with your sensory awareness exercises, but this time you are touching each other simultaneously. There is still a ban on kissing or sexual intercourse, but you can now use your tongue to explore one another's bodies, although not with the purpose of arousal. Now you must simultaneously focus your attention on touch and on the sensation of being touched. Explore each other's bodies with different types of strokes, using fingertips or palms, just as you have done in the previous exercises.

stage five: making love

Begin this stage of the programme with your whole-body touch, including sensual touching of the genital regions. However, during this phase, you can now move on to the first steps of resuming sexual intercourse. The man should lie on his back

and, as the woman, you should climb on top of him so that you are kneeling across his hips.

Carry your sensual awareness with you, and begin by just letting your genitals make contact. Absorb these sensations into yourself. Then, as the woman, take your partner's penis and gently guide its head into your vagina. Avoid any thrusting or deep penetration. Explore the different feelings which arise with each motion that you make. Gradually, you can deepen the depth of penetration and begin to move very slowly and gently, continuously focusing on your immediate physical experience, while having a greater awareness than ever before of the sensations your partner is experiencing.

You are now ready to resume your full sexual relationship, but with a completely heightened sensual awareness. This does not mean you cannot have passionate and wild sex again, but every once in while, go back to the exercises to enrich your intrinsic feeling senses.

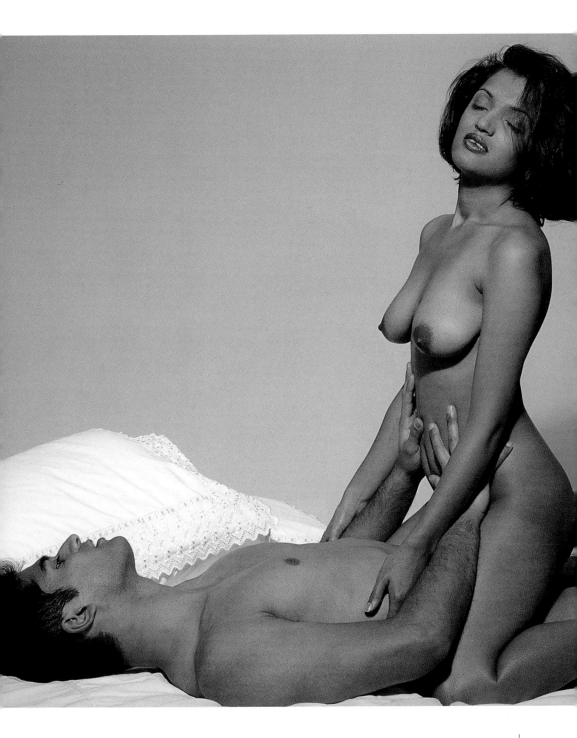

overcoming erection failure

A failure to get an erection or to maintain one during sexual activity happens to most men at some time in their lives. This may be the result of stress and tiredness, sexual boredom, lack of attraction to a partner, or ill health. This is usually temporary, and the man's arousal response will improve by itself, or when circumstances and events change for the better.

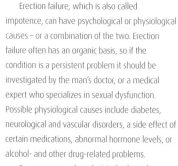

Erection failure, which is also called impotence, can have psychological or physiological causes – or a combination of the two. Erection failure often has an organic basis, so if the condition is a persistent problem it should be investigated by the man's doctor, or a medical expert who specializes in sexual dysfunction. Possible physiological causes include diabetes, neurological and vascular disorders, a side effect of certain medications, abnormal hormone levels, or alcohol- and other drug-related problems.

For many men, though, it is the fear of impotence and anxiety over performance that most often lead to consistent erection failure. A man may be putting himself under a lot of pressure to achieve super-stud status every time he makes love. Sometimes, a bad sexual experience, perhaps compounded by the unsympathetic comments of a sexual partner, has increased his anxiety about how well he is going to perform. This worry may then become a self-fulfilling prophecy in all future sexual relationships. If the man does not have a secure relationship, and so is constantly involved in new sexual situations, his fears about his performance in bed may become so extreme that the tension makes it virtually impossible to get an erection, or to keep one once he has started penetrative sex.

Alternatively, if a man has been orientated solely towards thrusting, penetrative sexual intercourse, driven along by high levels of excitement, and his relationship then becomes more companionable, he may be unable to achieve or sustain arousal in this new climate of intimacy.

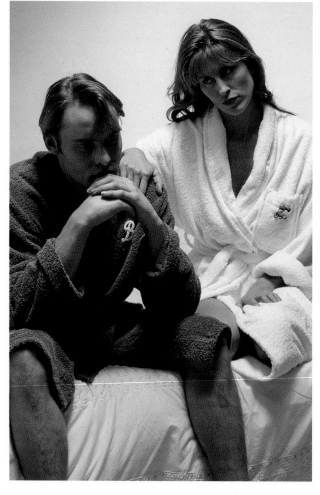

LEFT | Sometimes a man can go through a temporary period of impotence due to factors such as stress or anxiety, but with the understanding and loving support of his partner, he should eventually recover his enthusiasm and ability to achieve an erection.

When a man is struggling with the emotional and physical factors of erection failure, for whatever reasons, the best thing he can do is to take the pressure off the situation. Temporary abstinence from sex will give him the time he needs to unlink the connection between anxiety and performance. If he has a sympathetic partner, who is willing to assist him at this time, they can benefit from the sensate focus exercises described previously.

They should work through the programme step by step, not reaching the last stage until the man has been able to relax totally into sensual touching and receiving touch for its own sake, rather than to achieve a climax. Once the woman has started to touch his genitals, she should avoid focusing on them too closely. If an erection occurs it should not become central to the sensory experience of whole-body touching.

When the man begins to relax into his whole-body sensuality, the woman can stimulate him to an erection, either manually or orally, but should then allow the erection to subside while she concentrates on other areas of his body. When his penis has become softer, she can again stimulate him to an erection. At this stage, she should not try to bring him to an orgasm.

In this way, the man begins to realize that he can have an erection, lose it, and then regain it at a later time. The couple should practise this phase of the exercises for about three weeks, or for however long it takes for the man to accept the fluctuations of his erections without anxiety.

As the couple progress through the mutual touching and genital-to-genital contact stages of the sensate focus exercises, the man should continue to involve himself totally with touching and caressing the woman's body, and avoid focusing on whether or not he has an erection. The woman can help by continuing to touch and stroke his body and genitals without expecting something to happen. When the couple are able to reach the sensual lovemaking stage, the woman should begin by taking her partner's penis slowly into her vagina as described. If the penis becomes soft at any stage, both partners should simply

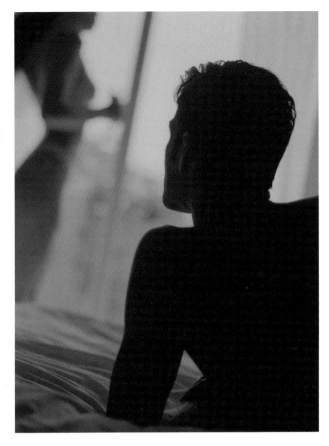

continue with their sensual touching, allowing the erection to return later, or not, as the case may be.

Gradually, with patience and loving support, the man may be able to break the cycle of anxiety which has inhibited his responses. By becoming less focused on his penis, and more involved in the pleasures of sensual contact with his partner, he will be able to relax and gain a new confidence in his sensuality and sexuality.

A single man who has anxieties about his performance should try to avoid casual sexual encounters which may confirm his insecurity. It is better to develop a secure and loving partnership where the sexual relationship has time to build slowly and where his sexual confidence is not immediately challenged.

ABOVE | Fears about performance with a new partner can create anxiety and tension.

overcoming premature ejaculation

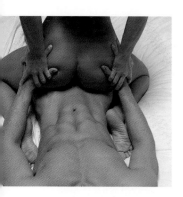

ABOVE | It will benefit the woman to learn to recognize the signals that indicate when her partner is close to ejaculation.

PREMATURE EJACULATION IS FAIRLY COMMON in younger men who have not yet learned to control and extend the plateau phase of their sexual response, which occurs just before orgasm. In all men, there is a point when ejaculation is inevitable. However, some men ejaculate almost immediately upon genital-to-genital stimulation, or even during the initial stages of physical contact. This is disappointing for both partners, but is particularly frustrating for the woman if she has no time to achieve orgasm herself.

A consistent pattern of premature ejaculation will cause anxiety because the man feels unable to control his bodily responses, and fears disappointing his partner. Such anxiety can lead to erection failure, or sex avoidance, especially if he is regularly criticized for "poor performance" in bed.

Fortunately, premature ejaculation can be successfully treated by sex therapy. Ideally this should involve both partners. If the couple have a good basis of communication, and are mutually willing to explore new sensual techniques to help change the man's habitual patterns of sexual response, they can benefit from the following self-help exercises using the "squeeze technique". However, if there are other fundamental problems within the relationship, the couple are better advised to seek professional help to improve their communication, and resolve the sexual problems.

In the self-help method, the couple must agree to abstain from intercourse during the period of time they are following the exercises until a certain stage of progress has been reached. However, the man can help his partner climax through oral or manual stimulation whenever she wants him to.

Having committed themselves to this programme, which should be held at least three times a week, the couple begin with manual stimulation. The woman masturbates the man, applying the "squeeze" to the top of the penis when he approaches his orgasm threshold. Once the erection has subsided slightly, she stimulates him again by hand, repeating this procedure up to three times. He is then allowed to ejaculate. After several sessions, which ought to be no more than two days apart, the man should begin to feel more confident in his ability to delay ejaculation.

At this point the couple can progress to genital-to-genital contact. The woman sits astride her partner and uses her hand to move his penis around her vaginal lips and clitoris, while applying the squeeze technique as necessary. Once both partners feel confident that the man has achieved some control over his ejaculatory process in this more intimate situation, they can apply the squeeze technique to the first stages of intercourse. The woman should position herself astride her partner and then guide his penis into her vagina. They should both then remain still.

If the woman senses her partner is close to ejaculating, she must lift off his penis and apply the squeeze technique. The couple can then repeat this procedure at least three times before allowing ejaculation to occur. If the man ejaculates prematurely, despite their efforts to delay it, neither partner should regard this as a disaster.

the squeeze technique

The basic squeeze technique is useful in helping a couple tackle the problem of premature ejaculation. The squeeze is applied by the woman who simultaneously presses her thumb pad against the frenulum, just below the head of the penis, and the pad of her first finger just above the coronal ridge on the top of the glans, while her second finger rests parallel to the first on the shaft of the penis. Pressure must come directly from the pads of the fingers and thumb (avoid a grasping squeeze) and needs to be maintained firmly for at least four seconds. It should not be applied to the sides of the penis. The man can indicate how much pressure feels comfortable if his partner is unsure. This pressure should cause the erection to subside slightly and delay the ejaculation. The procedure is carried out at least three times in one session, always just prior to the ejaculation phase. The woman should learn to recognize the signals that indicate when her partner is close to this level of arousal, or he can let her know himself.

Anxiety, expectation or criticism all work against the possibility of overcoming premature ejaculation. By persevering with the exercises, the man gradually builds up his confidence and ability to delay ejaculation.

If good progress is made after three or more sessions in the penetration phase described above, the woman can begin to move very gently while his penis is inside her. Again, as she becomes aware that her partner is reaching the point of no return, she should stop moving, lift up from his penis and apply the squeeze technique before resuming penetration and gentle movement.

The couple should continue with these exercises until the man is able to sustain his erection for up to 15 minutes inside his partner before ejaculating. The more the couple engage in this phase of the exercise, the more likely it is that the old patterns of sexual response will dissolve. They should not worry if the man occasionally ejaculates too soon, but should persevere.

Once the partners are able to sustain a longer period of intercourse, and feel confident enough to increase thrusting and movement, they can start to apply a different form of squeeze which does not necessitate the woman dismounting from the penis. The pressure is now applied, by either the man or the woman, to the base of the penis, with the thumb pad pressing on the area just above the scrotum, and the first two fingers parallel, applying pressure on the opposite side of the penis. Again, the penis should not be squeezed at the sides.

Eventually, the couple can experiment with other lovemaking positions, using the squeeze technique when necessary, especially if the man resumes the on-top position, which is more likely to lead to premature ejaculation. Many men may wish to prolong lovemaking without ejaculating before either they or their partners are ready. The sensate focus exercises will help them to relax more into sensual touching and intercourse and are bound to enrich their sexual relationship.

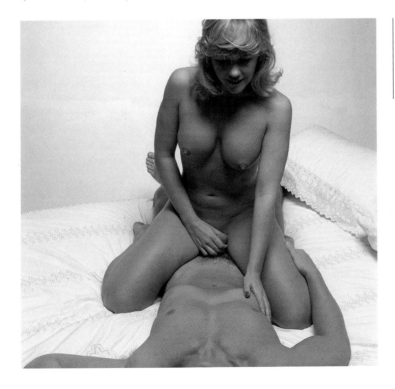

LEFT | Whenever you feel your partner is close to ejaculating, you can apply the squeeze technique so that his erection subsides slightly. Then you can begin to stimulate him again.

overcoming orgasmic difficulties

THERE ARE MANY REASONS WHY A WOMAN may have difficulty in reaching an orgasm, but most of these can be overcome by creating a new and more sensual attitude towards her body, and by the willingness of her and her partner to explore more mutually satisfying forms of lovemaking.

For a woman who has difficulty in achieving an orgasm, or who has lost this capacity altogether, the following self-help suggestions may enable her to attain sexual fulfilment.

She should learn to enjoy self-pleasuring, not only through masturbation, but also by becoming more sensually aware of her whole body. Self-massage, stroking and caressing herself, applying aromatic moisturizing creams to her skin, and learning to love her own body, will help to boost her body image and self-esteem. If she is shy, or has negative feelings about her genitals, self-exploration, using a mirror and her fingers, will help her to accept these most intimate parts.

Once she has established a better body image, she will benefit from self-masturbation, allowing herself to stroke, caress and rub her vaginal lips and clitoral area to discover the pressures and motions that are most arousing. The more sensual she makes this experience, the more enhanced

her responses are likely to be. She should dedicate time to regular self-pleasuring, letting her strokes involve her whole body, including her face, neck, breasts, belly, thighs, buttocks, mons and vulva.

To put herself in the right mood, she can bathe in an aromatic bath beforehand so that she feels totally relaxed both mentally and physically, and then moisturize her skin with lotion to leave it soft and glowing. She can then retire to a warm and private setting, perhaps lit by candles and with relaxing or sexy music playing in the background.

The woman can begin to let go into erotic fantasy, conjuring up whatever sexual pictures help to arouse her. Some women find it difficult to allow sexual fantasy, either because of guilt feelings or because they do not have an adequate source of erotic mental images. Women who feel guilty about having erotic fantasies should read Nancy Friday's book *My Secret Garden*. Here, the author's careful research reveals the rich diversity of women's fantasies, some funny, some bizarre, some lurid, but all giving testimony to the fertile, erotic female mind. The woman can also use a vibrator to explore her sexual responses.

Sometimes, a woman may block her orgasmic reactions because she is reluctant to really let go,

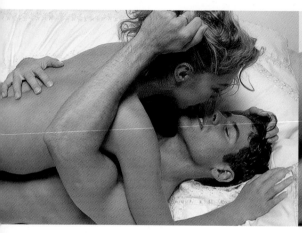
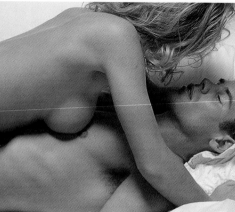

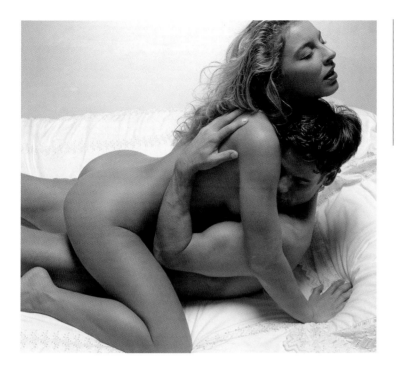

OPPOSITE AND LEFT | Once
you are able to fully relax into
your own body and sensual
and erotic feelings of pleasure
in touching and lovemaking,
without worrying about
performance or results, you
may find that your orgasmic
capacity increases.

fearful of losing control over her body. Enacting out an orgasmic response to the full, breathing deeply, writhing on the bed, sighing and crying out will give her more confidence to abandon herself freely when she is orgasmic with a lover.

Self-stimulation techniques allow the woman to become familiar with her own unique sexual responses, so she can regard herself as orgasmic in her own right, rather than as a result of what someone else does to her.

When a woman is experiencing orgasmic dysfunction within her sexual relationship, both she and her partner will benefit from the sensate focus exercises. They can learn or rediscover how to touch each other's bodies in a sensual rather than immediately sexual way. They can also benefit from the non-demanding genital contact exercises, during which the woman shows her partner how she prefers to masturbate herself.

Leisurely foreplay, including kissing, caressing, manual clitoral stimulation and oral-genital contact, all enjoyed for the sheer sake of pleasure, rather than focused purely towards orgasm, will help the woman to feel cherished and become more fully aroused before penetration occurs.

The woman should not feel she has to have an orgasm to soothe her partner's sexual ego, or to prove herself to be sexually responsive. This demand can create a mental and physical tension which is likely to block her natural responses.

It is also important for the couple to resolve their relationship conflicts before making love, because hidden resentments and other negative feelings may also affect the woman's ability to relax sexually. Choosing the right time to make love, when neither partner is tired or under stress, or when they are unlikely to be interrupted by their children, will enhance the sexual responses of both of them.

A woman who is unable to attain an orgasm by any means of stimulation – a condition known as anorgasmia – will benefit from the guidance of a qualified sex therapist if she wishes to become orgasmic.

treating vaginismus

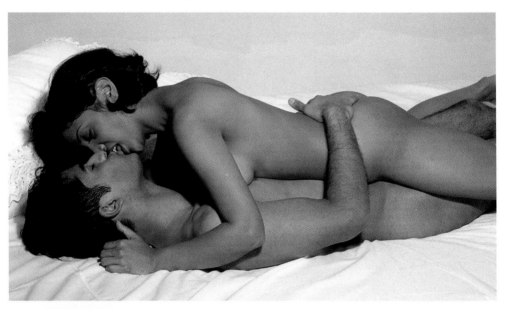

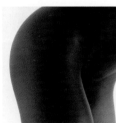

FOR SOME WOMEN, penetrative sex can be an uncomfortable or even painful experience. In rare cases, intercourse may be impossible because of involuntary contractions of the muscles surrounding the vagina – a condition known as vaginismus. Many sufferers may otherwise have completely normal sexual responses and desires, and may easily attain orgasm through non-penetrative sex such as masturbation or oral-genital contact.

Vaginismus occurs most commonly in young women. However, a woman may suffer this disorder at various times throughout her sexual life, and it can cause great distress to both her and her partner who may, in every other respect, enjoy a close relationship. The problem can be so serious that the woman is unable to insert a tampon, a pessary or even her own finger into her vagina, and a pelvic examination is an impossibility without sedation. If the woman has never been able to experience vaginal

penetration, the condition is known as primary vaginismus. If she has had penetrative sex in the past, but has consequently developed these distressing symptoms, the condition is called secondary vaginismus.

Vaginismus can result from a number of complex causes. If it is primary, the problem may stem from early childhood or adolescent conditioning, possibly due to parental or religious influences, which have created negative feelings about sexuality in general, or her genitals in particular.

Other causes include trauma due to rape, sexual or indecent assault or childhood sexual and physical abuse, a painful and insensitive gynaecological examination in adolescence, or an exaggerated fear of becoming pregnant or of contracting a sexually transmitted disease. Secondary vaginismus may occur as a result of a genital infection, a difficult childbirth, or other pathological causes which previously made intercourse painful and have consequently precipitated the involuntary muscular response. The woman may then become fearful of further pain on penetration.

Whatever the reasons for vaginismus, and sometimes they are complex and indefinable, a woman must first be examined by a sympathetic gynaecologist to discover whether there is an identifiable underlying cause, such as a physical abnormality or infection that can be treated easily. Vaginismus is almost always treatable once the woman and her partner, if she has one, decide to seek professional advice and receive sex therapy. The complexity of the psychological issues involved in vaginismus, and the need to ascertain whether the condition is a primary or secondary one, make it advisable that the woman's circumstances are assessed by a psychosexual counsellor. The therapist will then be able to carefully guide the woman and her partner through the treatment strategy that is most appropriate to her particular case.

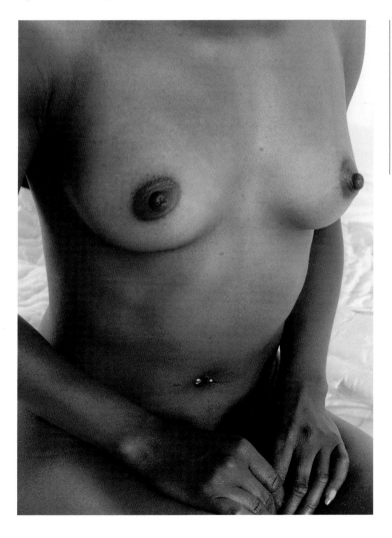

OPPOSITE AND LEFT | Through loving care, mutual support and the changing of existing patterns through simple exercises and techniques, problems such as premature ejaculation and vaginismus can be understood, coped with and hopefully overcome, especially with the aid of sympathetic counselling.

rape and abuse

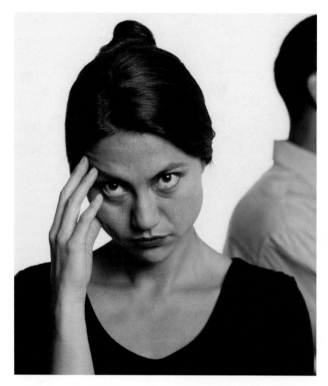

ABOVE | There is no magic formula for recovering from sexual or violent abuse. It is important to remember, however, that time and counselling are great healers. Most important of all, remind yourself that it was not your fault that it happened.

RAPE AND SEXUAL VIOLENCE are far more common than most people think, and anyone can be a victim: young women, old women, men, children – in short, people of all classes and all cultures. Most rape and sexual violence is carried out by men against women. The majority of women who have been raped know their attacker, because they are a current partner, ex-partner, family friend, neighbour or workmate: someone they trust.

why do men rape women?
Rape is not so much about sex as about power and control. For example, the notorious date rapes, of which young women under the age of 25 are the main victims, are carried out by men, often with the use of drugs such as Rohypnol which are

used to spike drinks. Many of the men questioned do not admit that their behaviour is wrong. All too often, the perpetrators have it in their minds that a woman saying no doesn't actually mean no. She wanted sex, she was gagging for it, they maintain, and feel they deserve something in return for the money and attention they have spent on her.

One of the most common arguments that men raise for forcing themselves on their wives, girlfriends or dates is that, in the midst of a heavy petting session, when the man is all ready to go, the woman decides she doesn't want to continue. She ends the session, leaving her partner frustrated. However, if a woman says no, it means no. If a woman wants to pull out at the last moment, that is her right. There is absolutely no biological or psychological reason why a man cannot stop.

why do men rape men?
In many countries, male rape has only recently become a crime. In Britain, Home Office statistics for 1999/2000 reported an increase of 19% in reported male rape. This is believed to be a huge under-representation of the true figure.

Although there has been less research on the subject than on female rape, and there are far fewer services for male victims, we know that a lot of men won't report being raped. This is also about power. It is prevalent in institutions, particularly prisons, and has only recently been taken seriously by the authorities. Many myths surround male rape: only gay men are raped; men are raped because they are weak; men are strong and should be able to defend themselves against their attackers. Heterosexual as well as gay men are raped and this can have the consequence of making them doubt their sexuality.

what to do if you are raped
If you are raped, whether you are a man or a woman, get to a safe place, call the police or a rape crisis centre, or phone a family member or

friend to help. You must see a doctor to have a medical check-up. You will also need medical evidence for any prosecution. Don't change your clothes, don't have a bath or shower, don't even comb your hair or adjust anything until you have been examined by the doctor, otherwise you could destroy evidence.

If you have been raped, or sexually abused by a family member, the most important thing to remember is that it is not your fault. Rapists are responsible for their own actions. It is a brutal and humiliating experience and you will need tender care afterwards. Therapy is often a necessity after such an ordeal.

While most rapes are carried out by men who are known to the victim, there are rapes that are completely random. People must be vigilant wherever they are, whether walking down a dark street at night, in an empty train carriage (coach) or even in a work situation. Keep your wits about you and, if you are planning to travel alone, think carefully about how you are going to get to your destination safely.

Many people feel suicidal, suffer from post-traumatic stress disorder and go into deep depressions when they have been raped. Therapy is probably the best long-term solution after such a horrendous ordeal.

One in four women will experience rape or attempted rape, and most will not report it to the police. The legal definition of rape varies from country to country, but if a man has sexual intercourse with a person who at the time does not consent to it, that is essentially rape. It is defined as the non-consensual penetration of the vagina or anus by a penis. Forced oral sex and the penetration of the vagina or anus by a foreign object are, at the very least, serious sexual assault. Touching and other kinds of unwanted sexual contact are also sexual assault.

abuse

This is an extreme form of control. While mostly carried out by men against women or children, it happens within gay relationships and violence by women against men appears to be on the

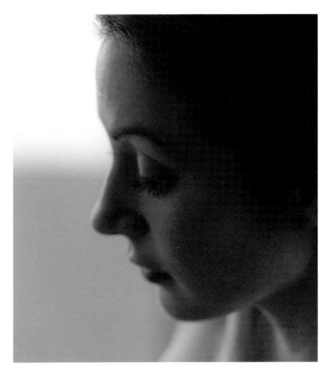

increase. The abuse can be both emotional and physical. A partner can be hit, kicked or beaten, humiliated in front of other people, threatened with death, or made to perform sexual acts that they do not want to do: in effect, rape. Even silent treatment, in which one partner refuses to communicate, is a form of abuse.

Being abused can cause depression, anxiety and illness, as well as injury. In many cases it can lead to homelessness and, in extreme cases, it results in murder. Many abusers don't understand the meaning and effect of emotional and verbal abuse, and need to be educated about what respectful behaviour towards a partner means. Many victims lose their self-esteem, and may even lose all control of their actions and lives.

Nobody should have to put up with it, so if you are being abused, seek help. Most people are acutely embarrassed by abuse and its consequences, but it is crucial that you seek the help of a professional to guide you through this time.

ABOVE | After a traumatic experience, don't suffer in silence, however ashamed or frightened you feel. Find someone you can trust who will support you, and find out about which organization to contact for help should you wish to.

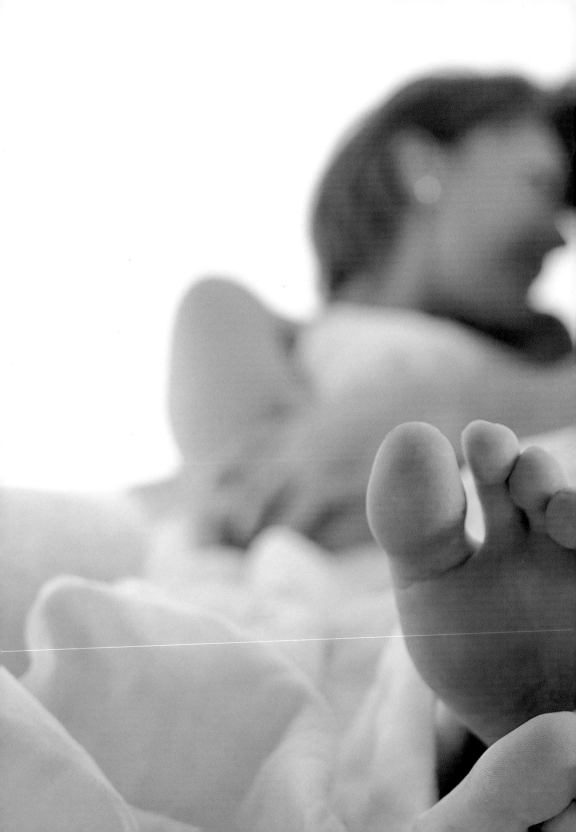

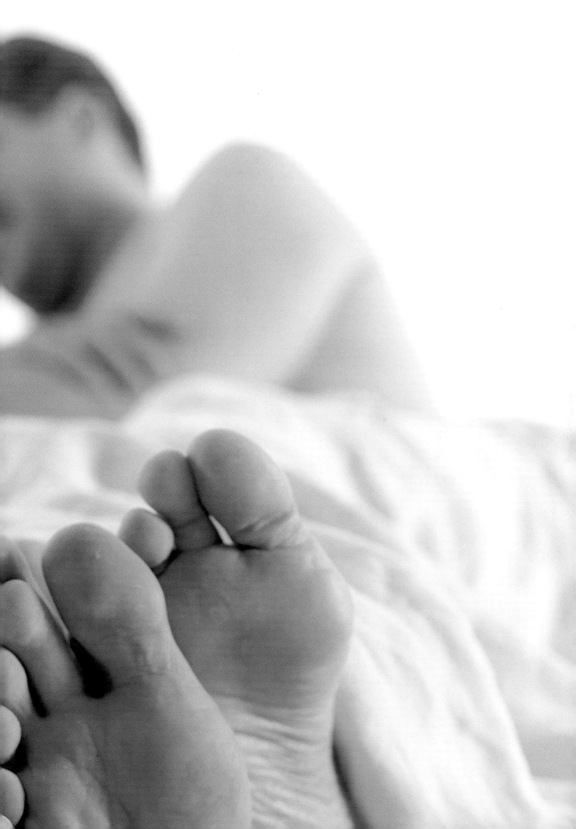

glossary

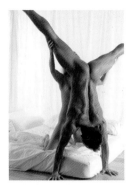

A spot The anterior fornex erogenous spot is the G spot's neighbour. Located about one-third of the way down the front vaginal wall.

adrenaline A hormone released after exercise which can increase the libido.

anal Relating to the anus, as in anal sex.

anal beads A string of beads placed up the anus and pulled out at the point of orgasm.

aphrodisiac An experience or substance that stimulates or enhances sexual desire.

B/D Bondage/discipline.

BDSM Bondage discipline and sadomasochism – the elements of dominance and submission.

bisexual A person who feels sexually aroused by people of both sexes.

blow job Oral sex done on a man; fellatio.

body modification Altering your body with tattoos, piercings and corsets.

bondage Sexual arousal by physical restrictions, such as handcuffs and rope restraints.

bottom The submissive half of a bondage duo. The dominant half is known as the top.

buggery Anal intercourse.

butt plug A diamond shaped or flared implement that is inserted up the anus and is usually made of silicone or plastic. It is used to create a feeling of fullness.

CAT Coital Alignment Technique – an intercourse technique where you roll rather than thrust.

cervical cap Birth control device that covers the cervix and acts as a barrier to prevent the sperm from entering.

cervix Opening of the uterus.

chakras Described in Tantric sex. These are the seven points in individuals which are believed to regulate different types of energy.

chlamydia A sexually transmitted infection that affects both men and women. It often displays no symptoms but can lead to infertility, highlighting the importance of regular check-ups. If found early it can be treated with antibiotics.

circumcision A small operation which is

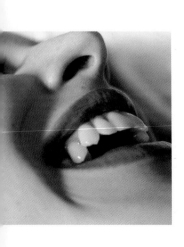

performed by either a doctor or a religious expert to remove the foreskin of the penis. It is usually performed either for medical reasons such as phimosis (a tight foreskin), for reasons of hygiene or for religious reasons.

clitoris The only organ in the human body whose sole function is pleasure. This little organ is located at the top of a woman's vulva. It is covered with a clitoral hood and becomes erect when the woman is sexually aroused.

cock ring A penis ring made of either rubber or leather that fits around the base of an erect penis to maintain an erection for longer by trapping blood in the organ. Never wear one for more than 20 or 30 minutes.

condom A latex sheath that fits snugly over the penis. The most commonly used form of barrier contraception.

Cowper's glands Small structures near the urethra inside the base of the penis, involved in the secretion of pre-seminal fluid.

crabs A sexually transmitted infection in the form of lice which inhabit the pubic hair.

cross-dressing When a member of one sex finds sexual gratification in wearing the clothes of and mimicking the opposite sex. NB: cross-dressers are by no means always gay.

cum Slang term for male ejaculate.

cunnilingus Oral sex on a woman. "Cunnus" is Latin for vulva and "lingere" is Latin for lick.

diaphragm Contraceptive barrier method which holds spermicidal jelly against the woman's cervical opening.

dildo Penis-shaped object, which can be inserted into the vagina or anus for sexual stimulation. Not to be confused with a vibrator, which is similar in structure but is battery operated and vibrates for extra stimulation.

dildo harness A device that can be worn with a dildo attached, allowing hands-free thrusting.

doggy style A sexual position where the woman is on all fours and the man enters from behind.

dom Dominatrix or dominator.

double dildo A dildo that can be used at both ends by two people at the same time.

double penetration A penis or dildo in the vagina and anus at the same time.

ectopic pregnancy When the developing embryo implants in the fallopian tubes and not the uterus. If not caught quickly it can lead to maternal death.

ejaculate The white fluid which usually accompanies male orgasm.

endorphins These are the body's feel-good hormones, neuro-transmitters which have a wide range of functions. They help regulate heart action, hormone function, the perception of pain and the mechanisms of shock from blood loss, and are thought to be involved in some way in controlling emotion, mood and motivation. Exercise, sex and chocolate are thought to stimulate production.

felching Licking male ejaculate out of either the anus or vagina.

fellatio Oral sex for the male; a blow job.

fetish A specific object or body part that an individual eroticizes for sexual gratification.

foreskin A flap of skin that extends from the shaft of the penis and over the head to maintain moisture and provide protection. In the circumcised male it is removed.

French kiss A mouth-open, tongue-twizzling kiss!

frenulum Located below the glans or head of the penis, on the side that faces away from the body, when erect. This is an extremely sensitive area.

frottage Simulating sex with your clothes on.

full hundred A Pilates-based exercise which you perform 100 times.

G spot Named after Ernest Grafenburg who claimed that an area on the roof of the vagina is potentially sexually stimulating for some women.

gender dysphoria When a person of a specific sex wishes to be of the opposite sex.

genitals Sex organs.

glans The head of the penis.

golden shower Urinating on your partner as a means of sexual stimulation.

gonad A sex gland.

hermaphrodite An individual who is born with both the male and female sex organs. This is

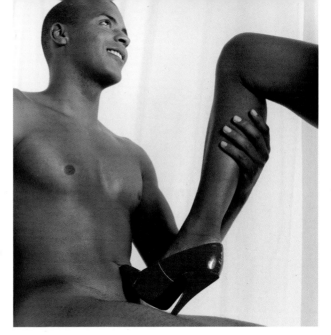

usually caused by an excess of the hormone androgen during pregnancy.

herpes A virus that can affect either the mouth or genitals. It forms a rash and can cause flu-like symptoms. Once infected, it remains in the body, usually in a relatively harmless dormant state. It is important to use barrier methods of contraception such as condoms if you are aware that you are a carrier, but especially if you are not 100 per cent confident that your partner is not.

impotence When a man is unable to get an erection on a regular basis.

IUD Formerly known as the coil, an intrauterine device is fitted into the uterus and prevents conception by stopping the egg implanting in the uterus wall.

Kama Sutra An Indian classical book on the technique and art of love and lovemaking.

Kegel exercises Squeezing and contracting your puboccygeus muscle. These help to make you more aware of sexual sensation and some say that they can result in more intense orgasms. Especially useful for women to regain genital strength after childbirth.

Kinsey average The amount of time researcher Alfred Kinsey estimated it took for the average male to reach orgasm during intercourse.

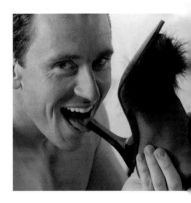

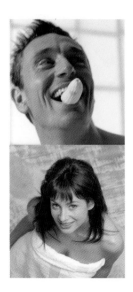

kundalini Derived from the Sanskrit word "kundal" meaning coiled up, which is normally represented as a coiled or sleeping serpent in Vedic and Tantric texts. An awareness of the presence of this energy within the human body was considered by the sages and saints to be the highest knowledge.

labia minora The inner lips of the vagina that are attached to the clitoris. Pink in colour and thinner than the outer lips (labia majora).

lesbian A woman who prefers sexual relationships with other women.

libido The desire that drives us to have a sexual relationship with another person.

lingham Sanskrit for penis, a definition used in Tantric texts.

maithuna A skill men use to suppress their orgasm in Tantric sex.

masochist A person who welcomes pain and finds sexual gratification in receiving it. Also known as a "bottom" or submissive.

masturbation Stimulating your own genitals to achieve sexual gratification.

merkin A wig made specifically for the pubic region, held on with glue.

missionary position The man and woman have sex in a horizontal position facing one another, with the man on top.

monilia A vaginal yeast infection (candida albicans) that can be painful and cause thick discharge together with intense itching.

mons pubis The fleshy mound on top of the vulva that pubic hair grows from.

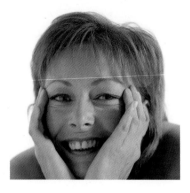

Montgomery glands Small bumps on the nipples.

morning-after pill Emergency contraception that comes in the form of two pills taken 12 hours after each other. Can be used up to 72 hours after unprotected sex.

mula bandha or root lock – a yoga position concentrating on the pelvic floor muscles.

nipple clamps A clip that is placed on the nipples during sex play. They come with varying degrees of pressure and are often used in BDSM.

nocturnal emission A wet dream, common in boys during puberty.

nonoxynol-9 Ingredient of most contraceptive foams and gels that changes the pH of male sperm and renders it infertile.

nonspecific urethritis An infection of the urinary tubes that is pretty common.

orgasm The sensations that ripple through your body at the climax of sexual excitement.

orgasmic platform The vulva and the first third of the vaginal passage where there is a concentration of nerve endings.

papervine A drug injected into the penis, which makes it hard and erect.

Pelvic Inflammatory Disease (PID) A bacterial infection that causes inflammation of the female sex organs, usually the fallopian tubes.

pelvic tilt An exercise to keep the muscles of the pelvis in trim.

perineum Sensitive area between the anus and the male or female genitals.

pessaries Spermicides in the form of small bullets which are inserted into the vagina.

Pilates A gentle form of exercise for the body inspired by Joseph Pilates.

polyamory Individuals who have a committed sexual relationship with more than one partner.

pranayama This is a breathing technique practised in yoga.

precum The fluid that leaks from an erect penis during sexual excitement. Its properties deacidify the urethra so that ejaculate has a greater chance of impregnating the female.

prepuce The foreskin of the penis.

priapism Named after the Greek God of male reproductive power Priapus, this is an often painful affliction that causes a "trapped" erection, i.e. one that will not go down. It is often necessary to seek medical assistance to prevent permanent damage.

Prince Albert A male genital piercing that goes through the urethral opening of the penis, coming out on the underside of the shaft.

prostate The gland that is responsible for a portion of the male ejaculate, it contracts seconds before orgasm. Located on the floor of the rectum.

puboccygeus (PC) muscle This holds the pelvic floor together.

rape Forced sex on either a male or female. A serious criminal offence that results in tremendous psychological damage to its victims.

rimming Kissing and licking the anus.

safe word Used in bondage, this is a prearranged expression that the bottom uses to tell the top either to stop, or to ease up.

safer sex It is important to take precautions against STIs, but there is no such thing as safe sex.

Sanskrit The ancient Indo-European literary language of India.

scissors A Pilates-based exercise holding the legs in the air and making a scissor action.

serotonin The neuro-transmitter and hormone 5-hydroxytryptamine (5-HT) which is found in many tissues, especially the brain, the intestinal lining and the blood platelets. Serotonin is concerned with controlling moods and levels of consciousness.

S&M Sexual scenarios where individuals act out submission and domination fantasies.

smegma Build-up of thick pungent substance

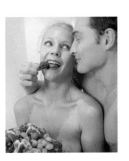

underneath the foreskin or clitoral hood.

sodomy Generally understood to mean anal penetration.

soixante-neuf (69) Where a couple perform oral sex on each other simultaneously.

spermicide A cream, gel or pessary that will kill sperm on contact, often added to condoms.

STI Sexually transmitted infection. Also known as STD (sexually transmitted disease) or, less commonly nowadays, VD (venereal disease).

swinging Husband-and-wife-swapping, often involving group sex or specific parties where couples swap and have sex with other partners.

switches People who participate in BDSM and alternate, being either the "top" or the "bottom".

Tantra A number of Hindu and Buddhist writings giving religious teaching and ritual instructions.

thrush A vaginal yeast infection caused by either candida or monilia fungus. Penile thrush can also occur in men but is less common.

tipped uterus A uterus that points towards the back as opposed to lying parallel to the spine. Can cause problems in conception.

top The master, mistress or dominator in BDSM.

toxic shock syndrome (TSS) A rare but potentially lethal infection associated with using tampons.

tubal ligation Permanent female sterilization, which involves surgically sealing the fallopian tubes.

urethral sponge Cushioned area that protects the urethra during intercourse.

vibrator An electrical vibrating device used most commonly by women for masturbation. Can be used vaginally or anally.

voyeurism A fetish involving individuals achieving sexual stimulation from watching other people undress or have sex.

vulva The external female genitalia.

wall slide An exercise to strengthen the thigh and stomach muscles.

yeast infection Fungal infections that particularly afflict moist areas such as between the toes, the vagina and penis.

yoga An ancient and holistic form of exercise suiable for all ages.

yoni The Sanskrit word for a woman's vulva, a term often used in Tantra.

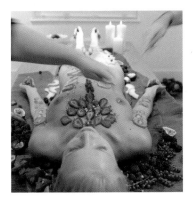

bibliography

Allende, Isabel, Aphrodite: The Love of Food and the Food of Love (Flamingo, UK, 1998)

Allison, Sadie, Tickle Your Fancy (Tickle Kitty Press, USA, 2002)

Alman, Isadora, Doing It (Conari Press, USA, 2001)

Anderson, Dan and Berman, Maggie, Sex Tips for Straight Women from a Gay Man (2nd edn, Thorsons, UK, 2002)

Blank, Joani, Still Doing It: Women and Men over 60 Write About their Sexuality (Down There Press, USA, 2000)

Burton, Sir Richard, The Kama Sutra of Vatsyayana and the Phaedrus of Plato (Kimber Editions, 1963)

Cattrall, Kim, and Levinson, Mark, Satisfaction: The Art of the Female Orgasm (Thorsons, 2002)

Comfort, Alex, The Joy of Sex (5th edn, Mitchell Beazley, UK, 1996)

D'Argy Smith, Marcelle, The Lover's Guide: What Women Really Want (Carlton Books, UK, 2002)

Davies, Dominic, Gillespie-Sells, Kath and Shakespeare, Tom, The Sexual Politics of Disability: Untold Desires (Cassell, UK and New York, USA 1996)

Delvin, David, The She Complete Guide to Sex and Loving (Ebury Press, UK, 1985)

Dennis, Wendy, Hot and Bothered (2nd edn, Grafton, UK, 1993)

Easton, Dossie and Hardy, Janet W., The New Bottoming Book (Greenery Press, USA, 2001)

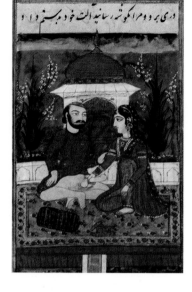

Friday, Nancy, My Secret Garden (Quartet Books Ltd, UK, 1975)

Hooper, Anne, Massage and Loving (Unwin Hyman Ltd, UK, 1988)

Joannides, Paul, Guide To Getting it On (2nd edn, Vermilion, UK, 2001)

Kriedman, Ellen, Light His Fire (Judy Piatkus Ltd, UK, 1990)

Lacroix, Nitya, Love, Sex and Intimacy (7th edn, Lorenz Books, UK, 2002)

Lacroix, Nitya, Tantric Sex: The Tantric art of Sensual Loving (2nd edn, Southwater, UK, 2000)

Lawson, Michael, The Better Marriage Guide, (Hodder & Stoughton Ltd, UK, 1998)

McConville, Brigid, My Secret Life: Sexual Revelations from Long-term Lovers (Thorsons, UK, 1998)

Paget, Lou, How To Give Her Absolute Pleasure (2nd edn, Judy Piatkus Ltd, UK, 2001)

Paros, Lawrence, The Erotic Tongue (2nd edn, Arlington Books Ltd, UK, 1988)

Powling, Suzy and Thoburn, Marj, The Relate

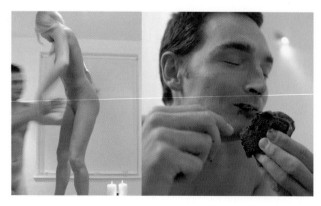

Guide to Loving In Later Life: How To Renew
Intimacy And Have Fun In The Prime Of Life (2nd
edn, Vermilion, UK, 2000)

Quilliam, Susan and Relate, Staying Together:
From Crisis to Deeper Commitment (2nd Edition,
Vermillion, UK 2001)

Reyes, Alina, The Butcher (3rd edn, Minerva,
UK, 1992)

Youngson, Dr Robert, The Royal Society of
Medicine Health Encyclopedia (3rd edn,
Bloomsbury Publishing Plc, UK)

articles

Campbell, Carolyn, Speed Dating: A New Form of
Matchmaking (Discovery Health Channel website)

Crisp, Charlotte, Talking Dirty (Cosmopolitan, May
2002, p.145)

Goleman, Daniel, Language of Love (New York
Times, February 14th 1995)

Guerra, Fred, What is Semen Made From?
(JakinWorld.com Science Corner)

Hill, Amelia, Women to Get Sex Toys on the NHS,
(The Observer website, September 29th 2002)

Kaylin, Lucy, The Porning of America (GQ, August
1997, pp.166–70)

Keyishian, Amy, The Complete Guide to Your
Clitoris (Cosmopolitan, May 2002, pp.137–140)

Mauro, Jim, Keeper of the Flame (Smoke, vol 11,
no.2, pp.84–91)

O'Connell, Sanjida, Follow Your Nose (Guardian
Unlimited, September 27th 2002)

Stewart, Fiona, R U RDY 4 THS? (iVillage.co.uk,

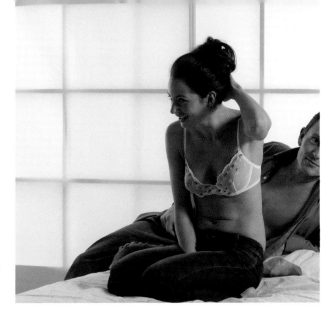

September 5th 2002)

Vincent, Sally, Everybody's Doing It (The Guardian
Weekend, August 10th 2002)

Whitfield, John, The Sweet Smell of the Immune
System (Nature News Service, March 7th 2002)

websites

www.cliterati.co.uk
The website that admits that women like sex too.

www.tantra.com
The resource for Tantra, sex and the Kama Sutra.

www.tantra.org
Church of Tantra and the text of the Kama Sutra.

www.tantraworks.com
Vatsayana's contribution.

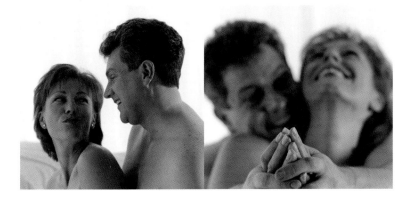

useful addresses

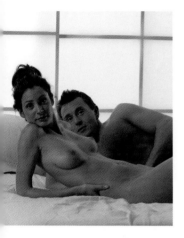

American Counseling Association
6101 Stevenson Avenue, Alexandria, Virginia 22304
(800) 347–6647
www.counseling.org

British Association for Sexual and Relationship Therapy (BASRT)
National charity with a list of therapists.
PO Box 13686, London SW20 9ZH
020 8543 2707
www.basrt.org.uk

British Pregnancy Advisory Service
03457 30 40 30
www.bpas.org

Dateable International
Social organization for people with disabilities.
15520 Bald Eagle School Road
Brandywine, MD 20613
(301) 657–3283
www.dateable.org

Disability Alliance BC
204–456 West Broadway, Vancouver,
British Columbia, Canada V5Y 1R3
(604) 875–0188
www.disabilityalliancebc.org

Education for Choice
Information about abortion, professional training and education.
50 Featherstone Street, London EC1Y 8RT
020 7284 6056
www.efc.org.uk

fpa (formerly the Family Planning Association)
50 Featherstone Street, London EC1Y 8QU
020 7608 5240
www.fpa.org.uk

Marie Stopes International
Sexual and reproductive health information.
www.mariestopes.org.uk
www.mariestopes.org.za
www.mariestopes.org.au

National Sexual Health Helpline
0300 123 7123

NHS 111
Call 111 when it's less urgent than 999.

Outsiders
Enabling the disabled to express their sexuality.
www.outsiders.org.uk

Rape, Abuse and Incest National Network, USA
National Sexual Assault Hotline 1.800.656.HOPE
rainn.org

Rape Crisis England & Wales
BCM Box 4444, London WC1N 3XX
Helpline: 0808 802 9999
www.rapecrisis.co.uk

Rape Prevention Education
PO Box 78 307, Grey Lynn, Auckland 1245
09 360 4001
www.rpe.org.nz

Relate – the relationship people
The UK's largest and most experienced relationship support organization.
Premier House, Carolina Court, Lakeside,
Doncaster DN4 5RA
0300 100 1234
www.relate.org.uk

Relationships Australia
1300 364 277
relationships.org.au

Shada (Sexual Health and Disability Alliance)
Trust@Outsiders.org.uk
077704 993 527

Survivors UK
Resources for men who have experienced any form of sexual violence.
Unit 1, Queen Anne Terrace, Sovereign Court,
The Highway, London E1W 3HH
020 3598 3898
www.survivorsuk.org

TLC Trust
www.tlc-trust.org.uk

World Health Organization
Avenue Appia 20, 1211 Geneva 27, Switzerland
(+ 41 22) 791 21 11
www.who.int

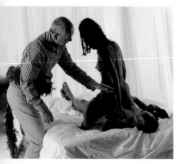

index

A

A spot 496
abortion 455
abuse 493
accentuate the positive,
 body language 35
accidents, sexual positions 219
acne 70
adrenaline 496
AFE zone 176–7
after-sex behaviour 181
afterglow 125
AIDS 442–5, 448
al fresco sex 139, 304–5
anal 496

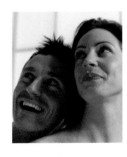

anal beads 496
anal sex 246–9
 dildos 289
 gay factor 247
 hygiene 244, 247
 law and 249
 strap-ons 248
anal stimulation 112
 during fellatio 238
ananga ranga 338–45
anorgasmia 177
antaha-samdansha 363
anterior fornix erotic zone
 (AFE) 176–7
anus

female body 76
male body 62
 see also anal sex
anvartha-nakhadana 342
aphrodisiacs 372–3, 496
Aphrodite's delight 359
arguments 403
armpits, erogenous zones 99
arousal, sexual 116
ascending position 344–5
ass position 362
atmosphere
 massage 253, 324–5
 meditation 351
attics, making love in 300
attraction 16–47
 art of wooing 46–9
 body language 30–43
 dating 28–9
 first encounters 40–3
 first impressions 16–47
 first moves 27
 flirting 26–7
 language of clothes 18–21
 next steps 44–5
 psychological exercise 22–5
availability, relaying 36–7

B

B/D 496
back (male), erogenous
 zones 105
back problems 146
back to back attunement 432–3
backward bow 55
bad breath 17
balanitis 438
balling, fellatio 239
baths 299, 308
 massage 326–7
BDSM 496

beards 16–17
bedrooms 403
belly, erogenous zones 104
bindhu-dashana 343
Bioenergetic Therapy 55
birth, sex after giving 391
bisexual 496
biting 342–3
blind dates 29
blow-jobs 236–41, 496
board games 265
body 51–87
 caring for yourself 52–3
 physical fitness 54–5
 skincare 56–8
body language 30–9
 accentuate the positive 35
 close contact 38
 confused signals 32–3
 displacement activity 38–9
 eye language 39
 negative signals 34–5
 relaying availability 36–7
 sexual signals 31–2
body modification 496

body piercing 283
bondage 274–80, 496
books 409
bottom 496
bras
 removing 96
 striptease 262
breasts
 cancer 440–1
 caring for 440–1
 checking 83
 erogenous zones 103
 female body 76–8
 foreplay 116
 male 70
 sexual arousal 116
 size and shape 78
breath, skin teasing 272–3
breathing 22–3
 exercises 418
 tantric sex 347
bridge, cunnilingus 245
bridge exercise 419
bud 359
buggery 496

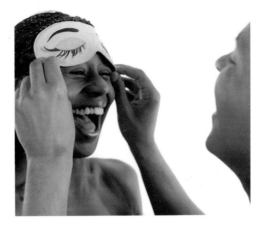

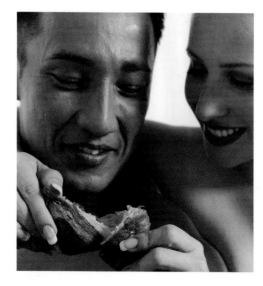

D

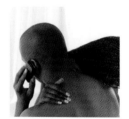

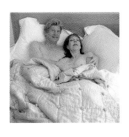

and illness 410–12
  effects of disability 410
  practical solutions 411
displacement activity,
  body language 38–9
divine sex 332–68
dog tantric position 362
doggy positions 222–8, 496
dom 497
domination 275, 276–7
double dildo 497
double penetration 497
dress 18–21
dressing up fantasies 266–7
dressing up games 264

E

e-mails 44–5
eating 52–3
ECPs 453
ectopic pregnancy 497
edge, cunnilingus 245
edging, fellatio 238
ejaculate 497
ejaculation
  delayed 475
  premature 177, 475, 486–7
  retrograde 475
  see also orgasm
elephant position 362
elephant woman 337
emergency contraception pills
  (ECPs) 455
endorphins 497
energy centres 352
epididymis 64, 67

erectile dysfunction 63
erections
  failure to maintain 177, 178
  male body 61, 68–9
  problems 468–9, 471, 480–1
  see also penis
erogenous zones 102–5
  seduction 98–9
erotica 250–90
  bondage 274–80
  cross-dressing 268–9, 283
  dressing up fantasies 266–7
  fantasies 254–7
  literature 290–1
  s&m 274–80
  sensuality 252–3
  sex games 264–5
  skin teasing 270–3
  spanking 275
  striptease 258–63
ESO 183
essential oils 319, 325
etiquette, dating 29
exercises 54–5, 414–33, 472
  games and 424–33
  increasing flexibility 422–3
  pelvic floor strengthening
    420–1
  sensate focus 472–8
  warming up 416–19
exhibitionism 311
extended sexual orgasm (ESO)
  183
eyes 147
  eye contact 26
  eye language 39

F

fabrics
  masturbation 187
  skin teasing 270–3
face
  erogenous zones 104
  massage 330–1
face sitting, cunnilingus 245

facial hair 16–17
faking orgasm 177
fallopian tubes 80–1
families
  middle years 394–5
  starting 390–1
  today 391
fan strokes, massage 123, 320–1
fantasies 284–5, 310–11
  bondage 276–7
  dominance 276–7
  dressing up 266–7
  femme fatale 267
  masturbation 186
  mutual masturbation 193
  sharing 254–7
  striptease 258–63
  temptress 266–7
feathering 309
feathers, skin teasing with 271
feel-good factor, exercises
  and 421
feet
  erogenous zones 104
  tactile stimulation 115
feet yoke 360

felching 497
fellatio 236–41, 497
  abstention 240
  objections 240–1
  swallowing semen 239
  tantric 363
  taste and smell 241
female body 74–87
  anus 76
  breast 76–8
  bulbs of vestibule 75
  clitoris 75
  erogenous zones 102–5
  internal sex organs 80–1
  labia 74
  mons pubis 74
  perineum 76
  self exploring 82–3
  urethral opening 76
  vagina 80
  vulva 74
female sexuality
  development 84–7
  sex education 86
  sexual experience 87
  sexual peak 87

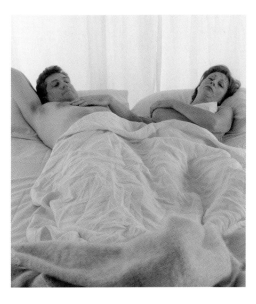

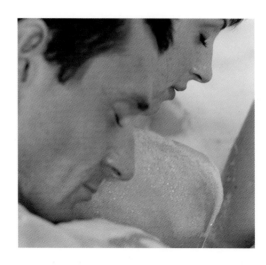

G

H

I

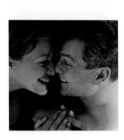

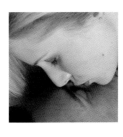

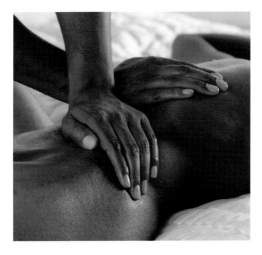

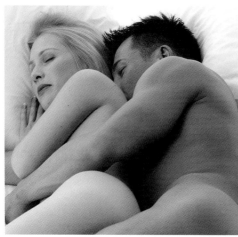

N

O

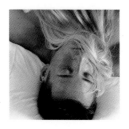

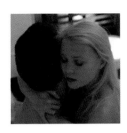

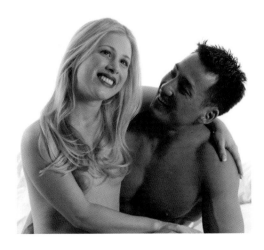

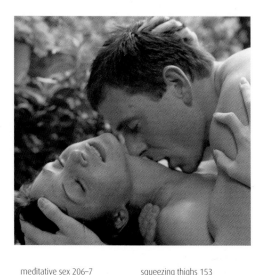

T

talking
  about sex 233, 404–5
  communication 404–7
  dirty 106, 107
tantra 499
tantric sex 107, 334, 346–68,
  352
  orgasm 174, 175, 183
tapping 189
taste, sensuality 253
tattooing 283
teasing 265
teeth, cleanliness 17
televisions, in the bedroom 403
temptress fantasies 266
tension, relieving 417
testicles (testes) 61
  orgasm and 175
testicular cancer 438
testicular self-examination
  (TSE) 67, 439
therapists 408–9, 472–3
thighs, erogenous zones 103, 104
thrush 499
tila-tandula 339
tipped uterus 499

tiryak kissing 341
toes
  erogenous zones 98–9, 104
  tactile stimulation 115
tomatoes 373
tongues
  skin teasing 272
  see also cunnilingus,
    fellatio *and* kissing
top 499
touch
  as a healing force 316
  see also massage
toxic shock syndrome 499
toys 286–8
tri-digit fidget 189
triangle, cunnilingus 245
tripod position 362
trust, developing 431
truth or dare games 264
TSE 67, 439
tubal ligation 499
turn and twist 187
turned on, men 152

U

U spot 176–7
uchchushita 363

uchun-dashana 343
underwear 21
  as gifts 404
  striptease 259, 260
undressing
  each other 94–7
  foreplay 107
urethra 61
  body 76
urethral sponge 499
urupaguha 339
uterus 80
uttaroshtha 341

V

vadavaka 359
vagina 80
  discharges 437
  large 337
  lubrication 474
  sexual arousal 116
vaginismus 177, 486–7
vas deferens 64
vasectomies 451, 453
vibrators 288, 499
  cunnilingus 244
  while restrained 280
victory roll 189
virginity, loss of 87
visualization techniques 24
vital energy, releasing 54–5
vitamins 381
voyeurism 311, 499
  mirrors 257
vrishadhirudha 339
vulnerability 470
vulva 499
  female body 74

W

wall slide 423, 499
warming-up exercises 416–19
watersports 283
wet dreams 63, 72, 498

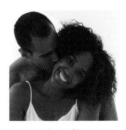

woman on top position
  137, 156–69
  becoming a better lover 160–9
  clitoral stimulation 162
  compatibility 134–5
  confidence 166–7
  different angles 167
  ecstatic moments 164
  edge of the bed 154
  heightened bodily contact 168
  intimacy 146
  sensate exercise 165
  slow entry 144
  slow motions 167
  stimulating strokes 168
  taking charge 165
  visual variations 168
  woman on top 137, 156–69
woman's orgasm 174–5, 181
  masturbation 184–5, 188–9
  response to 181
  see also orgasm
wooing, art of 46–9
work of man, kama sutra 336

X

x-factors 230–47
  anal sex 246–9
  cunnilingus 242–6
  fellatio 236–41

Y

yab-yum 361
yeast infections 448, 499
yoga 423, 499
yoni 336, 499

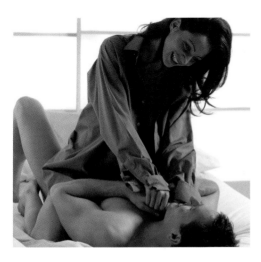

acknowledgements

The authors and publisher would like to thank the photographers Alistair Hughes, John Freeman and his assistant Alex Dow, and make-up artist Bettina Graham. And for using their bodies to illustrate the text, Katy and Nathan, Helen and Armani, Tino and Jennifer, Steve and Barbara, Jessica and Kitt, Justin and Abigail, Ralph Beck, Daz Crawford, Kay Marshall and Kerry Ann Martin. Apologies to those that may have been omitted. Marie Stopes provided the items for contraception. Sh! Women's Erotic Emporium, Coco de Mer and Myla were very kind to lend underwear, toys and other paraphernalia for photography. Thanks to The Terrence Higgins Trust, Stonewall, and Peta Heskell, director of the UK Flirting Academy, www.flirtcoach.com.

Judy Bastyra would like to say a special thank you firstly to Clare Spurrell, a budding writer and adventurer who has contributed greatly to the book both in research and editorially, and secondly to Tessa Swithinbank, who is a writer and close friend who was also a great support and contributor to this book. She would also like to thank Ruth Thomson, Tannis Taylor, Jonathan Hart, Emily Dubberley from cliterati.co.uk, Lynn Warner, Robert Page from *The Lovers' Guide*, Trilby Fairfax, Simon Parritt, Robert and Lynn Watson from Dateable, Dr Jane Roy from Relate and all those who were kind enough to discuss their sex lives and fantasies. Finally Judy would like to dedicate this book to all the men in her life who in their own way helped her write this book: her father and greatest supporter, Jessel, followed by many relatives, and much-loved friends past and present: Dominic, Stuart, John, Gil, Charlie, Robert, Roger and B.K.

Thanks to the following for the loan of props for photography:

The Cloth Shop
290 Portobello Road, London W10 5TE
020 8968 6001

Coco de Mer
23 Monmouth Street, London WC1
020 7836 8882
www.coco-de-mer.com

Ganesha London
3-4 Gabriel's Wharf, London SE1 9PP
020 7928 3444
www.ganesha.co.uk

Myla
Cabot Place West E14
020 7715 5374
www.myla.com

Sh!
57 Hoxton Square, London N1 6PB
03333 444 005
www.sh-womenstore.com

The White Company
4 Symons Street, London SW3 2TJ
020 8166 0199
www.thewhitecompany.com